T0314263

Controversies in
Neurosurgery II

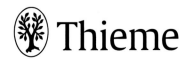

Controversies in Neurosurgery II

Ossama Al-Mefty, MD
Director of Skull Base Surgery
Brigham and Women's Hospital
Harvard School of Medicine
Boston, Massachusetts

Thieme
New York • Stuttgart

Thieme Medical Publishers, Inc.
333 Seventh Ave.
New York, NY 10001

Executive Editor: Kay Conerly
Managing Editor: Judith Tomat
Editorial Assistant: Genevieve Kim
Senior Vice President, Editorial and Electronic Product Development: Cornelia Schulze
Production Editor: Barbara A. Chernow
International Production Director: Andreas Schabert
Vice President, Finance and Accounts: Sarah Vanderbilt
President: Brian D. Scanlan
Cover illustrator: Jennifer Pryll
Compositor: Carol Pierson, Chernow Editorial Services, Inc.
Printer: Everbest Printing Co.

Library of Congress Cataloging-in-Publication Data

Controversies in neurosurgery II [edited by] Ossama Al-Mefty.
    p. ; cm.
  Includes bibliographical references and index.
  ISBN 978-1-60406-232-8 — ISBN 978-1-60406-233-5
  1. Al-Mefty, Ossama, editor of compilation.
  [DNLM: 1. Nervous System Diseases—surgery—Case Reports. 2. Nervous System Neoplasms—surgery—Case Reports.
3. Neurosurgical Procedures—methods—Case Reports.   WL 368]
  RD593
  617.4′8—dc23   2013020386

Important note: Medical knowledge is ever-changing. As new research and clinical experience broaden our knowledge, changes in treatment and drug therapy may be required. The authors and editors of the material herein have consulted sources believed to be reliable in their efforts to provide information that is complete and in accord with the standards accepted at the time of publication. However, in view of the possibility of human error by the authors, editors, or publisher of the work herein or changes in medical knowledge, neither the authors, editors, nor publisher, nor any other party who has been involved in the preparation of this work, warrants that the information contained herein is in every respect accurate or complete, and they are not responsible for any errors or omissions or for the results obtained from use of such information. Readers are encouraged to confirm the information contained herein with other sources. For example, readers are advised to check the product information sheet included in the package of each drug they plan to administer to be certain that the information contained in this publication is accurate and that changes have not been made in the recommended dose or in the contraindications for administration. This recommendation is of particular importance in connection with new or infrequently used drugs.

Some of the product names, patents, and registered designs referred to in this book are in fact registered trademarks or proprietary names even though specific reference to this fact is not always made in the text. Therefore, the appearance of a name without designation as proprietary is not to be construed as a representation by the publisher that it is in the public domain.

Printed in China

5 4 3 2 1

ISBN 978-1-60406-232-8

Also available as an e-book:
eISBN 978-1-60406-233-5

To Rami and Kaith
Keep the healer's spirit and the intellectual rigor

Contents

Preface

A flattering, but motivating, aura of enthusiasm and worthiness continues to embrace the first edition of *Controversies in Neurosurgery,* which Thomas C. Origitano, H. Lewis Harkey, and I edited more than 15 years ago. That volume fulfilled its goal of delivering a sound and stimulating discussion about the controversial subjects of that time. It was well received and is surprisingly still invaluable to my neurosurgical colleagues around the world, whether they are in training, in academia, or in private practice. Many of the "controversies" presented in that volume have been settled. Some vanished with the advent of new techniques or knowledge, but new ones have arisen and have become heated. As we urged the chapter authors of the first edition, I have urged the authors of this edition to be strong advocates in promoting their approach or technique.

As in the first edition, the expertise of the authors and scholarly moderators serves as the golden core of this volume. At the time of the first edition, this approach served to nurture innovative ideas and techniques so as to dispel the weight of conservative and established ones. Now, it serves to bring balance to overly promoted new developments. This attitude of accepting and learning the good "new" while retaining and defending the good "old," with scholarly and thoughtful discernment of the two, has been an attribute of practitioners of the healing arts throughout the ages. This balanced approach stems from their commitment to do what is best for the patient and is eloquently stated in a popular translation of the prayer of the physician Maimonides:

> Should those who are wiser than I wish to improve and instruct me, let my soul gratefully follow their guidance; for vast is the extent of our art. But if fools deride me, let my love for my profession allow me to withstand scorn, even by men of high stature. May truth illuminate my way, for any failing in my craft may bring death or illness upon thy creatures.

Acknowledgments

My profound gratitude goes to Julie Yamamoto, for without her dedicated, outstanding, and perfectionist editorial ability, this work simply would not have seen publication. She saved the project. Julie, you did it again!

This volume is the offspring of its predecessor, *Controversies in Neurosurgery,* in aim, form, and substance, and which Dr. T.C. Origitano and Dr. H. Lewis Harkey co-edited with their remarkable contributions.

I am indebted to all the contributors who provided excellent chapters advancing and substantiating their opinion. My gratitude also goes to Ms. Catherine Johnson for her assistance in the crushing hours and to Judith Tomat and Kay Conerly of Thieme Medical Publishers for their exemplary support and commitment to excellence.

Contributors

Mohamad Abolfotoh, MD
Consultant Neurosurgeon
Lecturer of Neurosurgery
Ain Shams University
Cairo, Egypt

Skull Base Clinical Research Associate
Brigham and Women's Hospital
Harvard Medical School
Boston, Massachusetts

Emad T. Aboud, MD
Arkansas Neuroscience Institute at St. Vincent
Little Rock, Arkansas

Pankaj K. Agarwalla, MD
Clinical Fellow in Surgery
Department of Surgery
Massachusetts General Hospital
Boston, Massachusetts

Kaith K. Almefty, MD
Neurosurgery Resident
Barrow Neurological Institute
Phoenix, Arizona

Ossama Al-Mefty, MD
Director of Skull Base Surgery
Brigham and Women's Hospital
Harvard School of Medicine
Boston, Massachusetts

Rami Almefty, MD
Barrow Neurological Institute
Phoenix, Arizona

Jorge E. Alvernia, MD, MSc
Neurosurgery Department
Glenwood Brain and Spine
West Monroe, Louisiana

Mario Ammirati, MD
Professor of Neurological Surgery
Department of Neurological Surgery
Wexner Medical Center
Ohio State University
Columbus, Ohio

Salah G. Aoun, MD
Postdoctoral Research Fellow
Department of Neurological Surgery
Northwestern University Feinberg School
   of Medicine
Chicago, Illinois

Kenan I. Arnautovic, MD
Semmes-Murphey Clinic
Memphis, Tennessee

Miguel A. Arraez, MD, PhD
Head of the Department of Neurosurgery
Carlos Haya University Hospital
Malaga, Spain

Ramsey Ashour, MD
Professor of Clinical Neurosurgery and
   Otolaryngology
University of Miami
Miami, Florida

Garni Barkhoudarian, MD
Saint John's Brain Tumor Center
Santa Monica, California

Alim Louis Benabid, MD, PhD
Clinatec Institute
Minatec Campus
CEA Grenoble
Grenoble Cedex, France

Bernard R. Bendok, MD
Associate Professor of Neurological Surgery
   and Radiology
Northwestern University
Feinberg School of Medicine
Chicago, Illinois

Mitchel S. Berger, MD
Professor and Chairman
Brain Tumor Research Center
Department of Neurological Surgery
University of California at San Francisco
San Francisco, California

Aditya Bharatha, MD
Division of Neuroradiology
Toronto Western Hospital
University Health Network
Toronto, Ontario, Canada

Markus Bookland, MD
Resident
Department of Neurosurgery
Temple University School of Medicine
Philadelphia, Pennsylvania

Frederick A. Boop, MD
Semmes-Murphey Neurologic and Spine
  Institute
Memphis, Tennessee

Luis A.B. Borba, MD, PhD
Department of Neurosurgery
Hospital Universitario Evangelico de Curitiba
Curitiba, Parana, Brazil

Jeffrey A. Brown, MD
Neurological Surgery, P.C.
Great Neck, New York

Kim J. Burchiel, MD
Oregon Health and Science University
Portland, Oregon

Paolo Cappabianca, MD
Federico II University
Department of Neurological Sciences
Division of Neurosurgery
Università degli Studi di Napoli Federico II
Naples, Italy

Daniel D. Cavalcanti, MD
Department of Neurosurgery
Paulo Niemeyer State Brain Institute
Rio de Janeiro, Brazil

Luigi Maria Cavallo, MD, PhD
Department of Neurological Sciences
Division of Neurosurgery
Università degli Studi di Napoli Federico II
Naples, Italy

Feres Chaddad, MD
Neurosurgical Assistant of the Discipline
  of Neurosurgery
Department of Neurology at State University
  of Campinas
Campinas, Brazil
Neurosurgeon of Instituto de Ciencias
  Neurologicas (ICNE)
São Paulo, Brazil

E. Antonio Chiocca, MD, PhD, FAANS
Neurosurgeon-in-Chief and Chairman
Department of Neurosurgery
Co-Director, Institute for the Neurosciences
Brigham and Women's/Faulkner Hospital
Surgical Director, Center for Neuro-oncology
Dana-Farber Cancer Institute
Professor of Surgery
Harvard Medical School
Boston, Massachusetts

Shakeel A. Chowdhry, MD
Division of Neurological Surgery
Barrow Neurological Institute
St. Joseph's Hospital and Medical Center
Phoenix, Arizona

Benedicto Colli, MD
Department of Surgery
Campus Universitario
University of São Paulo
São Paulo, Brazil

Roxana Contreras, MD
Chief, Division of Surgery
Hospital de Especialidades Centro Médico Nacional Siglo XXI
Mexico City, Mexico

William T. Couldwell, MD, PhD
Department of Neurosurgery
University of Utah
Salt Lake City, Utah

Mark J. Dannenbaum, MD
Department of Neurosurgery
University of Texas Houston Medical School
Mischer Neuroscience Institute/Memorial Hermann
  Hospital
Houston, Texas

Arthur L. Day, MD
Department of Neurosurgery
University of Texas Houston Medical School
Houston, Texas

Franco DeMonte, MD
Professor, Mary Beth Pawelek Chair in Neurosurgery
Department of Neurosurgery
University of Texas M.D. Anderson Cancer Center
Houston, Texas

Evandro de Oliveira, MD
Professor of the Discipline of Neurosurgery
Faculty of Medical Sciences
UNICAMP
Director of Instituto de Ciencias Neurologicas (ICNE)
São Paulo, Brazil

Doniel Drazin, MD
Department of Neurosurgery
Cedars Sinai Medical Center
Los Angeles, California

Colin L.W. Driscoll, MD
Departments of Otorhinolaryngology and
Neurologic Surgery
Mayo Clinic
Rochester, Minnesota

Rose Du, MD, PhD
Associate Surgeon
Instructor of Neurosurgery
Department of Neurosurgery
Brigham and Women's Hospital
Harvard Medical School
Boston, Massachusetts

Ian F. Dunn, MD
Brigham and Women's Hospital
Boston, Massachusetts

Christopher S. Eddleman MD, PhD
Department of Neurological Surgery and Radiology
University of Texas Southwestern Medical Center
Dallas, Texas

Tarek Y. el Ahmadieh, MD
Postdoctoral Research Fellow
Department of Neurological Surgery
Northwestern University Feinberg School
of Medicine
Chicago, Illinois

Samer K. Elbabaa, MD
Director of Pediatric Neurosurgery
Assistant Professor of Neurosurgery
Cardinal Glennon Children's Medical Center
St. Louis, Missouri

A. El Khamlichi, MD
Department of Neurosurgery
Mohammed V University
Hopital des Specialites
Rabat, Morocco

Robert E. Elliott, MD
Mainline Healthcare Neurosurgery
Newtown Square, Pennsylvania

Kadir Erkmen, MD
Assistant Professor of Neurosurgery and Neurology
Section of Neurosurgery
Dartmouth-Hitchcock Medical Center
Geisel School of Medicine at Dartmouth
Lebanon, New Hampshire

Felice Esposito, MD, PhD
Department of Neurological Sciences
Division of Neurosurgery
Università degli Studi di Napoli Federico II
Naples, Italy

José Maria de Campos Filho, MD
Neurosurgeon of Instituto de Ciencias
Neurologicas (ICNE)
São Paulo, Brazil

Ricardo B.V. Fontes, MD
Department of Neurosurgery
Rush University Medical Center
Chicago, Illinois

John L. Fox, MD
Little Rock, Arkansas

Kai U. Frerichs, MD
Departments of Radiology and Neurosurgery
Brigham and Women's Hospital
Boston, Massachusetts

Allan Friedman, MD
The Guy L. Odom Professor of Neurological
Surgery
Neurosurgeon-in-Chief
Duke University Medical Center
Durham, North Carolina

Venelin M. Gerganov, MD, PhD
International Neuroscience Institute-Hannover
Hannover, Germany

Rasha Germain, MD
St. Joseph's Hospital and Medical Center
Phoenix, Arizona

Atul Goel, MD
Professor and Head
Department of Neurosurgery
K.E.M. Hospital
Seth G.S. Medical College
K.E.M. Hospital
Parel, Mumbai, India

Pablo González-López, MD, PhD
Department: Department of Neurosurgery
Alicante University Hospital
Alicante, Spain

Cristian Gragnaniello, MD
Department of Neurosurgery
University of Arkansas for Medical Sciences
Little Rock, Arkansas

Bradley A. Gross, MD
Brigham and Women's Hospital
Boston, Massachusetts

Gerardo Guinto, MD
Chairman
Department of Neurosurgery
Hospital de Especialidades Centro Médico Nacional Siglo XXI
Hospital Angeles del Pedregal
Mexico City, Mexico

Stephen J. Haines, MD
Department of Neurosurgery
University of Minnesota
Minneapolis, Minnesota

P. Hallacq, MD
Department of Neurosurgery
Hopital Neurologique of Lyon
Lyon, France

Robert E. Harbaugh, MD
Director, Penn State Institute of the Neurosciences
University Distinguished Professor and Chair
Department of Neurosurgery
Professor, Engineering Science and Mechanics
Penn State Hershey Neurosurgery
Hershey, Pennsylvania

Toshinori Hasegawa, MD
Department of Neurosurgery
Gamma Knife Center
Komaki City Hospital
Komaki City, Aichi, Japan

Juha Hernesniemi, MD, PhD
Professor of Neurosurgery, Chairman
Helsinki University Central Hospital (HUCH)
Töölö Hospital
Helsinki, Finland

Kathryn L. Holloway, MD
Professor
Department of Neurosurgery
Harold F. Young Neurosurgical Center
Virginia Commonwealth University
Richmond, Virginia

L. Nelson Hopkins, MD
Professor and Chairman
Department of Neurosurgery
Professor of Radiology
Director, Toshiba Stroke Research Center
School of Medicine and Biomedical Sciences
University at Buffalo
Millard Fillmore Gates Hospital
Kaleida Health
State University of New York
Buffalo, New York

John A. Jane, Jr., MD
Department of Neurosurgery
University of Virginia Health System
Charlottesville, Virginia

Peter J. Jannetta, MD
Professor and Vice Chairman
Department of Neurosurgery
Allegheny General Hospital
Pittsburgh, Pennsylvania

Paulo Kadri, MD
Department of Neurosurgery
University of Arkansas School for Medical Sciences
Little Rock, Arkansas
Auxiliary Professor
Department of Neurosurgery
Federal University of Mato Groso do Sol
Director
El Kadri Neurological Institute
Campo Grande, Brazil

Hideyuki Kano, MD, PhD
Department of Neurological Surgery and the Center for Image-Guided Neurosurgery
University of Pittsburgh School of Medicine
Pittsburgh, Pennsylvania

Yucel Kanpolat, MD
Ankara, Turkey

Takeshi Kawase, MD, PhD
Department of Neurosurgery
Keio University School of Medicine
Tokyo, Japan

Ahmet Hilmi Kaya, MD
Department of Neurosurgery
Yeditepe University School of Medicine
Istanbul, Turkey

Osaama H. Khan, MD, MSc
Department of Surgery
Division of Neurosurgery
University of Toronto
Toronto, Ontario, Canada

Wesley A. King, MD
Department of Neurosurgery
Cedars Sinai Medical Center
Los Angeles, California

Engelbert Knosp, MD
Chairman of the Department of Neurosurgery
Medical University of Vienna
Vienna, Austria

Douglas Kondziolka, MD
Professor of Neurological Surgery
Department of Neurological Surgery and the Center for
    Image-Guided Neurosurgery
University of Pittsburgh School of Medicine
Pittsburgh, Pennsylvania

Miikka Korja, MD
Associate Professor
Department of Neurosurgery
Helsinki University Central Hospital
Helsinki, Finland

Timo Krings, MD, PhD
Division of Neuroradiology
Toronto Western Hospital
University Health Network
Toronto, Ontario, Canada

Ali F. Krisht, MD
Arkansas Neuroscience Institute
St. Vincent Infirmary
Little Rock, Arkansas

Abhaya V. Kulkarni, MD, PhD
Hospital for Sick Children
Toronto, Ontario, Canada

Sanju Lama, MD, PhD Candidate
Project NeuroArm
Health Research Innovation Center
Calgary, Alberta, Canada

Edward R. Laws, MD
Department of Neurosurgery
Brigham and Women's Hospital
Harvard School of Medicine
Boston, Massachusetts

Michael T. Lawton, MD
Department of Neurological Surgery
University of California at San Francisco
San Francisco, California

Elad I. Levy, MD
Department of Neurosurgery
School of Medicine and Biomedical Sciences
University at Buffalo
Millard Fillmore Gates Hospital
Kaleida Health
State University of New York
Buffalo, New York

Ning Lin, MD
Department of Neurosurgery
Brigham and Women's Hospital
Harvard Medical School
Boston, Massachusetts

Michael J. Link, MD
Departments of Neurologic Surgery and
    Otorhinolaryngology
Mayo Clinic
Rochester, Minnesota

Mark E. Linskey, MD
Department of Neurosurgery
University of California at Irvine Medical Center
Orange, California

Jay Loeffler, MD
Department of Radiation Oncology
Massachusetts General Hospital
Boston, Massachusetts

Christopher M. Loftus, MD, DHC (Hon.)
Professor and Chair
Department of Neurosurgery
Assistant Dean for International Affiliations
Temple University School of Medicine
Philadelphia, Pennsylvania

Donlin M. Long, MD
Johns Hopkins University Hospital
Baltimore, Maryland

Andres M. Lozano, MD, PhD, FRCS
Division of Neurosurgery
Toronto Western Hospital
Toronto, Ontario, Canada

L. Dade Lunsford, MD
Department of Neurological Surgery and the Center for
    Image-Guided Neurosurgery
University of Pittsburgh School of Medicine
Pittsburgh, Pennsylvania

Michael S. McKisic, MD
Department of Neurosurgery
University of Virginia Health Sciences Center
Charlottesville, Virginia

Aygül Mert, MD
Department of Neurosurgery
Medical University Vienna
Vienna, Austria

Brandon A. Miller, MD, PhD
Department of Neurosurgery
Emory University
Atlanta, Georgia

Basant K. Misra, MD
P.D. Hinduja National Hospital and Medical Research
    Centre
Mumbai, India

Stephen J. Monteith, MD
Department of Neurological Surgery
University of Virginia Health Sciences Center
Charlottesville, Virginia

Jacques J. Morcos, MD, FRCS(Eng), FRCS(Ed)
Professor of Clinical Neurosurgery and
Otolaryngology
University of Miami
Miami, Florida

Osman Arikan Nacar, MD
Department of Neurological Surgery
University of California, San Francisco

Jalal Najjar, MD
Consultant Neurosurgeon
Alameen Hospital
Homs, Syria

Peter Nakaji, MD
Neuroscience Publications
Barrow Neurological Institute
Phoenix, Arizona

Stephen V. Nalbach, MD
Department of Neurosurgery
Temple University Hospital
Philadelphia, Pennsylvania

G. Robert Nugent, MD
Robert C. Byrd Health Science Center North
Morgantown, West Virginia

Christopher S. Ogilvy, MD
Neurosurgical Service
Massachusetts General Hospital
Boston, Massachusetts

Kenji Ohata, MD, PhD
Professor and Chairman
Department of Neurosurgery
Osaka City University Graduate School
of Medicine
Osaka, Japan

Chima Oluigbo, MD
Department of Neurosurgery
Center for Neuroscience and Behavioral
Medicine
Children's National Medical Center
Washington, DC

T. C. Origitano, MD, PhD
Neuroscience and Spine Institute
Kalispell, Montana

Nelson Oyesiku, MD, PhD
Department of Neurosurgery
Emory University
Atlanta, Georgia

Koray Özduman, MD
Department of Neurosurgery
Acibadem University School of Medicine
Istanbul, Turkey

M. Necmettin Pamir, MD
Chairman and Professor of Neurosurgery
Department of Neurosurgery
Acibadem University School of Medicine
Istanbul, Turkey

Selcuk Peker, MD
Associate Professor of Neurosurgery
Department of Neurosurgery
Acibadem University School of Medicine
Istanbul, Turkey

Bruce E. Pollock, MD
Departments of Neurosurgery and Radiation Oncology
Mayo Clinic
Rochester, Minnesota

A. John Popp, MD
Department of Neurosurgery
Stanford University
Stanford, California

Ali Rezai, MD
Center for Neurological Restoration
Cleveland Clinic Foundation
Cleveland, Ohio

Ana Rodríguez-Hernández, MD
Department of Neurological Surgery
University of California, San Francisco
San Francisco, California

James T. Rutka, MD, PhD
Hospital for Sick Children
Toronto, Ontario, Canada

Madjid Samii, MD, PhD
International Neuroscience Institute-Hannover
Hannover, Germany

Duke Samson, MD
University of Texas Southwestern Medical Center
Dallas, Texas

Nader Sanai, MD
Department of Neurological Surgery
Barrow Brain Tumor Research Center
Barrow Neurological Institute
Phoenix, Arizona

Tejas Sankar, MDCM
Division of Neurosurgery
University of Alberta
Edmonton, Alberta, Canada

R. Michael Scott, MD
Professor, Department of Surgery (Neurosurgery)
Harvard Medical School
Neurosurgeon-in-Chief, Emeritus, and Fellows Family Chair
Boston Children's Hospital
Boston, Massachusetts

Jason P. Sheehan, MD, PhD
Department of Neurological Surgery
University of Virginia Health Sciences Center
Charlottesville, Virginia

Ali Shirzadi, MD
Department of Neurosurgery
Cedars Sinai Medical Center
Los Angeles, California

Adnan H. Siddiqui, MD, PhD
Department of Neurosurgery
School of Medicine and Biomedical Sciences
University at Buffalo
Millard Fillmore Gates Hospital
Kaleida Health
State University of New York
Buffalo, New York

Marc P. Sindou, MD, DSc
Hopital Neurologique
Pierre Wertheimer
Pinel/Groupement Hospital
Lyon, France

Edward R. Smith, MD
Associate Professor
Boston Children's Hospital
Boston, Massachusetts

Domenico Solari, MD
Department of Neurological Sciences
Division of Neurosurgery
Università degli Studi di Napoli Federico II
Naples, Italy

Volker K.H. Sonntag, MD
Barrow Neurosurgical Associates
Barrow Neurological Institute
Phoenix, Arizona

Robert F. Spetzler, MD
Division of Neurological Surgery
Barrow Neurological Institute
St. Joseph's Hospital and Medical Center
Phoenix, Arizona

Christopher J. Stapleton, MD
Department of Neurosurgery
Massachusetts General Hospital and Harvard Medical School
Boston, Massachusetts

Juraj Šteňo, MD
Comenius Universirt in Bratislava
Bratislava, Limbova, Slovakia

Rahadian Indarto Susilo, MD
Department of Neurosurgery
Osaka City University Graduate School of Medicine
Osaka, Japan

Garnette R. Sutherland, MD
Professor of Neurosurgery
University of Calgary
Health Research Innovation Centre
Calgary, Alberta, Canada

Daryoush Tavanaiepour, MD
Virginia Commonwealth University
Richmond, Virginia

Rabih G. Tawk, MD
Mayo Clinic/Neurosurgery
Jacksonville, Florida

Karel terBrugge, MD
Head, Division of Neuroradiology
University of Toronto
Toronto Western Hospital
University Health Network
Toronto, Ontario, Canada

Vincent C. Traynelis, MD
Director, Neurosurgery Spine Service
Vice Chairperson and Professor
Department of Neurosurgery
Rush University Medical Center
Chicago, Illinois

Uğur Türe, MD
Professor and Chairman
Department of Neurosurgery
Yeditepe University School of Medicine
Istanbul, Turkey

Urvashi Upadhyay, MD
Rotating Resident
Brigham and Women's Hospital
Department of Neurosurgery
Boston, Massachusetts

Shobhan Vachhrajani, MD
Division of Neurosurgery
University of Toronto
Toronto, Ontario, Canada

Scott D. Wait, MD
Director of Pediatric Neurosurgery
Levine Children's Hospital/Carolinas Medical Center
Carolina Neurosurgery and Spine Associates
Charlotte, North Carolina

Jeffrey H. Wisoff, MD
New York, New York

Stefan Wolfsberger, MD
Associate Professor
Department of Neurosurgery
University of Vienna
Vienna, Austria
Adjunct Professor
Department of Clinical Neurosciences and the Hotchkiss
    Brain Institute
University of Calgary
Calgary, Alberta, Canada

Esmiralda Yeremeyeva, MD
Department of Neurological Surgery
Mercy Medical Center
Des Moines, Iowa

Chapter 1

Surgical Removal of Tuberculum Sellae Meningioma: Endoscopic vs. Microscopic

Case

A 45-year-old woman has visual acuity of 20/800 in the right eye, 20/40 in the left eye, and an incongruous visual field defect.

Participants

Microsurgical Removal of Tuberculum Sellae Meningiomas: Franco DeMonte

Endoscopic Removal of Tuberculum Sellae Meningiomas: Paolo Cappabianca, Luigi Maria Cavallo, Felice Esposito, and Domenico Solari

Moderator: Surgical Removal of Tuberculum Sellae Meningiomas: Endoscopic vs. Microscopic: William T. Couldwell

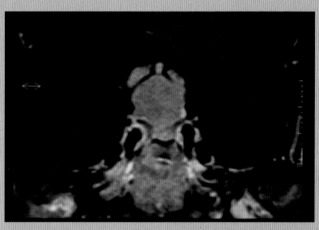

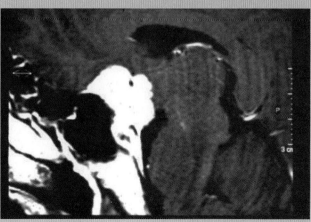

Microsurgical Removal of Tuberculum Sellae Meningiomas

Franco DeMonte

Meningiomas of the tuberculum sella account for 4 to 10% of meningiomas, and they almost universally present with varying degrees of visual loss.[1] These tumors arise from the tuberculum sellae, chiasmatic sulcus, limbus sphenoidale, and the diaphragma sellae, and usually displace the optic chiasm superiorly and posteriorly and the optic nerves laterally or anterolaterally and superiorly. They very commonly extend into one or both optic canals.[2–4] Early diagnosis and advances in microsurgical technique have essentially eliminated mortality in recent microsurgical series, but even contemporary studies continue to report up to a 20% rate of visual deterioration after surgery.[5–10]

There recently has been a proliferation of reports describing the transsphenoidal resection of tuberculum sellae meningiomas, with both microsurgical and endoscopic techniques, although the patients included in these reports represent a highly selected subset of these tumors.

Surgical Considerations

Crucial to the patient's visual outcome and the selection of the operative approach is the surgeon's ability to recognize the high rate of optic canal extensions of tuberculum sellae meningiomas (**Fig. 1.1**). Such extensions have been identi-

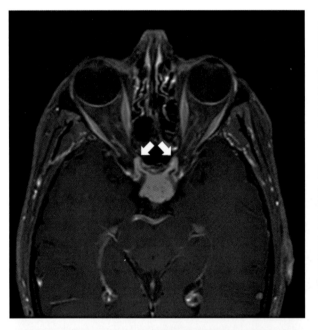

a

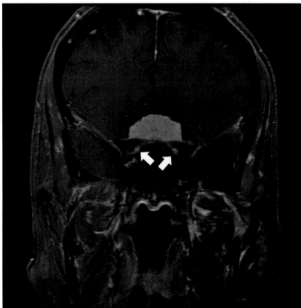

b

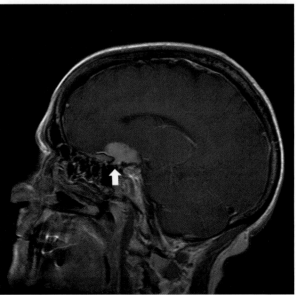

c

Fig. 1.1a–c Axial (**a**), coronal (**b**), and sagittal (**c**) T1-weighted postcontrast magnetic resonance imaging studies of a patient with a large tuberculum sella meningioma with bilateral extension into the optic canal (*arrows*). (Used with permission of the Department of Neurosurgery, the University of Texas M.D. Anderson Cancer Center.)

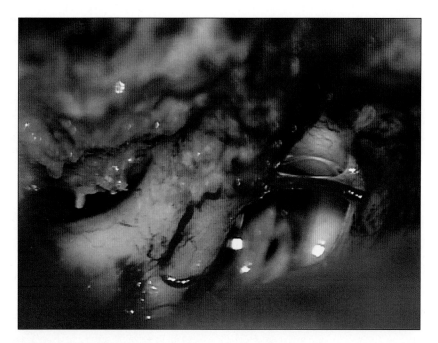

Fig. 1.2 Intraoperative photograph during resection of a tuberculum sella meningioma. Notice the preserved perforating vessel to the optic nerve and chiasm and the presence of tumor tissue superior and lateral to the right optic nerve. (Used with permission of the Department of Neurosurgery, the University of Texas M.D. Anderson Cancer Center.)

fied in 75% of patients or more,[2,4] and early optic canal decompression is an important factor in optimizing visual outcome.[2,3,9,11] Similarly crucial to visual outcome is the preservation of the small vessels to the inferior surface of the optic nerves and chiasm. These vessels are part of the superior hypophyseal arterial complex that arises from the medial wall of the internal carotid artery bilaterally[12,13] **(Fig. 1.2)**.

Vascular encasement, especially of the anterior cerebral arteries (ACAs) and the anterior communicating artery, must be addressed through careful, precise arachnoidal microdissection to prevent perforator injury.[1,12] Occasionally, contributions to the tumor's blood supply may come from small branches of the anterior cerebral and anterior communicating complex. This supply needs to be interrupted but the parent vasculature preserved.

The pituitary stalk is typically displaced posteriorly and is usually not difficult to dissect from the tumor. Liliequist's membrane tends to remain intact; thus, separating the posterior portion of the tumor is usually relatively straightforward even in the presence of marked posterior displacement of the basilar artery.[14]

Treatment of the Controversial Patient

This patient is a 45-year-old woman with significantly compromised vision and vascular encasement of the ACA and anterior communicating artery complex by a relatively large tuberculum sellae meningioma (see images at the beginning of the chapter). She is best served by the complete microsurgical resection of the tumor. The approach selected must accomplish several goals:

1. Allow for the circumferential decompression of, and tumoral dissection from, the optic nerves.
2. Preserve the microvasculature of the optic nerves and chiasm.
3. Allow precise arachnoidal microdissection to free the encased ACA and anterior communicating artery complex.
4. Allow access to, and removal of, the tumor, the dura of origin, and any hyperostotic bone.
5. Preserve the pituitary stalk and endocrinologic function.
6. Allow for reliable dural repair and reconstruction to avoid leakage of cerebrospinal fluid (CSF).

Given the degree of visual compromise and the vascular encasement, I would choose a right-sided fronto-orbital approach **(Fig. 1.3)**. In this approach, microdissection is used to separate the right olfactory tract from the inferior surface of the frontal lobe back to the olfactory trigone. The anterior falcine insertion is identified and used for midline orientation. Tumor devascularization begins in the midline, and careful tumor debulking is begun. The ipsilateral optic nerve is identified.

Before manipulating the optic nerve, the surgeon removes the dura overlying the optic canal (typically involved with tumor), and the bony optic canal is widely opened with a high-speed drill and diamond bur or ultrasonic bone curette and constant irrigation. The falciform ligament and the dura of the optic canal are opened to decompress the optic nerve. Tumor is removed from around the ipsilateral optic nerve, and the right internal carotid artery is identified. Care must be taken to avoid injuring the ophthalmic artery. Precise arachnoidal microdissection is used to remove tumor from around the ACA and anterior communicating

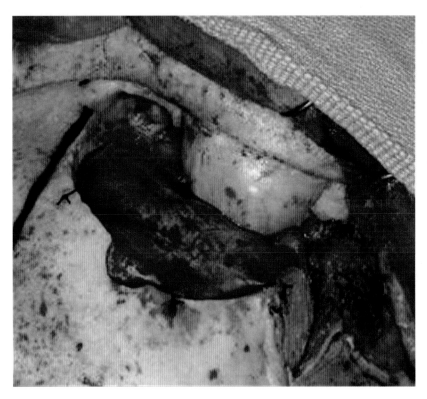

Fig. 1.3 Intraoperative photograph of the right supraorbital craniotomy used to approach tuberculum sella meningiomas. (Used with permission of the Department of Neurosurgery, the University of Texas M.D. Anderson Cancer Center.)

artery complex. The right optic nerve is followed to the chiasm, and the left optic nerve is subsequently identified. This nerve is then decompressed through opening of the bony and dural optic canal, and tumor is removed from around the left optic nerve. The final dural attachments are divided and the posterior margin of the tumor is dissected off the pituitary stalk and Liliequist's membrane. All of the involved dura is resected and any hyperostotic bone is drilled away.

Dural reconstruction is done with an intradural graft sewed to the dura of the base where possible. Vascularized pericranium is readily available to augment the reconstruction and to separate the sinonasal cavity from the intracranial space.

Discussion

The optimal treatment for a patient with a meningioma of the tuberculum sella is the complete removal of the tumor, normalization of the patient's vision, and freedom from surgical complications. Over the past decade, these outcomes have most commonly been achieved by using a transcranial route to access the tumor.[1–5,8–19] More recently, anterior-based approaches through the sinonasal cavities have been proposed and increasingly used to achieve these same goals through what is perceived to be a less morbid alternative to craniotomy.[20–31]

The transcranial, microsurgical resection of a tuberculum sellae meningioma, be it through subfrontal, interhemispheric, or pterional routes, has many advantages. It allows vascular control of the internal carotid artery, ACA, and middle cerebral artery; direct decompression and inspection of the optic canals, nerves, and chiasm; multiple local tissues (free and vascularized) for reconstruction; and a great degree of familiarity among neurosurgeons. Using these various transcranial routes, surgeons have reported gross total resection rates of 73 to 98%, with a mean rate of 90.5% (median 85%). The tumors described in these reports ranged from 0.5 to 8 cm but averaged 2.8 cm (median 2.7 cm).[2–13,15–19]

In contradistinction, a mean gross total resection rate of 76% has been reported when a transsphenoidal route is used, be it traditional or endoscopic (range 57 to 85%, median 83%), with tumors ranging from 1.2 to 3.7 cm (mean 2.2 cm, median 2.3 cm).[20,23,24,27,28,30] Thus, it seems that a less complete extent of resection is achieved with transnasally based approaches despite a population of patients with smaller tumors on average (selected patients).

Of primary concern when treating a patient with a tuberculum sellae meningioma is the patient's visual outcome. Often the optic nerves and chiasm are markedly compressed, distorted, and thinned. Many surgeons believe that the optic canals should be opened and the optic nerve decompressed before direct dissection of the nerves and

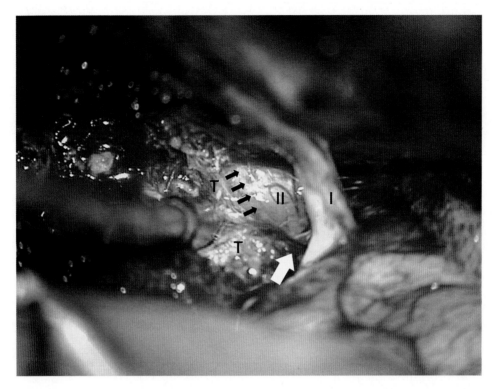

Fig. 1.4 Intraoperative photograph during a right supraorbital approach to a tuberculum sella meningioma. The olfactory (I) and optic (II) nerves are labeled, as is the tumor (T). Note the nearly indiscernible plane between the tumor and the medial edge of the optic nerve (*small black arrows*). Also note the tumor extending superolateral to the optic nerve (*white arrow*). (Used with permission of the Department of Neurosurgery, the University of Texas M.D. Anderson Cancer Center.)

chiasm takes place. Mathiesen and Kihlström[9] were able to achieve a 91% rate of visual improvement in their patients when proceeding in this manner. This figure can be compared with an overall mean rate of visual improvement of 59% reported in the microsurgical literature.[2–11,13,15–19] Unfortunately, this same body of literature reveals that visual worsening remains a significant problem, with a mean rate of visual decline of 13%.[2–11,13,15–19]

In the most typical arrangement, the optic nerves are elevated superiorly and laterally and the chiasm superiorly and posteriorly by the tumor. This pathological anatomy most favors an inferomedial approach for decompression as the approach least likely to require manipulation of the optic nerve or chiasm.[21,23,29] This is likely the reason for the improved visual outcome reported in the literature for anteriorly based surgical approaches. Rates of visual improvement ranging from 71 to 100% have been reported (mean 85%), whereas visual deterioration has been reported in less than 5%.[20,23,24,27,28,30] A drawback of this approach, however, is the inability to remove tumor extensions above or lateral to the optic nerves **(Fig. 1.4).**

Another unfortunate by-product of this inferomedial exposure of the optic nerves and chiasm is the direct communication of the intradural space with the sinonasal cavity and the paucity of reconstructive options available to achieve a watertight closure, let alone a primary closure.

Mean rates of CSF leaks of 30% have been reported, although meningitis does not seem to be common.[20,23,24,27,28,30] The transcranial microsurgical literature reports mean CSF leak rates of 4%.[2–11,13,15–19]

Finally, there is also a greater chance of trauma to the pituitary gland and stalk with the transnasally based approaches. The literature reports an almost twofold increase in the incidence of diabetes insipidus (6.4% vs. 3.5%) after surgery.[2–11,13,15–20,23–25,27,28,30]

Conclusion

Although great strides have been made in the use of transnasal techniques to access the anterior cranial base and sellar region, many questions remain about the indications for their use in the treatment of a patient with a tuberculum sellae meningioma. According to findings reported in the literature to date, the transcranial routes have the advantages of applicability to tumors of any size, a better extent of resection, lower rates of endocrinopathy and spinal fluid leakage, and, with early decompression of the optic nerves, impressive rates of visual improvement. Currently, these approaches most closely meet the ideals of complete tumor removal, normalization of vision, and freedom from surgical complications in patients with a tuberculum sellae meningioma.

Endoscopic Removal of Tuberculum Sellae Meningiomas

Paolo Cappabianca, Luigi Maria Cavallo, Felice Esposito, and Domenico Solari

Tuberculum sellae meningiomas account for 5 to 10% of all intracranial meningiomas. Such tumors often compress and sometimes encase neighboring neurovascular structures, namely the optic nerves and chiasm, the pituitary stalk, the hypothalamus, the third cranial nerve, and the internal carotid, anterior cerebral, and anterior communicating arteries. Hence, they have been historically managed through different and extensive transcranial approaches. During recent decades, however, with the contributions of microsurgery and especially the "keyhole surgery" concept, surgical techniques and the results of treatment have been significantly refined, with a tremendous improvement in terms of morbidity and mortality rates.

More recently, the evolution of endoscopic techniques has progressively reduced the invasiveness of transcranial approaches and stimulated new interest in transsphenoidal surgery. Indeed, the panoramic view offered by the endoscope has improved the safety of the transsphenoidal approach,[32–35] creating the possibility of passing through the nasal cavity to reach the brain and its neurovascular structures without parenchymal manipulation or retraction. Thus far, use of the endoscope has extended indications for such an approach, initially reserved for sellar or intra-suprasellar intradiaphragmatic lesions,[33,34,36,37] to different "pure" supradiaphragmatic lesions, including tuberculum sellae meningiomas.[20,23,24,27,29–31,38–41] This application had already been foreseen by Hardy[42] in the 1970s.

From the Sellae to the Tuberculum

The visualizing tool for this kind of approach is the same as that used during standard transsphenoidal surgery: a rigid 0-degree endoscope 18 cm in length and 4 mm in diameter (Karl Storz Endoscopy, Tuttlingen, Germany). Notwithstanding the close proximity of the sellar, suprasellar, and tuberculum-planum sphenoidal areas, the endoscopic endonasal approach requires some modifications from the standard approach traditionally adopted to access the sella. The endoscopic endonasal approach for the treatment of tuberculum sellae meningiomas should give surgeons the opportunity to proceed through the same surgical steps as those provided by the adoption of a classic bimanual microsurgical technique—devascularization, debulking, and dissection—that represent the backbone of meningioma surgery.

Because the surgical corridor routinely used in the standard approach to the sellar area is not sufficient, a wider, bi-nostril surgical corridor, attained by removing some nasal structures, must be established to increase the working space and the maneuverability of instruments, according to the basic rules for the extended endoscopic approaches to the skull base standardized by Kassam and associates.[43–45] Hence, the middle turbinate on one side (usually the right) and the posterior portion of the nasal septum are removed, and the middle turbinate in the other nostril is lateralized (sometimes even this turbinate can be removed).

If needed, the superior turbinate and the posterior ethmoid air cells on both sides can be removed to increase the working space. Thereafter, a wider anterior sphenoidotomy is performed; all the septa inside the sphenoid sinus are removed, and every irregularity of the bone and mucosa is flattened to increase the maneuverability of the endoscope and surgical instruments while working above the sella. Once the posterior wall of the sphenoid sinus is completely exposed, a series of protuberances and depressions (according to the grade of pneumatization) becomes visible: the sellar floor at the center, the sphenoethmoid planum above it, and the clival indentation below; the bony prominences of the intracavernous carotid artery and the optic nerves laterally; and between them the opticocarotid recess molded by the pneumatization of the optic strut of the anterior clinoid process. In such a way, it is possible to create a corridor that allows the surgeon to perform bimanual dissection through both nostrils while a coworker holds the endoscope, dynamically moving it along the surgical corridor and switching between the close-up and panoramic views of the surgical field on demand.

Once such a preliminary stage has been performed, additional bone is removed from the cranial base: the tuberculum sellae and the planum sphenoidale anteriorly, depending on the extension of the meningioma, up to the level of the posterior ethmoidal arteries and laterally up to both medial opticocarotid recesses. This aspect of such a bony depression, limited by the parasellar portion of both the intracavernous carotid arteries and the optic nerves, corresponds intracranially to the entrance of the optic canals.[43] Bone removal at this level can be extended more laterally up to the medial border of the lateral opticocarotid recess, which corresponds intracranially to the optic strut of the anterior clinoid process, to expose the optic canals. Superiorly, the bone opening can be widened over the planum because the optic nerve diverges, so that the resulting craniectomy resembles a chef's hat[46,47] (**Figs. 1.5, 1.6**). The neuronavigator has proved to be quite useful in better defining the limits of bone removal. Unlike with craniopharyngiomas, in the endoscopic endonasal approach for tuberculum sellae meningiomas, management of the superior intercavernous sinus is not so troublesome because the tumor itself often compresses and obliterates the sinus.

Lesion Management

At this point in the procedure, management of the lesion can begin. The fundamental steps of dissection and removal are tailored to each lesion, according to the standard prin-

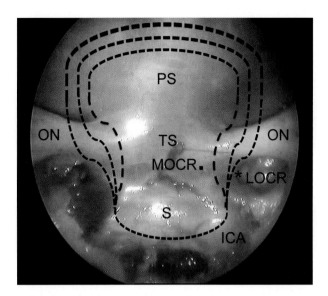

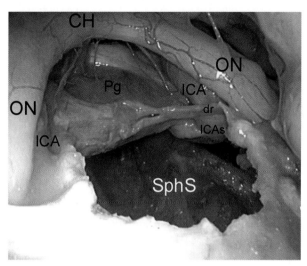

Fig. 1.5 Anatomic endoscopic endonasal transsphenoidal view showing the "chef's hat"–shaped bone and dural opening (*dashed lines*) to gain access to the suprasellar area. Such an opening can be tailored according to the lateral extension of the lesion. In the inferior portion, bone can be removed up to the medial border of the lateral opticocarotid recess, which corresponds intracranially to the optic strut of the anterior clinoid process so that even the optic canals can be exposed in their inferomedial aspects. The opening can be widened over the planum. ICA, internal carotid artery covered by the dura mater; LOCR, lateral opticocarotid recess; MOCR, medial opticocarotid recess; ON, optic nerve covered by the dura mater; PS, planum sphenoidale; S, sella; TS, tuberculum sellae; *, medial aspect of the lateral opticocarotid recess.

Fig. 1.6 Anatomic endoscopic transcranial view showing the skull-base opening achieved through the extended endoscopic endonasal approach to the suprasellar area. CH, chiasm; dr, distal dural ring; ICA, internal carotid artery; ICAs, parasellar tract of the internal carotid artery; ON, optic nerve; Pg, pituitary gland; SphS, sphenoid sinus cavity.

ciples of transcranial microsurgery. When approached from below, removal of a tuberculum sellae meningioma is preceded by coagulation of the dural attachment so that the tumor is devascularized early. Thereafter, the tumor is debulked safely and its capsule is finally dissected from the surrounding microvascular structures either with or without manipulation of the optic pathways.

Because of the intraoperative leakage of CSF, an accurate reconstruction of the skull-base defect is needed after the lesion is removed. First, a thin layer of fibrin glue is placed in the intradural space to create a barrier against the CSF. The osteo-dural defect is then closed with heterologous dural substitutes combined with an autologous septal or turbinate bone or even a synthetic, easy-to-shape bone substitute, according to the various techniques (intradural, extradural, or intra-extradural).[48] Multiple layers of dural substitute are placed to support the reconstruction and further reinforced with the mucoperichondrium of the middle turbinate, or a pedicled flap of septal mucosa (the Hadad-Bassagasteguy flap[49] popularized by the Pittsburgh group[50]), or both. Finally, the sphenoid sinus is filled with surgical glue (Tisseel, Duraseal, or both) to reduce the dead spaces and hold the reconstruction material in place. No lumbar drainage is required at the end of the procedure;

nevertheless, we advise our patients to remain on bed rest for 3 to 5 days, depending on the grade of pneumocephalus, while medical therapy with acetazolamide, laxatives, and wide-spectrum antibiotics is administered.

The Advantages of the Low Route

Like other meningiomas, those of the tuberculum sellae involve the subdural compartment, growing outside the arachnoid. Their development determines the compression of the chiasmatic cistern, which could be stretched over the tumor. The parachiasmatic cisterns provide a protective plane between a tuberculum sellae meningioma and the optic apparatus, pituitary stalk, vessels of the anterior circulation, and the hypothalamus so that an extra-arachnoidal route or, above all, an extracranial avenue such as from below, might be preferred to manage this type of tumor.[21–23]

The endoscopic endonasal approach, with the removal of the posterior part of the planum, tuberculum sellae, and upper half of the sella, provides a direct, median, and bilateral view of the neurovascular structures of the entire suprasellar region, with some additional advantages from the surgical route and the properties of the endoscope itself. Indeed, this technique provides a wider, close-up view of the surgical field that permits the identification of many surgical landmarks, in the sphenoid sinus and even intradurally, thus allowing safe dissection of the tumor from the neurovascular structures without any brain retraction or manipulation of the optic apparatus.

The key points in meningioma surgery are early identification and coagulation of the tumor's dural attachment with subsequent devascularization. Referring to the early devascularization of an anterior cranial fossa meningioma, Yasargil[51] reported that "turgor of the tumor is markedly reduced and the consistency becomes similar to that of a lipoma." This seems the most relevant advantage of the endoscopic endonasal technique—that it permits the complete devascularization of a meningioma before the surgeon enters the intradural compartment, thus providing the possibility of dealing with a lesion that seems to be a lipoma.

Hence, working through the "low route" can facilitate a Simpson grade I removal, defined as complete tumor removal with excision of the dural attachment and involved bone, because the approach itself requires the removal of skull-base bone and dura to expose the lesion.

Once a meningioma has been devascularized, the low route presents as a further advantage the opportunity to

debulk the lesion through a midline trajectory. Thereafter, the tumor is dissected from the neurovascular structures, namely the optic nerves and chiasm, in an opposite way compared with the transcranial route: all the dissection maneuvers are made to manipulate the tumor surface, as for convexity meningiomas, without touching any vascular structures. This ability presents an advantage during the dissection of the small vessels supplying the chiasm and the optic nerves or in the presence of severe A1–optic nerve neurovascular conflicts (**Fig. 1.7**). As a result, the risk of postoperative visual loss, which is strictly related to the integrity of the vascularization of the optic chiasm, seems to be reduced.

Another advantage of the endonasal route is the opportunity to manage a limited expansion of the tuberculum sellae meningioma into the optic canal. Lesions with a

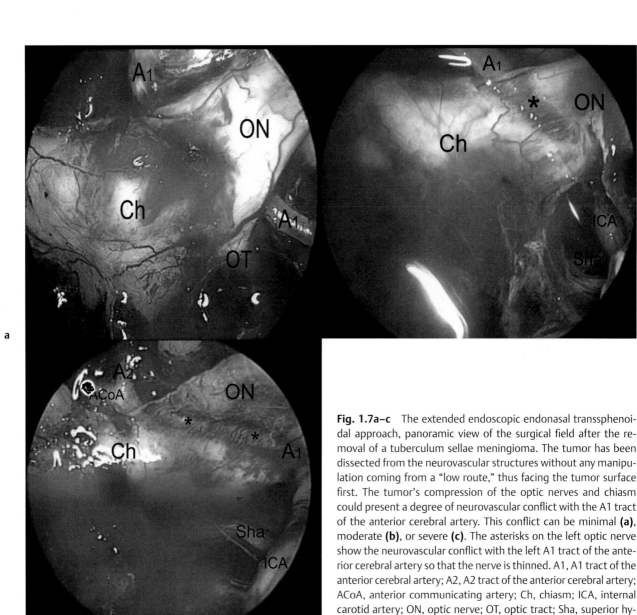

a

b

c

Fig. 1.7a–c The extended endoscopic endonasal transsphenoidal approach, panoramic view of the surgical field after the removal of a tuberculum sellae meningioma. The tumor has been dissected from the neurovascular structures without any manipulation coming from a "low route," thus facing the tumor surface first. The tumor's compression of the optic nerves and chiasm could present a degree of neurovascular conflict with the A1 tract of the anterior cerebral artery. This conflict can be minimal **(a)**, moderate **(b)**, or severe **(c)**. The asterisks on the left optic nerve show the neurovascular conflict with the left A1 tract of the anterior cerebral artery so that the nerve is thinned. A1, A1 tract of the anterior cerebral artery; A2, A2 tract of the anterior cerebral artery; ACoA, anterior communicating artery; Ch, chiasm; ICA, internal carotid artery; ON, optic nerve; OT, optic tract; Sha, superior hypophyseal artery.

wide dural attachment initially involve the inferomedial aspect of the optic canal, pushing the nerve upward, so that the endoscopic endonasal approach enables the removal of dura and lesion in the optic canal without manipulation of the nerve. Contrariwise, when the meningioma encases the optic nerve, this approach will not provide adequate access to deal with this component of the lesion.

The Disadvantages of the Low Route

Some drawbacks should be kept in mind when using this technique. First, it is technically demanding; thus, additional anatomic knowledge, experience, and dedicated surgical tools are needed because the anatomy is approached from a different and somewhat opposite point of view. In addition, an imaginative tridimensional concept for mental reconstruction of the lesion and the surrounding structures as seen from below is mandatory. Furthermore, some anatomic conditions could affect management of the lesion via the transsphenoidal route. If a well-pneumatized sphenoid sinus allows better visualization of all important landmarks, thus favoring surgical orientation, a conchal-type sphenoid sinus represents an obstacle. In addition, a small sella, with two close intracavernous carotids, could mandate a narrower approach, and a wider chiasmatic sulcus could facilitate the endonasal approach.

Problems concerning the control of bleeding from the main vessels in such a narrow space and the higher risk of postoperative CSF leak, as compared with the transcranial approaches, are still challenging. Regardless, the CSF leak rate is lower than that after endoscopic endonasal surgery for craniopharyngiomas. Meningiomas, especially when medium sized, compress the adjacent arachnoid cisterns, creating a natural barrier, which often is found intact even during transcranial surgery. Nevertheless, improvements in closure techniques and the use of new materials and dedicated instruments seem to further reduce such risks.

The successful use of such a technique requires careful patient selection. Appropriate indications include a small or medium-sized lesion without vascular encasement, with a dural attachment that does not extend beyond the optic canals, or without a broad attachment over the planum surface, and without lateral extension. Lesions that fit these criteria can be approached by means of such a technique so that the tumor can be exposed consistently to ensure that it is easily identified and removed.

Finally, it has to be kept in mind that adequate endoscopic equipment, image-guidance systems, dedicated instruments, and, above all, considerable experience with the endoscopic transsphenoidal technique are essential for the realization of this approach.[44] Nevertheless, further technological advancements in instrumentation, both optical and surgical, are expected to make such techniques safer and more feasible, therefore appropriately defining the indications for this approach and rendering it a viable alternative to be considered when dealing with a tuberculum sellae meningioma.

Moderator

Surgical Removal of Tuberculum Sellae Meningiomas: Endoscopic vs. Microscopic

William T. Couldwell

This case nicely exemplifies a timely controversy in skull-base surgery. Since Martin Weiss[52] first described the extended transsphenoidal approach, there has been a steady growth of interest in using the transnasal approach to remove an ever-expanding number of tumor types in the parasellar area and anterior skull base. The advantages of the endonasal endoscopic and transcranial microscopic approaches have been well discussed here by Cappabianca and DeMonte and their colleagues. I will briefly summarize my analysis of the advantages and disadvantages of these approaches before offering my opinion.

Endonasal Endoscopic Approach

Advantages

The advantages of the endonasal approach include ease and a lack of visible surgical incisions. The approach enables early devascularization of the tumor through removal of the tuberculum bony attachment and interruption of the tumor's blood supply. In addition, it offers the most direct access to the tumor and its bony attachment. The approach is midline and does not require any brain retraction for tumor exposure. Early indirect decompression is achieved with initial tumor removal. The olfactory nerves are at less risk of stretch injury than with a transcranial approach, as no brain retraction is necessary, and hyperostotic bone, usually an indication of tumor invasion, is removed. There are no blind spots during dissection, as all of the region medial to the carotid artery and optic nerve is visible, in contrast to a unilateral transcranial approach. Any tumor extending down into the sella may be easily removed through the endonasal transsphenoidal approach.

The visualization offered by the endoscope is superior to that of the microscope because it places the surgeon's eye at the level of the sella or anterior skull base and it provides the ability to look laterally around corners with appropriate angled endoscopes. This is particularly helpful in the present case to ensure there is no tumor lateral to the bony opening, which is limited by the carotid arteries and optic nerves.

Disadvantages

Because the endonasal endoscopic approach entails removal of the bone underlying the tumor, efforts to prevent a CSF leak are an important consideration. Any bone removal anterior to the tuberculum with an extended transsphenoidal approach is associated with a significantly higher risk of CSF fistulas than with a standard transsphenoidal approach to the sella.[20,21,53,54] This may be a significant risk and may necessitate a longer in-hospital course for management, including the adjuvant use of a lumbar drain. The techniques for reducing this operative risk vary,[20,53–55] but they all still result in a higher risk of postoperative fistulas than does a standard transcranial approach.

The other main disadvantage of the endonasal endoscopic approach is the difficulty in removing the tumor or its dural attachment over the optic nerve in the canal, or above and lateral to the anterior clinoid process. With the current instruments, the bimanual surgical technique is limited beyond the immediate direct view of the endoscope. That is, the surgeon is limited in his or her ability to work laterally despite the ability to visualize the tumor or its attachment. The recent advent of three-dimensional endoscopy may facilitate visualization, but the limitations of the instrumentation still remain.

Transcranial Microscopic Removal

Advantages

The advantages of an approach using the microscope are considerable in this case. First, it is a familiar approach. (I would choose a frontotemporal craniotomy for this case, although it may be amenable to a unilateral or bilateral subfrontal exposure.) It enables fine microsurgical dissection of the tumor from important cranial nerves (the optic nerves and chiasm here) and vascular structures (anterior cerebral and communicating arteries) under direct vision and with bimanual microsurgical control. The important

cranial nerves and arteries are identified early in the dissection in contrast to the endonasal endoscopic approach, during which they are identified near the end of tumor removal and may already have been manipulated if adherent to the tumor.

Another important advantage of the transcranial approach is the removal of the anterior clinoid process and any dural involvement over the clinoid and lateral to it. Removing the anterior clinoid allows complete decompression of the optic nerve and removal of tumor superior and lateral to this nerve, which is clearly difficult to achieve from below.

Disadvantages

Disadvantages of the approach include the obvious ones, such as a visible incision and the need for frontal lobe retraction. In addition, early devascularization of the tumor necessitates a basal approach designed to detach the tumor from the tuberculum early in the procedure. It may be necessary to partially remove the tumor to facilitate decompression of the optic nerves and chiasm before disconnecting the tumor from its attachment. Removal of the tumor in this case may therefore entail early blood loss. The other major disadvantage of the transcranial approach, if not performed in a midline fashion, is that tumor medial to the ipsilateral carotid artery and optic nerve may be difficult to visualize and remove. I have supplemented the frontotemporal approach with the use of an angled endoscope for this task, with good results.

The Verdict

Which approach would I choose? In this case, my experience has led me to increasingly favor a transcranial approach for such a tumor. Certainly, the mass can be removed through the transnasal approach, as has been well described by our group[20] and others.[21,22,27–29] However, removing the mass is only part of the goal of this surgery. Complete removal of these tumors should be the charge and should include all of the tumor plus its dural and bony attachments. This is accomplished most easily at the first operative intervention. To remove all tumor superior to the optic nerve in the optic canal, to adequately remove the clinoid if it is involved, and to remove the dural attachment above or lateral to the optic nerve is more easily and more certainly accomplished through a standard transcranial approach in my hands.

An example of the limitation of the endonasal endoscopic approach for this purpose is illustrated in the following case. A 54-year-old woman presented with visual loss from a tuberculum meningioma (**Fig. 1.8a,b**). After the tumor was completely resected through an endoscopic endonasal approach (**Fig. 1.8c,d**), she had a recurrence 3 years later with tumor lateral to the carotid artery and above the optic nerve in the region of the anterior clinoid process with compression of the left optic nerve (**Fig. 1.8e**). She required

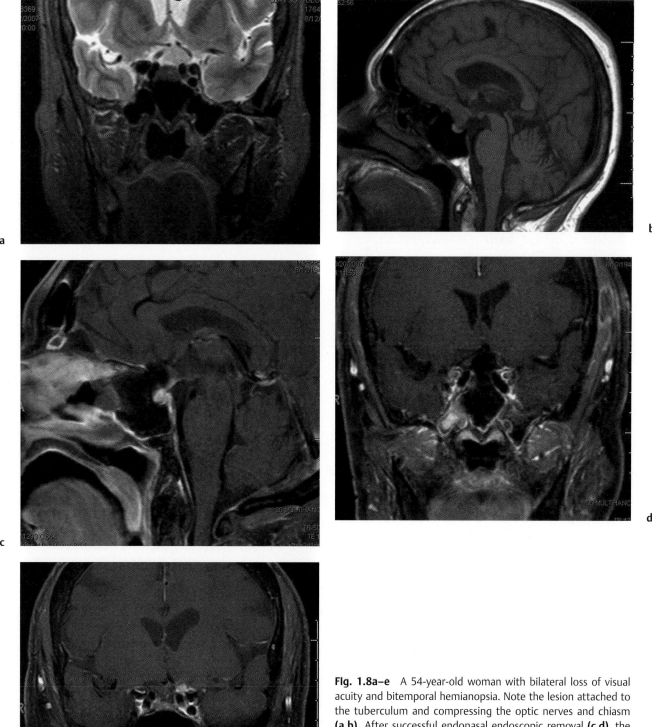

Fig. 1.8a–e A 54-year-old woman with bilateral loss of visual acuity and bitemporal hemianopsia. Note the lesion attached to the tuberculum and compressing the optic nerves and chiasm **(a,b)**. After successful endonasal endoscopic removal **(c,d)**, the fat-suppressed, contrast-enhanced T1-weighted magnetic resonance imaging studies showed no evidence of residual tumor. Three years after the tumor was removed, the patient presented again with recurrent visual loss in the left eye, with tumor above and lateral to the optic nerve **(e)**. The patient underwent transcranial surgery for removal.

a transcranial operation to remove the tumor, and surgery was complicated by extensive scarring in and around the optic nerve that we were attempting to decompress.

In the final analysis, there is a valid argument to be made for both approaches to the tumor. It will require long and careful follow-up of these cases to determine the optimal strategy for tumor control in the case of a meningioma. It may well be true that a meningioma, although a common skull-base lesion in this region, is not particularly well suited for endonasal removal, given the necessity for optimal Simpson-grade removal for long-term tumor control. Whether this can be achieved by an endonasal approach with improved instrumentation in the future remains to be determined. Optimal, safe, Simpson-grade removal should be the goal of surgery, and the choice of approach should be dictated with this goal in mind, when both approaches are safely performed by experienced hands.

References

1. Goel A, Muzumdar D. Surgical strategy for tuberculum sellae meningiomas. Neurosurg Q 2005;15:25–32
2. Nozaki K, Kikuta K, Takagi Y, Mineharu Y, Takahashi JA, Hashimoto N. Effect of early optic canal unroofing on the outcome of visual functions in surgery for meningiomas of the tuberculum sellae and planum sphenoidale. Neurosurgery 2008;62:839–844, discussion 844–846
3. Otani N, Muroi C, Yano H, Khan N, Pangalu A, Yonekawa Y. Surgical management of tuberculum sellae meningioma: role of selective extradural anterior clinoidectomy. Br J Neurosurg 2006;20:129–138
4. Schick U, Hassler W. Surgical management of tuberculum sellae meningiomas: involvement of the optic canal and visual outcome. J Neurol Neurosurg Psychiatry 2005;76:977–983
5. Bassiouni H, Asgari S, Stolke D. Tuberculum sellae meningiomas: functional outcome in a consecutive series treated microsurgically. Surg Neurol 2006;66:37–44, discussion 44–45
6. Chicani CF, Miller NR. Visual outcome in surgically treated suprasellar meningiomas. J Neuroophthalmol 2003;23:3–10
7. Kim TW, Jung S, Jung TY, Kim IY, Kang SS, Kim SH. Prognostic factors of postoperative visual outcomes in tuberculum sellae meningioma. Br J Neurosurg 2008;22:231–234
8. Li X, Liu M, Liu Y, Zhu S. Surgical management of Tuberculum sellae meningiomas. J Clin Neurosci 2007;14:1150–1154
9. Mathiesen T, Kihlström L. Visual outcome of tuberculum sellae meningiomas after extradural optic nerve decompression. Neurosurgery 2006;59:570–576, discussion 570–576
10. Park CK, Jung HW, Yang SY, Seol HJ, Paek SH, Kim DG. Surgically treated tuberculum sellae and diaphragm sellae meningiomas: the importance of short-term visual outcome. Neurosurgery 2006;59:238–243, discussion 238–243
11. Margalit N, Kesler A, Ezer H, Freedman S, Ram Z. Tuberculum and diaphragma sella meningioma—surgical technique and visual outcome in a series of 20 cases operated over a 2.5-year period. Acta Neurochir (Wien) 2007;149:1199–1204, discussion 204
12. Benjamin V, Russell SM. The microsurgical nuances of resecting tuberculum sellae meningiomas. Neurosurgery 2005;56(2, Suppl):411–417, discussion 411–417
13. Jallo GI, Benjamin V. Tuberculum sellae meningiomas: microsurgical anatomy and surgical technique. Neurosurgery 2002;51: 1432–1439, discussion 1439–1440
14. DeMonte F. Surgical treatment of anterior basal meningiomas. J Neurooncol 1996;29:239–248
15. Fahlbusch R, Schott W. Pterional surgery of meningiomas of the tuberculum sellae and planum sphenoidale: surgical results with special consideration of ophthalmological and endocrinological outcomes. J Neurosurg 2002;96:235–243
16. Goel A, Muzumdar D, Desai KI. Tuberculum sellae meningioma: a report on management on the basis of a surgical experience with 70 patients. Neurosurgery 2002;51:1358–1363, discussion 1363–1364
17. Nakamura M, Roser F, Struck M, Vorkapic P, Samii M. Tuberculum sellae meningiomas: clinical outcome considering different surgical approaches. Neurosurgery 2006;59:1019–1028, discussion 1028–1029
18. Pamir MN, Ozduman K, Belirgen M, Kilic T, Ozek MM. Outcome determinants of pterional surgery for tuberculum sellae meningiomas. Acta Neurochir (Wien) 2005;147:1121–1130, discussion 1130
19. Zevgaridis D, Medele RJ, Müller A, Hischa AC, Steiger HJ. Meningiomas of the sellar region presenting with visual impairment: impact of various prognostic factors on surgical outcome in 62 patients. Acta Neurochir (Wien) 2001;143: 471–476
20. Couldwell WT, Weiss MH, Rabb C, Liu JK, Apfelbaum RI, Fukushima T. Variations on the standard transsphenoidal approach to the sellar region, with emphasis on the extended approaches and parasellar approaches: surgical experience in 105 cases. Neurosurgery 2004;55:539–547, discussion 547–550
21. de Divitiis E, Cavallo LM, Esposito F, Stella L, Messina A. Extended endoscopic transsphenoidal approach for tuberculum sellae meningiomas. Neurosurgery 2007;61(5, Suppl 2):229–237, discussion 237–238
22. de Divitiis E, Esposito F, Cappabianca P, Cavallo LM, de Divitiis O. Tuberculum sellae meningiomas: high route or low route? A series of 51 consecutive cases. Neurosurgery 2008;62:556–563, discussion 556–563
23. de Divitiis E, Esposito F, Cappabianca P, Cavallo LM, de Divitiis O, Esposito I. Endoscopic transnasal resection of anterior cranial fossa meningiomas. Neurosurg Focus 2008;25:E8
24. Dusick JR, Esposito F, Kelly DF, et al. The extended direct endonasal transsphenoidal approach for nonadenomatous suprasellar tumors. J Neurosurg 2005;102:832–841
25. Dusick JR, Fatemi N, Mattozo C, et al. Pituitary function after endonasal surgery for nonadenomatous parasellar tumors: Rathke's cleft cysts, craniopharyngiomas, and meningiomas. Surg Neurol 2008;70:482–490, discussion 490–491
26. Fatemi N, Dusick JR, de Paiva Neto MA, Kelly DF. The endonasal microscopic approach for pituitary adenomas and other parasellar tumors: a 10-year experience. Neurosurgery 2008;63(4, Suppl 2):244–256, discussion 256
27. Gardner PA, Kassam AB, Thomas A, et al. Endoscopic endonasal resection of anterior cranial base meningiomas. Neurosurgery 2008;63:36–52, discussion 52–54

28. Jane JA Jr, Dumont AS, Vance ML, Laws ER Jr. The transsphenoidal transtuberculum sellae approach for suprasellar meningiomas. Semin Neurosurg 2003;14:211–218

29. Kitano M, Taneda M, Nakao Y. Postoperative improvement in visual function in patients with tuberculum sellae meningiomas: results of the extended transsphenoidal and transcranial approaches. J Neurosurg 2007;107:337–346

30. Laufer I, Anand VK, Schwartz TH. Endoscopic, endonasal extended transsphenoidal, transplanum transtuberculum approach for resection of suprasellar lesions. J Neurosurg 2007;106:400–406

31. Laws ER, Kanter AS, Jane JA Jr, Dumont AS. Extended transsphenoidal approach. J Neurosurg 2005;102:825–827, discussion 827–828

32. Carrau RL, Jho HD, Ko Y. Transnasal-transsphenoidal endoscopic surgery of the pituitary gland. Laryngoscope 1996;106:914–918

33. Jho HD, Carrau RL, Ko Y. Endoscopic pituitary surgery. In: Wilkins H, Rengachary S, eds. Neurosurgical Operative Atlas, vol. 5. Park Ridge, IL: American Association of Neurological Surgeons, 1996:1–12

34. Cappabianca P, Alfieri A, de Divitiis E. Endoscopic endonasal transsphenoidal approach to the sella: towards functional endoscopic pituitary surgery (FEPS). Minim Invasive Neurosurg 1998;41:66–73

35. Cappabianca P, Cavallo LM, Colao A, de Divitiis E. Surgical complications associated with the endoscopic endonasal transsphenoidal approach for pituitary adenomas. J Neurosurg 2002;97:293–298

36. Guiot G. Transsphenoidal approach in surgical treatment of pituitary adenomas: general principles and indications in nonfunctioning adenomas. In: Kohler PO, Ross GT, eds. Diagnosis and Treatment of Pituitary Adenomas. Amsterdam: Excerpta Medica, 1973:159–178

37. de Divitiis E, Cappabianca P, Cavallo LM. Endoscopic transsphenoidal approach: adaptability of the procedure to different sellar lesions. Neurosurgery 2002;51:699–705, discussion 705–707

38. Cook SW, Smith Z, Kelly DF. Endonasal transsphenoidal removal of tuberculum sellae meningiomas: technical note. Neurosurgery 2004;55:239–244, discussion 244–246

39. Cappabianca P, Cavallo LM, Esposito F, de Divitiis O, Messina A, de Divitiis E. Extended endoscopic endonasal approach to the midline skull base: the evolving role of transsphenoidal surgery. In: Pickard JD, Akalan N, Di Rocco C, et al, eds. Advances and Technical Standards in Neurosurgery. Vienna: Springer, 2008:152–199

40. Kim J, Choe I, Bak K, Kim C, Kim N, Jang Y. Transsphenoidal supradiaphragmatic intradural approach: technical note. Minim Invasive Neurosurg 2000;43:33–37

41. Prevedello DM, Thomas A, Gardner P, Snyderman CH, Carrau RL, Kassam AB. Endoscopic endonasal resection of a synchronous pituitary adenoma and a tuberculum sellae meningioma: technical case report. Neurosurgery 2007;60(4, Suppl 2):E401, discussion E401

42. Hardy J. Transsphenoidal hypophysectomy. J Neurosurg 1971;34:582–594

43. Kassam AB, Vescan AD, Carrau RL, et al. Expanded endonasal approach: vidian canal as a landmark to the petrous internal carotid artery. J Neurosurg 2008;108:177–183

44. Snyderman C, Kassam A, Carrau R, Mintz A, Gardner P, Prevedello DM. Acquisition of surgical skills for endonasal skull base surgery: a training program. Laryngoscope 2007;117:699–705

45. Prevedello DM, Kassam AB, Snyderman C, et al. Endoscopic cranial base surgery: ready for prime time? Clin Neurosurg 2007;54:48–57

46. de Divitiis E, Cavallo LM, Cappabianca P, Esposito F. Extended endoscopic endonasal transsphenoidal approach for the removal of suprasellar tumors: part 2. Neurosurgery 2007;60:46–58, discussion 58–59

47. Cavallo LM, de Divitiis O, Aydin S, et al. Extended endoscopic endonasal transsphenoidal approach to the suprasellar area: anatomic considerations: part 1. Neurosurgery 2007;61:ONS24–ONS34

48. Cavallo LM, Messina A, Esposito F, et al. Skull base reconstruction in the extended endoscopic transsphenoidal approach for suprasellar lesions. J Neurosurg 2007;107:713–720

49. Hadad G, Bassagasteguy L, Carrau RL, et al. A novel reconstructive technique after endoscopic expanded endonasal approaches: vascular pedicle nasoseptal flap. Laryngoscope 2006;116:1882–1886

50. Kassam AB, Thomas A, Carrau RL, et al. Endoscopic reconstruction of the cranial base using a pedicled nasoseptal flap. Neurosurgery 2008;63(1, Suppl 1):ONS44–ONS52, discussion ONS52–ONS53

51. Yasargil MG. Meningiomas. In: Yasargil MG, ed. Microneurosurgery: Microneurosurgery of CNS Tumors, vol. IV B. Stuttgart: Georg Thieme Verlag, 1996:140

52. Weiss MH. The transnasal transsphenoidal approach. In Apuzzo MLJ, ed. Surgery of the Third Ventricle. Baltimore: Williams & Wilkins, 1987:476–494

53. Cavallo LM, Messina A, Esposito F, et al. Skull base reconstruction in the extended endoscopic transsphenoidal approach for suprasellar lesions. J Neurosurg 2007;107:713–720

54. Hadad G, Bassagasteguy L, Carrau RL, et al. A novel reconstructive technique after endoscopic expanded endonasal approaches: vascular pedicle nasoseptal flap. Laryngoscope 2006;116:1882–1886

55. Couldwell WT, Kan P, Weiss MH. Simple closure following transsphenoidal surgery. Technical note. Neurosurg Focus 2006;20(3):E11

Management of Parasagittal Meningiomas Involving the Superior Sagittal Sinus: Partial Removal with Radiosurgery vs. Total Removal with Repair

Case

A 40-year-old right-handed woman presented with headache and a new onset of generalized seizures. A physical examination showed mild left hemiparesis.

Participants

Combined Surgical and Radiosurgical Treatment of Parasagittal and Falx Meningiomas with Superior Sagittal Sinus Invasion: M. Necmettin Pamir, Selcuk Peker, and Koray Özduman

Total Removal of Parasagittal Meningiomas Involving the Superior Sagittal Sinus: Marc P. Sindou, P. Hallacq, and Jorge E. Alvernia

Moderators: Management of Parasagittal Meningiomas Involving the Superior Sagittal Sinus: Partial Removal with Radiosurgery vs. Total Removal with Repair: Kenji Ohata and Rahadian Indarto Susilo

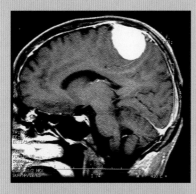

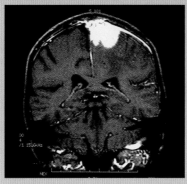

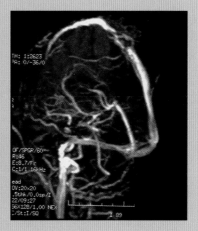

Combined Surgical and Radiosurgical Treatment of Parasagittal and Falx Meningiomas with Superior Sagittal Sinus Invasion

M. Necmettin Pamir, Selcuk Peker, and Koray Özduman

This patient's neurologic examination showed mild hemiparesis, and magnetic resonance imaging (MRI) demonstrated a left-sided parasagittal meningioma located in the middle third. Magnetic resonance venography showed partial occlusion or narrowing of the superior sagittal sinus (SSS). Our recommendation for this patient is surgical resection of the tumor outside the sinus and subsequent radiosurgery for the residual portion that invades the sinus.

Parasagittal meningiomas invading the SSS have long presented a problem for neurosurgeons. Most of the patients with this lesion have neurologic signs or symptoms, prompting some form of treatment, and even if asymptomatic, most of these tumors grow over time, infiltrating surrounding structures. But choosing the form of treatment is not so straightforward. The literature from the microsurgical era concentrates on two treatment options: conservative resection, and radical resection of both the tumor and the invaded sinus combined with reconstruction of the sinus. However, accumulating evidence has shown us that neither of these options provides a safe, effective, and long-lasting solution to the problem, and this lack of a solution has prompted a search for new and more effective treatment options.

General Considerations

Parasagittal and falx meningiomas make up a significant proportion of intracranial meningiomas, with reported rates ranging from 19.24 to 33.7%.[1-4] In early studies, these meningiomas were classified based on whether or not they showed hyperostosis. An anatomic classification into anterior, middle, and posterior locations was first devised by Olivecrona.[4] Anterior cases are located between the crista galli and the coronal suture, middle cases arise between the coronal and lambdoid sutures, and posterior cases are localized between the lambdoid suture and the torcular. Most of these lesions occur in the middle third, and the reported relative rates are 14.8 to 33.9%, 44.8 to 70.4%, and 9.2 to 29.6% in the anterior, middle, and posterior portions, respectively.[1,5-8]

Superior sagittal sinus involvement is reported in a significant proportion of the cases, with Simpson[9] noting a rate of 40%. The extent of venous involvement by the meningioma can range from invasion of the outer surface of the venous wall to complete invasion and obliteration of the sinus. Several authors have devised classification schemes for surgical decision making. The first detailed classification scheme of Krause was later modified by Merrem and then Bonnal and Brotchi.[10] This widely cited classification scheme was in turn later modified by Hakuba to include eight subtypes. The latest, simplified version by

Sindou and Alvernia[11] describes six types of parasagittal meningiomas classified according to the degree of sinus invasion:

> **Type I:** Invasion of the outer surface of the sinus wall
> **Type II:** Invasion of the lateral recess
> **Type III:** Invasion of the lateral wall
> **Type IV:** Invasion of the lateral wall and roof
> **Type V:** Total occlusion of the sinus with one wall free of tumor
> **Type VI:** Total occlusion of the sinus without one wall free of tumor

The reported rates of these types are 31%, 8%, 11%, 13%, 5%, and 32%, respectively.[11,12]

The anatomic classification into three segments along the anteroposterior axis is not merely of diagnostic significance but relates to the neurologic consequences of SSS closure at that segment. According to their terminal drainage, the superficial veins of the cerebral hemispheres are divided into superior sagittal, falcine, sphenoid, and tentorial groups.[13-15] These systems are interconnected by three large anastomotic veins: the vein of Trolard, the vein of Labbé, and the superficial sylvian vein. The superior sagittal group drains blood from both hemispheres into the SSS, the largest draining vein. The size of the SSS increases from anterior to posterior with the addition of veins from the frontal, parietal, and occipital lobes.[13-15] The terminal veins adjoin to form 1- to 2-cm free venous segments along the superior margin of the hemisphere in the subdural space. These terminal cortical veins can drain directly into the SSS or pass through lacunae before they drain into the sinus.[14]

The clinical consequences of acute occlusion, thrombosis, or sacrifice of the SSS were first documented in the first quarter of the 20th century,[13] and it was soon concluded that the site of closure is the dominant factor in the patient's neurologic outcome. Sacrifice of the anterior third is well tolerated, but some authors note that general slowing of the patient's thought process and activity, or even akinetic mutism, are reported after such sacrifice, although these phenomena are rare.[15] Sacrifice of the middle third causes hemiplegia, more prominent in the lower extremities, and akinesia.[15] The posterior third is the largest portion and receives the straight sinus, and acute occlusion or surgical sacrifice of this portion carries a significant risk of fatal brain edema and increased intracranial pressure.

Although acute obliteration of the sinus is associated with such serious consequences, a more gradual closure during tumor growth is usually well tolerated. One must bear in mind that the gradual closure from tumor invasion is not merely a closure of the sinus. The living organism reacts actively to changes in the "interior milieu," and gradual occlusion of the sinus is certainly accompanied by functional changes in venous drainage. Closure of the main drainage route does not necessarily lead to diversion of the venous drainage to other systems away from the SSS. In many cases, venous collaterals take over the role of the main channel, and sacrifice of these collaterals leads to morbidity similar to that of SSS sacrifice. Whether, or how much, the tumor contributes to venous drainage of the region is not known.[16]

Management Strategy

The goal in managing this type of "problem" meningioma is clear: keep the patient fully functional and prevent or provide long-term relief from problems associated with intracranial tumor growth. The availability of several alternative treatment possibilities indicates that there is still no single best form of treatment for meningiomas invading the SSS. The most straightforward treatment option is complete surgical excision. Meningiomas located in the anterior third are the least controversial with regard to treatment, and most authors recommend simple radical resection. Parasagittal meningiomas located in the middle third of the SSS are the most difficult to treat because of the abundance of afferent veins, the significant morbidity associated with their sacrifice, and the high risk of recurrence. Meningiomas in this group were early christened as "problem" meningiomas.[2] Total resection is technically demanding; it can be associated with significant morbidity in patients with invasion of the SSS. In some cases total resection is not possible. The general consensus for lesions that have limited sinus invasion is surgery followed by limited local reconstruction. Simple repair or patching with endogenous material (for example, muscle grafts) is adequate in most of these cases. If the invasion is more extensive, a radical excision necessitates venous reconstruction, but this entails a significant complication rate. Some authors have advocated more conservative resections to avoid this increased risk, but conservative approaches are associated with continued growth.

Authors who have advocated subtotal resection of these meningiomas resect the tumor outside the sinus and leave the invading portion untouched.[3,17] Surgery is planned to restore or preserve function in an attempt to combine the lowest possible risk with the maximum benefit to the patient, based on the notion that most meningiomas are slow-growing tumors and even subtotal resection provides long, progression-free periods. However, most of these patients survive for long periods and therefore regrowth is inevitable after such conservative resections.[18–20] Recurrences are managed through repeated conservative resections until the sinus is obliterated, when total resection becomes an option. Although this idea may sound attractive, it is well known that the efficacy of surgery decreases and the complication rate increases with each repeated sur-

gical intervention. The literature contains no solid scientific evidence on the long-term results of subtotal resection.

The high rate of regrowth after subtotal resection and the fact that complete surgical resection including the invaded structures is associated with lower rates of recurrence led several authors to develop techniques to resect the invaded sinus along with the tumor. As noted above, resecting part of a patent SSS can cause serious morbidity and mortality due to venous infarction and brain edema. Therefore, techniques have been developed to repair or reconstruct the sinus after the portion invaded by the meningioma is removed.[5,6,10–12,21–29] Most recent studies, however, indicate that such aggressive approaches are not necessarily associated with good surgical results or low recurrence rates, and they are still associated with significant morbidity.[25] Such a venous reconstruction is a formidable surgical challenge, and the literature contains only a few large series of SSS reconstruction totaling fewer than 200 cases.

Bonnal and Brotchi[10] were the leading authors advocating such procedures. In 1978, they published the results of 34 patients with SSS repair or reconstruction with venous allografts for parasagittal meningiomas. In nine patients, the surgeons were able to preserve the patency of the sinus without using a graft. In the other 25, they removed one or more walls of the SSS and then rebuilt the structure using a dural or venous graft. In one case, they needed to remove the entire SSS and then create a new sinus structure using a total vein graft.

Hakuba[23] also reported his results with 23 cases of parasagittal meningiomas. In six patients, he totally removed the tumor and the sinus. Seventeen patients had sinus involvement and, after total tumor excision, Hakuba repaired the sinus wall or reconstructed the sinus with a vein graft. In this group, 29% of patients had postoperative paresis.

On two occasions, Sindou and his colleague[11,12] reported their experience with the aggressive management of parasagittal meningiomas invading the SSS. The second study, of 100 meningiomas that invaded the dural sinuses, included 92 cases that were located in the SSS. Of these, 30.4% were in the anterior third in close relation to the precentral veins, 52.3% were in the middle third in relation to the postcentral veins, and 17.4% were in the posterior third.[11] The authors reported gross total removal in 93% of these patients (Simpson grade I or II) and radical excision combined with coagulation of a small amount of residual tumor (Simpson grade III) in the other 7%. The permanent neurologic morbidity rate was 8%, and the mortality rate was 3%. Looking back at those publications, one realizes that the techniques are not very efficient. In Bonnal and Brotchi's series, the immediate postoperative control angiogram showed a patent SSS in 87% of the 34 patients. This rate was 66% in Hakuba's[23] series and 64% in Sindou's[12] 2001 series, indicating that, in up to a third of cases, the venous reconstruction did not work.

Similarly, the recurrence rates after radical resection are not very impressive either. Regardless of the form of surgical treatment, recurrence is common in patients with meningiomas invading the SSS. This high risk of recurrence was originally documented by Simpson's[9] landmark study, which indicated a recurrence rate of 5% for Simpson grade I and 17% for Simpson grade II resections. This is most likely due to microscopic residuals undetected at the time of surgery. Mathiesen and colleagues[30] reported microscopic residual meningioma growth in dural resection margins in 41% of "radical" Simpson grade I operations. Authors who have not attempted sinus reconstruction have reported similarly high rates of recurrence in patients in whom radical resections were possible. Jääskeläinen[31] reported a recurrence rate of 21% after seemingly complete removal. At a mean follow-up of 25.4 years, Caroli and colleagues[5] reported a 9.3% recurrence rate after Simpson grade I and a 42.9% recurrence after Simpson grade II resections. The mean time to recurrence was 6.8 years after grade I removal and 4.7 years after grade II or III resections. These results indicate that a more radical resection can decrease but not eliminate the risk of recurrence in patients with parasagittal meningiomas invading the SSS. One can also conclude that a more radical resection does not significantly delay the time to recurrence either. Based on these findings, it is not surprising that, even in the hands of masterful surgeons, radical resection combined with SSS reconstruction are associated with considerable rates of recurrence. In 2003, Brotchi's research group[25] documented the long-term results for these cases. Of the 25 individuals who underwent partial or total SSS removal and sinus reconstruction, 15 had total tumor excision, and these patients had been followed for more than 10 years. Five of these 15 individuals (33%) developed a focal meningioma recurrence. The remaining 10 of the 25 patients underwent subtotal tumor excision, and eight of them had been followed for more than 10 years. Five of these eight patients (63%) developed local recurrence. Because of these outcomes, the authors questioned the efficacy of their approach and concluded that the optimal strategy for patients with meningiomas involving the SSS is gross tumor removal followed by monitoring, and radiosurgery if regrowth occurs.

In stark contrast, Sindou and Alvernia[11] reported a recurrence rate of 4% over a mean 8-year follow-up period (3–23 years). Such perfect results have not been replicated by any other master surgeon. Having analyzed the literature, we gave up the strategy of radical resection and reconstruction and started using a combination of surgery and the gamma knife.[8] Our rationale is based on our previous good results with the combination of surgery and radiosurgery for meningiomas in other locations[32] and the good results of other groups with this type of meningioma.[7]

The Role of Radiosurgery

The high complication rates of aggressive treatment strategies and the risk of recurrence after conservative treatment have created a need for alternative treatment strategies. Radiosurgical treatment of meningiomas has proven safe and effective, and this treatment modality for meningiomas has become very popular in recent years for the primary treatment of small meningiomas or as an adjuvant for residual or recurrent cases.[26,27] The reported tumor growth control rates range from 85 to 95%.[27] As in the case of cavernous sinus meningiomas, this relatively less-invasive treatment modality can potentially be used as an adjunct or alternative in patients with parasagittal meningiomas invading the SSS to achieve long-term control of tumor growth with little morbidity.[28]

Currently there is no definitive evidence to show the superiority of aggressive or less invasive treatment paradigms. Only two studies have been published to test the hypothesis that the gamma knife can be used effectively to treat parasagittal meningiomas that invade the SSS. Kondziolka and colleagues[7] conducted a multicenter study and documented treatment results for 23 such patients. Most of these meningiomas had invaded the middle or posterior region of the SSS, and the mean tumor volume was 10 cm[3]. Seventy-eight patients underwent radiosurgery as the primary therapy, with a 5-year actuarial tumor control rate of 93%, and none of the tumors smaller than 7.5 cc showed regrowth in the long term. For the 125 patients who had undergone surgery before gamma knife treatment, the 5-year control rate was only 60%. The authors reported that most cases of radiosurgery failure were due to remote tumor growth, as a precise definition of meningioma borders can be complicated in patients who have undergone previous surgery for SSS-invading meningiomas. In the 203 cases reported by Kondziolka and colleagues, the median marginal dose was 15 Gy. Sixteen percent of the patients developed symptomatic edema after radiosurgery. The authors analyzed the potential causes of this edema and found that the only factor correlated with this complication was previous neurologic deficit. In all cases, the edema resolved with medical therapy. The authors concluded that, in patients with a small meningioma (< 3 cm diameter) that has invaded the SSS but in whom the sinus is still patent, radiosurgery should be the primary surgical procedure. In patients in whom the tumor is larger, they recommend planned, second-stage radiosurgery.

In 2006, we reported our experience with gamma knife radiosurgery in 43 patients with parasagittal meningiomas that invaded the SSS.[8] Twenty-eight patients had undergone previous resection, and the follow-up period after radiosurgery ranged from 24 to 86 months (median 46 months). The median dose was 15 Gy. During this follow-up, 22 tumors (51%) decreased in size, 16 (37%) remained volumetrically unchanged, and five (12%) grew. The overall rate of tumor control with radiosurgery was 88%. Based on a minimum of 2 years' follow-up, our results show that radiosurgery provided successful tumor control in 13 of the 17 patients with recurrent meningiomas and 10 of the 11 patients with residual tumor tissue. The discrepancy relates to small tumor volumes in residual cases, resulting in possibly higher marginal doses. Our data also indicated that, at 2 years' follow-up, gamma knife radiosurgery controlled tumor growth 100% in virgin cases. We found that radiosurgery was ineffective in two patients with malignant meningiomas. We therefore do not recommend radiosurgery as the first-line treatment for these cases. The overall recurrence rate for the 24 residual or recurrent meningiomas with a typical histology was 8%, a rate comparable to the recurrence rates reported after gross total resection. Our surgical strategy for these tumors in the earlier years was total excision with removal of the affected SSS wall and grafting for repair. However, in 1997 we changed our policy. We now remove the gross mass of the tumor, coagulate the infiltrated portion of the sinus wall, and then assess with MRI within the first 24 hours.

Conclusion

Our management of parasagittal meningiomas is currently based on the following considerations:

1. Parasagittal and falx meningiomas invading the SSS are common, and frequently present with neurologic symptomatology. Most of these tumors grow at follow-up; therefore, treatment is indicated.

2. The general consensus for managing tumors in the anterior third is surgery regardless of sinus invasion. Radiosurgery is also an option for patients with small meningiomas.

3. Conservative resection is associated with a high rate of regrowth. The increased morbidity rates with each repeat surgery speak against this treatment option.

4. Radical surgical resection combined with sinus reconstruction is associated with significant morbidity, low efficiency, and similarly high recurrence rates.

5. Radiation treatment is associated with significant morbidity and is reserved as a salvage treatment in recurrent cases unresponsive to other treatment methods.

6. Radiosurgery is an exciting treatment strategy and can be used as a primary treatment in all patients with small parasagittal meningiomas, unless there is a significant mass effect or peritumoral edema. Radiosurgery can also be effectively administered as an adjuvant therapy after maximal surgical resection outside the sinus to decrease the risk of regrowth. Short- and medium-term results indicate that this is a safe and effective strategy. Long-term results are yet to be determined.

Total Removal of Parasagittal Meningiomas Involving the Superior Sagittal Sinus with Sinus Repair

Marc P. Sindou, P. Hallacq, and Jorge E. Alvernia

The presented case illustrates the difficulties of surgical decision making. The T1-weighted MRI shows that the tumor is located in the posterior part of the SSS, in the middle third, and invades at least the ipsilateral wall of the sinus, and perhaps also its roof. From these images and the venous MR angiogram, it seems impossible to ascertain whether the sinus lumen is totally or only subtotally occluded. The venous collateral circulation visible on the oblique image of the venous MR angiogram might be, in part, a still open (or recanalized) sinus lumen or, in part, satellite channels belonging to the afferent cortical veins. In addition, the picture shows (emissary) intradiploic drainage for the anterior third of the SSS. These paths of drainage contribute to the collateral circulation of the partially (or totally) occluded sinus.

For this otherwise healthy young woman, two surgical approaches are possible: gross tumor removal with coagulation of the invaded sinus walls leaving an intrasinusal fragment in place, or radical removal with or without restoration of the venous circulation. Our preference would be to first remove the extrasinusal portion of the meningioma

after debulking the tumor, with dissection of its so-called capsule from the brain cortex. We would then resect the invaded walls and restore circulation with a patch.

Case Discussion

To reduce the risk of recurrence of a parasagittal meningioma, our current attitude is to attempt whenever possible a total removal of the tumor, including the invaded walls or the occluded portion of the sinus. Such a decision to radically remove the tumor leads to an aggressive surgical approach, which implies restoration of the venous circulation.

In the "dangerous" case presented here, our decision to radically remove the tumor and restore the venous circulation is reinforced by the tumor's location within the province of rolandic outflow. Impairment in this location would probably cause hemorrhagic infarction in crucial sensorimotor territories. Because the meningioma in this patient likely does not invade the contralateral wall, it would be possible to restore flow with a patch.

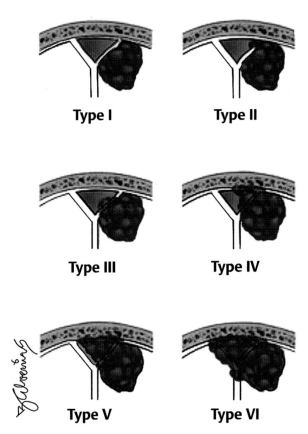

Type I   **Type II**

Type III   **Type IV**

Type V   **Type VI**

Fig. 2.1 The authors' classification of parasagittal meningiomas.[11,12,15,33] Type I: The meningioma is attached to the outer layer of the sinus wall. Type II: The lateral recess is invaded. Type III: The ipsilateral wall is invaded. Type IV: Both the ipsilateral wall and the roof of the sinus are invaded. Type V: The lateral wall and the roof are invaded and the lumen is occluded, but the contralateral wall is free of invasion. Type VI: All sinus walls are invaded and the sinus is totally occluded.

General Considerations

Classification

Our surgical experience comprises a series of 160 meningiomas involving the major dural venous sinuses.[11,12,15,33] This experience has led us to adopt the following surgical strategies based on the classification of these meningiomas into six types,[11,12,15,27,33] as shown in **Fig. 2.1**:

> **Type I:** The meningioma is attached to the sole outer layer of the sinus wall. The outer dural layer is resected and the site of attachment coagulated, leaving a clean and glistening dural surface.
> **Type II:** The lateral recess is invaded. The intrasinusal fragment is extracted and the dural defect repaired with either a simple running suture or a patch made of autologous aponeurosis (dura mater, periosteum, fascia lata, or, better, fascia temporalis).
> **Type III:** The ipsilateral lateral wall is invaded. The invaded wall is resected and repaired with a patch.

> **Type IV:** The ipsilateral wall and the roof are both invaded. The invaded walls are resected and the sinus is kept patent with a patch reconstruction.
> **Types V and VI:** The sinus is totally occluded. In Type V, one wall is free of tumor.

Although the current theory is to remove the invaded portion of the sinus without reestablishing venous circulation, our preference is to restore this circulation. In tumors of type V, circulation can be restored with a patch after the two invaded walls (or ipsilateral wall and roof) have been resected and the fragment that occludes the sinus extracted (**Fig. 2.2**). In tumors of type VI, restoration must be done with a bypass, which can be end-to-side before tumor removal or end-to-end after removal. For meningiomas in the posterior third of the SSS, the torcular or the lateral sinus, a sino-jugular bypass at the neck can be done before sacrifice of the invaded portion (**Fig. 2.3**).

Technical Considerations

Surgery of meningiomas invading the dural venous sinuses is facilitated when the following technical considerations are respected. Good venous return is best obtained by placing the patient in a semi-sitting (lounging) position, and the operative exposure should be as extensive as possible. The skin flap and craniotomy should extend across the midline to expose both sides of the sinus and some 3 cm proximal and distal to the margins of the invaded sinus. The operation should be stopped and the venous circulation evaluated if the brain swells, which can happen when the collateral venous pathways through the pericranium, diploë, or dura mater become impaired. Evaluation consists of determining the evolution of the swelling, taking Doppler measurements, and measuring intravascular venous pressure with a small needle[27] so that a decision can be made. The decision can be to defer further resection or pursue removal with venous reconstruction.

Because there might be discrepancies between the images and anatomic findings, the sinus should be explored through a short incision to evaluate the patency of the lumen and reveal any intrasinusal fragment. The temporary control of hemostasis is obtained rather easily by packing small pledgets of Surgicel within the lumen and at the ostia of afferent veins, if necessary. Vascular and aneurysm clips might crush or injure the sinus walls and tear the afferent veins. Balloons cannot be moved through the lumen because of septa inside. Furthermore, their use is dangerous as they might avulse the sinus endothelium.

Venous reconstruction can then be done with patches or bypasses. Continuous sutures (Prolene 8-0) complete the procedure. Although an autologous vein appears to be most suitable for a patch, harvesting a vein graft would be disproportionate. Dura mater, pericranium, fascia lata, or fascia

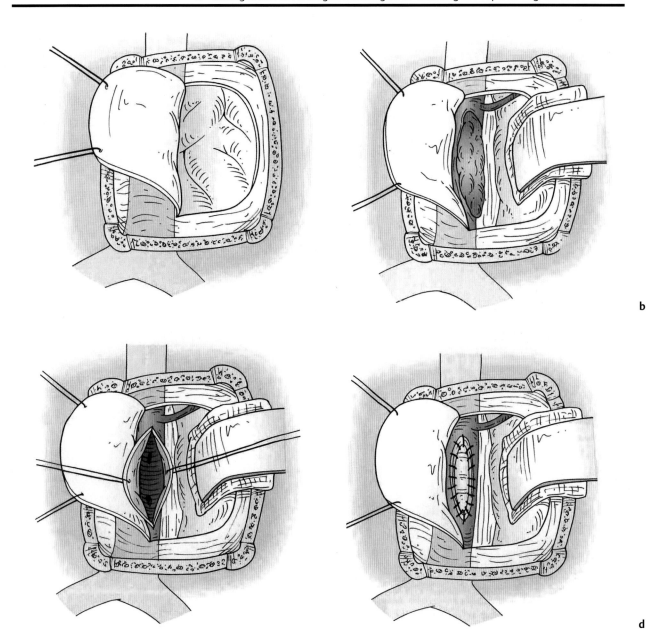

a

b

c

d

Fig. 2.2a–d The patching technique in the superior sagittal sinus (SSS) for a parasagittal meningioma that totally occludes the lumen of the sinus (type V) on the right side in the posterior third. **(a)** The meningioma is exposed. **(b)** Tumor outside the sinus is removed; the ipsilateral wall has been invaded. **(c)** The intraluminal fragment is removed. The inner aspect of the contralateral wall of the sinus is visible, and the wall is intact. The ostia of two afferent veins entering the sinus are also visible. Blood loss is controlled by packing with Surgicel (not shown). **(d)** Reconstruction of the resected (right) wall by means of a patch made of fascia temporalis sutured with two hemi-running sutures. (From Sindou M, Alvernia J. Intracranial venous revascularization. In: Abdulrauf S, ed. Cerebral Revascularization Techniques in Extracranial-to-Intracranial Bypass Surgery. Philadelphia: Elsevier Saunders, 2010:361. Reprinted by permission.)

temporalis may be used as patches; they have a structure rigid enough to allow blood to flow inside without collapse.

Patching

A patch can be used to maintain venous flow not only for tumors of types II, III, and IV, but also for type V to restore venous circulation. The best material is fascia temporalis, which is both soft and robust and can be harvested close to the surgical area. The patch is placed with two hemi-running continuous sutures made with 6-0 to 8-0 nylon thread. An illustration of the patch technique appears in **Fig. 2.2**.

Bypassing

Experimental studies and clinical assays have been performed to find the best material for bypasses in cerebral venous surgery.[21,29,34–36] Autologous veins grafts are taken

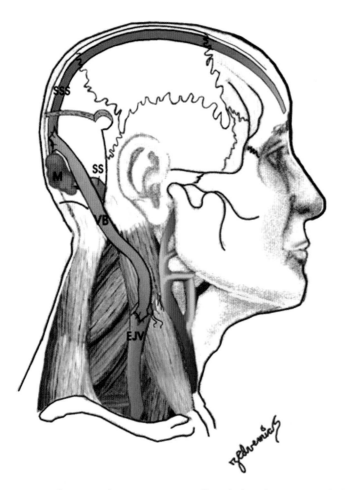

a

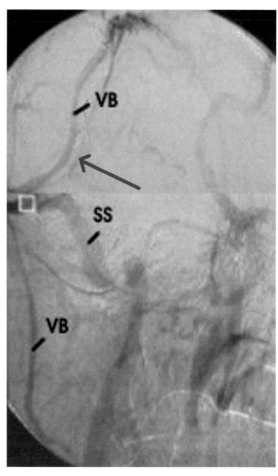

b

Fig. 2.3a,b A torcular meningioma totally occluding the venous confluence (type VI) with a long sino-jugular bypass. The patient's clinical presentation included the intracranial hypertension syndrome with headaches, papilledema, and dementia. **(a)** Venous hypertension was treated with an autologous venous bypass (VB) from the posterior third of the SSS to the external jugular vein (EJV) using a 20-cm graft from the median saphenous vein. M, meningioma; SS, straight sinus. **(b)** Two weeks after surgery, digital subtraction angiography showed that the bypass was patent (*arrows*).

either from the external jugular vein for a short graft, or from the internal saphenous vein when the bypass must be longer than 10 cm (**Fig. 2.3**). Thrombosis occurred in the bypass segments of all six of our patients in whom we used Gore-Tex, asymptomatically in five and with acute but fortunately transient intracranial hypertension in one.

Patency

The patency of the venous reconstruction can be checked at the end of the procedure with the so-called patency test with two forceps or, better, with a Doppler probe. The flow pattern reflects the equilibrium established between the anastomotic outflow of the collateral veins and the flow in the newly opened sinus. After surgery, it is important to maintain good blood volume and have the patient's head elevated to enhance intracranial drainage. To prevent clotting, we consider postoperative anticoagulation therapy to be mandatory for at least 3 months, until endothelialization occurs. This strategy did not increase hemorrhagic complications in our series. Heparin is administered as

soon as the morning after surgery and for 3 weeks following at dosages that double the coagulation time. Warfarin is then administered for the next 3 months until the (hypothetical) end of sinus, patch, or graft endothelialization.

The long-term patency of venous repair remains an unsolved problem (**Table 2.1**). The fact that all of our patients who had a graft that thrombosed (with the exception of one with a Gore-Tex tube) remained asymptomatic does not mean that the venous reconstruction was useless. It is possible that the venous repair allows time for compensatory venous pathways to develop. Importantly, the three patients who died of brain swelling all had type VI meningiomas with sinus invasion that had been totally resected without the restoration of venous flow.[11]

Conclusion

Meningiomas invading major dural sinuses raise a dilemma for the surgeon: leave the fragment invading the sinus and have a higher risk of recurrence, or attempt total removal with or without venous reconstruction and expose the pa-

Table 2.1 Patency of Sinus Reconstruction in Our Series[11]

Angiographic Control Surgical Modality	Total	Angio	Patent Yes	Patent No
Resection of intraluminal fragment within lateral recess + resuture	8	8	8	0
Resection of invaded wall + patch (fascia)	19	15	13	2
Resection of invaded portion + bypass with saphenous vein	11	10	7	3
Resection of invaded portion + bypass with external jugular vein	1	1	1	0
Resection of invaded portion + bypass with Gore-Tex	6	6	0	6
Total	45	40	29	11

tient to a potentially greater operative danger. Radical removal implies the need to preserve or repair the venous circulation.

Our study of long-term results in a series of 100 patients with meningiomas involving a major dural sinus, in whom we attempted radical removal and venous repair,[11] has led us to the following conclusions. The low recurrence rate of 4% with a mean follow-up of 8 years (range, 3 to 23 years) supports a decision to resect not only the tumor outside the sinus but also the fragment invading the sinus itself. When radical removal is attempted, we consider venous reconstruction mandatory when the sinus is incompletely occluded, and potentially useful even if there is complete occlusion. The traditional belief that radical removal of meningiomas totally occluding the sinus is not dangerous must be reconsidered because the compensatory collateral channels may be compromised during the approach. In our series, the three patients who died (all from brain swelling) had a meningioma that totally occluded the sinus and was removed *en bloc* without any restoration of the sinus circulation.[11] Because surgical access may destroy some or all of the collateral pathways that naturally develop to compensate for occlusion, restoring the venous circulation at the end of surgery reduces brain swelling.

To guide surgical decision making for patients with parasagittal meningiomas, we introduced a classification of six types simplified from the ones described by Merrem[37] and Bonnal and colleagues.[38] Finally, we emphasize that, during intracranial surgery, "dangerous" veins and sinuses must be scrupulously respected or reconstructed, if necessary, especially in tumor surgery. The prognosis for patients undergoing intracranial surgery lies in preserving not only the arterial supply but also venous drainage. Many other experienced neurosurgeons throughout the world share this view.[10,39–45]

Moderators

Management of Parasagittal Meningiomas Involving the Superior Sagittal Sinus: Partial Removal with Radiosurgery vs. Total Removal with Repair

Kenji Ohata and Rahadian Indarto Susilo

The optimal outcome for a patient with a newly diagnosed parasagittal meningioma includes complete removal of the tumor and its dural base, preservation of normal brain and associated vascular structures, and the absence of neurological deficits.[7] To manage an infiltrated but patent SSS, several different surgical options have been proposed in the recent literature:

1. Resection of only the extrasinusal portion with maximal safe tumor resection outside the involved sinus, and the use of the gamma knife for any residual tumor.
2. Maximal safe tumor resection outside the involved sinus, followed by gamma knife surgery only if the residual tumor regrows.

3. Aggressive surgical resection of the involved portion with subsequent venous reconstruction when the lumen is invaded.

Considerations

Parasagittal meningiomas often pose significant surgical obstacles because of their location and invasion into surrounding structures. These meningiomas have an intimate relationship with the sagittal sinus and with the cortical vein, with its critical tributary bridging vein. Invasion and involvement of the tributary bridging vein and the SSS present a significant challenge.

This type of meningioma has the highest postoperative recurrence rate (7.9 to 29%) of all meningiomas.[1] Recurrence not only complicates control of the neoplasm but also drastically increases the morbidity rate.[46] Well-established factors influencing the recurrence rate include the histopathological grade, the extent of resection, and the presence of biological markers.[46]

Although most of these tumors are benign, the concern about recurrence underscores the importance of achieving gross total resection (Simpson grade I or II). When managing parasagittal meningiomas, the surgeon and patient must make decisions after weighing the benefits and risks of each option against the long-term outcome, and these decisions are made based on the tumor's location, the degree of sinus involvement, and the cortical vein anatomy and collateral circulation. We would like to affirm that tumor resection must avoid any sacrifice of possible dominant or collateral bridging veins.

Preoperative Evaluation

In patients with parasagittal tumors, the venous patency and collateral anastomoses must be clearly defined for correct surgical planning, especially in patients with partially obstructive lesions. MRI can be used to assess the relevant anatomy. Catheter angiography is still considered the reference standard to evaluate the arterial and venous vasculature, but because of its invasiveness and potential complications, noninvasive techniques such as magnetic resonance (MR) venography and three-dimensional computed tomography (CT) venography are commonly preferred. Three-dimensional CT venography has a high sensitivity for depicting the intracerebral venous circulation as compared with digital subtraction angiography,[47,48] and it is a reliable method to determine the patency of the sinus, the extent of occlusion, and the number of collateral anastomoses close to the insertion of the meningioma.[49]

Contrast-enhanced MR venography allows excellent visualization of the venous morphology.[50] It discriminates between contrast in the patent sinus and the tumoral mass, providing good visualization of patency of the SSS and enabling the surgeon to accurately estimate the number of collateral anastomotic vessels, compared with phase-contrast MR angiography.

The radiographic findings suggestive of aggressiveness include marked peritumoral edema, a mushroom or lobulated shape, cystic changes, nonhomogeneous enhancement, an absence of calcification, and bone or brain invasion,[51] particularly for grade III meningiomas.[52] Perfusion MRI can provide useful information to aid the preoperative diagnosis of some subtypes of meningioma.[53] However, radiological features cannot reliably distinguish aggressive meningiomas from their benign counterparts.[52] They are only suggestive, not diagnostic. Nevertheless, when these features are present, aggressive surgical therapy should be considered as a primary approach in high-risk patients.

Aggressive Meningiomas

Although meningiomas are typically benign, they occasionally behave in an aggressive fashion, resulting in less favorable outcomes and higher rates of recurrence.[52] This aggressive variant is referred to as grade II or grade III, according to the World Health Organization (WHO) classification system.[54] Both types have a higher rate of recurrence and a poorer prognosis than grade I lesions, even if total surgical excision is achieved.[52]

A patient's recurrence-free survival, even after complete removal, greatly depends on the histological grade of the tumor. The 5-year recurrence rate after total resection is only 3 to 4% for benign meningiomas, but rises to 35 to 38% for atypical (WHO grade II) and 78 to 84% for anaplastic (WHO grade III) tumors. The malignant histological variant is a different and difficult disease, with median survival of only 1.5 years and a fatal outcome in most cases.[46] Complete surgical resection and the subsequent administration of adjuvant irradiation are crucial for long-term control.[55]

From a clinical standpoint, a major concern is the discrepancy that arises between the histological appearance of the tumor and its clinical behavior. The changes in the WHO grading system for meningiomas in the year 2000 have significantly improved the correlation between histological grade and tumor behavior. These changes significantly increased the number of meningiomas diagnosed as WHO grade II; thus, a greater proportion of surgically treated meningiomas have been identified as WHO grade II atypical lesions.[56] For example, Pearson and colleagues[57] described an increase from 4.4 to 35.5%, and Smith and colleagues[58] reported an increase from 18.3 to 23% after the introduction of the WHO criteria in the year 2000.

Biological Markers to Predict Clinical Behavior

Regardless of the treatment selected, the surgeon's main concern is how to predict recurrence. The cell proliferation index usually correlates with the aggressiveness of meningiomas,[46] and a high mitotic rate is usually associated with malignancy and can be measured by determining the mitotic index using K_i-67 or MIB-1. The MIB-1 antibody detects the same, or a similar, epitope as the original K_i-67 antibody, and has advantages over K_i-67 in that it can be used in frozen, paraffin-embedded, or decalcified tissue, and the results are easier to interpret. The MIB-1 concentration corresponds to the histological features of the tumor, increasing with malignancy grade and recurrence risk.[46,52] Unfortunately, the usefulness of the MIB-1 is limited because of variability in the results obtained by different laboratories due to differences in staining technique, counting methods, and the interpretation of results. For example, a different MIB-1 finding is obtained depending on whether the count is performed in the area of tissue showing the densest labeling or in randomly chosen fields. Some authors suggest that these findings be used as tie-breaker in cases of borderline atypia, with a cutoff value of 4.2%.[59] This biological marker can be used to determine the need for close radiological observation at shorter intervals or adjuvant radiotherapy in the early postoperative period.

Role of Radiotherapy

The use of radiation in the treatment of meningiomas is still controversial. Over the past two decades, indications for meningioma radiosurgery have expanded to include patients with newly diagnosed disease instead of being limited to those with recurrent or residual tumor after initial resection.[60]

The efficacy of stereotactic radiosurgery for meningiomas has been reported with long-term follow-up results. Kondziolka and associates[60] presented a comprehensive analysis of patients with meningiomas (at all sites) who were treated with stereotactic radiosurgery. They reported an overall control rate of 93% for benign lesions (WHO grade I) and a 15-year actuarial tumor control rate of 87%. However, for patients with WHO grade II and grade III tumors, the control rates were 50% and 17%, respectively, with median follow-up periods of 2 years and 15 months, respectively. The 5-year actuarial control rate was 40% for grade II tumors and 15% for grade III tumors.

The role of postoperative radiotherapy in patients undergoing first-time resection of WHO grade II and III meningiomas remains somewhat controversial. Several authors recommend postoperative radiation therapy for patients with WHO grade II and III meningiomas to control the invasive behavior of the tumor, regardless of the extent of resection.[52,56,61] A malignant meningioma recurring after conventional fractionated radiotherapy can be treated with radiosurgery.[62] Mair and colleagues[56] suggest that radiotherapy is not appropriate for patients with totally resected (Simpson grade I or II) WHO grade II meningiomas because 50% of patients undergoing gross total resection will ultimately remain free of recurrent disease. They advise that any tumor remnant seen on postoperative imaging should be treated with radiosurgery, and suggest that postoperative radiotherapy should be reserved for tumor remnants that are too large for radiosurgery and for which a second-stage operation is not planned. Sughrue and coworkers[61] recommended selective use of radiotherapy in patients with WHO grade II lesions, based on epidermal growth factor receptor (EGFR) staining and the MIB-1 labeling index. Their group uses radiotherapy to treat all incompletely resected and all gross-total resected tumors that are EGFR-negative or have elevated MIB-1 labeling (>10%), but they only observe patients with WHO grade II tumors that have positive wild-type EGFR staining and MIB-1 labeling of <10% who have undergone gross total resection.

Potential Risks of Radiosurgery

Radiosurgery may not always be the safest choice. Patients with a parasagittal meningioma treated with radiosurgery have been shown to be at risk for postoperative symptomatic peritumoral edema.[7,63–65] Once the edema develops, corticosteroids often ameliorate symptoms, but the need for their prolonged use may lead to such undesirable side effects that surgical resection of the tumor may become necessary.[65]

The potential side effects associated with stereotactic radiosurgery are not trivial. Kim and associates[63] documented that patients with parasagittal lesions had a tendency to develop severe post-radiosurgical edema. Chang and colleagues[64] also reported that patients with meningiomas in the convexity, parasagittal region, and falx cerebri that were deeply embedded in the cortex have a higher rate of peritumoral edema after radiosurgery than do patients with meningiomas at the skull base. Post-radiosurgical edema was found in 4 of 79 skull-base meningiomas (5%) in contrast to 26 of 52 hemispheric meningiomas (50%). Kondziolka and associates[7,60] documented that the rate of transient, symptomatic edema after gamma knife radiosurgery was 16% in 203 patients with parasagittal meningiomas, and that this complication was more common in patients with larger tumors within 2 years. Hasegawa and coworkers[66] reported that the rate of newly developed or increased peritumoral edema 3 to 12 months after gamma knife radiosurgery was 29 in 125 patients (28%) with convexity, parasagittal, and falcine meningiomas. The actuarial symptomatic radiation-induced rate of edema was 7%. Based on a chart review, 21 of these 29 patients (72%) had gamma knife radiosurgery as the initial treatment.

One reported actuarial rate for developing any post-radiosurgical injury reaction was 8.8% ± 3.0% at 5 and 10 years.[67] The risk of post-radiosurgery sequelae was lower in patients treated with stereotactic radiosurgery at lower doses, and tended to increase with treatment volume.[67]

Comment on Pamir and Peker's Section

Pamir and Peker explained the scientific reasons for combining conventional surgery and gamma knife surgery, and reported their experience with gamma knife surgery in 43 patients with parasagittal meningiomas that invaded the SSS, including 15 cases of virgin small tumors that showed complete growth control at 2 years of follow-up. Studies by Kondziolka and associates[60] in patients with benign meningiomas showed similar results. Therefore, the authors conclude that radiosurgery could be the primary treatment for all small parasagittal meningiomas unless there is a significant mass effect or peritumoral edema. The authors also suggest that complete resection is contraindicated in the case of sinus invasion.

The application of radiosurgery is effective for the primary treatment of small parasagittal meningiomas, and several studies also support its role in the treatment of incompletely resected tumors.[57,61,66,68] In their series of 203 parasagittal meningiomas, Kondziolka and associates[60] showed that treatment with radiation on initial presentation was effective for patients with tumors smaller than

3 cm in diameter. However, because most patients present with symptomatic tumors of a larger size, radiation is not usually practical as initial treatment.[69] We agree with the suggestion that significant mass effect or peritumoral edema is a contraindication for radiosurgery. Cai and colleagues[65] reported that preexisting peritumoral edema has a 77% chance of increasing after radiosurgery.

We suggest that total removal with venous reconstruction is indicated in patients with aggressive meningiomas. Surgical resection is an independent prognostic factor for survival in these patients, and complete tumor removal is the main positive prognostic factor for those with grade II or clinically aggressive meningiomas.[70]

Comment on Sindou and Colleagues' Section

Sindou and his colleagues support the aggressive resection of tumors with sinus reconstruction or venous bypass. The authors report their series of 100 meningioma cases involving a major dural sinus. The recurrence rate was low (4%), with a mean follow-up period of 8 years (range, 3–23 years).[11]

We want to emphasize that preserving the cortical vein is a primary concern. The appropriateness of sinus reconstruction is dictated primarily by the patient's ability to tolerate temporary occlusion and the significance of cortical veins that empty into the involved segment. Reconstruction is done not only of the sinus but also of the cortical vein.

When discussing the rationale for radical versus limited surgery, the benefits and risks of adjuvant radiosurgery must be considered. The ability to reconstruct the venous sinus to totally remove a parasagittal meningioma needs to be considered together with recent evidence that small, benign (WHO grade I) residual tumors remain unchanged for several years and that their growth may be further slowed by radiosurgery.[60] We suggest that total removal coupled with time-consuming and technically demanding venous reconstruction is indicated only for aggressive meningiomas.

Moderators' Viewpoint

We continue to suggest that surgery must be the first-line treatment for patients with parasagittal meningiomas, to confirm the definitive pathology and to reduce the tumor size, except in high-risk older patients or in those with medical comorbidities.

A complete tumor resection requires reconstruction of the sagittal sinus and cortical veins. Total resection of the tumor and the invaded sinus, by destroying more or less of the venous channel coursing through subcutaneous, periosteal, osseus, and dural tissue, compromises the progressively developed anastomotic drainage of the brain.

Our strategy for treating patients with a grade I meningioma that partially invades the sinus consists of an attempt at maximal tumor removal without sacrificing critical structures, and subsequently following any residual tumor with serial imaging studies. We use the gamma knife to control the residual disease in these patients only if there is tumor regrowth. When the postoperative pathology results reveal a WHO grade II or III tumor, we suggest a second-stage surgery to completely remove the invaded portion of sinus and reconstruct the sinus including the involved cortical veins.

Our strategy for patients with WHO grade II and III lesions has been to achieve gross total removal (Simpson grade I or II) with venous reconstruction, especially of the cortical and collateral veins, because surgical resection is an independent prognostic factor for survival in these patients. Complete tumor removal is the main prognostic factor in grade II meningiomas.[70] We believe that this must also be true for clinically aggressive meningiomas that have been classified as WHO grade I. A grade I meningioma can invade surrounding tissues, such as bone and soft tissue. Although this invasion makes resection more difficult, it does not change the grade. The invasion of brain tissue, on the other hand, results in a prognosis equivalent to that of an atypical meningioma, even if the tumor appears otherwise benign.[59] We agree with the opinion of Roser and colleagues[71] that MIB-1 is an important tool in addition to routine histological evaluation, but a combination of clinical factors and particularly the extent of surgical resection, along with the biological features of the tumor, should influence the surgeon's decision regarding the patient's follow-up.

Another important consideration is the intraoperative evaluation of the bridging vein. Sacrificing the bridging vein causes focal venous engorgement and decreases vascular flow, which can cause venous stasis and resultant thrombosis.[69,72] Parasagittal meningiomas may encase several large cortical veins, and the patency of venous flow can be evaluated during procedures with indocyanine green fluorescent microscope–integrated angiography.[73] To avoid their occlusion, cortical veins encased by a meningioma can be anastomosed, regardless of the flow direction.[26]

When the SSS is opened or sacrificed, parasagittal meningiomas involving this sinus raise concerns of hemorrhage, sinus occlusion, and corticovenous thrombosis.[21] Whether a bypass is justified every time a total resection is attempted, or only in selected patients with proven high venous pressure, remains a debatable issue.[11] For WHO grade II or III meningiomas invading the SSS, we favor attempting total removal, but sinus reconstruction in patients with incomplete invasion of the lumen depends on the intrasinus venous pressure measurements anterior to the surgical site, before and after the application of clips.[21,27] The rationale behind our strategy is to minimize immediate morbidity and mortality through the judicious selection of patients. The high rate of delayed thrombosis after venous sinus reconstruction (23–36%) presents a major concern regarding any attempt to replace the sagittal sinus.[10,28] If the intrasinus venous pressure does not increase after clip placement, and adequate collateral venous flow is developed and preserved during surgery, then sinus reconstruction might present additional risks and prolong the operating time without providing definite benefits.

References

1. Colli BO, Carlotti CG Jr, Assirati JA Jr, Dos Santos MB, Neder L, Dos Santos AC. Parasagittal meningiomas: follow-up review. Surg Neurol 2006;66(Suppl 3):S20–S27, discussion S27–S28

2. Cushing H, Eisenhardt L. Meningiomas: Their Classification, Regional Behavior, Life History and Surgical End Results. Springfield, IL: Charles C. Thomas, 1938

3. Ojemann RG, Ogilvy CS. Convexity, parasagittal and parafalcine meningiomas. In: Apuzzo MLJ, ed. Brain Surgery: Complication Avoidance and Management. New York: Churchill Livingstone, 1993:187–202

4. Olivecrona H. The parasagittal meningiomas. J Neurosurg 1947;4:327–341

5. Caroli E, Orlando ER, Mastronardi L, Ferrante L. Meningiomas infiltrating the superior sagittal sinus: surgical considerations of 328 cases. Neurosurg Rev 2006;29:236–241

6. DiMeco F, Li KW, Casali C, et al. Meningiomas invading the superior sagittal sinus: surgical experience in 108 cases. Neurosurgery 2004;55:1263–1272, discussion 1272–1274

7. Kondziolka D, Flickinger JC, Perez B; Gamma Knife Meningioma Study Group. Judicious resection and/or radiosurgery for parasagittal meningiomas: outcomes from a multicenter review. Neurosurgery 1998;43:405–413, discussion 413–414

8. Pamir MN, Peker S, Kilic T, Sengoz M. Efficacy of gamma-knife surgery for treating meningiomas that involve the superior sagittal sinus. Zentralbl Neurochir 2007;68: 73–78

9. Simpson D. The recurrence of intracranial meningiomas after surgical treatment. J Neurol Neurosurg Psychiatry 1957;20:22–39

10. Bonnal J, Brotchi J. Surgery of the superior sagittal sinus in parasagittal meningiomas. J Neurosurg 1978;48:935–945

11. Sindou MP, Alvernia JE. Results of attempted radical tumor removal and venous repair in 100 consecutive meningiomas involving the major dural sinuses. J Neurosurg 2006; 105:514–525

12. Sindou M. Meningiomas invading the sagittal or transverse sinuses, resection with venous reconstruction. J Clin Neurosci 2001;8(Suppl 1):8–11

13. Andrews BT, Dujovny M, Mirchandani HG, Ausman JI. Microsurgical anatomy of the venous drainage into the superior sagittal sinus. Neurosurgery 1989;24:514–520

14. Oka K, Rhoton AL Jr, Barry M, Rodriguez R. Microsurgical anatomy of the superficial veins of the cerebrum. Neurosurgery 1985;17:711–748

15. Sindou M, Auque J, Jouanneau E. Neurosurgery and the intracranial venous system. Acta Neurochir Suppl (Wien) 2005;94:167–175

16. Oka K, Go Y, Kimura H, Tomonaga M. Obstruction of the superior sagittal sinus caused by parasagittal meningiomas: the role of collateral venous pathways. J Neurosurg 1994;81:520–524

17. Wilkins RH. Parasagittal meningiomas. In: Al-Mefty O, ed. Meningiomas. New York: Raven, 1991:329–344

18. Marks SM, Whitwell HL, Lye RH. Recurrence of meningiomas after operation. Surg Neurol 1986;25:436–440

19. Mirimanoff RO, Dosoretz DE, Linggood RM, Ojemann RG, Martuza RL. Meningioma: analysis of recurrence and progression following neurosurgical resection. J Neurosurg 1985;62:18–24

20. Naumann M, Meixensberger J. Factors influencing meningioma recurrence rate. Acta Neurochir (Wien) 1990;107: 108–111

21. Bederson JB, Eisenberg MB. Resection and replacement of the superior sagittal sinus for treatment of a parasagittal meningioma: technical case report. Neurosurgery 1995; 37:1015–1018, discussion 1018–1019

22. Buster WP, Rodas RA, Fenstermaker RA, Kattner KA. Major venous sinus resection in the surgical treatment of recurrent aggressive dural based tumors. Surg Neurol 2004;62: 522–529, discussion 529–530

23. Hakuba A. Reconstruction of dural sinus involved in meningiomas. In: Al-Mefty O, ed. Meningiomas. New York: Raven, 1991:371–382

24. Hakuba A, Huh CW, Tsujikawa S, Nishimura S. Total removal of a parasagittal meningioma of the posterior third of the sagittal sinus and its repair by autogenous vein graft. Case report. J Neurosurg 1979;51:379–382

25. Hancq S, Baleriaux D, Brotchi J. Surgical treatment of parasagittal meningiomas. Semin Neurosurg 2003;3:203–210

26. Murata J, Sawamura Y, Saito H, Abe H. Resection of a recurrent parasagittal meningioma with cortical vein anastomosis: technical note. Surg Neurol 1997;48:592–595, discussion 595–597

27. Schmid-Elsaesser R, Steiger HJ, Yousry T, Seelos KC, Reulen HJ. Radical resection of meningiomas and arteriovenous fistulas involving critical dural sinus segments: experience with intraoperative sinus pressure monitoring and elective sinus reconstruction in 10 patients. Neurosurgery 1997;41: 1005–1016, discussion 1016–1018

28. Sindou M, Hallacq P. Venous reconstruction in surgery of meningiomas invading the sagittal and transverse sinuses. Skull Base Surg 1998;8:57–64

29. Steiger HJ, Reulen HJ, Huber P, Boll J. Radical resection of superior sagittal sinus meningioma with venous interposition graft and reimplantation of the rolandic veins. Case report. Acta Neurochir (Wien) 1989;100:108–111

30. Mathiesen T, Lindquist C, Kihlström L, Karlsson B. Recurrence of cranial base meningiomas. Neurosurgery 1996;39: 2–7, discussion 8–9

31. Jääskeläinen J. Seemingly complete removal of histologically benign intracranial meningioma: late recurrence rate

and factors predicting recurrence in 657 patients. A multivariate analysis. Surg Neurol 1986;26:461–469

32. Pamir MN, Kiliç T, Bayrakli F, Peker S. Changing treatment strategy of cavernous sinus meningiomas: experience of a single institution. Surg Neurol 2005;64(Suppl 2):S58–S66

33. Sindou M, Auque J. The intracranial venous system as a neurosurgeon's perspective. Review Adv Tech Stand Neurosurg 2000;26:131–216

34. Sindou M, Mazoyer JF, Fischer G, Pialat J, Fourcade C. Experimental bypass for sagittal sinus repair. Preliminary report. J Neurosurg 1976;44:325–330

35. Sindou M, Mercier P, Bokor J, Brunon J. Bilateral thrombosis of the transverse sinuses: microsurgical revascularization with venous bypass. Surg Neurol 1980;13:215–220

36. Sekhar LN, Tzortzidis FN, Bejjani GK, Schessel DA. Saphenous vein graft bypass of the sigmoid sinus and jugular bulb during the removal of glomus jugulare tumors. Report of two cases. J Neurosurg 1997;86:1036–1041

37. Merrem G. Parasagittal meningiomas. Fedor Krause memorial lecture. Acta Neurochir (Wien) 1970;23:203–216

38. Bonnal J, Brotchi J, Stevenaert A, Petrov VT, Mouchette R. Excision of the intrasinusal portion of rolandic parasagittal meningiomas, followed by plastic surgery of the superior longitudinal sinus. Neurochirurgie 1971;17:341–354 [in French]

39. Donaghy RM, Wallman LJ, Flanagan MJ, Numoto M. Sagittal sinus repair. Technical note. J Neurosurg 1973;38:244–248

40. Kapp JP, Gielchinsky I, Deardourff SL. Operative techniques for management of lesions involving the dural venous sinuses. Surg Neurol 1977;7:339–342

41. Yasargil MG. Microneurosurgery, vol. 1. Stuttgart: Thieme, 1984

42. Schmidek HH, Auer LM, Kapp JP. The cerebral venous system. Review. Neurosurgery 1985;17:663–678

43. Hakuba A, ed. Surgery of the Intracranial Venous System. Proceedings of the First International Workshop on Surgery of the Intracranial Venous System, Osaka, September 1994. Tokyo: Springer-Verlag, 1996

44. Al-Mefty O, Krisht AF. The dangerous veins. In: Hakuba A, ed. Surgery of the Intracranial Venous System. Proceedings of the First International Workshop on Surgery of the Intracranial Venous System, Osaka, September 1994. Tokyo: Springer-Verlag, 1996:36–42

45. Auque J, ed. Venous sacrifice in neurosurgery: risk, assessment and management. Neurochirurgie 1996;42(Suppl 1) [in French]

46. Al-Mefty O, Kadri PA, Pravdenkova S, Sawyer JR, Stangeby C, Husain M. Malignant progression in meningioma: documentation of a series and analysis of cytogenetic findings. J Neurosurg 2004;101:210–218

47. Suzuki Y, Ikeda H, Shimadu M, Ikeda Y, Matsumoto K. Variations of the basal vein: identification using three-dimensional CT angiography. AJNR Am J Neuroradiol 2001;22:670–676

48. Lee JM, Jung S, Moon KS, et al. Preoperative evaluation of venous systems with 3-dimensional contrast-enhanced magnetic resonance venography in brain tumors: comparison with time-of-flight magnetic resonance venography

and digital subtraction angiography. Surg Neurol 2005;64:128–133, discussion 133–134

49. Zhen J, Liu C, Jiang B, He J, Pang Q, Wang G. Preoperative evaluation of venous systems with computed tomography venography in parasagittal meningiomas. J Comput Assist Tomogr 2008;32:293–297

50. Bozzao A, Finocchi V, Romano A, et al. Role of contrast-enhanced MR venography in the preoperative evaluation of parasagittal meningiomas. Eur Radiol 2005;15:1790–1796

51. Ildan F, Erman T, Göçer AI, et al. Predicting the probability of meningioma recurrence in the preoperative and early postoperative period: a multivariate analysis in the mid-term follow-up. Skull Base 2007;17:157–171

52. Engenhart-Cabillic R, Farhoud A, Sure U, et al. Clinicopathologic features of aggressive meningioma emphasizing the role of radiotherapy in treatment. Strahlenther Onkol 2006;182:641–646

53. Zhang H, Rödiger LA, Shen T, Miao J, Oudkerk M. Preoperative subtyping of meningiomas by perfusion MR imaging. Neuroradiology 2008;50:835–840

54. Louis DN, Ohgaki H, Wiestler OD, et al. The 2007 WHO classification of tumours of the central nervous system. Acta Neuropathol 2007;114:97–109

55. Dziuk TW, Woo S, Butler EB, et al. Malignant meningioma: an indication for initial aggressive surgery and adjuvant radiotherapy. J Neurooncol 1998;37:177–188

56. Mair R, Morris K, Scott I, Carroll TA. Radiotherapy for atypical meningiomas. J Neurosurg 2011;115:811–819

57. Pearson BE, Markert JM, Fisher WS, et al. Hitting a moving target: evolution of a treatment paradigm for atypical meningiomas amid changing diagnostic criteria. Neurosurg Focus 2008;24:E3

58. Smith SJ, Boddu S, Macarthur DC. Atypical meningiomas: WHO moved the goalposts? Br J Neurosurg 2007;21:588–592

59. Commins DL, Atkinson RD, Burnett ME. Review of meningioma histopathology. Neurosurg Focus 2007;23:E3

60. Kondziolka D, Mathieu D, Lunsford LD, et al. Radiosurgery as definitive management of intracranial meningiomas. Neurosurgery 2008;62:53–58, discussion 58–60

61. Sughrue ME, Rutkowski MJ, Shangari G, Parsa AT, Berger MS, McDermott MW; Clinical Article. Results with judicious modern neurosurgical management of parasagittal and falcine meningiomas. Clinical article. J Neurosurg 2011;114:731–737

62. Ojemann SG, Sneed PK, Larson DA, et al. Radiosurgery for malignant meningioma: results in 22 patients. J Neurosurg 2000;93(Suppl 3):62–67

63. Kim DG, Kim ChH, Chung HT, et al. Gamma knife surgery of superficially located meningioma. J Neurosurg 2005;102(Suppl):255–258

64. Chang JH, Chang JW, Choi JY, Park YG, Chung SS. Complications after gamma knife radiosurgery for benign meningiomas. J Neurol Neurosurg Psychiatry 2003;74:226–230

65. Cai R, Barnett GH, Novak E, Chao ST, Suh JH. Principal risk of peritumoral edema after stereotactic radiosurgery for intracranial meningioma is tumor-brain contact interface area. Neurosurgery 2010;66:513–522

66. Hasegawa T, Kida Y, Yoshimoto M, Iizuka H, Ishii D, Yoshida K. Gamma knife surgery for convexity, parasagittal, and falcine meningiomas. J Neurosurg 2011;114:1392–1398

67. Flickinger JC, Kondziolka D, Maitz AH, Lunsford LD. Gamma knife radiosurgery of imaging-diagnosed intracranial meningioma. Int J Radiat Oncol Biol Phys 2003;56:801–806

68. Kondziolka D, Lunsford LD, Coffey RJ, Flickinger JC. Stereotactic radiosurgery of meningiomas. J Neurosurg 1991;74: 552–559

69. Raza SM, Gallia GL, Brem H, Weingart JD, Long DM, Olivi A. Perioperative and long-term outcomes from the management of parasagittal meningiomas invading the superior sagittal sinus. Neurosurgery 2010;67:885–893, discussion 893

70. Durand A, Labrousse F, Jouvet A, et al. WHO grade II and III meningiomas: a study of prognostic factors. J Neurooncol 2009;95:367–375

71. Roser F, Samii M, Ostertag H, Bellinzona M. The Ki-67 proliferation antigen in meningiomas. Experience in 600 cases. Acta Neurochir (Wien) 2004;146:37–44, discussion 44

72. Fries G, Wallenfang T, Hennen J, et al. Occlusion of the pig superior sagittal sinus, bridging and cortical veins: multistep evolution of sinus-vein thrombosis. J Neurosurg 1992; 77:127–133

73. Killory BD, Nakaji P, Maughan PH, Wait SD, Spetzler RF. Evaluation of angiographically occult spinal dural arteriovenous fistulae with surgical microscope-integrated intraoperative near-infrared indocyanine green angiography: report of 3 cases. Neurosurgery 2011;68:781–787, discussion 787

Management of Petroclival Meningiomas: Subtotal Resection and Radiosurgery vs. Total Removal

Case

A 50-year-old woman has mild diplopia and trigeminal neuralgia that responded well to medical treatment.

Participants

Management of Petroclival Meningiomas: The Role of Excision and Radiosurgery: Basant K. Misra

Total Removal of Petroclival Meningiomas: Ian F. Dunn, Rami Almefty, and Ossama Al-Mefty

Moderator: Management of Petroclival Meningiomas: Total Removal vs. Subtotal Resection and Radiosurgery: Kadir Erkmen

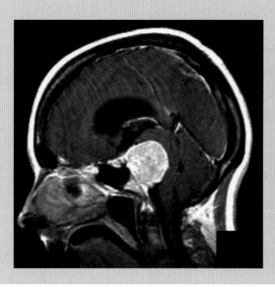
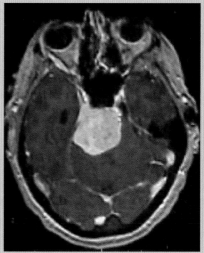

Management of Petroclival Meningiomas: The Role of Excision and Radiosurgery

Basant K. Misra

As meningiomas are potentially curable, their treatment is a gratifying surgical exercise when the tumor is avascular and occurs in the convexity. But when the tumor is firm and arising deep at the base of the skull, it presents one of the most formidable challenges in neurosurgery. Petroclival meningiomas fall in this latter category. For this discussion, clival and petroclival meningiomas are considered as one entity—those meningiomas arising from the upper two thirds of the clivus and those originating at the clivus and petroclival junction medial to the trigeminal nerve.[1–3]

Up to 1970, petroclival meningiomas were considered inoperable, as only 10 of the 26 patients reported in the literature survived surgery and only one had a total excision.[3] Parallel advances in microneurosurgery and the introduction of innovative skull-base approaches in the late 1980s led to a renewed enthusiasm about radical excision of petroclival meningiomas, and several successful series were published.[4–10] Many neurosurgeons practicing skull-base surgery (including this author) were carried away by the possibility of total excision with a very low mortality rate and a great postoperative scan, and accepted the accompanying morbidity as inevitable. Only a few wise men dared to question this approach lest they be frowned upon as incompetent.[11]

But the seeds of doubt were sown and led to soul-searching and rethinking at first by a few and then by the majority. Reports of the successful control of meningiomas through gamma knife radiosurgery further dampened enthusiasm for the high-risk radical surgery of petroclival meningiomas.[12] There remains, however, a minority of brilliant neurosurgeons who achieve total excision in the majority of patients with petroclival meningiomas. I am a convert to radiosurgery, not one of the brilliant neurosurgeons who always achieve total excision. In this section of the chapter, I address two principal issues based on personal experience and evidence from the literature.

Total or Subtotal Excision of Petroclival Meningiomas

The objective of surgery in patients with a meningioma is total removal of the tumor, including the dural attachment and involved bone. The completeness of surgical removal is the single most important prognostic factor for tumor recurrence. However, when total removal entails unacceptable risks of morbidity or mortality, it is prudent to be satisfied with subtotal excision. Sound judgment in choosing the best treatment depends on a high level of clinical acumen, for the best treatment is that which is best for the patient, not necessarily what is best for the tumor!

Another related question to ask is, What constitutes total excision? Total excision, including the dural attachment and bone (Simpson grade I), is not always possible in patients with petroclival meningiomas. By the time patients present to the surgeon, most petroclival meningiomas have reached a large size with a wide attachment, and the tumor often invades the exit foramina of multiple cranial nerves. Total excision of the tumor with its dura and bony attachment is not possible in such cases without significant risks and unacceptable morbidity. In several cases, the difficulty of excision is further compounded by arterial and brainstem involvement.[3,13–15] A review of the literature clearly demonstrates the trend toward less aggressive surgery and an emphasis on the functional outcome, as reported in various series (**Table 3.1**). The total excision rates dropped over the years from a high of 70 to 80% to less than 40%. The total excision rates in the earlier literature reported by Samii and colleagues,[5] Al-Mefty and Smith,[2] Misra and coworkers,[8] Kawase and colleagues,[7] and Bricolo and associates,[9] were 71%, 83%, 82%, 70%, and 79%, respectively. The total excision rates for petroclival meningiomas in the recent reported series are much lower: 20% by Jung and colleagues,[16] 40% by Little and associates,[14] and 41% by Mathiesen and coworkers.[17] The total excision rate in the series of Sekhar and associates[6,13] dropped from a high of 78% in 1990 to 32% in 2007. Similarly, the group from Barrow Neurological Institute reported a total excision rate of 91% in 1992 but only 43% in 2007.[10,18]

The trend toward a less radical approach in almost all recent series is aimed at a better quality of life for the patient. That this attempt is successful is proven by lower post-

Table 3.1 Petroclival Meningiomas: Rate of Total Excision

Authors (Year)	No. of Pts.	Gross Total Resection (%)
Samii et al (1989)[5]	24	71
Sekhar et al (1990)[6]	41	78
Al-Mefty and Smith (1991)[2]	18	83
Misra et al (1991)[8]	11	82
Kawase et al (1991)[7]	10	70
Bricolo et al (1992)[9]	33	79
Spetzler et al (1992)[10]	46	91
Jung et al (2000)[16]	49	20
Little et al (2005)[14]	137	40
Mathiesen et al (2007)[17]	29	41
Natarajan et al (2007)[13]	150	32
Bambakidis et al (2007)[18]	46	43

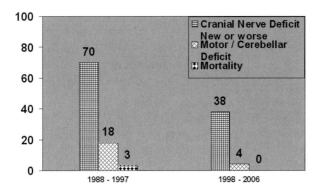

Fig. 3.1 The trend in complications after microsurgery in patients with petroclival meningiomas in the author's series from 1988 through 1997 and then from 1998 to 2006.

operative morbidity rates reported in the recent series. I have had a similar experience, operating on 81 patients with petroclival meningiomas, mostly large and giant, between 1988 and 2008. Of the 70 patients treated up to 2006, 58 underwent microsurgery; six of these had adjunct gamma knife radiosurgery, and primary gamma knife radiosurgery was the modality used for 12 patients. A comparison of postoperative function of patients in my series between those operated on before 1997 (radical excision) and those operated on in 1997 or later (safe excision with gamma knife radiosurgery) demonstrated that the morbidity was significantly lower in the latter group (**Fig. 3.1**).

What happens, then, to the patients with subtotally excised petroclival meningiomas? One needs to study the natural history of these lesions, both untreated and partially excised, before arriving at any conclusion, but there are conflicting data in the literature. The growth pattern of untreated petroclival meningiomas is unpredictable and variable, with a radiological progression of 58 to 76%.[19,20] But radiological progression does not always correlate with clinical worsening. Moreover, the clinical progression, when it did occur, was often mild and not disabling.[19] The growth rate of subtotally resected petroclival meningiomas without adjunct treatment seems to be low, and there is a suggestion that recurrence and growth rates are higher if a large residual tumor is left behind and in younger patients.[13,14,16] The recurrence rate after complete and incomplete excision was almost the same, 4% and 5%, respectively, in the series of Natarajan and colleagues,[13] although a large number of patients with incomplete resection had adjunct radiation. In summary, many committed skull-base surgeons have a significant number of patients with petroclival meningiomas in their series who undergo subtotal excision, resulting in reduced overall postoperative morbidity. The recurrence rate after near-total or subtotal excision is not alarming.

Another equally important question is, What constitutes near-total, subtotal, or partial excision and radical decompression? Although some authors have tried to quantify

these terms, there is no consensus about the use of the terminology. One surgeon's subtotal resection may be near-total for another. Although it is critical to have unambiguous definitions so that meaningful comparisons can be made across groups, unless these definitions are made based on the volume of the residual tumor, a fallacy remains. Dogmatic dictums are not going to work, as each surgeon must discover how far he or she can go without damaging the patient; hence, the concept of safe radical decompression. Each series, then, should be followed up with a mention of residual volume.

Is there a place for "total" excision of petroclival meningiomas then? Yes. An attempt at total excision can be made in less than 50% of patients. A moderate-sized petroclival meningioma with a good plane of cleavage from the adjacent neurovascular structures and without a wide attachment can be totally excised, as was done in the patient illustrated in **Fig. 3.2**. A planned subtotal excision is the way to go when the imaging findings suggest an excessive adhesiveness of neurovascular structures, a pial breach, brainstem edema, or a wide en plaque attachment of the tumor involving the exit foramina of multiple cranial nerves (**Fig. 3.3**). Similarly, the author recommends leaving an intracavernous extension of the tumor (**Fig. 3.4**). Despite all the recent advances in imaging, surprises during surgery are not uncommon. A seemingly difficult meningioma may occasionally be totally excised, whereas an "easy" tumor may be only subtotally excised, mainly because of excessive adhesiveness and infiltration of neurovascular structures.

The Role of Radiosurgery

Radiosurgery has become an accepted modality of treatment for patients with petroclival meningiomas, both as an adjunct to microsurgery and as a primary modality.[13,16,17,21–27] Long-term follow-up data now confirm the tumor control rate of more than 90% reported in earlier series with shorter follow-up. Zachenhofer and associates[26] reported a tumor control rate of 94% in patients with skull-base meningiomas treated with gamma knife radiosurgery after a mean follow-up of 103 months. Tumor shrinkage and clinical improvement continued during the longer follow-up period. Kreil and colleagues[22] reported long-term follow-up of one of the largest series of benign skull-base meningiomas treated with gamma knife radiosurgery. In a series of 200 patients with a follow-up of 5 to 12 years, 99 were treated with a combination of microsurgery and gamma knife radiosurgery and 101 patients underwent primary gamma knife radiosurgery. The authors reported an actuarial progression-free survival rate of 98.5% at 5 years and 97.2% at 10 years.[23] The neurologic status improved in 41.5%, remained unaltered in 54%, and deteriorated in 4.5% of patients, whereas only five patients (2.5%) required repeated microsurgical resection. Iwai and associates,[24] reporting the long-term results of low-dose treatment in patients with

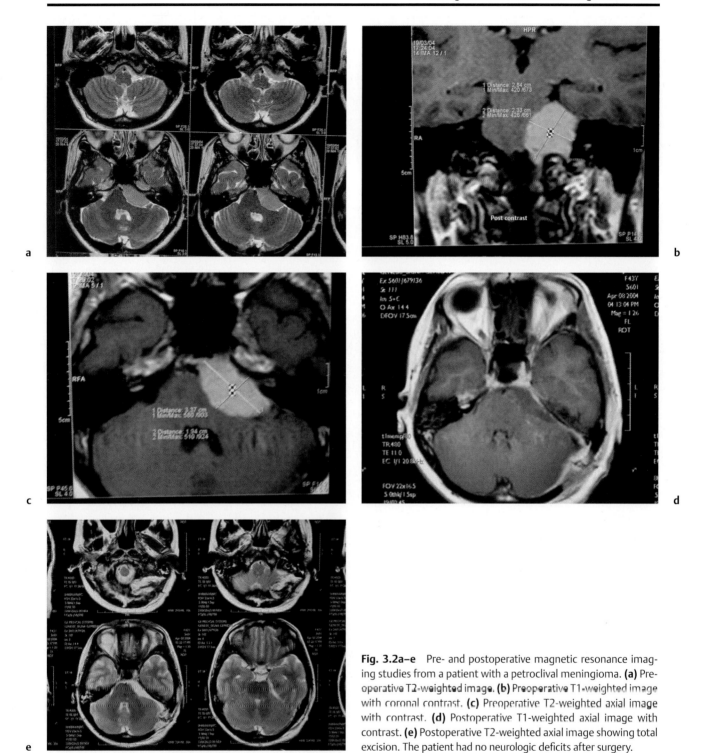

Fig. 3.2a–e Pre- and postoperative magnetic resonance imaging studies from a patient with a petroclival meningioma. **(a)** Preoperative T2-weighted image. **(b)** Preoperative T1-weighted image with coronal contrast. **(c)** Preoperative T2-weighted axial image with contrast. **(d)** Postoperative T1-weighted axial image with contrast. **(e)** Postoperative T2-weighted axial image showing total excision. The patient had no neurologic deficits after surgery.

skull-base meningiomas with gamma knife radiosurgery, reported a slightly lower actuarial progression-free survival rate of 93% at 5 years and 83% at 10 years.

Some cynics ascribe the control rate of skull-base meningiomas after radiosurgery to a mere function of the natural history and low growth rate of many skull-base meningiomas. Yet the same surgeons do not hesitate to advocate early surgery for small skull-base meningiomas

for better functional outcome. If a pathological entity has a 10-year progression-free survival rate of more than 95% as its natural history, it definitely needs no treatment! It is true that many petroclival meningiomas grow slowly and may remain static for long periods. I believe it is prudent to offer a period of observation to asymptomatic or minimally symptomatic patients with petroclival meningiomas, especially elderly ones, and do neither microsurgery nor

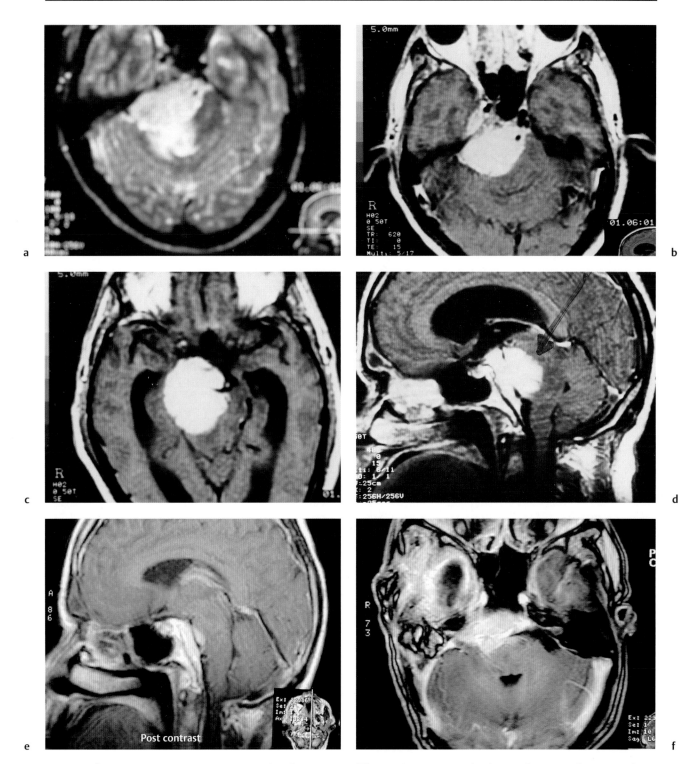

Fig. 3.3a–f Magnetic resonance imaging studies from a patient with a huge petroclival meningioma. **(a)** Preoperative T2-weighted axial image showing brainstem edema. **(b,c)** Preoperative T1-weighted axial images with contrast showing the engulfed basilar artery and its branches and the cavernous sinus extension.

(d) Preoperative T1-weighted sagittal image with contrast showing an irregular margin of the tumor (*red arrow*), suggesting pial invasion. **(e,f)** Postoperative T1-weighted sagittal and axial images with contrast showing residual tumor, which was treated through gamma knife radiosurgery.

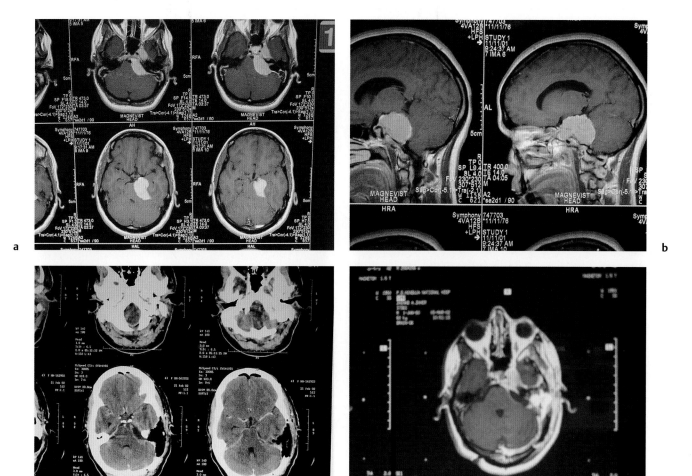

Fig. 3.4a–d **(a,b)** Preoperative T1-weighted axial and sagittal MRIs with contrast showing a large sphenopetroclival meningioma. **(c,d)** Postoperative contrast-enhanced images showing total excision of the intradural component. The residual intracavernous component was treated through gamma knife radiosurgery.

radiosurgery. However, a symptomatic patient with a large petroclival meningioma who has had a subtotal excision presents a completely different situation and is better treated up front with radiosurgery for the residual tumor.[17] These patients were symptomatic enough to need surgery in the first place, and second, very importantly, poor follow-up in many referral centers led to patients again presenting with a large recurrence requiring a repeated microsurgery. For a minimal residual tumor after surgery and in elderly patients, a watchful-waiting policy rather than up-front radiosurgery is an equally acceptable option. Similarly, a patient who has had a petroclival meningioma for many years before requiring surgery, reflecting a slow growth rate, can be followed with a scan-and-watch policy after subtotal excision.

What about primary radiosurgery for petroclival meningiomas? I am not a great fan of this approach because there is the possibility of a wrong diagnosis and the inability to grade the meningioma. However, I do advise primary gamma knife radiosurgery in selected patients with a classic imaging morphology, especially in elderly or medically infirm patients with progressive cranial nerve deficits and a small-volume tumor based on the bone and dura or presenting en plaque (**Fig. 3.5**).

What are the risks of radiosurgery? The two main concerns are neurologic worsening and the risk of malignancy. Radiation-induced worsening is often delayed, requires active medication, and, hence, requires long-term follow-up. Tissue tolerance to radiosurgery is often dose dependent, and recent series show that lower dose treatment has reduced the complication rates significantly.[17,22,25,28] There still remains a finite, though small, percentage of patients who develop neurologic deficits ascribable to radiosurgery. These instances range from 0 to 6% and occur mainly in the form of cranial nerve deficits.[22–26] Thus, it is critical that the tumor volume is reduced through safe microsurgery, the brainstem is decompressed, and any small residual volume is treated with radiosurgery to achieve the optimal outcome.[17,21]

The other concern is that of malignancy after radiosurgery, but there is no evidence of this phenomenon other than what is seen in the general population.[25,29]

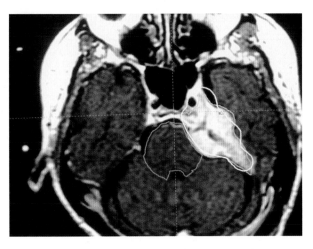

Fig. 3.5 T1-weighted axial MRI with contrast enhancement from a 62-year-old woman who had primary gamma knife radiosurgery. Her intractable facial pain disappeared after 4 weeks of treatment. Four years after treatment, she remains free of pain and the tumor is stable.

Conclusion

Not all patients with petroclival meningiomas need microsurgical or radiosurgical treatment. Many who come to the neurosurgeon, however, have advanced disease and need intervention, though not always without a period of observation. In fewer than half the patients, the meningioma can be excised totally without aggravating neurologic deficits. The rest are better managed through subtotal excision. A majority of patients who have had a subtotal excision are better treated through up-front adjunct radiosurgery (especially if they were operated on for a large symptomatic tumor). Some petroclival meningiomas may never need intervention, and a select group of patients with petroclival meningiomas is better treated with primary gamma knife radiosurgery. A flexible approach of individualizing the treatment protocol for a given patient goes a long way toward satisfying the patient and freeing the surgeon from guilt. I think I would be comfortable with this paradigm if I were the patient!

Total Removal of Petroclival Meningiomas

Ian F. Dunn, Rami Almefty, and Ossama Al-Mefty

Case

The contrast-enhanced axial and sagittal magnetic resonance imaging (MRI) of this patient show what appears to be a petroclival meningioma. There is typical displacement of the brainstem in the contralateral and posterior direction and posterior and contralateral displacement of the brainstem. There is also an extension into the posterior cavernous sinus. This patient's ventricular system above the aqueduct appears enlarged on the sagittal view, and her right temporal horn is prominent. Her diplopia is likely from compression of the abducens nerve and her trigeminal neuralgia from lateral displacement of the fifth nerve, characteristics consistent with the known growth pattern of these tumors. Clinically, the status of the patient's hearing in the ipsilateral ear is unknown, as is her handedness as a surrogate for hemispheric dominance. Radiographically, the patient's venous architecture, an important consideration for selecting the approach, cannot be ascertained from these images, and the basilar artery is difficult to discern. Moreover, the tumor's calcification and water content, features that help the physician infer the tumor's consistency, are difficult to judge from the images provided.

The Case for Surgery

Petroclival meningiomas are rare, accounting for less than 0.5% of intracranial tumors[30] and their surgical anatomy is also complex. They arise at the petroclival junction, medial to the trigeminal nerve, and compress the brainstem and the basilar artery and its perforators to the contralateral side. They displace the middle cranial nerves and often span the middle and posterior fossae, occasionally extending into the cavernous sinus. Consequently, the surgeon's management of these technically challenging lesions is usually refined over time.

The first decision is whether or not to treat this likely menopausal patient, whose tumor growth may be slowed. Although mild diplopia and medically responsive facial pain are fairly benign and may be managed nonsurgically, a further clinical decline is inevitable; worsening cranial neuropathies, symptoms of brainstem compression, and manifestations of hydrocephalus will ensue. The patient is young and treatment of the tumor is most certainly indicated.

The tumor is too large for radiation therapy alone and as yet there are no meaningful chemotherapeutic treatments. Contemporary treatment options are radical surgical resection, or a more conservative decompression or debulking followed by radiation therapy to the residual tumor. Although early reports have shown the feasibility of surgically resecting these formidable tumors,[4,31] an emerging body of literature has endorsed more conservative surgical approaches coupled with radiotherapy to preserve the patient's quality of life. The strategy of using subtotal resection and radiosurgery rests upon the assumption that the immediate surgical risk and likelihood of cranial neuropathies are reduced and that radiosurgery is an equal surrogate for surgery in the long-term management of intentionally unresected tumors. Although some reports are sanguine about the results,[13,14,16,18,32–34] this approach ultimately fails to recognize the serious issue of the long-term failure to control the tumor after radiosurgery and the potentially aggressive growth pattern of recurrent or residual tumors.[35] The detection of a recurrence as late as 14 years after the initial radiation treatment highlights the need for extended long-term follow-up in these patients.[35]

Anecdotally, we are seeing a surge in recurrent tumors in patients from various centers around the world who were treated initially through planned subtotal resection followed by radiation and who may then have undergone additional surgery and radiation. In these patients, the surgical landscape is so treacherous, with scar tissue from previous surgery and radiation vasculopathy, that the chance of cure is essentially lost. Other centers may also be able to attest to the difficulty of managing tumor growth after subtotal surgery and radiation. A residual meningioma may remain stable for some time,[36] but some reports suggest that radiation therapy for a residual meningioma offers inadequate long-term control, with a recurrence rate of up to 75% in one series.[37]

For this patient, we favor surgery with complete resection as the therapeutic goal, in accordance with Simpson's ageless mandate that the likelihood of a meningioma recurrence is directly related to the extent of surgical resection.[38]

Surgery

Multiple surgical approaches have been promoted to attack these formidable lesions. Essential to the safe and successful removal of these tumors in the petroclival region is the ability to visualize the tumor and the critical adjacent neural and vascular structures, direct access to which is obscured by the petrous temporal bone. General unfamiliarity with this bony anatomy among neurosurgeons has led to the use of the more traditional suboccipital and pterional approaches to petroclival tumors.[18,39,40] However, lateral skull-base approaches through the petrous bone have among their advantages a decreased operative distance to the tumor and neurovascular structures, improved visualization and illumination, and decreased brain retraction.[41] In addition, the access for dissection is improved because of the lateral and anterior projection to the brainstem. Specific approaches through the petrous bone include removing the petrous apex in the middle fossa approach, resecting the presigmoid retrolabyrinthine petrous bone in the posterior petrosal approach,[4,31] and complete petrosectomy.

Clinical and radiographic factors combine to influence the choice of the optimal surgical approach. Small tumors above the internal auditory canal may well be accessed through an anterior petrosal approach (**Fig. 3.6**). A posterior petrosal approach is ideal for larger tumors extending below the internal auditory canal when the patient's hearing is serviceable (**Fig. 3.7**). Should a larger tumor extend

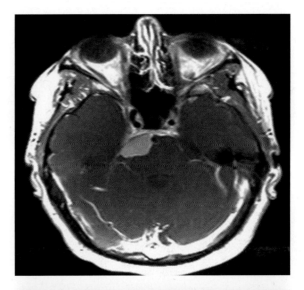

a

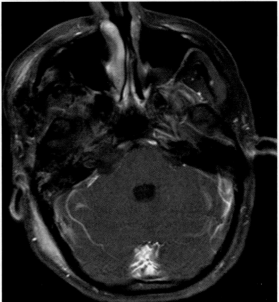

b

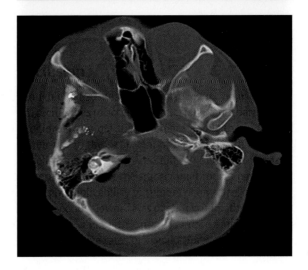

c

Fig. 3.6a–c A petroclival meningioma of the upper clivus. Use of the anterior petrosal approach facilitated its safe and total removal. **(a)** Preoperative MRI. **(b)** Postoperative MRI. **(c)** Postoperative computed tomography scan showing the bone removal.

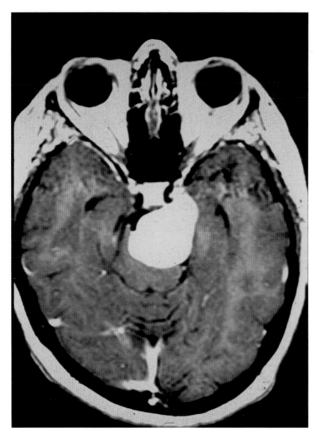

a

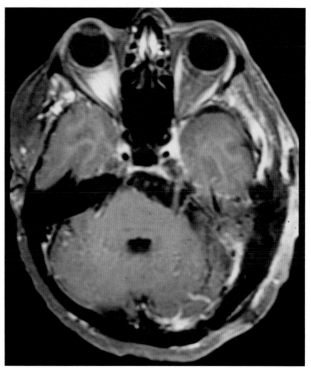

b

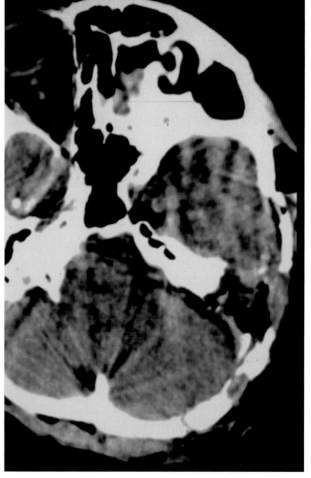

c

Fig. 3.7a–c A large posterior fossa meningioma extending below the internal auditory canal in a patient with intact hearing. Use of the posterior petrosal approach facilitated its safe and total removal. **(a)** Preoperative MRI. **(b)** Postoperative MRI showing total removal. **(c)** Postoperative computed tomography scan showing the extent of bony mastoid removal.

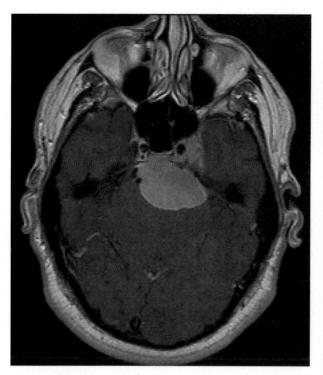

a

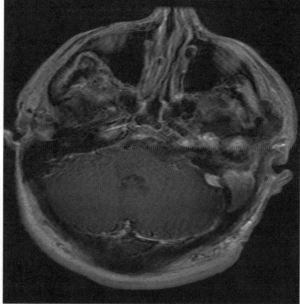

b

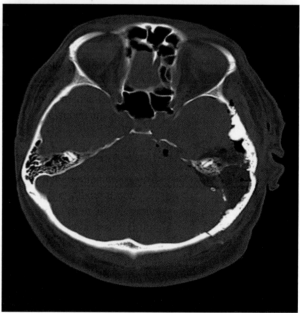

c

Fig. 3.8a–c A large petroclival meningioma extending across the midline in a patient with intact hearing. Use of the combined petrosal approach facilitated its safe and total removal.

across the clival midline or into the anterior cavernous sinus, a combined anterior and posterior petrosal approach may be used (**Fig. 3.8**). If the patient's hearing is lost, additional exposure may be afforded by a complete petrosectomy, sacrificing the labyrinth and cochlea (**Fig. 3.9**). The tumor's consistency may be inferred by the appearance of calcium on computed tomography scans or by the brightness of the mass on T2-weighted MRI, as an indicator of water content. Additionally, brainstem edema may suggest invasion of the brainstem pial plane. A rim of T2 signal between the brainstem and tumor may suggest an intact arachnoid plane for dissection.

As the tumor in this patient is large and extends to the contralateral aspect of the clivus and into the posterior portion of the cavernous sinus, a combined anterior and

posterior petrosal approach is an appropriate operative strategy in the absence of information regarding the patient's hearing status. The patient is positioned supine with the head turned to the opposite side and the ipsilateral shoulder raised. For this combined approach, the skin incision begins at the zygoma in front of the ear and arcs anteriorly, curving behind the ear to below the mastoid. The skin is reflected anteriorly with the temporalis fascia, and the zygomatic arch is cut anteriorly and posteriorly, allowing maximal inferior reflection of the temporalis muscle. Posteriorly, the temporalis fascia is taken in continuity with the sternocleidomastoid muscle, and this combined flap is taken off the mastoid and posterior fossa. Four bur holes are made to straddle the transverse sinus, exposing the sigmoid-transverse junction, and a combined posterior

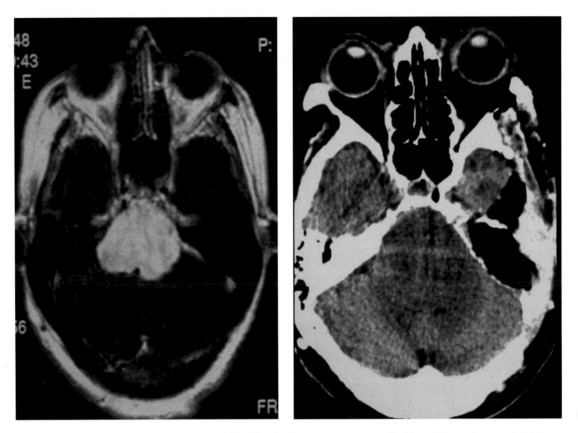

Fig. 3.9a,b   A large clival meningioma in a patient who had hearing loss. A petrosectomy facilitated the total removal. **(a)** Preoperative MRI. **(b)** Postoperative MRI showing the absence of the tumor and the extent of bony removal.

and middle fossa craniotomy is done. The mastoid cortex is removed, after which a mastoidectomy is done to expose the presigmoid dura. The labyrinth is kept intact if hearing is to be preserved. The facial nerve should be monitored throughout this drilling. The sigmoid sinus is then skeletonized to the bulb. After the middle meningeal artery is coagulated, the dura may be elevated from the middle fossa floor. The petrous apex is exposed after elevating the dura from the third division of the fifth cranial nerve and exposing the trigeminal ganglion. The petrous apex, from the trigeminal impression to the internal auditory canal medial to the carotid, is drilled to expose the dura of the posterior fossa.

The dura is opened along the inferior temporal lobe, and the surgeon can then identify the vein of Labbé and open the presigmoid dura. The superior petrosal sinus is coagulated and divided and the tentorium cut, with care, parallel to the petrous ridge to the incisura to avoid the trochlear nerve. In a combined approach, the tentorium may also be incised anterior to the incisura, behind the insertion of the trochlear nerve, to meet the posterior cut. A careful study of the venous anatomy is critical in this case. Greater risk may be incurred in patients with a dominant or isolated sigmoid or transverse sinus on the side of the tumor or with venous drainage through the tentorium. In the latter scenario, should the vein of Labbé drain into the tentorium or superior petrosal sinus before the sigmoid-transverse

junction, the tentorial incision must be made anterior to the insertion of Labbé, with sparing of the petrosal sinus.[4,42]

Results

In a recent review of 55 patients with true petroclival tumors followed on average for 4 years—excluding midclival, sphenopetroclival, and posterior petrosal tumors—gross-total resection was achieved in 35 patients, including a 72% gross-total resection rate in patients with a cavernous sinus extension. A posterior petrosal approach was most commonly used, followed by, in order of decreasing frequency, the combined petrosal approach, the anterior petrosal approach, and total petrosectomy. The average preoperative Karnofsky Performance Scale score was 88; the average at follow-up was 89.

Cranial neuropathy is often noted when surgical debulking is conservative. In our series, 50% of patients experienced a new postoperative cranial nerve deficit, and 11% experienced deterioration of a preexisting deficit. Of the patients with new deficits, nearly 25% had no deficits on follow-up. Specifically, two of three patients with oculomotor deficits, neither of two patients with trochlear deficits, one of three patients with a trigeminal deficit, five of nine patients with abducens deficits, and five of 11 patients with facial nerve palsies were improved on follow-up. These results suggest that petroclival tumors, with or without a cavernous sinus extension, can be resected with consistency and that, although postoperative cranial deficits are a frequent complication, they are often transient and may not be as detrimental to a patient's quality of life as some believe.

Patients with residual tumor were followed expectantly. Among 20 patients with residual tumors, 30% showed progressive growth managed with either radiation or surgery. Of the 35 patients with gross-total resection, four had tumor recurrence, one of which was treated with surgery and one with radiation. Of 55 patients, 52 had a grade I tumor, and three had grade II and were treated postoperatively with radiation.

Conclusion

Once treatment is indicated, meningiomas in the petroclival region should be held to the same standard Simpson grade applied to all meningiomas: that is, that complete resection mitigates recurrence. One must accept that not all petroclival meningiomas may be completely removed, but this should not alter the surgeon's goal to fully resect these tumors. Residual tumor can be followed initially; subsequent growth or an aggressive pathology may prompt radiotherapeutic consideration.

Moderator

Management of Petroclival Meningiomas: Total Removal vs. Subtotal Resection and Radiosurgery

Kadir Erkmen

The role of surgical resection in treating petroclival meningiomas has evolved over the course of neurosurgery. Originally, these tumors were thought to be unresectable because of the extremely high rates of mortality.[2] At that time, radiosurgery was not available as an alternative technique for treatment, and most patients succumbed to the tumor or the surgery that aimed to resect it. Since then, microsurgical techniques and skull-base approaches have revolutionized the treatment of tumors that were once considered inoperable. Indeed, many published series have shown the feasibility of resection with rare mortality. These series measured the rates of complete resection, as well as rates of morbidity, including cranial neuropathies, vascular and brainstem injury, and cerebrospinal fluid leakage.[2,4–6,9,17,31,43–49] Progressive series have shown varying rates of complete resection and surgical morbidity.

The most recent development with regard to treating these tumors has once again changed the paradigm. The idea of "safe resection and radiosurgery" has become commonplace and is increasing in popularity.[12,24,50–57] The rationale for such an approach, as detailed in Basant Misra's section of this chapter, is that subtotal resection followed by radiosurgery controls the tumor while minimizing morbidity. The alternative approach is to totally resect these tumors, optimizing patient outcomes by improving surgical techniques and technologies.

I have been asked to referee the discussion of whether petroclival meningiomas are best treated with the goal of complete resection or with the goal of safe resection followed by radiosurgery. This is a difficult task because there is no consensus on the topic and there are no long-term studies comparing large numbers of patients treated with

these approaches that evaluate and compare morbidity rates, the risk of recurrence, and the quality of life for patients. In essence, all arguments made in favor of either side of the argument are based on the vast personal experience of the senior authors of the chapters and cannot be "proven" with clear evidence from the literature. Misra's section of this chapter discusses the change in his approach based on changing trends in the literature, as well as a change seen in the results of his personal series of patients in more recent years since he adopted the new paradigm. He reviews the rates of recurrence of residual meningiomas and discusses the published control rates of meningiomas with radiosurgery. Ian F. Dunn and colleagues' section describes the approach to these tumors based on results and a critical evaluation of side effects in their series of patients, and reviews skull-base approaches for resecting these tumors.

I will first identify the areas of agreement between the authors before their differing views diverge. I will then identify where the authors disagree and consider the rationale for their views. Finally, I will describe my approach to these tumors, and try to justify these ideas through the arguments presented.

Misra and Dunn very clearly and carefully identify the salient points of both views. Both state that complete resection of the tumor is optimal when it is possible. This idea was clearly demonstrated in 1957, in the landmark paper by Simpson,[38] which noted that the risk of recurrence of meningiomas is directly correlated with the extent of resection. The importance of complete resection to minimize the risk of recurrence has been shown in more recent series as well.[58–61]

Misra and Dunn also agree that the complete resection of petroclival meningiomas is not always feasible because of the involvement of critical neurovascular structures or the lack of resectability of the tumor. These characteristics vary between tumors and are usually not predictable on preoperative studies. As Misra stated, some tumors that seem to be complex on preoperative MRI studies are surprisingly resectable, whereas some tumors that appear to be straightforward are not. The degree of resectability relates primarily to the firmness of the tumor as well as to its adherence to cranial nerves and vascular structures. With these ideas as common ground, we can evaluate where the authors differ in opinion.

The Goal of Surgery

Dunn and Al Mefty argue that the goal of surgery should always be complete resection, whereas Misra argues that the goal of surgery should be safe debulking or subtotal resection. This is a difficult idea to referee because it truly represents the surgeons' philosophy toward their patients with this complex tumor. If we consider the idea that the authors agree on as a basis for discussion, that complete removal is optimal but not always possible, then I disagree with all of them regarding their philosophy. First, because complete removal is not always possible, as Dunn and Al-Mefty show in their series, the idea that complete resection should be done for all patients does not follow. Having worked closely with Al-Mefty, I am aware that his approach is not to remove the entire tumor regardless of morbidity or cost to the patient, but to attempt a complete resection for every patient by optimizing the surgical conditions. He does this by establishing extensive surgical corridors, utilizing available technologies including neuronavigation, neuromonitoring, and endoscopy, and performing delicate microsurgery based on a mastery of anatomy, physiology, and biology. Conversely, because we agree that complete tumor removal is optimal, an approach that starts with the idea of subtotal resection does not give the patient the benefit of an attempted complete resection. Although I realize that Misra is not arguing for subtotal resection in all patients, even when a complete resection is possible, the primary goal before surgery should not be subtotal resection.

The unintended consequences of such an approach are that neurosurgeons who read these chapters may believe that complete resection is not required, and thus neither is formal training in skull-base surgery or a mastery of the anatomy and approaches required to do these surgeries safely. The dangerous trend I see with this way of thinking is not the outcomes in patients when treated by experienced skull-base surgeons such as Misra, but the outcomes that occur when less-experienced surgeons, or those who do not have an understanding of the anatomy, biology, and skull-base techniques, feel liberated to take on these challenging cases because the expectation and acceptable goal of surgery is debulking of the tumor. This paradigm leads to inappropriate surgery by inexperienced surgeons. Over the years, I have seen an increasing number of patients referred for postoperative radiosurgery after debulking of a petroclival meningioma who have had significant morbidity without the benefit of a complete resection, or who have merely had a glorified biopsy and would not be acceptable candidates for radiosurgery because of persistent brainstem compression by the tumor. In these scenarios of major residual tumor, a repeated surgery is often required before radiosurgical alternatives can be considered (**Fig. 3.10**). Surgical complexity and morbidity increases significantly in patients who have had prior surgery, and thus the patient is exposed to the additional risks of a second surgical procedure under suboptimal conditions because the initial treating surgeon misunderstood the concept of subtotal resection followed by radiosurgery.

A Compromise Approach

As a compromise between viewpoints, I propose the following as a philosophy or approach to these tumors, to maximize surgical resection (**Fig. 3.11**). This idea requires that an attempt be made at complete resection using all of the advantages available for skull-base surgery as detailed above, but with the recognition that it is not possible to completely resect the tumor safely in all patients[62] (**Fig. 3.12**). Whether this approach results in complete resection in 40% or 80% of patients is not important, because each case is unique and referral patterns and tumor types vary between centers and surgeons. What this idea cautions against is surgery to debulk a tumor that might be completely resectable by experienced hands or surgery for these tumors without preparation or optimized conditions with the excuse that complete resection is not required.

In Misra's hands, this approach is safe, but when surgery is done by inexperienced surgeons without skull-base techniques or an understanding of the anatomy, with the goal of simply debulking the tumor, I would argue that surgery is not safe. Surgery in these situations exposes the patient to risks, as in the case shown in **Fig. 3.10**, in which a patient with preoperative signs of brainstem compression from a large petroclival meningioma was treated through a suboccipital approach for a tumor with ventral compression of the brainstem. The surgeon's rationale for not using a petrosal or other appropriate skull-base approach was that it would take too long and that his goal was to debulk the tumor before radiosurgery. In reality, the likely reason was that the surgeon was not familiar with such approaches because treating petroclival tumors was not a typical part of his practice. The surgery was done through suboptimal exposure by a surgeon without the necessary knowledge and experience who felt able to do this surgery as the goal was to "safely" debulk the tumor.

The idea that optimal treatment involves "safe" surgery followed by radiosurgery is also misleading. I would argue that all surgery should be safe regardless of the extent of resection. Indeed, multiple series have shown that petroclival meningioma surgery can be done safely.[4,5,9,43–45,48,49]

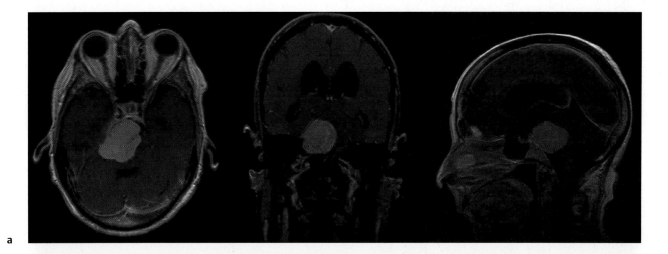

a

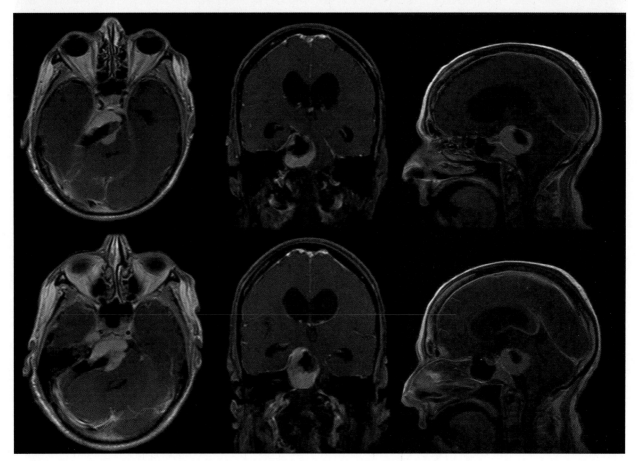

b

Fig. 3.10a,b   Preoperative **(a)** and postoperative **(b)** MRI scans from a patient with a large petroclival meningioma after partial resection through a retrosigmoid approach. The patient was referred for radiosurgery to treat the residual tumor. Based on the significant residual tumor and compression of the brainstem, this patient required a repeated surgical resection, at which time the tumor was completely removed.

The most common morbidity that remains in petroclival surgery done with modern techniques is cranial neuropathies. A patient who has a large petroclival meningioma who has undergone complete resection and who has a temporary sixth nerve palsy has indeed had "safe" surgery. In most cases, new cranial neuropathies are temporary, as stated by Dunn and Al-Mefty, and complete resection of the tumor in these cases represents safe surgery. The most frequent preoperative symptom in these patients is cranial neuropathy, and most patients who have subtotal resection followed by radiosurgery also have either preoperative or postoperative cranial neuropathies, or both.[28,53,54,57]

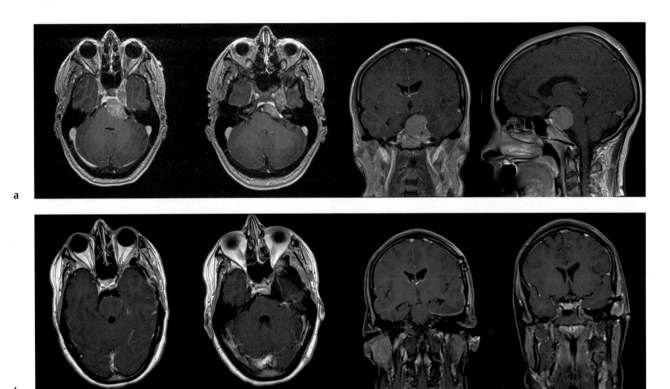

Fig. 3.11a,b Preoperative **(a)** and postoperative **(b)** MRI scans from a patient with a large petroclival meningioma who had complete resection. The patient had no neurologic deficits postoperatively. The patient was referred for evaluation with an "inoperable" tumor because of a cavernous sinus extension. At surgery, the tumor was found to be expanding Meckel's cave and was completely resectable without initiating cranial neuropathy. This patient benefited from the maximal surgical resection paradigm and would not need radiation. A "safe surgery and radiosurgery" approach would likely have left residual tumor, and the patient would have had the added risk of radiation and possible delayed recurrence.

Risk of Recurrence

The next point of discussion involves the risk of recurrence of small residual meningiomas after resection. Meningiomas in the skull base, including petroclival tumors, grow slowly and are more likely to be benign than are convexity or parasagittal meningiomas. Small residual tumors after maximal resection likely would behave similarly. Indeed, the risk of recurrence of small residual meningiomas over long-term follow-up is low.[36] Recurrence is seen in patients with rare tumors that recur and grow in an unrelenting pattern and continue to grow despite radiation. The radiosurgical literature shows that the recurrence rate of postsurgical meningiomas is higher than for those treated up front.[53,54] Some of the proponents of radiosurgery argue that this difference results from the difficulty in targeting postoperative meningiomas. Alternative reasonable conclusions are that tumors that grow to the point of needing resection may have a propensity to grow, and that the residual after surgery has the same propensity. The results of up-front radiosurgery likely define much of the natural history of meningiomas. A high percentage of meningiomas do not grow on serial imaging, and if one were to treat all meningioma patients with radiosurgery, the results would be biased to demonstrate the success of treatment because a large number of cases have a benign course of no growth. Thus, I agree with Misra's statement that radiosurgery is not optimal as the initial treatment of a meningioma. I disagree, however, with his use of the control rates quoted in radiosurgical articles to justify subtotal resection. Closer examination of these articles reveals lower rates of control with postsurgical cases, and these rates in fact are not significantly different from the control rates of postsurgical cases without postoperative radiosurgery.[36] Recently presented data also show that meningiomas that grow before radiosurgical treatment have poor control rates, significantly worse than treated tumors without prior evidence of growth.[63] Petroclival meningiomas that require surgical resection are typically growing preoperatively and would likely be in the category of tumors that have poor control rates with radiosurgery. Based on all of these data, I would not advocate radiosurgery as the frontline treatment for patients with meningiomas, and because the control rates with radiosurgery are poor in postoperative and in growing meningiomas, I would not advocate intentional subtotal resection with a plan to rescue with radiosurgery.

Radiosurgery is also not without complications of its own. The treatment of residual tumor with radiosurgery subjects the cranial nerves and brainstem to risk.[28,29,35,64–73]

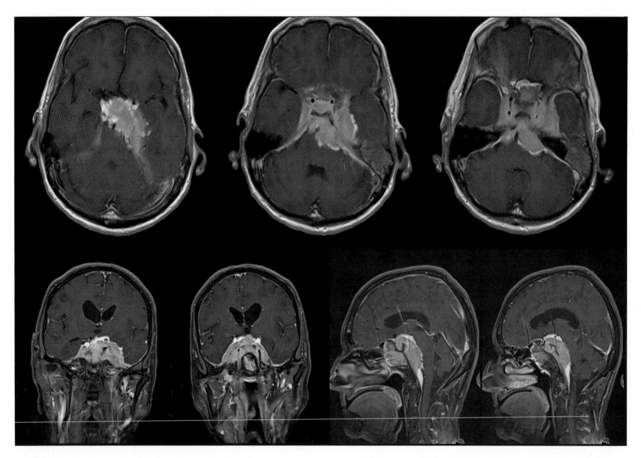

Fig. 3.12 Multiple plane MRI scans of a patient with an unresectable meningioma. The patient presented with bilateral sixth nerve palsy, a visual field deficit in the left eye, and panhypopituitarism. In this patient, the surgeon should not attempt total resection because the bilateral carotid arteries and basilar artery are encased and the bilateral cavernous sinuses are involved. Because complete resection is not possible, the goal of surgery for this patient is to decompress the brainstem and optic apparatus to prevent visual loss.

In fact, these risks may be increased in postoperative patients. The difference may lie in the fact that most radiosurgical complications are delayed months to years after treatment, whereas deficits after surgery are immediate and improve over the ensuing months and years. The treatment paradigm that incorporates "safe" surgery followed by radiosurgery may be trading risks on the day of surgery for delayed complications. Longer term studies are required to fully elucidate the long-term effects of radiosurgery in these patients. In addition, the location of residual tumor in patients who had deliberate subtotal resection is likely to be a high-risk location for radiosurgery. Indeed, the surgeon who performs a subtotal resection of a petroclival meningioma will leave the residual in the highest risk locations and those most difficult to reach. These include the cavernous sinus, the clivus, the interface with the brainstem, the basilar artery, or cranial nerves. These same locations are the sites of highest risk for radiosurgery, with well-studied maximum tolerated doses at the brainstem, optic apparatus, and cavernous sinus. Although the overall volume of the tumor may be decreased, the highest radiation risk locations remain for radiosurgery.

Outcome Studies

Recently, the published literature on the treatment of petroclival meningiomas has indeed shifted toward the paradigm of incomplete resection and radiosurgery. The fact that more papers are published with this idea does not justify the idea. A study comparing long-term outcomes in patients treated with both approaches would be the only data that could show the superiority of one paradigm over the other. Such a study is unlikely to be performed, and thus a definitive answer seems undeterminable.

The radiosurgical literature is also changing over time. Proponents cite high control rates that were seen in studies performed when higher doses of radiosurgery treatment were standard. In those series, however, complication rates were higher.[12,17,53,54,57] Over the years, as radiosurgery treatment has evolved, patients are being treated with lower radiation doses to minimize risks and complications. At the same time, it is likely that control rates will decrease with the lower doses. It is important to consider both control rates and complications in patients who have had the same dose of radiation. Proponents of radiosurgical treatment often cite the control rates of higher dose radiosurgery series while using the safety parameters with more recent reports of lower dose radiosurgery.

With these arguments, I am not a proponent of deliberate subtotal resection with the goal of using radiosurgery for residual disease. This does not mean, however, that there is no role for radiosurgery or radiation therapy in the treatment of petroclival meningiomas. For patients with residual disease after attempted maximal resection, our practice has been to follow these patients closely with serial MRIs. For the small percentage of patients who have growth of a residual meningioma after surgical resection, radiosurgery is a good adjunct to treatment. A large series of skull-base meningiomas with this treatment paradigm showed that only a small percentage of residual meningiomas progress after resection.[36] The reason for this is unclear because most of these tumors showed growth preoperatively, prompting surgical resection. One hypothesis is that, with maximal resection, the areas of residual tumor may have lost their vascular supply because of the resection of involved tentorium, hyperostotic bone, or other structures. In effect, the surgery removes the large mass and has an effect on controlling the residual tumor. This hypothesis has not been proven, however, but seems plausible as a description of the mechanism of rare growth in postoperative tumors. Residual tumors that do show growth on follow-up imaging may be optimal to treat with radiosurgery.

Radiation therapy also has a role in treating atypical and malignant meningiomas after resection. These tumors have a high recurrence rate despite maximal surgery and patients benefit from postoperative radiotherapy.

Conclusion

There is no clinical trial that answers the question of whether radical surgery or deliberate subtotal resection followed by radiosurgery is the optimal treatment plan for patients with petroclival meningiomas. I propose the middle road, in which maximal resection is done with the goal of complete resection when possible. This approach requires training, knowledge, and skill in skull-base and microvascular techniques to achieve optimal outcomes for patients.[62] For patients in whom complete resection is not possible, I would favor close radiographic follow-up of residual disease, with radiosurgery reserved for patients with atypical or anaplastic tumors or those with demonstrated growth of residual disease on follow-up MRIs. This approach provides patients with the benefit of attempted complete resection, and exposes them to radiation only in the rare scenario of a growing residual meningioma. Further research is needed to improve the care of these patients with this complex problem. This research may be in the form of new surgical techniques or novel surgical approaches or the increasing understanding of tumor biology and genetics.

References

1. Yasargil MG, Mortara RW, Curcic M. Meningiomas of the basal posterior cranial fossa. In: Krayenbühl H, ed. Advances and Technical Standards in Neurosurgery, vol. 7. Vienna: Springer, 1980:1–115

2. Al Mefty O, Smith RR. Clival and petroclival meningiomas. In: Al-Mefty O, ed. Meningiomas. New York: Raven Press, 1991: 517–537

3. Misra BK. Intracranial meningioma. In: Ramamurthi B, Tandon PN, eds. Textbook of Neurosurgery, 2nd ed. New Delhi: Churchill Livingstone, 1996:1077–1110

4. Al-Mefty O, Fox JL, Smith RR. Petrosal approach for petroclival meningiomas. Neurosurgery 1988;22:510–517

5. Samii M, Ammirati M, Mahran A, Bini W, Sepehrnia A. Surgery of petroclival meningiomas: report of 24 cases. Neurosurgery 1989;24:12–17

6. Sekhar LN, Jannetta PJ, Burkhart LE, Janosky JE. Meningiomas involving the clivus: a six-year experience with 41 patients. Neurosurgery 1990;27:764–781, discussion 781

7. Kawase T, Shiobara R, Toya S. Anterior transpetrosal-transtentorial approach for sphenopetroclival meningiomas: surgical method and results in 10 patients. Neurosurgery 1991;28:869–875, discussion 875–876

8. Misra BK, Rout D, Rao VRK, Rout A. Petroclival Meningioma: Surgical Experience with 11 Cases. Abstracts. 40th Annual Conference, Neurological Society of India, Manipal, India, 1991:25

9. Bricolo AP, Turazzi S, Talacchi A, Cristofori L. Microsurgical removal of petroclival meningiomas: a report of 33 patients. Neurosurgery 1992;31:813–828, discussion 828

10. Spetzler RF, Daspit CP, Pappas CT. The combined supra- and infratentorial approach for lesions of the petrous and clival regions: experience with 46 cases. J Neurosurg 1992;76:588–599

11. Ojemann RG. Skull-base surgery: a perspective. J Neurosurg 1992;76:569–570

12. Subach BR, Lunsford LD, Kondziolka D, Maitz AH, Flickinger JC. Management of petroclival meningiomas by stereotactic radiosurgery. Neurosurgery 1998;42:437–443, discussion 443–445

13. Natarajan SK, Sekhar LN, Schessel D, Morita A. Petroclival meningiomas: multimodality treatment and outcomes at long-term follow-up. Neurosurgery 2007;60:965–979, discussion 979–981

14. Little KM, Friedman AH, Sampson JH, Wanibuchi M, Fukushima T. Surgical management of petroclival meningiomas: defining resection goals based on risk of neurological morbidity and tumor recurrence rates in 137 patients. Neurosurgery 2005; 56:546–559, discussion 546–559

15. Adachi K, Kawase T, Yoshida K, Yazaki T, Onozuka S. ABC Surgical Risk Scale for skull base meningioma: a new scoring system for predicting the extent of tumor removal and neurological outcome. J Neurosurg 2009;111:1053–1061

16. Jung HW, Yoo H, Paek SH, Choi KS. Long-term outcome and growth rate of subtotally resected petroclival meningiomas: experience with 38 cases. Neurosurgery 2000;46:567–574, discussion 574–575

17. Mathiesen T, Gerlich A, Kihlström L, Svensson M, Bagger-Sjöbäck D. Effects of using combined transpetrosal surgical

approaches to treat petroclival meningiomas. Neurosurgery 2007;60:982–991, discussion 991–992

18. Bambakidis NC, Kakarla UK, Kim LJ, et al. Evolution of surgical approaches in the treatment of petroclival meningiomas: a retrospective review. Neurosurgery 2007;61(5, Suppl 2):202–209, discussion 209–211

19. Bindal R, Goodman JM, Kawasaki A, Purvin V, Kuzma B. The natural history of untreated skull base meningiomas. Surg Neurol 2003;59:87–92, discussion 92

20. Van Havenbergh T, Carvalho G, Tatagiba M, Plets C, Samii M. Natural history of petroclival meningiomas. Neurosurgery 2003;52:55–62, discussion 62–64

21. Misra BK. Management of central skull base tumors. In: Sindou M, ed. Practical Handbook of Neurosurgery: From Leading Neurosurgeons, vol. 2. New York: Springer, 2009:115–128

22. Kreil W, Luggin J, Fuchs I, Weigl V, Eustacchio S, Papaefthymiou G. Long term experience of gamma knife radiosurgery for benign skull base meningiomas. J Neurol Neurosurg Psychiatry 2005;76:1425–1430

23. Roche PH, Pellet W, Fuentes S, Thomassin JM, Régis J. Gamma knife radiosurgical management of petroclival meningiomas results and indications. Acta Neurochir (Wien) 2003;145:883–888, discussion 888

24. Iwai Y, Yamanaka K, Ikeda H. Gamma knife radiosurgery for skull base meningioma: long-term results of low-dose treatment. J Neurosurg 2008;109:804–810

25. Takanashi M, Fukuoka S, Hojyo A, Sasaki T, Nakagawara J, Nakamura H. Gamma knife radiosurgery for skull-base meningiomas. Prog Neurol Surg 2009;22:96–111

26. Zachenhofer I, Wolfsberger S, Aichholzer M, et al. Gamma-knife radiosurgery for cranial base meningiomas: experience of tumor control, clinical course, and morbidity in a follow-up of more than 8 years. Neurosurgery 2006;58:28–36, discussion 28–36

27. Misra BK. Surgical approaches to petroclival region. Prog Clin Neurosci 1999;14:183–192

28. Morita A, Coffey RJ, Foote RL, Schiff D, Gorman D. Risk of injury to cranial nerves after gamma knife radiosurgery for skull base meningiomas: experience in 88 patients. J Neurosurg 1999;90: 42–49

29. Rowe J, Grainger A, Walton L, Silcocks P, Radatz M, Kemeny A. Risk of malignancy after gamma knife stereotactic radiosurgery. Neurosurgery 2007;60:60–65, discussion 65–66

30. Diluna ML, Bulsara KR. Surgery for petroclival meningiomas: a comprehensive review of outcomes in the skull base surgery era. Skull Base 2010;20:337–342

31. Hakuba A, Nishimura S, Jang BJ. A combined retroauricular and preauricular transpetrosal-transtentorial approach to clivus meningiomas. Surg Neurol 1988;30:108–116

32. Park CK, Jung HW, Kim JE, Paek SH, Kim DG. The selection of the optimal therapeutic strategy for petroclival meningiomas. Surg Neurol 2006;66:160–165, discussion 165–166

33. Zentner J, Meyer B, Vieweg U, Herberhold C, Schramm J. Petroclival meningiomas: is radical resection always the best option? J Neurol Neurosurg Psychiatry 1997;62:341–345

34. Abdel Aziz KM, Sanan A, van Loveren HR, Tew JM Jr, Keller JT, Pensak ML. Petroclival meningiomas: predictive parameters for transpetrosal approaches. Neurosurgery 2000;47:139–150, discussion 150–152

35. Couldwell WT, Cole CD, Al-Mefty O. Patterns of skull base meningioma progression after failed radiosurgery. J Neurosurg 2007;106:30–35

36. Erkmen K, Pravdenkova S, Al Mefty-O. Growth rate of residual meningiomas: observation without stereotactic radiosurgery (SRS). American Association of Neurological Surgeons Meeting, New Orleans, LA, 2005

37. Mathiesen T, Kihlström L, Karlsson B, Lindquist C. Potential complications following radiotherapy for meningiomas. Surg Neurol 2003;60:193–198, discussion 199–200

38. Simpson D. The recurrence of intracranial meningiomas after surgical treatment. J Neurol Neurosurg Psychiatry 1957;20: 22–39

39. Goel A, Muzumdar D. Conventional posterior fossa approach for surgery on petroclival meningiomas: a report on an experience with 28 cases. Surg Neurol 2004;62:332–338, discussion 338–340

40. Spallone A, Makhmudov UB, Mukhamedjanov DJ, Tcherekajev VA. Petroclival meningioma. An attempt to define the role of skull base approaches in their surgical management. Surg Neurol 1999;51:412–419, discussion 419–420

41. Erkmen K, Pravdenkova S, Al-Mefty O. Surgical management of petroclival meningiomas: factors determining the choice of approach. Neurosurg Focus 2005;19:E7

42. Hafez A, Nader R, Al-Mefty O. Preservation of the superior petrosal sinus during the petrosal approach. J Neurosurg 2011; 114:1294–1298

43. al-Mefty O, Ayoubi S, Smith RR. The petrosal approach: indications, technique, and results. Acta Neurochir Suppl (Wien) 1991;53:166–170

44. Cho CW, Al-Mefty O. Combined petrosal approach to petroclival meningiomas. Neurosurgery 2002;51:708–716, discussion 716–718

45. Couldwell WT, Fukushima T, Giannotta SL, Weiss MH. Petroclival meningiomas: surgical experience in 109 cases. J Neurosurg 1996;84:20–28

46. Goel A. Extended lateral subtemporal approach for petroclival meningiomas: report of experience with 24 cases. Br J Neurosurg 1999;13:270–275

47. Hakuba A, Nishimura S, Tanaka K, Kishi H, Nakamura T. Clivus meningioma: six cases of total removal. Neurol Med Chir (Tokyo) 1977;17(1 Pt 1):63–77

48. Samii M, Tatagiba M. Experience with 36 surgical cases of petroclival meningiomas. Acta Neurochir (Wien) 1992;118:27–32

49. Tahara A, de Santana PA Jr, Calfat Maldaun MV, et al. Petroclival meningiomas: surgical management and common complications. J Clin Neurosci 2009;16:655–659

50. Eldebawy E, Mousa A, Reda W, Elgantiry M. Stereotactic radiosurgery and radiotherapy in benign intracranial meningioma. J Egypt Natl Canc Inst 2011;23:89–93

51. Flannery TJ, Kano H, Lunsford LD, et al. Long-term control of petroclival meningiomas through radiosurgery. J Neurosurg 2010;112:957–964

52. Kondziolka D, Flickinger JC, Perez B; Gamma Knife Meningioma Study Group. Judicious resection and/or radiosurgery for parasagittal meningiomas: outcomes from a multicenter review. Neurosurgery 1998;43:405–413, discussion 413–414

53. Kondziolka D, Levy EI, Niranjan A, Flickinger JC, Lunsford LD. Long-term outcomes after meningioma radiosurgery: physician and patient perspectives. J Neurosurg 1999;91:44–50

54. Kondziolka D, Mathieu D, Lunsford LD, et al. Radiosurgery as definitive management of intracranial meningiomas. Neurosurgery 2008;62:53–58, discussion 58–60

55. Linskey ME, Davis SA, Ratanatharathorn V. Relative roles of microsurgery and stereotactic radiosurgery for the treatment

of patients with cranial meningiomas: a single-surgeon 4-year integrated experience with both modalities. J Neurosurg 2005; 102(Suppl):59–70

56. Stafford SL, Pollock BE, Foote RL, et al. Meningioma radiosurgery: tumor control, outcomes, and complications among 190 consecutive patients. Neurosurgery 2001;49:1029–1037, discussion 1037–1038

57. Starke RM, Williams BJ, Hiles C, Nguyen JH, Elsharkawy MY, Sheehan JP. Gamma knife surgery for skull base meningiomas. J Neurosurg 2012;116:588–597

58. Adegbite AB, Khan MI, Paine KW, Tan LK. The recurrence of intracranial meningiomas after surgical treatment. J Neurosurg 1983;58:51–56

59. Ayerbe J, Lobato RD, de la Cruz J, et al. Risk factors predicting recurrence in patients operated on for intracranial meningioma. A multivariate analysis. Acta Neurochir (Wien) 1999;141: 921–932

60. Mahmood A, Qureshi NH, Malik GM. Intracranial meningiomas: analysis of recurrence after surgical treatment. Acta Neurochir (Wien) 1994;126:53–58

61. Mathiesen T, Lindquist C, Kihlström L, Karlsson B. Recurrence of cranial base meningiomas. Neurosurgery 1996;39:2–7, discussion 8–9

62. Erkmen K, Pravdenkova S, Al-Mefty O. Surgical management of petroclival meningiomas: factors determining the choice of approach. Neurosurg Focus 2005;19:E7

63. Mathiesen T. Control rate of meningiomas with radiosurgery. World Federation of Neurosurgical Societies Meeting, Granada, Spain, November 19–20, 2012

64. Attia A, Chan MD, Mott RT, et al. Patterns of failure after treatment of atypical meningioma with gamma knife radiosurgery. J Neurooncol 2012;108:179–185

65. Cai R, Barnett GH, Novak E, Chao ST, Suh JH. Principal risk of peritumoral edema after stereotactic radiosurgery for intracranial meningioma is tumor-brain contact interface area. Neurosurgery 2010;66:513–522

66. Chen CH, Shen CC, Sun MH, Ho WL, Huang CF, Kwan PC. Histopathology of radiation necrosis with severe peritumoral edema after gamma knife radiosurgery for parasagittal meningioma. A report of two cases. Stereotact Funct Neurosurg 2007;85: 292–295

67. Fujimoto A, Matsumura A, Maruno T, Yasuda S, Yamamoto M, Nose T. Normal pressure hydrocephalus after gamma knife radiosurgery for cerebellopontine angle meningioma. J Clin Neurosci 2004;11:785–787

68. Hsieh CT, Tsai JT, Chang LP, Lin JW, Chang SD, Ju DT. Peritumoral edema after stereotactic radiosurgery for meningioma. J Clin Neurosci 2010;17:529–531

69. Igaki H, Maruyama K, Tago M, et al. Cyst formation after stereotactic radiosurgery for intracranial meningioma. Stereotact Funct Neurosurg 2008;86:231–236

70. Kajiwara M, Yamashita K, Ueba T, Nishikawa T. Normal pressure hydrocephalus after radiosurgery for sphenoid ridge meningioma. J Clin Neurosci 2009;16:162–164

71. Kwon Y, Ahn JS, Jeon SR, et al. Intratumoral bleeding in meningioma after gamma knife radiosurgery. J Neurosurg 2002;97 (5, Suppl):657–662

72. Lee HS, Kim JH, Lee JI. Glioblastoma following radiosurgery for meningioma. J Korean Neurosurg Soc 2012;51:98–101

73. Yu JS, Yong WH, Wilson D, Black KL. Glioblastoma induction after radiosurgery for meningioma. Lancet 2000;356:1576–1577

Chapter 4

Management of Incidental Meningiomas

Case

A 39-year-old woman came to medical attention with headache. The magnetic resonance images show a meningioma of 1.5 cm in the maximum diameter.

Participants

Observation of Incidental Meningiomas: Mohamad Abolfotoh and Ossama Al-Mefty

Stereotactic Radiosurgery for Small Meningiomas: Toshinori Hasegawa

The Role of Microsurgery in the Management of Small Skull-Base Meningiomas: Luis A.B. Borba and Daniel D. Cavalcanti

Moderator: Management of Incidental Meningiomas: E. Antonio Chiocca

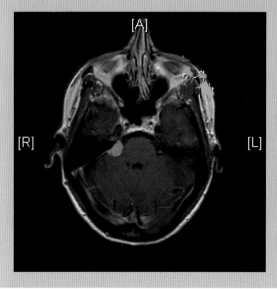
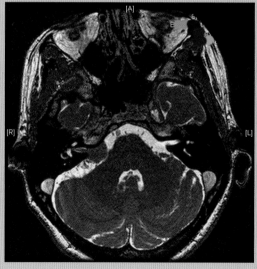

Observation of Incidental Meningiomas

Mohammad Abolfotoh and Ossama Al-Mefty

Images of the Presented Case

The magnetic resonance imaging (MRI) study of the patient presented shows a small enhanced lesion in the cerebellopontine angle (CPA) cistern measuring 10.5 × 16 mm in axial views. This lesion is dural based and isointense on T2-weighted images, excluding the possibility of a vestibular schwannoma or any of the rapidly growing lesions that might mimic a meningioma. According to the available clinical and radiological data, this lesion is likely to be an incidentally discovered CPA meningioma.

Incidentally Discovered Meningiomas

Although the exact definition of (asymptomatic) incidentally discovered meningiomas (IDMs) remains unclear,[1] the term refers to meningiomas discovered during a brain workup for any reason other than a known specific clinical presentation of a detected tumor,[2–5] related to neurofibromatosis type 2, present as a part of multiple meningiomas, or induced by radiation.[5] The rate of incidence of asymptomatic meningiomas has increased in the past decade, clearly because of the availability of, and advances in, diagnostic techniques.[1,6] These meningiomas now account for almost half of diagnosed meningiomas.[5]

Clinical Picture of the Presented Case

As this patient had only a headache, we could not immediately determine that this small lesion was the cause of her symptoms. Headache is a common presentation for relatively large CPA meningiomas[7] but is uncommon for smaller, premeatal, or intracanalicular ones.[8,9] Headache has never been postulated to be the specific or the main presentation for small CPA meningiomas.[7–9] The meningioma in the images appears to be a premeatal type of CPA meningioma, which is nearly always discovered early and is consequently small at the time of diagnosis. It does not commonly present with headache, but instead with symptoms of fifth, seventh, and eighth cranial nerve involvement.[7,10,11]

Headache and dizziness are the most common reasons for brain imaging that leads to the discovery of IDMs.[2–4] Many authors investigating IDMs believe them unlikely to cause headache, as these tumors are always small without causing mass effect.[2–4,12] Thus, for this patient, our approach would be based on the diagnosis of an IDM.

Conservative Treatment

With the exception of IDMs in certain locations such as the tuberculum sellae, we recommend conservative follow-up for asymptomatic IDMs, especially many skull-base IDMs, as some reports indicate that most are World Health Organization (WHO) grade I and are indolent in nature.[13–15] This recommendation is based on experience and a review of the literature. To the best of our knowledge, studies of IDMs overwhelmingly have recommended conservative close follow-up.[1–3,12,16–22] Recent criteria for managing IDMs have suggested observation for asymptomatic lesions in patients regardless of age, but for growing lesions in patients age 65 years or younger, surgery is recommended regardless of the size of the tumor.[6]

The rationale for conservative treatment of IDMs is that it defers the risks of intervention in asymptomatic patients.[23] However, although the risk is lower in young patients with relatively small lesions, like the patient described here, it is still not negligible. Nakamura and colleagues[3] concluded that most asymptomatic meningiomas show only minimal growth and may be observed without any surgical intervention, but close observation is recommended in young patients because of the higher tumor growth rates in this age group.

Conservative management (observation) is the initial treatment option for elderly patients, for medically unstable patients with small tumors and mild, stable symptoms, and for those who are unwilling to undergo surgery.[7] The dilemma for neurosurgeons is the treatment of young people who are medically fit for surgery. Asymptomatic young persons (such as the present patient) can be followed, with intervention necessary only when symptoms appear or when progressive growth is documented.

Follow-Up Protocol

The radiological diagnosis of meningiomas is usually straightforward. Other more aggressive lesions can mimic meningiomas, however, so close clinical and radiological follow-up is mandatory when giving the patient the conservative option of observation.[4,6]

Once a meningioma is discovered, we schedule follow-up scans at 3 and 9 months, and then yearly or perhaps every other year if the patient's condition is stable for 5 years. The importance of the early first MRI (after 3 months) is to exclude rapidly enlarging meningiomas or any other aggressive lesion that may mimic a meningioma. This follow-up protocol is more or less similar to other protocols reported in the literature.[4,16] It is critical to compare the last study to the previous ones, particularly the original or even an earlier prediagnostic study. Comparing the latest study to only the preceding one might be misleading and could miss significant changes that have taken place over time. During the follow-up period, if the lesion has begun to enlarge but is still asymptomatic, we do an MRI study every 6 months; if the lesion shows significant progressive growth, we proceed with surgical treatment (**Fig. 4.1**). At

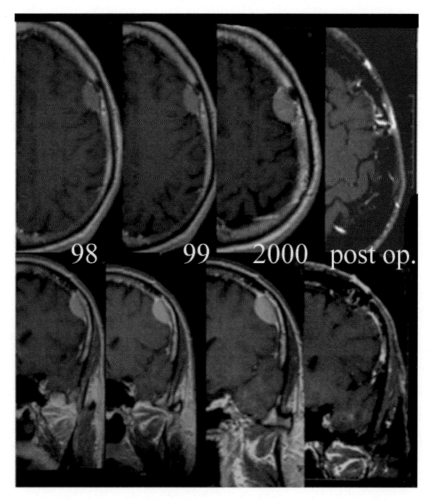

Fig. 4.1 Enhanced serial axial and coronal magnetic resonance imaging (MRI) studies of a 50-year-old man showing the progressive growth of a left frontal incidentally discovered meningioma (IDM) over 2 years. This progression led to the decision for surgical excision.

any time during the period of observation, if specific symptoms appear **(Fig. 4.2)** or progressive growth is documented **(Fig. 4.3),** we prefer to proceed with surgery, but many untreated lesions might show no growth over a long period of time **(Figs. 4.4, 4.5).**

Discussion

Before treating IDMs, one should understand their natural history and rate of growth, along with other factors that might influence the decisions regarding management. We

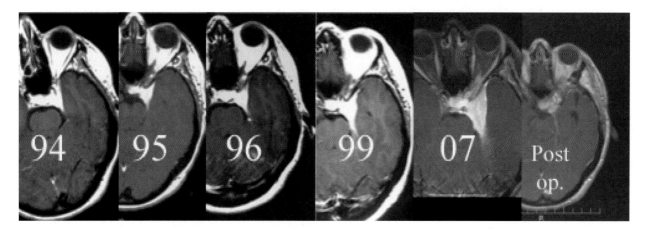

Fig. 4.2 Enhanced serial axial MRI studies of a meningioma in the left cavernous sinus of a 42-year-old woman show progressive growth of the tumor, which became symptomatic and has been operated on.

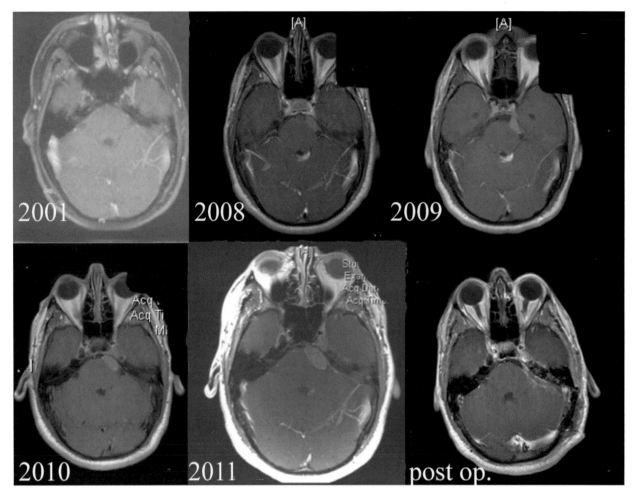

Fig. 4.3 Enhanced serial axial MRI studies of an IDM in a 24-year-old man. The tumor related to the petrous apex and showed rapid growth over a period of 2 years, requiring close follow-up and then surgery. The MRI study done in 2001 for nonspecific symptoms showed no abnormalities.

classify factors affecting the management of IDMs into three groups:

1. Patient factors: the patient's age, overall health, and fitness for surgery
2. Tumor factors: the location, size at diagnosis, radiological aspects, natural history, and rate of growth
3. Circumstances: the experience of the neurosurgeon and the availability of treatment facilities, which increase the chance of a good outcome and minimize morbidity.

Nonetheless, the management of IDMs should be determined on an individual basis, case by case, because all these factors must be considered in the decision-making process.[17] The age of the patient is the most important factor because the growth rate of IDMs in the elderly is very slow.[1,3,4,6,16–19] Rubin and colleagues[12] found that older age was significantly related to a low rate of tumor growth; every additional year in the patient's age decreases the risk of tumor growth by 8%, a fact that agrees with most previous studies.[1,3,18,20]

In addition, the risks associated with surgery are much greater in older patients. Awad and associates[24] reported

on 75 patients older than 60 years who underwent surgical resection of intracranial meningiomas, 21% of which were asymptomatic. Perioperative morbidity was 48% and operative mortality was 6.6%. Thus, there is agreement among neurosurgeons that conservative management is the first choice of treatment for elderly patients with IDMs that are asymptomatic or even those that cause mild, stable symptoms.[6,7,18]

The debate is about how to manage asymptomatic IDMs in younger patients, as it is now well known that higher growth rates of meningiomas are associated with the patient's young age.[5,6,12,16] Nevertheless, for us, this fact is not sufficient to warrant radiation or surgery. Understanding the natural history of the growth of IDMs is key to making the decision.

In young people with asymptomatic lesions, although the risks associated with surgery are fewer than in the elderly, conservative management is still our initial choice, as IDMs rarely become symptomatic within a follow-up period of 2 years or less.[5] Many authors have found observation acceptable if a patient has an asymptomatic IDM, is under the age of 60, and is reluctant to undergo surgery or

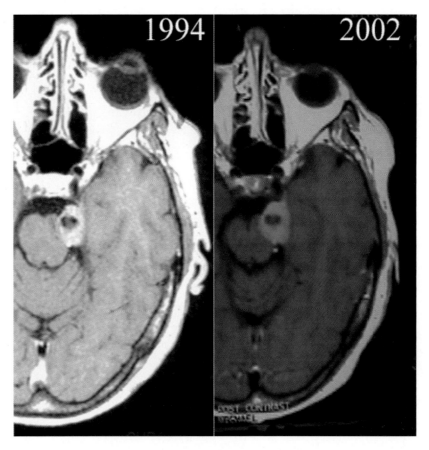

Fig. 4.4 Enhanced axial MRI studies of a small IDM in a 63-year-old woman. The tumor relates to the petrous apex and has a large central area of calcification. It showed no growth over a period of 8 years.

is not in optimal medical condition, as even tumor growth is usually not associated with morbidity.[2,4,12,18,25]

Before the turn of the 21st century, we knew little about the natural history of IDMs. Now the picture is getting clearer **(Table 4.1)**, but the definition and methods of calculating tumor growth still vary. In volume measurement studies, an annual growth rate of more than 1 cm^3 per year or a volume increase of greater than 15% are considered to

indicate tumor growth. In diameter measurement studies, growth has been defined as a change in tumor size of 2 or 5 mm, or even *any* measurable change.[5] In early studies, a large diameter was used to determine tumor size. This method may be useful for judging the treatment response of gliomas to adjuvant therapy, but it is not accurate for evaluating the exact increase in the volume of skull-base meningiomas because of their complex shape; these tu-

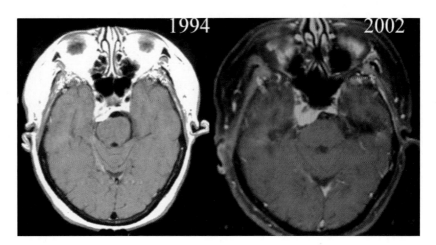

Fig. 4.5 Enhanced axial MRI studies of a right posterior cavernous IDM in a 68-year-old woman. The tumor showed no growth over a period of 8 years.

Table 4.1 Reported Rates of Tumor Growth, Initial Size, Rate of Symptomatic Change, and Predictive Factors for Tumor Growth for Untreated Incidentally Discovered Meningiomas (IDMs)

Author, Year	No. of Cases	Initial Tumor Size (Range)	Patients Becoming Symptomatic (%)	Significant Factors Related to Tumor Growth	Methods	Growth Cases (%)	Average Follow-Up Year (Range)	Tumor Growth Rate Per Year
Firsching et al[2] (1990)	17	4.7 cm³	ND		Volume	ND	1.8 (0.2–7.4)	3.60% (0.5–21.0%)
Olivero et al[4] (1995)	45	2.15 cm (0.5–5 cm)	None		Maximum diameter	10 (22.2)	2.7 (0.5–15)	0.24 cm
Braunstein and Vick[27] (1997)	5	ND	1 (20.0)		Three diameters	1 (20.0)	7.9 (3.3–11.5)	2.43 cm³
Go et al[20] (1998)	32	2.06 cm (1–7 cm)	1 (3.1)	Calcification	Maximum diameter	4 (12.5)	5.1 (0.4–15.2)	12% (1.2–25.6%)
Kuratsu et al[28] (2000)	63	9.75 cm³	ND	Calcification	Volume	20 (31.7)	2.3 (1.0–8.0)	ND
Niiro et al[18] (2000)	40[a]	2.60 cm	5 (12.5)	Tumor size, T2 signal, calcification	Maximum diameter	14 (35.0)	3.2 (0.5–8.1)	0.08 cm
Yoneoka et al[21] (2000)	37	ND	2 (5.4)	Age, volume of tumor	Volume	9 (24.3)[b]	4.2 ± 0.7 (0.5–17)	5.3 ± 2.1 cm³
Nakamura et al[3] (2003)	41	9.0 cm³	ND	Age, calcification, T2 signal	Volume	ND[c]	3.6 (0.5–8.8)	0.796 cm³
Herscovici et al[17] (2004)	44	17 ± 8 mm (3–45 mm)	ND	Age	Maximum diameter	16 (36.4)	5.6	3.9 ± 3 mm
Nakasu et al[26] (2005)	5	6.56 cm (0.27–17.4 cm)	ND	Calcification	Volume	2 (40.0)[b]	5.9 (4.2–8.7)	0.31 cm³ (0.22–0.40)
Yano et al[25] (2006)	67	2.40 cm (0.5–6.6 cm)	11 (16.4%)	Calcification	Maximum diameter	25 (37.3)	7.8 (5.0–13.6)	1.9 mm (0.42–11.47)
Hashiba et al[1] (2009)	70	10.4 cm (0.63–69.2 cm)	0.0	Calcification	Volume	44 (62.9)	3.3 (1.0–10.3)	15–25%
Rubin et al[12] (2011)	56 (63 tumors)	18 ± 11 mm (3–70 mm)	None	Age	Maximum diameter	38 (60.3)	5.4 ± 2.8 (1.2–10.4)	4 mm
Oya et al[16] (2011)	244 (273 tumors)	19.8 ± 10.9 mm (4–7 mm)	ND	Age, calcification, T2 signal, peritumoral edema	Maximum diameter[d]	120 (44.0)	3.8[e]	0.54 cm³ <60 years 0.83 cm³ >60 years[f]

Abbreviation: ND, no data (the variant was not done in the study).

[a] Patients were older than 70 years.

[b] Growth was defined as an increase of tumor volume of more than 1 cm³ per year.

[c] 66% of growth rates were less than 1 cm³ per year.

[d] Volume in 154 tumors.

[e] Only for group showing linear growth, and at least 1 year of follow-up of all patients.

[f] The number of growing lesions was larger for patients under the age of 60 years.

Source: Adapted from Yano S, Kuratsu JI. Natural course of untreated meningiomas. In DeMonte F, McDermott MW, Al-Mefty O, eds. Al-Mefty's Meningiomas, 2nd ed. New York: Thieme, 2011:63–67.[5] Reprinted by permission.

mors may grow in any direction.[1,4,18] Volumetry appears to reflect the tumor's size more accurately than does measuring the diameter because it is applicable to irregularly shaped tumors. For that reason, it has been used in recent studies to evaluate lesion size.[1,3,16,21,26] In practice, we still usually rely on measuring the maximum tumor diameter in two directions. This method is practical and less time-consuming than volumetry in the clinical setting; we also believe that a very small increase (even in diameter) can cause symptoms and may change the treatment options.

Herscovici and associates[17] found that 32 of 51 IDMs showed no growth at the end of follow-up (mean 67 months). However, the percentage of patients who showed tumor growth by the end of follow-up ranges from 0 to 44% across the literature **(Table 4.1)**.[27,28]

The IDMs do not always follow an exponential growth pattern, but always exhibit complex patterns of growth **(Fig. 4.6)**. Nakasu and associates[26] reported that benign meningiomas grow exponentially, linearly, or not at all. Hashiba and colleagues[1] noticed similar results in their large series of IDMs, also suggesting that some tumors show a complex pattern of growth throughout follow-up. Thus, a tumor might grow exponentially in its early stages, linearly in the intermediate stage, and finally reach a plateau at the terminal stage **(Fig. 4.6)**.

This argument means that the tumor doubling time or annual growth rate calculated by observation over a short period of time may not predict the growth potential and natural history of a tumor over the life of the patient.[1,22] For this reason, we do not start intervention for asymptomatic IDMs until after the appearance of new, specific symptoms or if the tumor shows a progressive and significant increase in size on serial follow-up scans.

In the published literature, neither the patient's sex nor the tumor location was found to predict the growth of an IDM; however, it is well known that skull-base IDMs grow slowly. Van Havenbergh and colleagues[19] retrospectively studied the natural history of 21 conservatively treated petroclival meningiomas and indeed found them to be slowly growing tumors. Growth rates were higher among patients with small meningiomas, although the growth index was not significantly correlated with the tumor's diameter or volume at the time of diagnosis. The site of the tumor is important in the decision for intervention. For example, tuberculum sellae meningiomas are known to be associated with visual deterioration within a relatively short time, even when the tumor is less than 2 cm,[5] which justifies resection at their discovery. The surgical removal of a convexity meningioma is associated with minimal risk, which indicates the need to proceed with surgical excision at discovery or whenever the meningioma shows enlargement in young patients **(Fig. 4.1)**. A concern over the probable aggressive nature of falcine meningiomas (particularly in males) is also indicative of early intervention.

The predictive value of a larger tumor size at diagnosis remains controversial.[12,19] Nakamura and associates[3] concluded that the initial tumor size is not a predictive factor

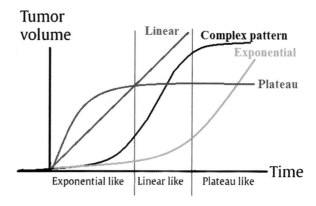

Fig. 4.6 A simple schematic diagram showing the different growth patterns of meningiomas: linear growth (*red line*), plateau (*blue line*), exponential (*green line*), and complex pattern (*black line*). (Adapted from Hashiba T, Hashimoto N, Izumoto S, et al. Serial volumetric assessment of the natural history and growth pattern of incidentally discovered meningiomas. J Neurosurg 2009;110:675-684. Reprinted by permission.)

for tumor growth, but the tumor's size at presentation is considered a risk factor for the development of new symptoms, as meningiomas smaller than 2.5 cm usually remain silent during the next 5 years of follow-up.[12,29]

Calcification may be the most significant predictive factor of slow tumor growth.[5] Many authors have pointed out that meningiomas without calcification on imaging are more likely to progress than are calcified meningiomas.[1,3,18,20,25,26] Herscovici and colleagues[17] found that 10 out of 28 nongrowing tumors had calcification. Thus, calcification allows a more conservative approach[12] **(Fig. 4.4)**. Oya and coworkers[16] analyzed data on 244 patients with 273 conservatively treated tumors; their results suggest that hyperintensity on T2-weighted MRI is associated with a higher rate of tumor growth.

The question is, Why do we not recommend primary radiosurgery for such tumors? In reviewing the literature, we found that the control rate of meningiomas after stereotactic radiosurgery does not look much different from the natural history of untreated IDMs. Moreover, the growth pattern of such meningiomas after failed control with radiosurgery is worse than the natural history of untreated meningiomas.[30] It has been confirmed that the long-term follow-up of radiosurgery shows a continuous decline in control rates over time. A study of the Kaplan-Meier curve provided in the large series of radiosurgery for posterior fossa meningiomas by Starke and associates[31] demonstrates that the control rate is 50% or lower by 15 years. A retrospective study comparing the Sheffield, England, database of radiosurgery-treated patients with national mortality and cancer registries showed an actuarial mortality of 47% at 15 years among patients treated with the gamma knife, with the progression of the meningioma listed as the cause of death in 69% of patients.[32] These results indicate that the effect of radiosurgery at best (the term effect) is *x* number of years of delaying the progression of these meningiomas.

Kondziolka and colleagues[33] have one of the largest series of stereotactic treatment of meningiomas over a period of 20 years. They treated younger patients with minimal symptoms and those who were asymptomatic but decided against observation. Unfortunately, the outcomes in these two groups were not separately identified. In our experience, surgery after failed radiosurgery is not as straightforward as surgery on untreated tumors, but confirmatory reports are not found in the literature. In our practice, surgery after radiation is always associated with a higher risk of complications (especially cranial nerve palsies) and the lower success of tumor resection because of loss of the arachnoidal plane and adhesions to vital structures. So we recommend observing IDMs until they need intervention,

at which point we recommend surgical resection if the patient is in good medical condition and has agreed to surgery after discussing other options.

Conclusion

Based both on an intensive review of the literature and on our own experience, we recommend beginning with conservative management for patients with asymptomatic IDMs, with some exceptions. Because radiosurgery is not without risks (including associated morbidity), and its benefits are time-limited, we are not in favor of the primary treatment of IDMs with radiosurgery when progression has not been documented.

Stereotactic Radiosurgery for Small Meningiomas

Toshinori Hasegawa

Treatment Options

The presented case is that of a 39-year-old woman with headache, indicating an incidentally found small petrous meningioma. The treatment strategy for this case includes three options: wait-and-see, microsurgery, and stereotactic radiosurgery. The aim of treatment is not to eliminate this tumor but to achieve tumor control during her lifetime without any neurologic deficits.

The Wait-and-See Strategy

Because this patient has no neurologic deficit at presentation, the wait-and-see strategy with periodic radiological studies can be a reasonable treatment option. When the tumor shows growth on the follow-up studies or causes neurologic deficits, it should be treated through either a craniotomy or radiosurgery. Jo and colleagues[34] showed that 24 of 77 patients (31.2%) with asymptomatic meningiomas had their tumors progress during a mean follow-up period of 5 years. In their series, the 5-year actuarial tumor progression rate was 38%. Van Havenbergh and colleagues[35] also reported the natural history of 21 patients with petroclival meningiomas, observing that 76% of patients had tumor growth during the follow-up period of 48 to 120 months, and 63% of the growing tumors caused functional deterioration. Considering the patient's age and the natural history of meningiomas, early intervention may be recommended because the risk of morbidity after treatment is considered higher in patients with symptomatic meningiomas than in those with asymptomatic ones. Thus, to avoid morbidity either microsurgery or radiosurgery should be

done before the progressive infiltration of cranial nerves or major vessels.

Microsurgery

Surgical resection is the most common treatment for young patients harboring meningiomas. The recent results of surgical resection have improved with the introduction of microsurgery, refinements in microsurgical techniques, and the use of navigation and monitoring systems, in addition to the development of various neuroimaging modalities, such as MRI, since Simpson[36] published the postoperative recurrence rates of intracranial meningiomas in 1957. Most recently, Sughrue and associates[37] documented the results of 373 patients who underwent initial resection for meningiomas of WHO grade I. With modern microsurgical techniques, the 5-year recurrence and progression-free survival was 95%, 85%, 88%, and 81% for patients achieving Simpson grades I, II, III, and IV resections, respectively, with a median follow-up of 3.7 years. Even patients who underwent Simpson grade I resection by experienced neurosurgeons have a 5-year recurrence risk of 5%. The duration of follow-up is too short to evaluate the true recurrence rate of benign meningiomas in this series, and the recurrence and progression rates are actually predicted to increase over time. The advantage of surgical resection is the ability to confirm the lesion with histological examination.

In recent decades, stereotactic radiosurgery has emerged as a minimally invasive treatment for patients with intracranial lesions. Pollock and colleagues[38] compared the tumor control between surgical resection ($n = 136$) and stereotactic radiosurgery ($n = 62$) in 198 patients with small to medium-

Table 4.2 Characteristics of the 149 Patients Treated with Gamma Knife Radiosurgery at the Author's Institute

Variables	No.	%
Age (years)	Range 15–91	Median 54
Men/women	41:108	28: 72
No. of prior surgeries		
0	70	47
1	52	35
2	16	11
≥ 3	11	7
Follow-up (months)	Range 3–193	Median 126
≥ 5 years	106	74
≥ 10 years	82	57

Table 4.3 Tumor Locations in Patients Treated with Gamma Knife Radiosurgery at the Author's Institute

Location	No.	%
Parasagittal	8	4.9
Falx	9	5.6
Cerebral convexity	9	5.6
Sphenoid ridge	15	9.3
Olfactory groove	2	1.2
Optic sheath	2	1.2
Tuberculum sellae	3	1.9
Lateral ventricle	8	4.9
Third ventricle	1	0.6
Cavernous sinus	29	17.9
Tentorial	13	8.0
Falcotentorial	1	0.6
Cerebellopontine angle	29	17.9
Petroclival	28	17.3
Clivus	4	2.5
Cerebellar convexity	1	0.6
Total	162	100.0

sized benign meningiomas. The progression-free survival after radiosurgery was equivalent to that after Simpson grade I resection, whereas radiosurgery provided higher progression-free survival than Simpson grade II, III, and IV resections. Furthermore, additional treatments were more commonly required in patients who underwent surgical resection. Contrary to the complication rate of 10% in patients treated with radiosurgery, 22% of those who underwent surgical resection developed some kind of complications.

Stereotactic Radiosurgery: Our Experience

Between May 1991 and April 1997, a consecutive 149 patients with meningiomas, excluding atypical or anaplastic meningiomas, were treated with gamma knife radiosurgery (GKRS) at our institute. Of these, nine patients had multiple lesions. A total of 162 lesions were treated. Five patients (five lesions) were lost to follow-up. The patients' characteristics are shown in **Table 4.2**. Seventy patients (47%) underwent GKRS as the initial treatment, and the disease was diagnosed on the basis of neuroimaging findings alone. Tumor locations are shown in **Table 4.3**, and tumor sizes and irradiation doses at the time of treatment are shown in **Table 4.4**. The median follow-up period was 126 months (range 3–193 months). During the follow-up period, 17 patients died—five from meningioma progression, and 12 from other diseases.

The 10-year survival rate to death from a brain tumor after GKRS was 95%. A total of 157 lesions were evaluated with follow-up imaging studies. In-field or out-of-field treatment failure was found in 29 lesions. The actuarial 3-, 5-, and 10-year progression-free survival rates were 96%, 89%, and 77%, respectively. A multivariate analysis of factors affecting progression-free survival showed that infratentorial lesions were successfully treated significantly ($p = 0.045$). Of the 157 lesions, 19 had in-field treatment failure, including two lesions with symptomatic peritumoral edema, indicating that the actuarial 3-, 5-, and 10-year local tumor control rates were 98%, 93%, and 84%, respectively. Five

patients experienced adverse radiation effects, two of whom had severe perifocal edema. Both of them had large supratentorial meningiomas with a tumor volume of 28 cm^3 and 50 cm^3. Other complications included oculomotor palsy in one patient with a cavernous sinus lesion, facial numbness in one with a CPA lesion, and a transient visual defect in one with a cavernous sinus lesion. In our experience, none of 29 patients with CPA meningiomas, like the patient described here, experienced treatment failure. In addition, if the results are limited to those whose tumors were 2 cm or less in mean diameter and who underwent initial treatment, 27 of 28 patients (96%) achieved good tumor control with a median follow-up of 130 months. Only one patient with a cavernous sinus lesion experienced in-field treatment failure at 70 months, requiring a repeated craniotomy and radiosurgery. These results encourage us to use stereotactic radiosurgery as the initial treatment for young patients with incidentally found meningiomas.

Table 4.4 Radiosurgical Techniques Used in Patients Treated with Gamma Knife Radiosurgery at the Author's Institute

Variables	Range	Median
Diameter (mm)	7.8–44.4	24.8
Volume (cm^3)	0.3–50.4	10.4
Max. dose (Gy)	18.6–50.0	29.9
Marg. dose (Gy)	10.0–25.0	14.8
No. of isocenters	1–21	6

Illustrative Case

A 50-year-old woman with left facial numbness underwent partial resection of a petrous tumor diagnosed as a WHO grade I meningioma (**Fig. 4.7a**). GKRS was directed to the residual tumor with maximum and marginal doses of 32 Gy and 16 Gy, respectively. The tumor volume had markedly decreased 15 years after treatment (**Fig. 4.7b**), and the patient did not develop any neurologic deterioration after radiosurgery.

Long-Term Tumor Control

For patients harboring WHO grade I meningiomas, long-term tumor control is essential. So far, numerous investigators have documented the safety and efficacy of radiosurgery for benign meningiomas.[38–47] But there is little information regarding long-term tumor control or late adverse radiation effects such as tumorigenesis more than 20 years after radiosurgery. In other words, it may not be uncommon to develop treatment failure or a secondary neoplasm several decades after treatment. This issue is the reason why radiosurgery for young patients remains controversial. The only way to resolve this issue is to keep following the patients who underwent radiosurgery.

In their large radiosurgical series of 972 patients harboring meningiomas in various locations with a mean follow-up period of 48 months, Kondziolka and associates[43] reported that the actuarial 5- and 10-year tumor control rates were 93% and 87%, respectively. They delivered a mean marginal dose of 14 Gy to the tumors with a mean volume of 7.4 cm³. The overall tumor control rates depended on the confirmed histology of the tumor, with 97% in tumors without previous histological confirmation, 93% in WHO grade I tumors, 50% in grade II tumors, and 17% in grade III tumors. The actuarial tumor control rates past 10 years were 91% and 95% in grade I tumors and in those without previous histological confirmation, respectively. In our experience, 19 patients developed in-field tumor progression 14 to 151 months after GKRS. Two of 82 patients (2.4%) who were followed longer than 10 years had in-field tumor progression, indicating that treatment failure past 10 years is uncommon. In another radiosurgical series of 200 patients harboring skull-base meningiomas, Kreil and associates[44] showed that the actuarial 5- and 10-year tumor control rates were 98.5% and 97%, respectively. Their median marginal dose was 12 Gy and the median tumor volume was 6.5 cm³. As described in our experience, most commonly, patients with skull-base meningiomas achieve higher tumor control rates than those with supratentorial meningiomas when treated with radiosurgery. Conversely, the complete resection of skull-base meningiomas without any morbidity is definitely more difficult than that of supratentorial meningiomas such as convexity or falx lesions. Thus, a higher long-term tumor control rate with radiosurgery is expected with a lower morbidity rate than surgical resection for the illustrative case of the 39-year-old presented at the beginning of this section.

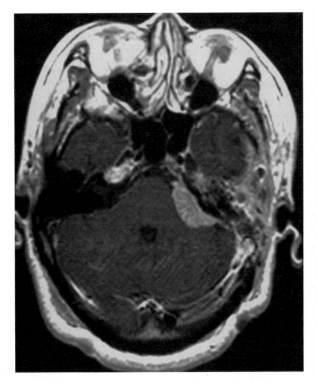
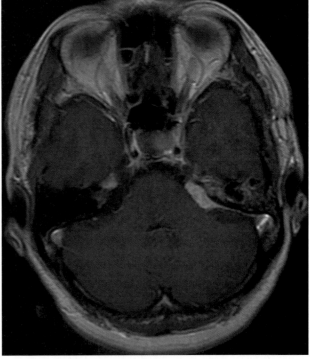

a   b

Fig. 4.7a,b **(a)** T1-weighted image with gadolinium enhancement showing a well-enhanced petrous meningioma at the time of gamma knife radiosurgery. **(b)** T1-weighted image with gadolinium enhancement showing that the tumor had decreased markedly 15 years after treatment.

Adverse Radiation Effects

Functional Outcomes

If a recent, optimum dose of 12 to 14 Gy were delivered to the tumor margin in the 39-year-old patient described in the illustrative case, the risk of neurologic deterioration caused by radiation injury would be extremely low. In our experience of 109 patients with cavernous sinus meningiomas treated at a mean marginal dose of 13 Gy, 4% had neurologic worsening as adverse radiation effects.[40] Similarly, Kreil and associates[44] found a complication rate of 2.5%, of which 2% was transient and 0.5% was persistent, in their series of 200 patients with benign skull-base meningiomas treated with GKRS. According to recent literature,[39–44,46–48] complication rates after radiosurgery for meningiomas ranged from 2.5% to 13%, indicating that such rates seem lower than those after surgical resection.

Radiation-Induced Peritumoral Edema

In cases of large meningiomas, especially with a volume of more than 10 cm³, the possibility of radiation-induced edema should be taken into consideration. Generally, patients with convexity, parasagittal, and falcine meningiomas are more likely to develop radiation-induced peritumoral edema than are those with skull-base tumors.[47] In patients with skull-base meningiomas, this complication is relatively rare as long as the tumors do not severely compress the brainstem, and especially when recent, reduced doses are used. In their series of 179 meningiomas, Chang and associates[48] noted postradiosurgical edema in four of 79 skull-base meningiomas (5%) compared with 26 of 52 hemispheric meningiomas (50%). The development of brain edema is considered to be associated with various factors, such as impairment of the blood–brain barrier, vascular endothelial growth factor affecting vascular permeability, mass effect with brain ischemia, and impaired venous drainage.[42] In particular, the development of peritumoral edema in meningiomas is considered to be strongly related to the pial blood supply.[49,50] Meningiomas with a greater pial blood supply tend to have peritumoral edema because vascular endothelial growth factor is strongly expressed.[50] Accordingly, skull-base meningiomas surrounded by the cistern are less likely to develop radiation-induced edema because of a lesser pial blood supply compared with convexity, parasagittal, or falcine meningiomas.

Radiosurgery-Induced Malignancy

Radiosurgery-induced secondary neoplasms are extremely rare. Rowe and associates[51] evaluated the risk of radiosurgery-induced malignant transformation or secondary neoplasms in their retrospective study of approximately 5,000 patients and 30,000 patient-years of follow-up. They found only one new astrocytoma suspected to be radiosurgery induced. They concluded that there was no evidence of an increased risk of intracranial malignancy compared to that

in the normal population. Kondziolka and colleagues[52] also reported no radiosurgery-induced tumor, with a median follow-up of 10 years, in 285 patients who underwent GKRS for benign intracranial tumors. On the other hand, two reports describe a secondary malignancy after radiosurgery for meningiomas. Yu and colleagues[53] documented a radiosurgery-induced glioblastoma multiforme 7 years after radiosurgery for a convexity meningioma, and Sanno and associates[54] described the development of an osteosarcoma after radiosurgery for a falx meningioma. Considering that 70,000 meningioma patients in the world had been treated with GKRS between 1991 and 2009, however, such an occurrence seems to be extremely rare.

To more correctly predict the risk of radiosurgery-induced malignancy, we assessed a limited number of meningiomas treated at 55 gamma knife units in Japan from 1991 to 2006. Except for patients treated within the past 5 years (to allow for a sufficient latency interval), the estimated risk is 0.011% (1 of 8753 cases). Furthermore, as the literature and our experience shows, a total of seven radiosurgery-induced malignancies have been reported in Japan[55–59] (**Table 4.5**). Seven (0.02%) of 34,201 patients with benign tumors and vascular lesions treated in Japan between 1991 and 2006 developed radiosurgery-induced malignancies during the 20-year GKRS experience. Although these calculations may underestimate the risk because of the possibility of underreporting, such a risk would be much less than 0.1% at worst. Consequently, the risk of a radiosurgery-induced secondary malignancy must be acceptable because such risk is much lower than postoperative mortality rates. Nonetheless, further long-term follow-up data should be collected to justify the use of radiosurgery for benign tumors or vascular lesions, particularly in younger patients with a long life expectancy, because the history of radiosurgery is too short to enable us to reach conclusions about this critical issue.

On the other hand, some patients with treatment failure experience atypical or anaplastic changes despite a previously confirmed benign histological process.[41] It is unclear whether such a malignant change is truly related to radiosurgery, because it is not uncommon for previously resected meningiomas to recur over time with atypical or anaplastic features.[60,61]

Conclusion

In the case of the 39-year-old patient, the choice of treatment between open surgery, radiosurgery, and a wait-and-see strategy depends on the patient's preference. Stereotactic radiosurgery for this incidental, deep-seated meningioma is an acceptable treatment option with a high rate of long-term tumor control as well as a low risk of adverse radiation effects. As this patient is young, however, a complete resection must undoubtedly be the best treatment if there is no risk of postoperative morbidity. Even so, there is no guarantee that complete resection of this tumor is absolutely safe even in the hands of experienced neurosurgeons.

Table 4.5 Radiosurgery-Induced Malignancies in Patients Treated with Gamma Knife Radiosurgery in Japan

Author, Year	Age/Sex	Initial Diagnosis	Prior Surgery	Target Volume (cm³)	Dose (Gy)	Latency Period (Years)	Final Histology
Kaido et al[55] (2001)	14/M	AVM	No	NA	40/20	6.5	GBM
Hanabusa et al[56] (2001)	57/F	VS	Yes	3.4	30/15	0.5	MPNST
Shin et al[57] (2002)	26/F	VS	Yes	NA	34/17	6	MPNST
Sanno et al[54] (2004)	56/F	Meningioma	Yes	NA	60/30	4	Osteosarcoma
Hasegawa et al[58] (2005)	56/F	VS	No	4.0	23/12.7	5	MPNST
Akamatsu et al[59] (2010)	67/F	VS	Yes	5.1	24.4/12	8	MPNST
Personal case	25/F	Acromegaly	Yes	3.7	32/16	14.5	High-grade sarcoma

Abbreviations: AVM, arteriovenous malformation; GBM, glioblastoma multiforme; MPNST, malignant peripheral nerve sheath tumor; NA, not available; VS, vestibular schwannoma.

Similarly, in the treatment choice of radiosurgery, it is possible that the patient may develop adverse radiation effects during her long life span, including cranial nerve impairment such as facial numbness or hearing loss, or a radiosurgery-induced secondary malignancy. Although such a risk would be extremely low, the possibility of long-term adverse radiation effects should be explained to all patients who hope to receive stereotactic radiosurgery for incidentally discovered benign tumors.

The Role of Microsurgery in the Management of Small Skull-Base Meningiomas

Luis A.B. Borba and Daniel D. Cavalcanti

Meningiomas are common intracranial tumors, encountered in 2.3% of autopsy studies,[62] and it has been suggested that 3% of individuals older than 60 years may harbor an asymptomatic meningioma. With improved health and rising longevity, added to the widespread availability of neuroimaging techniques, incidental meningiomas have been diagnosed more often.[3,62] Moreover, the current practice is to diagnose lesions at an initial stage based on subtle symptomatology.[6]

Too much debate has focused on the management of small lesions: Should treatment include observation, resection, or irradiation? Several points should be considered in the decision-making process for patients with small skull-base meningiomas:

1. The natural history of these tumors
2. The patient's clinical status
3. The tumor location and extension
4. The clinical symptoms
5. The radiological findings
6. The potential morbidity related to the therapy to be applied.

The Natural History of Meningiomas

The natural history of a particular intracranial tumor is the single most important variable to be analyzed to safely and ethically indicate either a treatment method or observation. By 1938, Cushing and Eisenhardt[63] had already classified meningiomas as lesions with a progressive growth pattern. Recently, Oya and associates[16] reported a seminal description of the natural history of meningiomas after managing conservatively 244 patients with 273 intracranial meningiomas. They found that 44% of the tumors grew linearly in an average time of 3.8 years. When the growth rate was assessed through volumetric analysis, the number of evolving lesions increased to 74% (114 of 154 tumors). In patients younger than 60 years, the absence of tumor calcification, an initial tumor diameter greater than 25 mm, hyperintensity on T2-weighted MRI studies, and the development of surrounding edema represent significant risk factors for tumor growth and better support a therapeutic option.

In another assessment of natural history, Van Havenbergh and colleagues[19] followed patients with initially untreated petroclival meningiomas; 50% had cranial nerve deficits, and 24% had cerebellar signs or gait disturbances. In about 80% of the patients, the tumor proved to be growing, and all patients with small petroclival tumors (< 2 cm) experienced enlargement in a mean follow-up of 82.2 months. Mean annual growth rates were 1.10 cm^3 in volume and 1.16 mm in diameter. In a series consisting of residual petroclival meningiomas, Jung and colleagues[64] estimated that the annual growth rate was about 5 cm^3 in volume and 0.37 cm in diameter; tumors doubled in size at a mean of 8 years. Age has been shown to significantly impact growth rate. Despite the absence of some of these predicting factors such as edema and a smaller size, as in the case presented in this chapter, we believe that enlargement of the tumor with potentially devastating consequences is just a matter of time, and that the patient should be treated with microsurgery, easing dissection around critical neurovascular structures.

The Patient's Clinical Status

This chapter's case is a 39-year-old healthy woman with a single history of headache, without any neurologic deficit or other symptoms. With the extensive increase in patient longevity, the large number of computed tomography (CT) scans and MRIs ordered to screen patients with headaches, and the assessment of traumatic brain injuries and paranasal sinus disease, asymptomatic meningiomas have been diagnosed more and more often. In these cases, the patient's medical status related to associated conditions must be considered, and sometimes represents the main issue in the decision-making process.

Associated severe comorbidities constitute a contraindication to treating patients with a benign lesion characterized by a potential low growth rate that is sometimes oligosymptomatic. We suggest surgical treatment in the elderly population only for symptomatic patients presenting with a lesion that causes neurologic deficits, who have elevated intracranial pressure (ICP), or who have severe edema related to the tumor mass.

Regarding the case in discussion, the patient's age and the tumor's potential rate of growth are, in our opinion, the main points favoring surgical management.

Tumor Location and Extension

The tumor location and its potential extension affecting surrounding neurovascular structures constitute another strong argument favoring microsurgical treatment. Van Havenbergh and associates[19] showed that, in patients with petroclival meningiomas, up to 50% of initially asymptomatic patients developed some cranial nerve deficit during the follow-up interval of conservative management. The meningioma in question is located on the anterior border of the internal anterior meatus with an extension to the midclivus, a lesion that we name a medial petrosal meningioma (see the figures at the beginning of the chapter).

Despite the intricate location and the well-known low growth rate of meningiomas, we believe that small lesions with little enlargement, many times only perceptible on serial MRI studies, should be approached surgically. For example, an en plaque extension of a small and untreated lesion extending into the internal auditory meatus, jugular foramen, or Dorello's canal can be associated with a high morbidity rate if surgical removal is attempted. Additionally, such potentially slow, asymptomatic growth of meningiomas is the main obstacle related to the impossibility of further radical removal.

This patient, a 39-year-old woman with a long life expectancy, will need surgical removal of that mass at some point in her life. The optimal surgical approach is the retrosigmoid avenue, with the patient placed in the left lateral position. We strongly believe that the better the patient's conditions, the better will be the outcome.

Clinical Symptoms

In the era before CT scans, the patient's symptoms and signs were taken into consideration not only to guide treatment but also as critical tools for diagnosing intracranial tumors. The symptoms in patients with small meningiomas represent a very important issue in their management, but are not the only or the main point to be considered.

Except in skull-base meningiomas affecting cranial nerves or in supratentorial meningiomas that can be diagnosed by the presence of seizures, long-tract deficits, or increased ICP, the great majority of skull-base meningiomas are oligosymptomatic until they reach a large size or affect eloquent neurologic structures. Most importantly, preoperative symptoms are directly related to the surgical outcome.

Radiological Findings

With the advent of MRI, small asymptomatic lesions have been diagnosed, even though large extensions through the dural base of the skull (the "dural tail") have been documented associated with these lesions. It is not uncommon for a dural tail or an en plaque extension of tumor to the skull-base foramina or cavernous sinus to be discovered without any related symptoms.

Today, preoperative MRI studies are crucial not only in the diagnosis and surgical planning but also to aid in determining the prognosis of patients with skull-base meningiomas. In the series of Oya and colleagues,[16] imaging features such as the presence of calcification, hyperintensity on T2-weighted images, surrounding edema, and an initial tumor diameter greater than 25 mm were associated with a higher annual growth.

Potential Morbidity Related to the Therapy

Any surgical decision should balance morbidity and the natural history. The experience of the surgical team is crucial in such decisions. In the beginning of the last century, Horsley[65] already believed that "all tumors which, growing from the meninges, penetrate the brain, or which are encapsulated ... can all be excised with a good permanent result." And Cushing[66] declared that meningiomas are "the most favorable type of tumor for operation."

Evolutions in microsurgical and skull-base techniques associated with improvements in illumination and neuroanesthesia have yielded increasingly better results in the surgery of meningiomas. Nevertheless, a high morbidity in patients with small meningiomas should not be accepted now. Indeed, surgical morbidity should be very small.[67] In this type of case, the most common morbidity is temporary trigeminal nerve dysfunction. Severe morbidity such as facial nerve palsy, hearing loss, or swallowing dysfunction are extremely uncommon, and should be close to 0%. Thus,

series with a 39.9% rate of morbidity related to the surgical resection of tumors in this area should be considered prohibitive.[67–69]

The role of radiosurgery in the treatment of meningiomas has been very well discussed in past years.[70] Starke and colleagues[71] recently reviewed a series of 255 patients with skull-base meningiomas treated with stereotactic radiosurgery. Radiosurgery was the primary treatment in 109 patients and adjuvant in 146 patients. After a median follow-up of 6.5 years (range 2–18 years), 86% of the tumors shrank or had no change in size. Progression-free survival at 3, 5, and 10 years was 99%, 96%, and 79%, respectively. The clinical status at the last follow-up showed no change or improvement in 90%, and clinical deterioration was observed in 10% of patients. Despite these authors' conclusion of high efficacy, radiosurgery has proven to delay tumor growth but does not provide a "cure," that is, complete resolution of the tumor mass.

Illustrative Case

A 44-year-old woman with headaches underwent an MRI after multiple consultations with ophthalmologists, otorhinolaryngologists, and neurologists. The MRI study revealed a small, homogeneously enhancing lesion arising on

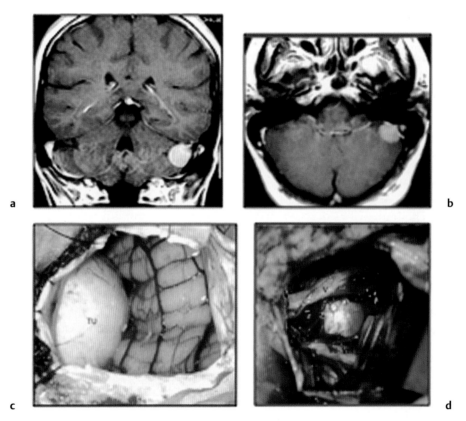

Fig. 4.8a–d (a,b) Contrast-enhanced axial and coronal T1-weighted MRI studies revealing a small posterior petrous meningioma. **(c)** Intraoperative view of an already devascularized round tumor (TU) located on the petrous bone posterior to the internal auditory canal and slightly compressing the cerebellar hemisphere. **(d)** At the end of resection, the trigeminal nerve (V) and facial-vestibulocochlear complex (VII-VIII) are seen dissected free at the cerebellopontine angle.

the right petrous bone posterior to the internal auditory canal, with small mass effect (**Fig. 4.8a,b**). We again stress the early management of these lesions before an en plaque extension develops or the tumor grows into the skull-base foramina.

In this patient, we used a right-sided retrosigmoid approach with facial nerve monitoring. The patient was placed in a left lateral position, an axillary roll was used to protect the brachial plexus, and the left arm was suspended. A semi-curved incision arching posteriorly was made two finger-breadths posterior to the mastoid tip, extending from the superior occipital line to two finger-breadths below the mastoid tip. Fishhooks were used to retract the scalp flap and the muscle layer anteriorly, exposing the intersection of the parietal and occipital bones and the mastoid. A bur hole was made on the parietomastoid suture 1 cm beyond the asterion, reaching the sigmoid-transverse junction. A line at the mastoid was drilled inferiorly starting at the bur hole to expose the posterior aspect of the sigmoid sinus down to the jugular bulb. A craniotomy was done, extending approximately 3 cm medially.

The dura was opened along the edge of the posterior sigmoid sinus wall and the superior edge of the craniotomy (**Fig. 4.8c**). The cisterna magna was opened to ensure the drainage of cerebrospinal fluid and relaxation of the cerebellum, thereby easing dissection. Such dissection should be carried within an arachnoid plane bordering the interface between the tumor and cerebellum. Finally, the tumor insertion on the posterior petrous region was coagulated extensively, devascularizing the lesion. The tumor was progressively dissected free of the cranial nerves and removed en bloc (**Fig. 4.8d**).

Conclusion

Microsurgical resection is the only curative treatment for this particular patient, and in the near future it will be performed. It is just a matter of time.

Moderator
Management of Incidental Meningiomas
E. Antonio Chiocca

The above three sections illustrate and advocate the views of the neurosurgeons Abolfotoh, Al-Mefty, Hasegawa, Borba, and Calvacanti, supported by studies cited in the literature and by extensive personal experience in their three management approaches to incidentally found meningiomas. With the widespread use of CT and MRI, more of these lesions are being discovered, and the patients are being referred to the neurosurgeon for consultation. Patients and their families increasingly use online resources to gather information and frequently come to the neurosurgical consultant with an array of questions and opinions. What is the best course of action?

Abolfotoh and Al-Mefty advocate the "wait-and-see" approach. They exclude meningiomas of the tuberculum sellae from this approach because of the possibility that future small growth could end up rapidly affecting vision irreparably. They base their opinion on a majority of studies showing that the natural history of incidentally discovered meningiomas (IDMs) is generally benign and indolent. This recommendation is definitely applied in older individuals, in those who are medically unstable, or in those who do not desire surgery. The authors describe the dilemma of the younger patient who presents with a IDM because some of the cited studies suggest a less indolent course. But they still advocate conservative management, reserving surgery for proven growth or for symptoms that are directly attrib-

utable to the lesion. The authors' management algorithm thus calls for follow-up scans at 3 and 9 months, followed by yearly MRIs and, after 5 years, MRIs every 2 years. Intervention is reserved for lesions with significant growth or symptoms attributable to the lesion. For lesions with a slow rate of growth, the authors follow with scans every 6 months, and imply that, if growth is documented with multiple successive scans, then they would intervene. Finally, they do not recommend radiosurgery or other radiation treatments, based on the finding that radiated lesions that continue to grow become more difficult to treat surgically.

Hasegawa makes the argument for radiosurgery as a treatment option for the IDM. He is also able to cite literature that shows excellent growth control with minimal morbidity for the IDM, although long-term follow-up periods of more than 20 years are still not available. He summarizes the data for growth control that appears to be as good as a Simpson grade I resection and the data on adverse outcomes (peritumoral edema, progression to anaplasia/malignancy, and radiation-induced damage to normal brain structures) showing a low incidence. He thus provides the argument for offering radiosurgery to the patient with the IDM rather than waiting or resecting.

Borba and Calvacanti instead advocate surgical resection of IDMs. They cite several studies, including Cushing's, in which a large percentage of tumors do indeed grow with time. Thus, they conclude: "Microsurgical resection is the only curative treatment . . . and in the near future it will be performed. It is just a matter of time." They make the compelling argument that the IDM is easily removed with microsurgery and a small craniotomy, and the likelihood of complications is minimal. They do not advocate surgery for a IDM in patients with severe comorbidities or in elderly patients with no or minimal symptoms.

Like most controversies in the management of neurosurgical diseases, we do not have level 1 or 2 evidence to support any one of these three positions. We are thus forced to use subjective experience, the experience of our teachers and colleagues, and the knowledge gained from the multiple retrospective studies published that, like most retrospective studies, may have considerable bias built in. I agree with all five authors that the elderly patient, the patient with significant comorbidities that are likely to lead to operative or perioperative complications, and the patient who has no symptoms or symptoms that he or she does not believe are affecting quality of life should be provided with a strong recommendation for "wait-and-see." I also agree with all five authors that serially growing lesions or lesions that are causing symptoms that compromise the patient's quality of life should be treated.

However, this is not where the controversy lies. The controversy is about the healthy individual with a IDM. In my opinion, this is an area where the opinion of the informed patient and the family should hold considerable weight and sway. Assuming that the neurosurgeon is highly comfortable (and perhaps has even accumulated data from personal practice to back this level of comfort!) with his or her ability to remove the IDM microsurgically or to treat with radiosurgery without disturbing brain function, and with the likelihood that the risk of morbidity would be low, then an informed discussion should be undertaken with the patient that includes the following information:

1. The lesion seen on MRI is most likely a IDM, although there is a rare possibility that other lesions could mimic it (lymphoma, metastatic tumor, solitary fibrous tumor).
2. Small incidental meningiomas are indolent or grow slowly, and the large majority of patients are followed conservatively.
3. Microsurgery and radiosurgery are two options for treatment. In both options and in experienced hands, the risk of complications is minimal but is not zero.

Based on this information, the neurosurgeon, the patient, and the family should agree on a plan of action: wait-and-see, surgery now, or radiosurgery now. In my practice, I tend to suggest the wait-and-see approach, and my impression is that the large majority of patients are highly comfortable with this. However, I remain open to the opinion, body language, gestures, and comfort level of the patient and family regarding the wait-and-see approach. I have encountered several patients who are concerned that the IDM may actually be a more serious lesion and do not wish to wait for the 3-month successive scan, as advocated by Abolfotoh and Al-Mefty, or are unlikely to comply with the practice of serial MRIs, or who cannot psychologically handle the knowledge that the presumed IDM may grow at a future date and that they may not be ready for treatment at that time. In these instances, I am comfortable with the decision to proceed with microsurgery or radiosurgery based on the knowledge that risks are minimal.

In conclusion, this is an area of controversy for which a prospective clinical trial comparing wait-and-see with treatment may be of benefit. This trial may also provide a socioeconomic benefit to society. It would provide data to show whether a lifelong course of serial imaging is more cost-effective than treatment followed by a shortened time frame or not-as-frequent period of serial imaging to ensure that the tumor does not recur.

References

1. Hashiba T, Hashimoto N, Izumoto S, et al. Serial volumetric assessment of the natural history and growth pattern of incidentally discovered meningiomas. J Neurosurg 2009;110:675–684
2. Firsching RP, Fischer A, Peters R, Thun F, Klug N. Growth rate of incidental meningiomas. J Neurosurg 1990;73:545–547
3. Nakamura M, Roser F, Michel J, Jacobs C, Samii M. The natural history of incidental meningiomas. Neurosurgery 2003;53:62–70, discussion 70–71
4. Olivero WC, Lister JR, Elwood PW. The natural history and growth rate of asymptomatic meningiomas: a review of 60 patients. J Neurosurg 1995;83:222–224
5. Yano S, Kuratsu JI. Natural course of untreated meningiomas. In: DeMonte F, McDermott MW, Al-Mefty O, eds. Al-Mefty's Meningiomas, 2nd ed. New York: Thieme, 2011:63–67
6. Chamoun R, Krisht KM, Couldwell WT. Incidental meningiomas. Neurosurg Focus 2011;31:E19
7. Samii M, Gerganov VM. Cerebellopontine angle meningiomas. In: DeMonte F, McDermott MW, Al-Mefty O, eds. Al-Mefty's Meningiomas, 2nd ed. New York: Thieme, 2011:262–269
8. Bacciu A, Piazza P, Di Lella F, Sanna M. Intracanalicular meningioma: clinical features, radiologic findings, and surgical management. Otol Neurotol 2007;28:391–399
9. Kunii N, Ota T, Kin T, et al. Angiographic classification of tumor attachment of meningiomas at the cerebellopontine angle. World Neurosurg 2011;75:114–121
10. Schaller B, Merlo A, Gratzl O, Probst R; Two Distinct Clinical Entities. Premeatal and retromeatal cerebellopontine angle meningioma. Two distinct clinical entities. Acta Neurochir (Wien) 1999;141:465–471
11. Nakamura M, Roser F, Dormiani M, Matthies C, Vorkapic P, Samii M. Facial and cochlear nerve function after surgery of cerebellopontine angle meningiomas. Neurosurgery 2005;57:77–90, discussion 77–90
12. Rubin G, Herscovici Z, Laviv Y, Jackson S, Rappaport ZH. Outcome of untreated meningiomas. Isr Med Assoc J 2011;13:157–160
13. Hashimoto N, Rabo CS, Okita Y, et al. Slower growth of skull base meningiomas compared with non-skull base meningio-

mas based on volumetric and biological studies. J Neurosurg 2012;116:574–580

14. Sade B, Chahlavi A, Krishnaney A, Nagel S, Choi E, Lee JH. World Health Organization grades II and III meningiomas are rare in the cranial base and spine. Neurosurgery 2007;61:1194–1198, discussion 1198

15. Bindal R, Goodman JM, Kawasaki A, Purvin V, Kuzma B. The natural history of untreated skull base meningiomas. Surg Neurol 2003;59:87–92, discussion 92

16. Oya S, Kim SH, Sade B, Lee JH. The natural history of intracranial meningiomas. J Neurosurg 2011;114:1250–1256

17. Herscovici Z, Rappaport Z, Sulkes J, Danaila L, Rubin G. Natural history of conservatively treated meningiomas. Neurology 2004; 63:1133–1134

18. Niiro M, Yatsushiro K, Nakamura K, Kawahara Y, Kuratsu J. Natural history of elderly patients with asymptomatic meningiomas. J Neurol Neurosurg Psychiatry 2000;68:25–28

19. Van Havenbergh T, Carvalho G, Tatagiba M, Plets C, Samii M. Natural history of petroclival meningiomas. Neurosurgery 2003; 52:55–62, discussion 62–64

20. Go RS, Taylor BV, Kimmel DW. The natural history of asymptomatic meningiomas in Olmsted County, Minnesota. Neurology 1998;51:1718–1720

21. Yoneoka Y, Fujii Y, Tanaka R. Growth of incidental meningiomas. Acta Neurochir (Wien) 2000;142:507–511

22. Zeidman LA, Ankenbrandt WJ, Du H, Paleologos N, Vick NA. Growth rate of non-operated meningiomas. J Neurol 2008; 255:891–895

23. Oya S, Sade B, Lee JH. Benefits and limitations of diameter measurement in the conservative management of meningiomas. Surg Neurol Int 2011;2:158

24. Awad IA, Kalfas I, Hahn JF, Little JR. Intracranial meningiomas in the aged: surgical outcome in the era of computed tomography. Neurosurgery 1989;24:557–560

25. Yano S, Kuratsu J; Kumamoto Brain Tumor Research Group. Indications for surgery in patients with asymptomatic meningiomas based on an extensive experience. J Neurosurg 2006; 105:538–543

26. Nakasu S, Fukami T, Nakajima M, Watanabe K, Ichikawa M, Matsuda M. Growth pattern changes of meningiomas: long-term analysis. Neurosurgery 2005;56:946–955, discussion 946–955

27. Braunstein JB, Vick NA. Meningiomas: the decision not to operate. Neurology 1997;48:1459–1462

28. Kuratsu J, Kochi M, Ushio Y. Incidence and clinical features of asymptomatic meningiomas. J Neurosurg 2000;92:766–770

29. Sughrue ME, Rutkowski MJ, Aranda D, Barani IJ, McDermott MW, Parsa AT. Treatment decision making based on the published natural history and growth rate of small meningiomas. J Neurosurg 2010;113:1036–1042

30. Couldwell WT, Cole CD, Al-Mefty O. Patterns of skull base meningioma progression after failed radiosurgery. J Neurosurg 2007;106:30–35

31. Starke RM, Nguyen JH, Rainey J, et al. Gamma knife surgery of meningiomas located in the posterior fossa: factors predictive of outcome and remission. J Neurosurg 2011;114:1399–1409

32. Rowe J, Grainger A, Walton L, Silcocks P, Radatz M, Kemeny A. Risk of malignancy after gamma knife stereotactic radiosurgery. Neurosurgery 2007;60:60–65, discussion 65–66

33. Kondziolka D, Mathieu D, Madhok R, Flickinger JC, Lunsford LD. Stereotactic radiosurgery for meningiomas. In: Lunsford LD,

Sheehan JP, eds. Intracranial Stereotactic Radiosurgery. New York: Thieme, 2009:58–62

34. Jo KW, Kim CH, Kong DS, et al. Treatment modalities and outcomes for asymptomatic meningiomas. Acta Neurochir (Wien) 2011;153:62–67, discussion 67

35. Van Havenbergh T, Carvalho G, Tatagiba M, Plets C, Samii M. Natural history of petroclival meningiomas. Neurosurgery 2003; 52:55–62, discussion 62–64

36. Simpson D. The recurrence of intracranial meningiomas after surgical treatment. J Neurol Neurosurg Psychiatry 1957;20: 22–39

37. Sughrue ME, Kane AJ, Shangari G, et al. The relevance of Simpson grade I and II resection in modern neurosurgical treatment of World Health Organization Grade I meningiomas. J Neurosurg 2010;113:1029–1035

38. Pollock BE, Stafford SL, Utter A, Giannini C, Schreiner SA. Stereotactic radiosurgery provides equivalent tumor control to Simpson grade 1 resection for patients with small- to medium-size meningiomas. Int J Radiat Oncol Biol Phys 2003;55: 1000–1005

39. DiBiase SJ, Kwok Y, Yovino S, et al. Factors predicting local tumor control after gamma knife stereotactic radiosurgery for benign intracranial meningiomas. Int J Radiat Oncol Biol Phys 2004;60:1515–1519

40. Hasegawa T, Kida Y, Yoshimoto M, Koike J, Iizuka H, Ishii D. Long-term outcomes of gamma knife surgery for cavernous sinus meningioma. J Neurosurg 2007;107:745–751

41. Iwai Y, Yamanaka K, Ikeda H. Gamma knife radiosurgery for skull base meningioma: long-term results of low-dose treatment. J Neurosurg 2008;109:804–810

42. Kollová A, Liscák R, Novotný J Jr, Vladyka V, Simonová G, Janousková L. Gamma knife surgery for benign meningioma. J Neurosurg 2007;107:325–336

43. Kondziolka D, Mathieu D, Lunsford LD, et al. Radiosurgery as definitive management of intracranial meningiomas. Neurosurgery 2008;62:53–58, discussion 58–60

44. Kreil W, Luggin J, Fuchs I, Weigl V, Eustacchio S, Papaefthymiou G. Long term experience of gamma knife radiosurgery for benign skull base meningiomas. J Neurol Neurosurg Psychiatry 2005;76:1425–1430

45. Sheehan JP, Williams BJ, Yen CP. Stereotactic radiosurgery for WHO grade I meningiomas. J Neurooncol 2010;99:407–416

46. Stafford SL, Pollock BE, Foote RL, et al. Meningioma radiosurgery: tumor control, outcomes, and complications among 190 consecutive patients. Neurosurgery 2001;49:1029–1037, discussion 1037–1038

47. Hasegawa T, Kida Y, Yoshimoto M, Iizuka H, Ishii D, Yoshida K. Gamma knife surgery for convexity, parasagittal, and falcine meningiomas. J Neurosurg 2011;114:1392–1398

48. Chang JH, Chang JW, Choi JY, Park YG, Chung SS. Complications after gamma knife radiosurgery for benign meningiomas. J Neurol Neurosurg Psychiatry 2003;74:226–230

49. Bitzer M, Wöckel L, Luft AR, et al. The importance of pial blood supply to the development of peritumoral brain edema in meningiomas. J Neurosurg 1997;87:368–373

50. Yoshioka H, Hama S, Taniguchi E, Sugiyama K, Arita K, Kurisu K. Peritumoral brain edema associated with meningioma: influence of vascular endothelial growth factor expression and vascular blood supply. Cancer 1999;85:936–944

51. Rowe J, Grainger A, Walton L, Silcocks P, Radatz M, Kemeny A. Risk of malignancy after gamma knife stereotactic radiosurgery. Neurosurgery 2007;60:60–65, discussion 65–66

52. Kondziolka D, Nathoo N, Flickinger JC, Niranjan A, Maitz AH, Lunsford LD. Long-term results after radiosurgery for benign intracranial tumors. Neurosurgery 2003;53:815–821, discussion 821–822

53. Yu JS, Yong WH, Wilson D, Black KL. Glioblastoma induction after radiosurgery for meningioma. Lancet 2000;356:1576–1577

54. Sanno N, Hayashi S, Shimura T, Maeda S, Teramoto A. Intracranial osteosarcoma after radiosurgery—case report. Neurol Med Chir (Tokyo) 2004;44:29–32

55. Kaido T, Hoshida T, Uranishi R, et al. Radiosurgery-induced brain tumor. Case report. J Neurosurg 2001;95:710–713

56. Hanabusa K, Morikawa A, Murata T, Taki W. Acoustic neuroma with malignant transformation. Case report. J Neurosurg 2001; 95:518–521

57. Shin M, Ueki K, Kurita H, Kirino T. Malignant transformation of a vestibular schwannoma after gamma knife radiosurgery. Lancet 2002;360:309–310

58. Hasegawa T, Fujitani S, Katsumata S, Kida Y, Yoshimoto M, Koike J. Stereotactic radiosurgery for vestibular schwannomas: analysis of 317 patients followed more than 5 years. Neurosurgery 2005;57:257–265, discussion 257–265

59. Akamatsu Y, Murakami K, Watanabe M, Jokura H, Tominaga T. Malignant peripheral nerve sheath tumor arising from benign vestibular schwannoma treated by gamma knife radiosurgery after two previous surgeries: a case report with surgical and pathological observations. World Neurosurg 2010;73:751–754

60. Jääskeläinen J, Haltia M, Laasonen E, Wahlström T, Valtonen S. The growth rate of intracranial meningiomas and its relation to histology. An analysis of 43 patients. Surg Neurol 1985;24:165–172

61. Al-Mefty O, Kadri PAS, Pravdenkova S, Sawyer JR, Stangeby C, Husain M. Malignant progression in meningioma: documentation of a series and analysis of cytogenetic findings. J Neurosurg 2004;101:210–218

62. Nakasu S, Hirano A, Shimura T, Llena JF. Incidental meningiomas in autopsy study. Surg Neurol 1987;27:319–322

63. Cushing HW, Eisenhardt L. Meningiomas: Their Classification, Regional Behaviour, Life History and Surgical End Results. Springfield, IL: Charles C. Thomas, 1938

64. Jung HW, Yoo H, Paek SH, Choi KS. Long-term outcome and growth rate of subtotally resected petroclival meningiomas: experience with 38 cases. Neurosurgery 2000;46:567–574, discussion 574–575

65. Horsley V. On the technique of operations on the central nervous system. BMJ 1906;2:411–423

66. Cushing HW. Surgery of the head. In: Keen WW, ed. Surgery: Its Principles and Practice. Philadelphia: WB Saunders, 1908: 17–276

67. Ramina R, Neto MC, Fernandes YB, Silva EB, Mattei TA, Aguiar PH. Surgical removal of small petroclival meningiomas. Acta Neurochir (Wien) 2008;150:431–438, discussion 438–439

68. Reinert M, Babey M, Curschmann J, Vajtai I, Seiler RW, Mariani L. Morbidity in 201 patients with small sized meningioma treated by microsurgery. Acta Neurochir (Wien) 2006;148: 1257–1265, discussion 1266

69. Strang RD, al-Mefty O. Small skull base meningiomas. Surgical management. Clin Neurosurg 2001;48:320–339

70. Subach BR, Lunsford LD, Kondziolka D, Maitz AH, Flickinger JC. Management of petroclival meningiomas by stereotactic radiosurgery. Neurosurgery 1998;42:437–443, discussion 443–445

71. Starke RM, Williams BJ, Hiles C, Nguyen JH, Elsharkawy MY, Sheehan JP. Gamma knife surgery for skull base meningiomas. J Neurosurg 2012;116:588–597

Management of a Vestibular Schwannoma in a Single Hearing Ear of a Patient with Neurofibromatosis Type 2

Case

A 45-year-old woman with neurofibromatosis type 2 previously underwent resection of a right giant acoustic tumor and is deaf in the right ear. In the left ear, she currently has serviceable hearing with 75% discrimination at 30 dB.

Participants

Microsurgical Removal of Acoustic Tumors in a Single Hearing Ear of Patients with Neurofibromatosis Type 2: Madjid Samii and Venelin M. Gerganov

Stereotactic Radiosurgery for an Acoustic Neuroma in the Only Hearing Ear: Michael J. Link, Colin L.W. Driscoll, and Bruce E. Pollock

Conservative Treatment of Acoustic Tumors in Patients with a Single Hearing Ear: Donlin M. Long

Moderator: Preserving Hearing in the Last Hearing Ear of Patients with Neurofibromatosis Type 2: Stephen J. Haines

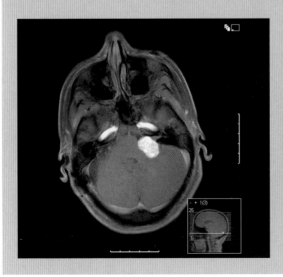
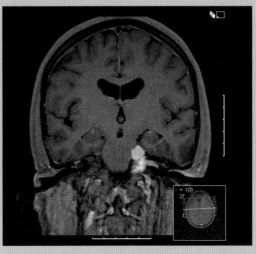

Microsurgical Removal of Acoustic Tumors in a Single Hearing Ear of Patients with Neurofibromatosis Type 2

Madjid Samii and Venelin M. Gerganov

The treatment of patients with neurofibromatosis type 2 (NF2) represents one of the most difficult challenges in neurosurgery. The patient's lifelong propensity to develop new tumors in the central nervous system predetermines the impossibility of definitive cure for these patients.[1] Treatment is focused on prolonging life, preserving or restoring neurologic function, and maintaining the patient's quality of life.[2–4] Vestibular schwannomas associated with NF2 differ in several ways from sporadic unilateral tumors, and the major concerns are the disabling consequences of acquired deafness.

In the presented case, the giant vestibular schwannoma on the right side was initially removed. The patient has useful hearing on the left side and a tumor in the left cerebellopontine angle with the characteristics of a vestibular schwannoma. The lesion is centered in the internal auditory canal and forms an acute angle with the posterior surface of the petrous bone. It extends into the internal auditory canal and shows homogeneous contrast enhancement. The sagittal image shows that the tumor has a significant caudal extension, which has been correlated with a worse outcome regarding at least the facial nerve function.[5]

In such cases, optimal results are obtained if the treatment is individualized and guided by the attitude and expectations of patients and their families. Decision making depends on several factors related to the tumor and to the clinical and psychological condition of the patient. The options are initial observation or early active treatment. Close collaboration with patients and their families is essential. The major issue is whether the patient is willing to take the risk of complete hearing loss from early active treatment or prefers to postpone treatment until hearing is lost through progression of the disease.

The possibility of preserving hearing depends on the size of the tumor, the patient's preoperative hearing level, and the quality of the brainstem auditory evoked potentials (BAEPs). With regard to the first two factors in the current case, the chance of preserving functional hearing is approximately 50%. But there is no information about the quality of BAEP, an examination we perform routinely. During surgery, BAEP monitoring provides essential feedback about the function of hearing pathways every 30 to 90 seconds.[6,7] Changes from traction or injury of the cochlear nerve and the interruption of vascular supply or compression of the brainstem are readily detected. A loss of wave V is most frequently associated with deafness, either temporary or permanent, but this loss is usually preceded by changes in waves I and III. This information enables the surgeon to modify the approach accordingly, for example, the degree of cerebellar retraction. When surgery is done on the only hearing side, the operation may even be interrupted. If the BAEP is of low quality, with loss of waves or considerable prolongation of intervals, this feedback is not available. In such a case, we would not recommend early surgery.

Once the decision for active treatment is made and a good BAEP wave form is available, the next task is to choose the best treatment option: surgery or radiosurgery. Our experience has shown that surgery of vestibular schwannomas via the retrosigmoid approach leads to the best outcome, especially with respect to hearing.[7] The advantages of this approach have been described in multiple publications.[8–10] Placing the patient in the semi-sitting position allows the surgeon to use both hands for tumor dissection because there is no need for constant suction. The assistant irrigates continuously with saline, which obviates the need to coagulate during tumor removal.

To preserve hearing, the structures of the inner ear must be preserved during drilling of the internal auditory canal. A careful study of thin-slice bone-window computed tomography scans of the pyramid before surgery allows the surgeon to plan the extent of safe bone removal. If the location of the inner ear precludes wide opening of the internal auditory canal, an angled endoscope can be used to inspect the most lateral portion of the canal.

Another critical issue is the dissection technique. The nerve should always be dissected from the tumor in the arachnoid plane, and dissection begins only after sufficient debulking of the tumor mass. The stretching of neural structures in one direction for a long time should be avoided. These steps should be constantly related to the BAEP input and modified accordingly. If the patient is in the semi-sitting position, coagulation is required only in cases of major bleeding.[8]

Vestibular schwannomas associated with NF2 differ from sporadic vestibular schwannomas and are more challenging for the surgeon.[11,12] Approximately 40% of them are multilobular, and the nerves and vessels may pass between the tumor lobules. The tumor can infiltrate the fibers of individual nerves, a phenomenon seldom found in unilateral tumors. In these cases, subtotal tumor removal may be done to prevent functional deficits.

When the BAEPs are unstable and even slight microsurgical maneuvers are followed by severe deterioration of the waveform, attempting complete tumor removal may endanger the patient's hearing. In this case, the surgeon may choose partial tumor removal and decompression of the cochlear nerve in the internal auditory canal during surgery. The senior author (M.S.) used this strategy in 23 patients, which led to long-term preservation of hearing in 15 of them.[3]

If the patient decides against surgery, the tumor should be followed and removed when hearing loss occurs or tumor progression leads to serious neurologic symptoms. For such patients, the surgeon should plan to restore hearing with an auditory implant during the same surgery or several weeks later. Such central auditory prostheses—the auditory brainstem implants, or, more recently, the auditory midbrain implants—help patients receive environmental sounds and enhance their lip-reading ability for better communication.[13–16]

Radiotherapy is another treatment option for the patient presented here. Published series show that it leads to tumor control in up to 81% of patients at 10 years.[17,18] The rate of hearing preservation is 33 to 43%, although some deterioration occurs during the ensuing years. In a recent study, Phi and colleagues[19] have shown that the rates of actual serviceable hearing preservation fall from 50% in the first year to 45% in the second year and to 33% in the fifth year. Postirradiation edema may lead to a transient increase in the tumor volume. When tumors compress the brainstem, as in the presented case, this possibility and the related risks should also be considered. In pa-

tients with vestibular schwannomas associated with NF2 on the only hearing side, an additional advantage of surgery compared with radiosurgery is the possibility of interrupting tumor removal if the BAEP changes and, thus, preserving the available hearing. In our experience, radiosurgery is best reserved for patients who have particularly aggressive tumors, those with medical contraindications for microsurgery, patients who refuse surgery, and the elderly.[3,4,11]

Over the past 35 years, the senior author (M.S.) has operated on more than 175 patients with NF2; the total number of vestibular schwannoma surgeries in these patients was 225. Total removal was achieved in 86% of the operated tumors. In the remaining 14%, total removal was impossible because of infiltration of the nerves or the risk of functional loss. Hearing was preserved in 65% of patients with useful preoperative hearing. In patients with vestibular schwannomas of a size similar to the one presented here, the cochlear preservation rate was 82% and the hearing preservation rate was 52%.

Stereotactic Radiosurgery for an Acoustic Neuroma in the Only Hearing Ear

Michael J. Link, Colin L.W. Driscoll, and Bruce E. Pollock

Under consideration is the case of a 45-year-old woman with NF2 who has previously undergone successful resection of a giant right acoustic neuroma and who has no hearing in that ear. As shown by the single axial and coronal images available, she has a left acoustic neuroma of 2.5 cm (the greatest posterior fossa diameter measured parallel to the petrous temporal bone). She is reported as having a speech discrimination score of 75% at 30 dB on the left. Thus, she likely has American Academy of Otolaryngology–Head and Neck Surgery (AAO-HNS) class A hearing in only her left ear.[20] Following the guiding principles for NF2 patients of preserving the quality of life and conserving or rehabilitating function, especially hearing, we discuss our approach to similar patients and the advisability of stereotactic radiosurgery (SRS) to treat her left acoustic neuroma.

In general, intervention for a lesion involving the only hearing ear can be considered in the following circumstances:

1. The predicted natural history of the disease is relatively rapid loss of the remaining hearing.
2. Substantial or life-threatening brainstem compression has developed.
3. Intervention may improve hearing or carries a relatively low risk of hearing loss.[21]

But none of these criteria apply to this patient at this time.

We would have placed an auditory brainstem implant on the right side when the giant right acoustic neuroma was removed, assuming that the tumor was so large there was no hope of preserving the cochlear nerve to allow placement of a cochlear implant. We would then follow the left acoustic neuroma in the only hearing ear with biannual magnetic resonance imaging (MRI) and audiology examinations, and intervene if hearing progressively deteriorates or the tumor shows sustained growth.

Lars Leksell[22] is deservedly credited with introducing SRS in 1951, and the first published report of SRS to treat an acoustic neuroma appeared in 1971.[23] Thus, we have had over 40 years to evaluate the potential, efficacy, and complications of this modality, and the technique and dose-planning software have changed dramatically during this time. In the last 15 to 18 years in particular, tumor marginal doses have been reduced to attempt to preserve cranial nerve function without sacrificing tumor control. In addition, the availability of high-resolution, multiplanar, thin-slice MRI scanning to assist in planning has resulted in more conformal treatment plans. Tumor control rates of 93 to 98% and hearing preservation rates of 33 to 78% have been reported with SRS for sporadic vestibular schwan-

Table 5.1 Published Experience of Gamma Knife Radiosurgery to Treat Vestibular Schwannoma in Patients with Neurofibromatosis Type 2

Institution or City	No. of Tumors	Mean Follow-Up (Mos.)	Margin Dose (Gy)	Tumor Control (%)	Hearing Preservation (%)	VII Weakness (%)
Marseille[33]	35	32	13	74	57	3
Komaki[37]	20	34	13	100	33	0
Pittsburgh[17]	74	53	14	85/81[a]	42	8
Sheffield[35]	92	NA	13.4	79/52[b]	38	5
Wake Forest[36]	12	48	12	92/75[c]	50	33
Seoul[19]	36	36.5	12.1	66[d]	33[d]	3

Abbreviation: NA, not available.

[a]Actuarial local control rates at 5 (85%) and 15 years (81%), respectively, with tumor control defined as a lack of the need for an additional intervention.

[b]Kaplan-Meier control rates at 8 years depending on whether control is defined as the lack of a need for additional intervention (79%) versus any sustained symptomatic growth (52%).

[c]Local control (92%) with one tumor failing and also calculated 5-year progression-free survival (75%).

[d]5-year actuarial rates for tumor control and hearing preservation.

nomas in many large, recently published series.[24-30] A comprehensive review of the literature published in 2009, encompassing 5,825 patients in 74 publications, reported an overall hearing preservation rate of 57% after SRS for vestibular schwannoma.[31] In this review, a marginal dose of less than 12.5 Gy was the only statistically significant factor for preserving hearing. Neither the patient's age nor the tumor size was significant. Several groups have found that a maximum dose of less than 4 or 4.2 Gy to the cochlea is associated with better hearing preservation rates after SRS or fractionated radiotherapy,[25,26,28,32] whereas at least one group has reported the dose to the cochlear nucleus to be the important prognostic variable.[29]

Although these data seem encouraging, there is much concern that vestibular schwannomas in patients with NF2 do not respond as well as sporadic vestibular schwannomas to SRS.[33,34] There are significantly fewer reports in the literature regarding the use of SRS to treat vestibular schwannomas associated with NF2[17,19,33-37] (**Table 5.1**). The largest and most recently reported experience is from Sheffield, England.[35] In this study, Rowe and colleagues report on their results in 92 tumors using current techniques (MRI localization) and doses (mean marginal dose of 13.4 Gy). The mean age of the patient at treatment was 29 years. Based on a Kaplan-Meier plot, if failure is defined as the need for an additional procedure, 79% of tumors were successfully controlled at 8 years. However, if a stricter definition of failure is defined as any progressive growth with increasing symptoms possibly attributed to a growing vestibular schwannoma, the control rate falls to 52% at 8 years.[35] The tumor volume at the time of treatment was the most significant determinant of failure ($p < 0.001$), with tumors larger than 10 cm³ correlating to a statistically higher likelihood of failure. Overall, 23 of 61 patients (38%) who had serviceable hearing before treatment maintained their hear-

ing grade, whereas 42% had some deterioration of their hearing, and 20% became completely deaf. Permanent facial weakness occurred in 5% of patients, and 2% developed permanent trigeminal dysfunction related to the SRS.[35]

Our results at the Mayo Clinic are similar. We treated 29 vestibular schwannomas in 24 patients with NF2 between 1999 and 2007. At a median follow-up of just over 3 years, 20 tumors have remained stable or decreased in volume at the last MRI follow-up, four tumors have shown progressive enlargement at more than one imaging follow-up, and no imaging follow-up could be obtained for five tumors. Depending on the outcome of these last five tumors, we would classify our tumor control rate as 69 to 86%. The affected ear in 15 patients had measurable hearing before SRS and 14 patients were profoundly deaf in the affected ear. Six maintained their pretreatment hearing, seven progressed to class D hearing, and no audiometry follow-up could be obtained for two. Thus, our hearing preservation rate is 46%.

Based on our experience and that reported in the literature, we would counsel the patient presented here that, if she elects to have SRS to treat the 2.5-cm vestibular schwannoma in her only hearing ear, there is an 80% chance that she will not require another intervention for that tumor 5 years after treatment. Furthermore, there is a 40% chance of maintaining useful hearing in that ear and a less than 5% risk of any permanent facial weakness or numbness.

Stereotactic radiosurgery also offers another potential significant advantage to this patient. If she does lose hearing after treatment, there is still a very high chance that her hearing could be rehabilitated with a cochlear implant.[38] We have implanted this device in three patients with NF2 after SRS for a vestibular schwannoma. The mean age of these patients was 68 years, and they had been profoundly deaf in the affected ear for 1 to 10 years before the cochlear

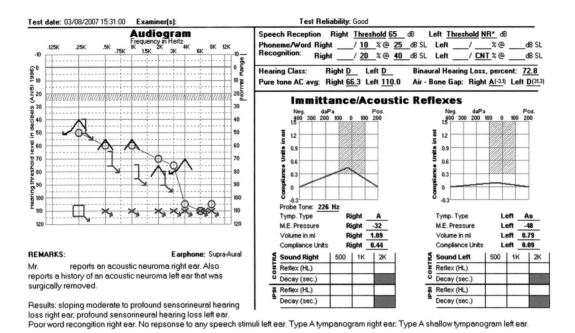

Test date: 03/08/2007 15:31:00   Examiner(s):

Test Reliability: Good

Audiogram
Frequency in Hertz

REMARKS: Earphone: Supra-Aural

Mr. _____ reports an acoustic neuroma right ear. Also reports a history of an acoustic neuroma left ear that was surgically removed.

Results: sloping moderate to profound sensorineural hearing loss right ear; profound sensorineural hearing loss left ear.
Poor word recongition right ear. No repsonse to any speech stimuli left ear. Type A tympanogram right ear; Type A shallow tympanogram left ear.

Speech Reception   Right   Threshold <u>65</u>   dB   Left   Threshold <u>NR*</u> dB
Phoneme/Word Right ____ / <u>10</u> % @ <u>25</u> dB SL   Left ____ / ____ % @ ____ dB SL
Recognition: Right ____ / <u>20</u> % @ <u>40</u> dB SL   Left ____ / <u>CNT</u> % @ ____ dB SL

Hearing Class: Right <u>D</u>   Left <u>D</u>   Binaural Hearing Loss, percent: <u>72.8</u>
Pure tone AC avg: Right <u>66.3</u> Left <u>110.0</u>   Air - Bone Gap: Right <u>A</u>(-3.1) Left <u>D</u>(31.3)

Immittance/Acoustic Reflexes

Probe Tone: **226 Hz**

Tymp. Type	Right	**A**
M.E. Pressure	Right	**-32**
Volume in ml	Right	**1.09**
Compliance Units	Right	**0.44**

Tymp. Type	Left	**As**
M.E. Pressure	Left	**-48**
Volume in ml	Left	**0.79**
Compliance Units	Left	**0.09**

	Sound Right	500	1K	2K
CONTRA	Reflex (HL)			
	Decay (sec.)			
IPSI	Reflex (HL)			
	Decay (sec.)			

	Sound Left	500	1K	2K
CONTRA	Reflex (HL)			
	Decay (sec.)			
IPSI	Reflex (HL)			
	Decay (sec.)			

Fig. 5.1 The pretreatment audiogram reveals profound left-sided hearing loss after a prior translabyrinthine removal of a left vestibular schwannoma. There is also severe right-sided hearing loss with a pure tone average of 65 dB. The patient's word recognition score was 20% at 40 dB.

implant. The mean tumor volume treated was 1 cm³. All patients experienced a significant restoration of hearing after receiving the cochlear implant.

For example, a 64-year-old man had previously undergone translabyrinthine resection of a left vestibular schwannoma in 1989 without complication. He then began to develop significant right-sided hearing loss 10 years later, and by 2007 he had a pure tone average of 65 dB and only 10 to 20% word recognition in the right ear (**Fig. 5.1**). His MRI showed a 1.1-cm right vestibular schwannoma and postoperative changes from his left-sided surgery (**Fig. 5.2**). At the last follow-up, 2 years after undergoing SRS and receiving a cochlear implant, his tumor had decreased to 0.8 cm in the posterior fossa diameter (**Fig. 5.3**), and his cochlear implant was working very well. He was achieving 85 to 87% on the hearing-in-noise test (HINT), which uses

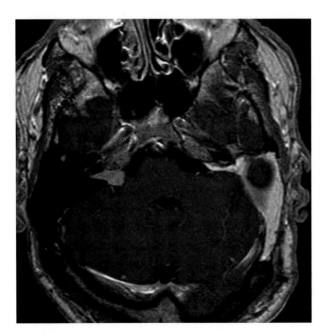

Fig. 5.2 The pretreatment magnetic resonance imaging shows postoperative fat packing from a prior left translabyrinthine surgery and a 1.1-cm right vestibular schwannoma.

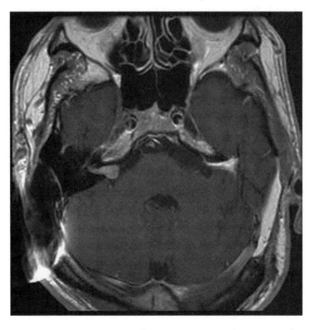

Fig. 5.3 An MRI 2 years after stereotactic radiosurgery. The tumor has decreased in size by 2 mm in the largest posterior fossa diameter.

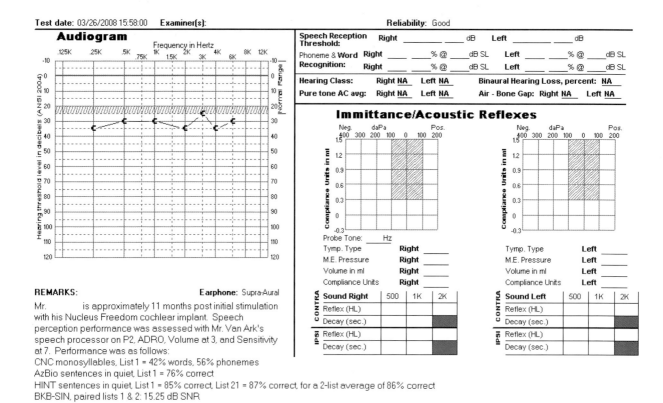

Fig. 5.4 An audiogram 1 year after cochlear implantation. The pure tone average has improved to 30 dB and the patient was consistently getting 85% correct on sentence testing.

sentence testing, and he achieved 42% correct on consonant-vowel-consonant (CNC) word testing. His pure tone average with the cochlear implant was 30 dB (**Fig. 5.4**).

Our other patients have had similarly good clinical results following cochlear implant after SRS. One of our patients, however, had sustained growth of a tumor after SRS but still had good cochlear implant function despite the tumor growth. Ultimately, the tumor had to be resected and the cochlear implant was removed and converted to an auditory brainstem implant. This device gives the patient environmental sound awareness but does not provide nearly as good hearing as his cochlear implant did.

There are three main concerns with treating vestibular schwannomas in NF2 patients with SRS. The first is that it will not be effective, and we have presented the results as reported in the literature with good evidence that NF2 tumors do not respond as well as sporadic ones, but still 80% of the tumors will be controlled at 5 years. Whether this is sufficient in a 45-year-old woman is a difficult decision. A related, valid concern is that, if the treatment does fail and the tumor requires surgical removal, it will be a more difficult operation due to scarring from the radiation. It has indeed been our limited experience that surgery after SRS is more challenging, and other groups have also reported this fact.[39,40]

A second concern is that hearing rehabilitation with either a cochlear implant or an auditory brainstem implant

will be less effective after SRS. This assumption has not been borne out in our experience or in the literature.[38,41] Both cochlear and auditory brainstem implants seem equally effective whether the tumor has been surgically removed or treated with SRS. In fact, the chance of getting a functioning cochlear implant, particularly in a patient with a tumor larger than 2.0 cm, is likely much higher after SRS compared with microsurgery because there is no surgical manipulation of the cochlear nerve.

Finally, there has been concern that even single-fraction, conformal SRS could induce malignancy in NF2 patients who already have a mutation in a tumor-suppressor gene.[44] There are only 14 potential cases of histologically verified intracranial malignancy arising in a stereotactically irradiated field (SRS and fractionated therapy), and in four of these cases the patient had NF2.[43–46] Although the concern of secondary malignancy should always be discussed, overall there has not been any evidence of an increased risk of malignancy in NF2 patients after SRS.[35]

Stereotactic radiosurgery is a reasonable option to treat this 2.5-cm vestibular schwannoma in the only hearing ear in a patient with NF2. If the patient loses hearing after treatment (a 60% chance) despite radiographic tumor control, her hearing could likely be rehabilitated to a high level with a cochlear implant. There is about an 80% chance of the patient not requiring another intervention for this tumor at 5 years. If the tumor does not respond to SRS and requires surgical removal, surgery will be technically more difficult. An auditory brainstem implant could be placed at the time of tumor removal, if that becomes necessary, with the expectation that it would function in an equiva-

lent manner to auditory brainstem implants in NF2 patients who do not undergo irradiation.

Unfortunately, the decision making for patients with NF2 remains difficult and controversial.

Conservative Treatment of Acoustic Tumors in Patients with a Single Hearing Ear

Donlin M. Long

The treatment of the patient with bilateral acoustic neuromas is one of the most perplexing conundrums in neurosurgery. To understand various possibilities for treatment and their rationale, it is worthwhile to review the preservation of hearing in patients undergoing surgery for acoustic neuroma.

Preserving Hearing

I recently reviewed studies comprising more than 10,000 reported cases of the so-called acoustic neuromas. Hearing preservation was deemed possible in about one quarter and successful in only about 10%. However, this general observation requires a more detailed analysis. Hearing preservation in patients with larger tumors, certainly those above 3 cm, is extremely unusual; only a few such cases have been reported. Lost hearing has been restored so infrequently that, based on any material available in the literature, it cannot be considered a goal with larger tumors.

On the other hand, the successful preservation of hearing in patients with smaller tumors is now recognized, and this success is gradually being reported in the literature. It appears that intracanalicular tumors can be removed, with hearing preservation approaching 50%. A few surgeons are reporting success rates in the 80% range. Although these reports are encouraging, this level of hearing preservation has not yet been documented with rigorous studies of preserved high-level hearing threshold and speech discrimination. Certainly, this success does not reflect the general experience and remains the province of a few of the most experienced surgeons.

With extracanalicular tumors greater than 1 cm but less than 3 cm, the success rate falls dramatically. The current experience available for review suggests that no more than one third of these patients will have satisfactory hearing. The chance of preservation is apparently directly related to the tumor size. Stereotactic radiosurgical techniques were initially unsuccessful, particularly in patients with neurofibromatosis, and tumors larger than 1 cm were not successfully radiated. However, reports are now appearing with newer techniques that allow radiation of even large

tumors. The initial reports generally covered only short follow-up periods. Now the results of radiating larger tumors are appearing. In patients with preserved hearing, functional hearing is retained in up to 60%.

My review of the current literature leads me to believe that, in the hands of the most accomplished surgeons, hearing preservation is predictable only with small tumors. If the tumor is within the canal or less than 1 cm in size, the success rate for hearing preservation may be as high as 80%, but is probably closer to 50%. The higher success rate of some surgeons suggests that, with greater experience, the 80% level may be achievable. Preserving hearing in patients with these small tumors is currently the greatest challenge of acoustic neuroma surgery. Preserving hearing in those with larger tumors (from 1 to 2.5 or 3 cm) is possible in no more than 30 to 50%, and is probably lower than either of these figures for tumors at the upper end of this range. Beyond 3 cm, the chance of hearing preservation is extremely small, certainly no greater than 10% at present.

Stereotactic radiosurgical techniques can now compete with the suboccipital approach to preserve hearing in patients with small and medium-sized tumors. With small tumors, hearing is retained at a functional level in 60 to 80% of patients, depending on the report. With medium-sized tumors, however, the outcome of radiation is typically better for preserving hearing. Sparing functional hearing in patients with large tumors is accomplished more frequently with radiation, but at the cost of substantially lower tumor control.

Treatment Options

In discussing treatment options, it must be emphasized that the most optimistic surgical reports indicate hearing preservation in no more than 80% of patients with acoustic tumors. This means a 20% failure rate as the best that can be envisioned currently, and with all but the most favorable circumstances, this figure falls precipitously.

The goal of surgery with these tumors is threefold: first, cure the tumor; second, preserve all possible neurologic function; and third, preserve functional hearing for as long as possible. But other factors must also be considered. Most patients with NF2 are prone to developing additional neoplasms: meningiomas, neurofibromas, schwannomas, and intrinsic gliomas. Tumors at the cerebellopontine angle may be multiple and may be on cranial nerves other than the vestibular portion of the acoustic nerve. Neurofibromas on these nerves are rare, but certainly not unknown. Therefore, the surgeon who decides to operate on one of these tumors cannot automatically assume that the tumor is a simple schwannoma of the vestibular nerve. All of these factors must be considered in planning a therapeutic course.

Treatment Strategy

When the only visible tumors are bilateral acoustic tumors, I make my decisions based on the size of the tumors and the state of the patient's hearing. If both threshold and discrimination are normal bilaterally and the tumors are small, the patient can be followed safely. However, rapid loss of hearing is common and regular evaluations are required. Because the growth potential of the tumors is not known when they are first found, I use the following strategy. Images of the tumors are taken every 3 months during the first year by using MRI with gadolinium enhancement. I obtain a complete hearing evaluation every 3 months, so that the patient is undergoing imaging or hearing tests every 6 weeks during that year. If no growth has occurred during the second year, I reduce the imaging studies to two, but continue hearing examinations every 3 months. If no changes occur, I reduce the imaging examinations to yearly and reduce the hearing tests to every 6 months, but I tell the patient to consciously alternate ears when using the telephone and to notify me if he or she has any difficulty using the telephone with either ear. I have followed one elderly patient for nearly 20 years who has had no apparent change in tumor size or in hearing function. On the other hand, I have seen patients whose tumors have changed rapidly over 6 to 9 months. Therefore, all patients need to be assessed regularly. The need for reevaluation in the event of any apparent change should be made clear to the patient.

With these patients and all others with bilateral acoustic tumors, I make the assumption that eventually the worst will happen and deafness will occur. Therefore, as soon as the diagnosis is made, I insist that the patient begin to learn sign language and take advantage of this period of good hearing to do so.

The next scenario is usually the patient with bilateral small tumors but significant hearing loss on one or both sides. In my experience, once hearing loss begins, it is usually progressive, and therefore I wish to act to preserve hearing. If hearing is still functional on both sides, I choose the largest tumor to be treated first and SRS is typically my treatment of choice. If hearing is failing in one ear and not the other, I treat the ear with the greatest hearing loss first. I then follow the patient and check hearing bilaterally on a regular basis, typically every 3 months. I treat the

remaining tumor only if there is evidence of growth or if hearing begins to fail in that ear. If there are indications for treatment, I typically use radiation in the second ear if the radiotherapist believes the appropriate doses can be given. If not, I proceed to microsurgery on the second ear as soon as there is a clinical indication of hearing loss. Some patients prefer surgery. Then, I choose either the smallest tumor or the tumor side in which hearing has begun to decline. Usually I operate on all tumors that are causing degradation of hearing. Both the middle fossa or suboccipital approach can be used, and a major goal of surgery is preservation of hearing. This includes constant intraoperative monitoring. If everything goes well on the most symptomatic side, I delay surgery on the other side until tumor growth is shown or some decline in hearing occurs. Then, I have the option of either radiation or surgery. I still insist that the patient begin to learn sign language even before any treatment has begun. I do not withhold treatment, but I encourage the patient to begin the process just in case.

Case Analysis

The case in point illustrates a common situation. One tumor was of giant size and was removed, and the patient has lost some hearing on the other side. I would make every effort to preserve the remaining hearing, expecting that it would be lost. I would have the patient begin learning sign language and wait to operate on the second side until that educational process is complete. My indication for surgery on the second tumor is growth demonstrated on an imaging study or declining hearing function. In this situation, the patient now has 75% speech discrimination at 30 dB. This is still satisfactory hearing function.

In my experience, once this hearing loss begins, it progresses steadily. When hearing has declined below the level of 50 dB and 50% speech discrimination, it is probably no longer functional. We need to do something to preserve hearing before that time, but we hope for the patient to be proficient in sign language before running the risk of deafness. Ideally, this patient began the educational process shortly after the previous right-sided tumor was removed. If not, I would begin that process immediately and institute an evaluation program that would include repeated hearing studies in 6 weeks, 3 months, and then at 3-month intervals while sign language is being learned. If rapid deterioration occurs, I would operate on this patient through the suboccipital route and attempt to preserve hearing; if it does not, I would stage the surgery to proceed as soon as the patient is proficient in sign language.

Delaying Surgery

An argument can be made for simply delaying surgery until functional hearing is lost, in this way guaranteeing the patient the longest possible period of hearing preservation. Those who advocate this view are pessimistic about the reported preservation of hearing, and point out that most of the reports do not clearly document hearing preservation at a functional level. The more optimistic will say that hearing can be preserved at least one third of the time in patients with tumors like this, and that some report 50 to 80% rates of hearing salvage. Because the eventual outcome of not treating this tumor will almost certainly be deafness, they argue that even the 30% chance is better than the virtual certainty of deafness, and that preserving hearing in the interim is less important than the chance of preserving lifelong hearing.

The most comprehensive studies of patients with expectant management of acoustic tumors are the extensive evaluations done in Denmark. Over a 10-year period, up to 60% of patients did not demonstrate progression of disease, though some of those patients did lose hearing. A spectrum of papers suggests that, over an extended period, between 40 and 60% of patients with demonstrated acoustic tumors will not have a progression of symptoms. Thus, it is reasonable to follow a patient who has a known acoustic tumor but no symptoms. This is particularly true when the tumor is in the single hearing ear. However, some authors have reported less good outcomes with expectant nontreatment of patients with acoustic tumors. Even though some loss of hearing can occur, I think it is reasonable to simply observe patients with asymptomatic or minimally symptomatic tumors in the single hearing ear until tumor growth begins or some evidence of hearing loss occurs. The patient does need to know that some hearing loss is a possibility with this approach, and the chance of preserving hearing with any of the treatment options should be discussed with the patient as well.

The use of cochlear implants has improved dramatically in the past few years. The cochlear implant now provides an excellent way to restore lost hearing to a functional level, which is far superior to deafness. If at all possible during surgery, an anatomically intact auditory nerve should be preserved. The use of cochlear implants is a great advance in the treatment of these patients in whom the prevention of complete deafness is very important. I still ask that these patients learn sign language, but the use of cochlear implants has made this much less of a necessity than it was in the past.

Choosing the Conservative Approach

At present, I still take a relatively conservative role with these patients. The first goal must be to protect the patient's life and vital neurologic function. When these are not at risk, preserving hearing is the most important factor in decision making. I want to plan treatment so that the patient has been given adequate time to learn sign language and the tumors are treated at a time when preserving functional hearing is still a possibility. This approach means that tumors involving nonfunctional ears can be removed immediately. Hearing should be preserved for as long as possible to allow the patient to become proficient in sign language and begin the rest of the education that a potential life of deafness requires. The cochlear implant has the possibility of restoring enough functional hearing that the patient will not need sign language. I still ask the patients to learn whenever possible, but the implants can prevent deafness in many patients.

Stereotactic radiosurgery and microsurgery both offer the patient an excellent chance for satisfactory treatment when surgery becomes necessary. In the hands of experienced surgeons, microsurgical removal of small and medium-sized tumors offers the best chance of cure and hearing preservation, and retained hearing appears to be in the 50 to 60% range. Radiosurgery is equally satisfactory. Cure rates are lower, but recently reported rates of hearing preservation are higher, at 60 to 80%. Increasingly, SRS is the first choice for patients with small or medium-sized tumors, particularly those with functional hearing in the affected ear. I believe the data for larger tumors still favors direct surgery, and hearing preservation is rarely an important issue for these patients. The data concerning nontreatment of these tumors is less clear, and the largest series suggest that a significant number of patients harboring acoustic tumors will not have a significant change in function over the first 10 years at least. Some reports are less optimistic. Therefore, I follow patients with careful hearing examinations and MRI on a regular basis until I am satisfied that tumor growth or some change in hearing is occurring. Once either is apparent, I proceed to treatment in the ways that I have outlined. I prefer to be conservative and watch these tumors for as long as possible to give the patient the greatest period of functional hearing without the risk of deafness.

Treating Giant Tumors

One other situation that is extremely difficult and requires attention is a giant bilateral tumor, which is found in a few of these patients. In these circumstances, the issue is preservation of life and general function. The surgeon can rarely take a conservative approach in these patients. Most of these giant tumors have already caused deafness. If they have not, I routinely operate on the side in which hearing is less satisfactory and hope that surgery will not be required on the opposite side until the patient learns sign language. No one has presented data indicating that hearing can be preserved in patients with larger tumors and, at present, deafness must be considered the virtually certain consequence of the removal of bilateral large tumors. For that reason, I remove the tumor on the side with the less adequate hearing or the one producing the more significant symptoms, and hope to leave the other until the patient can be prepared for deafness.

Conclusion

Preserving hearing is our greatest challenge in patients undergoing acoustic tumor surgery. It is now possible in some patients, which is a considerable step forward, and continued improvements in surgical technique may make the preservation of hearing in patients with functional ears

the rule rather than the exception. Until then, observation is an appropriate approach only for some of these patients.

Preserving Hearing in the Last Hearing Ear of Patients with Neurofibromatosis Type 2

Stephen J. Haines

This patient has the misfortune of suffering from a condition for which there is no consensus regarding the most appropriate treatment, but for which each form of treatment offers the tantalizing prospect of success. She has obtained quite different recommendations from internationally recognized experts with a great deal of experience in the treatment of her condition. My task is to help her choose among the options.

The choice cannot be made on the basis of data comparing the treatment options, for no such scientifically acceptable data exist. We will have to rely on the far less accurate method of interpreting the existing experience with the proposed methods of treatment in the light of logic, our own experience, and the patient's preference with regard to the likely outcomes. Although this is not a highly satisfactory way of resolving controversy, it is our only option in the absence of good data comparing treatments.

It will help if we separate the two primary goals for a patient in this situation: cure of her tumor and preservation of her hearing. We will also assume that we wish to minimize the morbidity of whatever form of treatment she chooses.

Our experts have proposed two quite different forms of treatment: immediate microsurgical resection with attempted hearing preservation or radiosurgery, possibly with the subsequent placement of a cochlear implant when hearing is lost. A third option always exists: to avoid active therapy until such time as tumor or symptom progression make treatment mandatory.

The First Goal: Curing the Tumor

In patients with NF2, "cure" is a term that does not apply. Even a complete resection of one vestibular schwannoma without recurrence does not leave the patient free of tumor. The strength of the argument favoring curative procedures over those that "control" tumors is lost in the setting of NF2.

The Second Goal: Preserving Hearing

Therefore, the primary goal in this case is maximal preservation of hearing. There is little doubt that, for short-term

preservation of hearing, the most conservative approach has the best outcome. On any given day, the probability that hearing will be preserved at its present level for the next 24 hours is highest if no therapeutic intervention is undertaken. The authors of this chapter have acknowledged that there is a clinically important risk of hearing loss associated with the form of therapy they have recommended, and that hearing loss occurs at different times after therapy and at different rates. Assessing the lifetime impact of 3 years of gradually progressive hearing loss to AAO-HNS class D hearing compared with 15 years of class C hearing is not something we can objectively do. The patient's preference is the overriding factor in making this choice.

The understanding of the impact on hearing between surgery and radiosurgery on a 2.5-cm vestibular schwannoma in a patient with NF2 requires excellent data with reliable audiograms of patients followed for 5 or more years after treatment. This information would have to be compared with natural history information of equal quality. Unfortunately, information of the necessary quality and duration simply does not exist.

We are therefore left with questionable comparisons of the best follow-up data available for the treatment options. These data generally come from single-institution series followed for variable periods of time. They are plagued with selection bias (in referral and surgeon decision making) and a lack of generalizability. (They are most frequently reported by the most experienced teams with results that they hope will set them apart from others.) It is the best available data and it is what the authors have used to make their recommendations.

Samii and Gerganov propose operating on this patient's only hearing ear if, in addition to the data provided, the auditory brainstem response is "good" according to their own institutional criteria.[3] Using this criterion and assuming the patient's willingness "to take the risk of complete hearing loss related to an early active treatment," they suggest that there is an 86% chance of complete tumor removal and a 65% chance of hearing preservation (in patients with NF2 who had "useful" preoperative hearing). Their 1997 publication[2] suggests that the cochlear nerve can be preserved in 59% of NF2 patients when anatomically intact preoperatively. Unfortunately, the definition of hearing preservation in this context is not clarified. In the authors' cited studies, this is generally determined according to their unique institutional classification of hearing (based solely on the measured decibels of hearing loss without reference to word recognition), which does not allow for direct translation into the internationally accepted AAO-HNS classification system.

These authors are extraordinarily good surgeons, but a realistic assessment of the likelihood that hearing of functional quality can be preserved is not possible from their published data. Furthermore, the fate of the hearing that is preserved over time is not well described. Once surgically preserved, does hearing decline faster, slower, or at the age-expected rate of decline in the general population? We simply do not know.

Neither can they provide us with any special insight into the rate of loss of useful hearing that this patient can expect or the likelihood that the slowly growing vestibular schwannoma will cause neurologic dysfunction at any particular time in the future. To make a decision, we are left, then, to trust their judgment and rely on the patient's personal philosophy: take the risk up front, accepting the loss of hearing if it happens, as opposed to delaying the loss of hearing as long as possible, accepting that it will gradually go away and that the eventual operation may be somewhat more difficult.

Link, Driscoll, and Pollock, who are also very good technical surgeons, interpret the same existing data and provide an alternative recommendation: treat the tumor now with SRS and expect that the patient has a 20% chance that surgical intervention will be required and a 60% chance of becoming functionally deaf sometime in the next 5 years. These authors rely on a combination of their own and reported experience with tumor growth after radiosurgery to produce the 20% surgical intervention estimate. They also acknowledge that the surgery is sometimes technically more difficult (and therefore of somewhat higher risk) when done after radiation. There is clearly a subjective component to the decision to operate when tumor growth is seen after radiosurgery, so this estimate must be taken with some uncertainty. The hearing preservation rate, based on the AAO-HNS classification system, is more objective and has been reproduced at several centers and can be considered relatively reliable.

They point out that some degree of hearing rehabilitation may be possible with a cochlear implant if the cochlear nerve remains intact, although it is difficult to compare the quality of that hearing directly with preoperative hearing classified according to the AAO-HNS scheme. This possibility should also exist for patients in whom the cochlear nerve is anatomically preserved surgically (59% in Samii's series[2]).

As posed by our authors, this is a decision between early aggressive therapy and delaying tactics. The aggressive approach, when successful, may preserve hearing at a better level than will eventually be achieved by the alternative, and may prevent subsequent neurologic compromise from a growing cerebellopontine angle tumor. However, there are small risks of very serious complications and a significant risk of losing useful hearing at the time of surgery. Delay clearly exposes fewer patients to sudden loss of the hearing they have at the time of diagnosis and, supplemented by radiosurgery, offers approximately a four in five chance that no other intervention will be required in the 5 years that follow treatment. However, in those 5 years, 60% of patients will become functionally deaf. It is not known if radiosurgery slows the rate of hearing loss in patients with vestibular schwannoma.

The best available untreated cohort is that of Stangerup and colleagues.[47] These are not patients with NF2. Of 491 patients presenting with speech discrimination scores of 70% or better, 59% remained at 70% or better after a mean of 4.7 years of follow-up. The worst prognostic group consisted of patients with less than 100% speech discrimination at presentation; 38% of them retained hearing at or above 70% speech discrimination. That figure is very similar to the rate of preservation quoted by Link, Driscoll, and Pollock, although the comparison is flawed by the incomplete measurement of hearing quality, nonsystematic dropouts in all series, and the eternal question of whether or not results in patients with sporadic vestibular schwannoma can be applied reliably to patients with NF2.

So how would I advise this patient? In our clinic, we have discussions very similar to those posed by the authors here. We discuss what is known about the natural history and the treated prognosis with radiosurgery and surgery. We try to extol the benefits of each approach and expose the flaws. We talk about the personal philosophy of the patient, and we answer questions. Often the patient asks what we would personally do—the surgeon, radiosurgeon, and patient-managing physician, which in our case are all the same doctor. We help the patient to a personally individualized decision among three reasonable and viable options (watchful waiting, radiosurgery, and microsurgery), and make sure the patient understands that any of the three management approaches may be appropriate for a given patient at a given time.

I would love to be able to tell the patient that there is one right approach, but the state of our understanding and the quality of data available simply make this impossible to do with integrity. I think that the patient is best served by consulting a center at which each of the three major options is readily available, ensuring that there are no inappropriate biases that would induce the treating team to force the patient in one direction. In the end, this patient must decide on a strategy that allows her to accept excellent results if they are achieved but also accept problems if they occur. This can only happen if the patient is fully informed of all the options and the uncertainty that remains in the data that support them.

References

1. Asthagiri AR, Parry DM, Butman JA, et al. Neurofibromatosis type 2. Lancet 2009;373:1974–1986
2. Samii M, Matthies C, Tatagiba M. Management of vestibular schwannomas (acoustic neuromas): auditory and facial nerve function after resection of 120 vestibular schwannomas in patients with neurofibromatosis 2. Neurosurgery 1997;40: 696–705, discussion 705–706
3. Samii M, Gerganov V, Samii A. Microsurgery management of vestibular schwannomas in neurofibromatosis type 2: indications and results. Prog Neurol Surg 2008;21:169–175
4. Baser ME, R Evans DG, Gutmann DH. Neurofibromatosis 2. Curr Opin Neurol 2003;16:27–33
5. Gerganov VM, Klinge PM, Nouri M, Stieglitz L, Samii M, Samii A. Prognostic clinical and radiological parameters for immediate facial nerve function following vestibular schwannoma surgery. Acta Neurochir (Wien) 2009;151:581–587, discussion 587
6. Matthies C, Samii M. Management of vestibular schwannomas (acoustic neuromas): the value of neurophysiology for evaluation and prediction of auditory function in 420 cases. Neurosurgery 1997;40:919–929, discussion 929–930
7. Samii M, Matthies C. Management of 1000 vestibular schwannomas (acoustic neuromas): hearing function in 1000 tumor resections. Neurosurgery 1997;40:248–260, discussion 260–262
8. Samii M, Gerganov VM. Surgery of extra-axial tumors of the cerebral base. Neurosurgery 2008;62(6, Suppl 3):1153–1166, discussion 1166–1168
9. Fischer G, Fischer C, Rémond J. Hearing preservation in acoustic neurinoma surgery. J Neurosurg 1992;76:910–917
10. Mohr G, Sade B, Dufour JJ, Rappaport JM. Preservation of hearing in patients undergoing microsurgery for vestibular schwannoma: degree of meatal filling. J Neurosurg 2005;102:1–5
11. Brackmann DE, Fayad JN, Slattery WH III, et al. Early proactive management of vestibular schwannomas in neurofibromatosis type 2. Neurosurgery 2001;49:274–280, discussion 280–283
12. Neff BA, Welling DB. Current concepts in the evaluation and treatment of neurofibromatosis type II. Otolaryngol Clin North Am 2005;38:671–684, ix
13. Maini S, Cohen MA, Hollow R, Briggs R. Update on long-term results with auditory brainstem implants in NF2 patients. Cochlear Implants Int 2009;10(Suppl 1):33–37
14. Lenarz T, Moshrefi M, Matthies C, et al. Auditory brainstem implant: part I. Auditory performance and its evolution over time. Otol Neurotol 2001;22:823–833
15. Otto SR, Brackmann DE, Hitselberger WE, Shannon RV, Kuchta J. Multichannel auditory brainstem implant: update on performance in 61 patients. J Neurosurg 2002;96:1063–1071
16. Samii A, Lenarz M, Majdani O, Lim HH, Samii M, Lenarz T. Auditory midbrain implant: a combined approach for vestibular schwannoma surgery and device implantation. Otol Neurotol 2007;28:31–38
17. Mathieu D, Kondziolka D, Flickinger JC, et al. Stereotactic radiosurgery for vestibular schwannomas in patients with neurofibromatosis type 2: an analysis of tumor control, complications, and hearing preservation rates. Neurosurgery 2007;60:460–468, discussion 468–470
18. Subach BR, Kondziolka D, Lunsford LD, Bissonette DJ, Flickinger JC, Maitz AH. Stereotactic radiosurgery in the management of acoustic neuromas associated with neurofibromatosis Type 2. J Neurosurg 1999;90:815–822
19. Phi JH, Kim DG, Chung HT, Lee J, Paek SH, Jung HW. Radiosurgical treatment of vestibular schwannomas in patients with neurofibromatosis type 2: tumor control and hearing preservation. Cancer 2009;115:390–398
20. Committee on Hearing and Equilibrium guidelines for the evaluation of hearing preservation in acoustic neuroma (vestibular schwannoma). American Academy of Otolaryngology–Head and Neck Surgery Foundation, Inc. Otolaryngol Head Neck Surg 1995;113:179–180
21. Driscoll CL, Jackler RK, Pitts LH, Brackmann DE. Lesions of the internal auditory canal and cerebellopontine angle in an only hearing ear: is surgery ever advisable? Am J Otol 2000;21: 573–581
22. Leksell L. The stereotaxic method and radiosurgery of the brain. Acta Chir Scand 1951;102:316–319
23. Leksell L. A note on the treatment of acoustic tumours. Acta Chir Scand 1971;137:763–765
24. Chopra R, Kondziolka D, Niranjan A, Lunsford LD, Flickinger JC. Long-term follow-up of acoustic schwannoma radiosurgery with marginal tumor doses of 12 to 13 Gy. Int J Radiat Oncol Biol Phys 2007;68:845–851
25. Kano H, Kondziolka D, Khan A, Flickinger JC, Lunsford LD. Predictors of hearing preservation after stereotactic radiosurgery for acoustic neuroma. J Neurosurg 2009;111:863–873
26. Timmer FC, Hanssens PE, van Haren AE, et al. Gamma knife radiosurgery for vestibular schwannomas: results of hearing preservation in relation to the cochlear radiation dose. Laryngoscope 2009;119:1076–1081
27. Kim KM, Park CK, Chung HT, Paek SH, Jung HW, Kim DG. Long-term outcomes of gamma knife stereotactic radiosurgery of vestibular schwannomas. J Korean Neurosurg Soc 2007;42: 286–292
28. Régis J, Tamura M, Delsanti C, Roche PH, Pellet W, Thomassin JM. Hearing preservation in patients with unilateral vestibular schwannoma after gamma knife surgery. Prog Neurol Surg 2008;21:142–151
29. Paek SH, Chung HT, Jeong SS, et al. Hearing preservation after gamma knife stereotactic radiosurgery of vestibular schwannoma. Cancer 2005;104:580–590
30. Tamura M, Carron R, Yomo S, et al. Hearing preservation after gamma knife radiosurgery for vestibular schwannomas presenting with high-level hearing. Neurosurgery 2009;64:289–296, discussion 296
31. Yang I, Aranda D, Han SJ, et al. Hearing preservation after stereotactic radiosurgery for vestibular schwannoma: a systematic review. J Clin Neurosci 2009;16:742–747
32. Thomas C, Di Maio S, Ma R, et al. Hearing preservation following fractionated stereotactic radiotherapy for vestibular schwannomas: prognostic implications of cochlear dose. J Neurosurg 2007;107:917–926
33. Roche PH, Régis J, Pellet W, et al. [Neurofibromatosis type 2. Preliminary results of gamma knife radiosurgery of vestibular schwannomas]. Neurochirurgie 2000;46:339–353, discussion 354
34. Rowe JG, Radatz MW, Walton L, Soanes T, Rodgers J, Kemeny AA. Clinical experience with gamma knife stereotactic radiosurgery in the management of vestibular schwannomas

secondary to type 2 neurofibromatosis. J Neurol Neurosurg Psychiatry 2003;74:1288–1293

35. Rowe JG, Radatz M, Kemeny A. Radiosurgery for type II neurofibromatosis. Prog Neurol Surg 2008;21:176–182

36. Wentworth S, Pinn M, Bourland JD, et al. Clinical experience with radiation therapy in the management of neurofibromatosis-associated central nervous system tumors. Int J Radiat Oncol Biol Phys 2009;73:208–213

37. Kida Y, Kobayashi T, Tanaka T, Mori Y. Radiosurgery for bilateral neurinomas associated with neurofibromatosis type 2. Surg Neurol 2000;53:383–389, discussion 389–390

38. Lustig LR, Yeagle J, Driscoll CI, Blevins N, Francis H, Niparko JK. Cochlear implantation in patients with neurofibromatosis type 2 and bilateral vestibular schwannoma. Otol Neurotol 2006;27:512–518

39. Roche PH, Khalil M, Thomassin JM, Delsanti C, Régis J. Surgical removal of vestibular schwannoma after failed gamma knife radiosurgery. Prog Neurol Surg 2008;21:152–157

40. Friedman RA, Brackmann DE, Hitselberger WE, Schwartz MS, Iqbal Z, Berliner KI. Surgical salvage after failed irradiation for vestibular schwannoma. Laryngoscope 2005;115:1827–1832

41. Kalamarides M, Grayeli AB, Bouccara D, et al. Hearing restoration with auditory brainstem implants after radiosurgery for neurofibromatosis type 2. J Neurosurg 2001;95:1028–1033

42. Baser ME, Evans DG, Jackler RK, Sujansky E, Rubenstein A. Neurofibromatosis 2, radiosurgery and malignant nervous system tumours. Br J Cancer 2000;82:998

43. Carlson ML, Babovic-Vuksanovic D, Messiaen L, Scheithauer BW, Neff BA, Link MJ. Radiation-induced rhabdomyosarcoma of the brainstem in a patient with neurofibromatosis type 2. J Neurosurg 2010;112:81–87

44. Bari ME, Forster DM, Kemeny AA, Walton L, Hardy D, Anderson JR. Malignancy in a vestibular schwannoma. Report of a case with central neurofibromatosis, treated by both stereotactic radiosurgery and surgical excision, with a review of the literature. Br J Neurosurg 2002;16:284–289

45. Norén G. Long-term complications following gamma knife radiosurgery of vestibular schwannomas. Stereotact Funct Neurosurg 1998;70(Suppl 1):65–73

46. Thomsen J, Mirz F, Wetke R, Astrup J, Bojsen-Møller M, Nielsen E. Intracranial sarcoma in a patient with neurofibromatosis type 2 treated with gamma knife radiosurgery for vestibular schwannoma. Am J Otol 2000;21:364–370

47. Stangerup SE, Thomsen J, Tos M, Cayé-Thomasen P. Long-term hearing preservation in vestibular schwannoma. Otol Neurotol 2010;31:271–275

Chapter 6

Management of Trigeminal Schwannoma: Microsurgical Removal vs. Radiosurgery

Case

A 40-year-old patient comes for medical treatment for facial pain and numbness with mild hypoalgesia and hypoesthesia in V_2 and V_3.

Participants

Total Removal of Trigeminal Schwannomas: Cristian Gragnaniello and Ossama Al-Mefty

Stereotactic Radiosurgery for Trigeminal Schwannomas: Douglas Kondziolka, Hideyuki Kano, and L. Dade Lunsford

Moderator: Management of Trigeminal Schwannoma: Microsurgical Removal vs. Radiosurgery: Takeshi Kawase

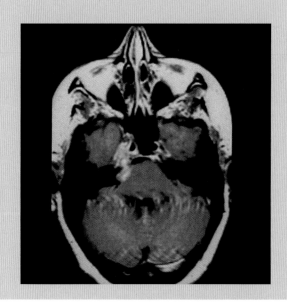

Total Removal of Trigeminal Schwannomas

Cristian Gragnaniello and Ossama Al-Mefty

Case Presentation

The imaging study shows a dumbbell-shaped right-sided skull-base lesion with a large component in the middle fossa that extends into the posterior fossa. It is highly enhancing and further extends into the cavernous sinus anteriorly and toward the brainstem in its posterior component. The imaging study shows a certain degree of bony erosion of the petrous bone. This patient presented with facial pain and numbness, hypoalgesia, and hypoesthesia in V_2 and V_3. The clinical presentation and the radiological findings are consistent with the diagnosis of a trigeminal schwannoma rather than a neurofibroma; neurofibromas most likely involve the cavernous sinus but do not typically extend posteriorly further than Meckel's cave.[1]

Trigeminal schwannomas are rare, benign lesions accounting for 0.07 to 0.5% of all intracranial tumors and 0.8 to 10% of all schwannomas. They arise from the Schwann cells of the nerve sheath and therefore may be located anywhere along the entire course of the nerve. As reported in the literature, 20% of trigeminal schwannomas emerge from the cisternal segment, 50% from Meckel's cave, and 5% from the distal intracranial segment. On magnetic resonance imaging (MRI), schwannomas are usually iso- or hypointense on T1-weighted images and hyperintense on T2-weighted images, and when contrast is administered they show either homogeneous or rim enhancement.[1]

Surgical Approach

The surgical approach for such a tumor is tailored to each patient, and proper selection is important to achieve total removal, improve preoperative neurologic deficits, and alleviate postoperative deficits **(Fig. 6.1)**. Trigeminal schwan-

nomas often involve the cavernous sinus space and extend to the posterior fossa. Therefore, skull-base approaches have shown many advantages for treatment, such as shortening the distance to the lesion, eliminating retraction of the brain, and facilitating the possibility of working below the temporal lobe, while protecting the draining veins below the intact dura. In particular, the extradural zygomatic middle fossa approach allows the removal of large dumbbell-shaped trigeminal schwannomas and offers a multiplicity of working angles to reach the tumor in its infratemporal, intramaxillary, intrasphenoidal, or intraorbital extension and in the cavernous sinus. Furthermore, the portion extending into the posterior fossa and compressing the brainstem can also be reached through the expanded Meckel's cave **(Fig. 6.2)**.[2,3]

The patient is placed in the supine position with the ipsilateral shoulder elevated and the head rotated to the contralateral side, with the zygoma almost parallel to the floor. The skin incision is carried 1 cm anterior to the tragus in a curvilinear fashion, behind the hairline, to the superior temporal line. The superficial temporal artery and the frontotemporal branches of the facial nerve are preserved. The skin flap is dissected anteriorly and the thick areolar tissue is left with the pericranial flap. At this stage, to preserve the facial nerve, an incision is made 1 cm posterior and parallel to its course along the zygomatic arch, keeping the nerve protected between the superficial and deep temporal fascia and the fat pad. The two fascias and the fat pad are then reflected anteriorly with the skin flap. A subperiosteal dissection of the temporal muscle, incised posteriorly to the superficial temporal artery, is carried from the root of the zygoma forward to protect the middle temporal artery.

With the B1 attachment, the zygoma is detached with oblique anterior cuts through the malar eminence and

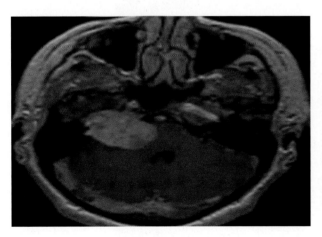

a

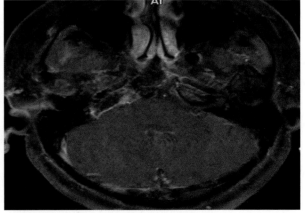

b

Fig. 6.1a,b Axial contrast-enhanced magnetic resonance imaging (MRI) studies depicting a trigeminal schwannoma that expands into Meckel's cave and extends in a dumbbell shape into both the middle and posterior fossae. **(a)** Preoperative image. **(b)** Postoperative image showing total removal.

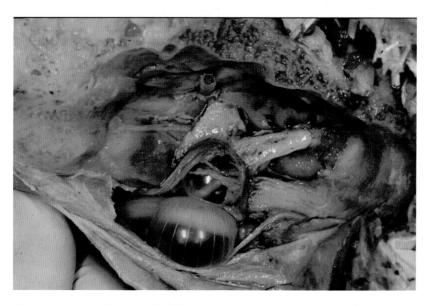

Fig. 6.2 Photograph of an anatomic model of a dumbbell-shaped tumor that expands into the orifice of Meckel's cave and compresses the trigeminal rootlet and ganglion.

through the root, posteriorly. The temporal muscle is detached at the level of the superior temporal line and reflected down with the zygoma to access the middle fossa. A bur hole is made at the level of the temporal fossa floor, a temporal craniotomy is designed, and the flap is elevated (**Fig. 6.3**). The surgeon should localize important landmarks in the middle fossa to prevent injury to the neurovascular structures. The dura of the middle fossa is elevated from the temporal fossa floor to expose and divide the middle meningeal artery at the foramen spinosum with a posterior-to-anterior and lateral-to-medial dissection to prevent injury of the greater superficial petrosal nerve, which could result in facial palsy. This nerve exits the facial

hiatus and runs in a groove on the floor of the middle fossa in an anteromedial direction, passing under Meckel's cave to reach the foramen lacerum, where it joins the deep petrosal nerve to form the vidian nerve. The greater superficial petrosal nerve is also an important landmark for locating the petrous segment of the internal carotid artery and gaining proximal control over the cavernous internal carotid artery.

The foramen rotundum and the maxillary division of the trigeminal nerve are identified lateral and posterior to the superior orbital fissure. The foramen ovale is located 1 cm posterior and lateral to the rotundum and transmits the mandibular division of the nerve. The outer dural layer

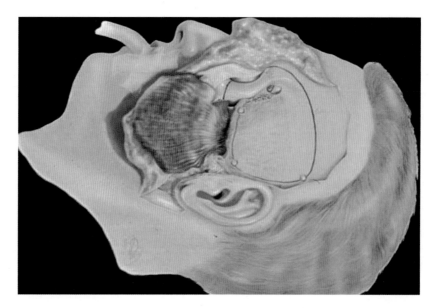

Fig. 6.3 Artist's illustration of the middle fossa zygomatic approach, including the skin incision, preserving the facial branches, sectioning of the zygoma, and the bone flap.

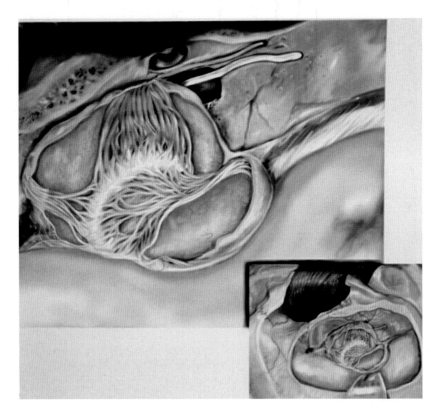

Fig. 6.4 Artist's illustration of the surgeon's extradural middle fossa view of a dumbbell-shaped trigeminal schwannoma with exposure of the petrous carotid artery, the three divisions and ganglion of the fifth cranial nerve, and entry into the expanded Meckel's cave. (From Al-Mefty O, Ayoubi S, Gaber E. Trigeminal schwannomas: removal of dumbbell-shaped tumors through the expanded Meckel cave and outcomes of cranial nerve function. J Neurosurg 2002;96:453-463. Reprinted by permission.)

over the trigeminal division is elevated to expose the lower cavernous sinus and peeled medially to expose the tumor in that location **(Fig. 6.4)**. The lesion can be reached between the divisions of the nerve or behind the ganglion. The tumor is carefully debulked with suction because of its soft consistency, and it is followed posteriorly through the expanded Meckel's cave. Once debulked, it is carefully dissected from the roots, ganglion, and divisions to save the fascicles that are not involved with the tumor.

There is no need to drill the petrous apex or section the tentorium because the enlarged mouth of Meckel's cave offers a natural pathway between the middle and posterior fossae to follow the lesion into the posterior fossa. If needed, the mouth can be enlarged with an upward incision toward the superior petrosal sinus, which might require coagulation and sectioning of its most anterior part. In the posterior fossa, the lesion can be safely dissected from the brainstem, rootlets, and basilar artery if an intra-arachnoidal plane of dissection is maintained **(Fig. 6.5)**. Fragments of the tumor may be present in the infratemporal and pterygoid fossae; these can be excised after the floor of the middle fossa is removed between the foramen ovale and the rotundum. Fragments along the superior orbital fissure can be extirpated to remove the middle fossa floor between the foramen rotundum and the superior orbital fissure. If the middle fossa floor is drilled, it can be reconstructed with a vascularized temporal muscle flap to prevent cerebrospinal fluid leaks.[3]

Discussion

Trigeminal schwannomas are benign and slow-growing lesions; however, their location has been the cause of morbidity in the past. These tumors can arise from any segment of the nerve (root, ganglion, or any one of the three divisions) and extend into more than one compartment, resulting in a more challenging treatment. This is particularly true in the case described here.

The first classification of trigeminal schwannomas proposed by Jefferson in 1959 was modified by Day and Fukushima[4] and others to include different features of the tumor, such as the degree of extension into the multiple fossae and the degree of bony erosion of the petrous apex[4,5] **(Table 6.1) (Figs. 6.6, 6.7)**. In earlier cases, these lesions were removed through conventional approaches but with high morbidity and recurrence reaching 70% and 65%, respectively.[6,7] Some authors have noted the difficulty in removing dumbbell-shaped schwannomas via the subtemporal and retrosigmoid approaches.[8]

The introduction of skull-base approaches and, more recently, extradural approaches has proved helpful in tackling the intradural portions of the lesion. The additional

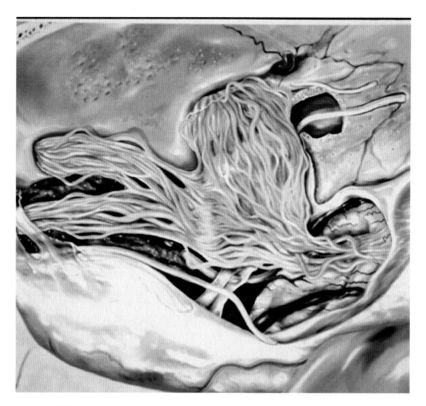

Fig. 6.5 Artist's illustration of the surgeon's view after the posterior fossa extension of the tumor has been reached and removed through Meckel's cave, exposing the basilar artery and the brainstem. (From Al-Mefty O, Ayoubi S, Gaber E. Trigeminal schwannomas: removal of dumbbell-shaped tumors through the expanded Meckel cave and outcomes of cranial nerve function. J Neurosurg 2002;96:453-463. Reprinted by permission.)

extradural approach used by Dolenc[9] and Day and Fuku-shima[4] enhanced the results of previous series. We found the zygomatic middle fossa approach and the zygomatic osteotomy, respectively, advantageous in achieving extradural total removal and minimizing retraction on the temporal lobe while providing multiple working angles. The zygomatic middle fossa approach exposes the tumor in every location, even in the posterior fossa. We maintain, however, that a different approach is needed for the very caudal extension of the tumor below the facial and acoustic nerves.[3]

Because this lesion is benign, it does not invade neural or vascular structures that are only displaced. Dissection from the fibers of the trigeminal nerve is possible with microsurgical techniques to preserve and improve nerve func-

tion (75% improvement of facial pain and 80% improvement of trigeminal motor function). The introduction of skull-base approaches to the treatment of trigeminal schwannomas offers the possibility of total removal with very good outcomes and low morbidity. During skull-base procedures, intraoperative neurophysiological monitoring offers the surgeon additional safety in removing lesions that involve and displace cranial nerves. More specifically, this type of monitoring allows the surgeon to locate the involved cranial nerves, which confirms nerve function during surgery and forecasts the surgical outcome.

In a previous report, the senior author (O.A.) analyzed the microsurgical total resection of 25 trigeminal schwannomas, of which only 24% involved the middle fossa alone and 76% involved both the middle and posterior fossae. All tumors involved the cavernous sinus. After surgery, all preoperative deficits of the cranial nerves (rather than just the trigeminal nerve) and all brainstem and cerebellar symptoms were alleviated. There was a remarkable improvement in 75% of patients who presented with facial pain, 80% of those suffering from motor trigeminal weakness, and 44% of those with facial numbness. Only 13% of the lesions recurred and 12% of patients had worsening or new deficits in trigeminal function. The mean age of the patients at the time of treatment was 44 years.[3]

Pamir and colleagues[10] reported on a series of 18 patients in which 50% of the lesions were Jefferson type C tri-

Table 6.1 Jefferson's Classification of Trigeminal Schwannomas

Type	Description
A	Tumors located mainly in the middle fossa that arise from the gasserian ganglion
B	Tumors located predominantly in the posterior fossa that arise from the root of the trigeminal nerve
C	Tumors with significant components in both middle and posterior fossae
	Dumbbell-shaped tumors

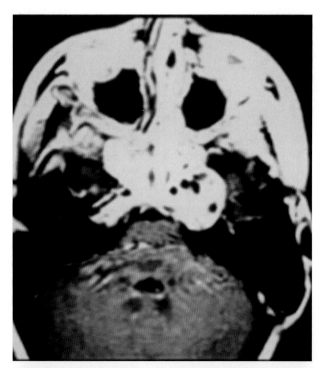

a

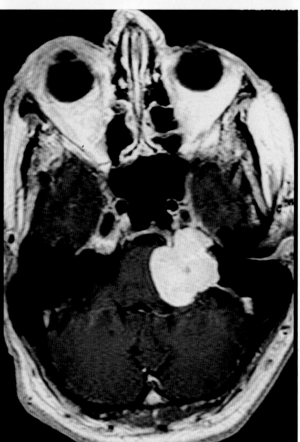

b

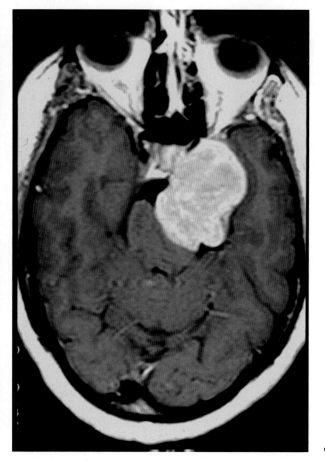

c

Fig. 6.6a–c MRI studies depicting the three types of trigeminal schwannomas in the Jefferson's classification. **(a)** Tumor located mainly in the middle fossa that arise from the gasserian ganglion. **(b)** Tumor located predominantly in the posterior fossa that arise from the roots of the trigeminal nerve. **(c)** Tumor with significant components in both middle and posterior fossae (dumbbell-shaped) tumors.

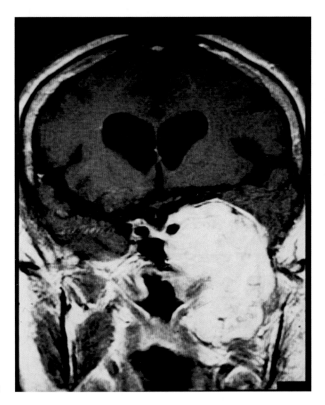

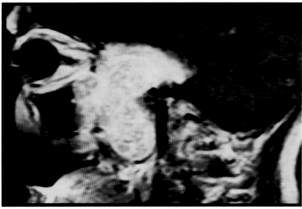

Fig. 6.7a,b   Contrast-enhanced MRI studies of a giant trigeminal schwannoma that extends into the infratemporal fossa along the division. **(a)** Coronal image. **(b)** Sagittal image.

geminal schwannomas and only two patients had a tumor smaller than 2 cm. They reported one recurrence and one subtotal removal, and 16 patients were free of tumor at 134 months. Zhou and associates[11] described a series of 57 cases of dumbbell-shaped Jefferson type C trigeminal schwannomas (50% more than 40 mm in diameter and 26% more than 50 mm). They reported a total removal rate of 87% and only one recurrence at a mean follow-up of 10 years. The neurologic function of cranial nerves improved in 93% of patients with facial numbness, 83% with deteriorating trigeminal motor function, 80% with palsy of the sixth and seventh nerves, and 75% with palsy of the ninth and tenth nerves and cerebellar or brainstem signs. They treated 38 patients with the gamma knife with a 65-month follow-up, and reported that 83% of the tumors decreased in size, 5.7% remained stable, and 8.6% increased with worsening trigeminal function in 25% of patients. They also reported four patients in whom surgical removal was incomplete but the residual tumor did not grow during long-term follow-up. In only one case (25%), it grew after 5 years, requiring further treatment.

In 2006, Moffat and colleagues[12] reported a small series of eight patients surgically treated. This report is important because of the characteristics of the lesions, which were more similar to those routinely radiated (50% Jefferson type A). The outcome was excellent: 100% of facial pain and 62.5% of facial numbness resolved. Sarma and associates[13] reported on 26 trigeminal schwannomas with a gross total resection in 100% of patients and the preservation of cranial nerve function, which reflects our experience. It is important to emphasize that, in 100% of patients, they

were able to dissect the tumor from the trigeminal nerve, preserving its function in all patients with a medium-sized tumor (2.5 cm or less). Yoshida and Kawase[8] reported a comprehensive series of trigeminal schwannomas involving multiple fossae. The lesions operated on through skull-base approaches were totally removed in 15 of 18 patients. Two of the recurrences, representing 11% of the series, had been treated first at other institutions. Only four patients had tumors of 3.5 cm or less whereas the others had a mean diameter of 4.9 cm (range 3.5 to 8 cm). In the small series of five trigeminal schwannomas reported by Mariniello and associates,[14] all the tumors were located in the cavernous sinus. The authors observed an improvement of facial pain in all patients with no recurrences or complications.

Recently, different series of stereotactic radiosurgery (SRS) have shown good control of tumor growth in patients with small trigeminal schwannomas (less than 3 cm in diameter) with a short follow-up. It is very difficult to compare the results of surgery and radiosurgery in the treatment of trigeminal schwannomas for multiple reasons, including the different size of treated lesions, the different times of onset of complications, and the short follow-up for radiosurgery. Regardless, it is the comparison between the two modalities that is the focus of the controversy. Hasegawa and colleagues[15] treated 37 patients affected with trigeminal schwannomas using the gamma knife. The mean dose delivered to the tumor was 27.9 Gy and the marginal dose was 14.2 Gy. Only 22% of the tumors were type C (dumbbell shaped) and only 16% of the patients had compression of the brainstem with deviation of the fourth ventricle. At 54 months of follow-up, there was good tumor growth control in 84% of patients whereas 14% suffered from an enlargement of the lesion or uncontrollable facial pain with radiation-induced edema that required surgical extirpation. There was no difference in the outcome of patients who underwent gamma knife surgery as a first treatment or after previous surgery. The functional outcome of the cranial nerves improved in 40% of the patients, with worsening or the onset of new symptoms in 14%.

Phi and associates[16] treated 22 patients and reported at 2-year follow-up. Eleven tumors were dumbbell shaped and 82% of patients underwent radiosurgery as a first treatment. The outcome showed persistence in trigeminal pain in 27% of patients, facial hypoesthesia in 63%, motor trigeminal weakness in 15%, and sixth nerve palsy in 50%. Facial dysesthesia was permanent in 13.6% of patients and 4.5% experienced worsening of preexisting trigeminal pain. New deficits were observed in 27% of patients. Overall, there was good tumor growth control, with only 4.5% of patients having uncontrolled lesions. The most interesting data in the series relates to the presence of tumor in the cavernous sinus, with the development of new deficits in 42.8% of patients. Pan and associates[17] reported on a series of 56 patients treated with the gamma knife, with results that overlap those of other reports for the same technique. The data from patients with uncontrolled tumors show an increase in recurrence in those affected by tumors with a diameter greater than 30 mm compared with those affected by tumors of 30 mm in diameter or less by a 3:1 ratio. Huang and colleagues[18] examined a series of 16 patients whose tumors were well controlled at 44-month follow-up and found no worsening of preexisting symptoms and improvement of 31. In a series of 23 patients treated for trigeminal schwannomas, Nettel and coauthors[19] reported tumor growth in 9% of patients at follow-up, 9% with a new onset of symptoms, and 4.3% with peritumoral changes.

Radiation-induced changes in neural tissue are well known and often have an insidious onset, especially in the long term. Trigeminal schwannomas mostly occur in the third and fourth decades of life in patients with a long life expectancy, but have also been reported in children and young adults.[15–17,19] Radiation-induced injuries to small

brain vessels are known to manifest shortly after treatment. Radiation vasculopathy of larger vessels, however, is not well recognized, and there are few reports that suggest reconsidering its incidence even with small doses of radiation, as in gamma knife surgery, especially when treating the cavernous sinus and brainstem for benign lesions. We focused on the possibility of dissecting the tumor from the fascicles of the trigeminal nerve using microsurgical techniques. Morita and colleagues[20] have suggested that 19 Gy is a safe dosage to be delivered to the trigeminal nerve. When the nerve is affected by the tumor, it is difficult on a radiological image to discern the tumor from the normal healthy nerve while delivering, in most cases, a mean dose of 27 Gy to the tumor.

As we have noted previously, the use of the gamma knife after failed surgery is as safe and effective as its use in patients who were never surgically treated. But this statement is not valid when we analyze data from patients undergoing surgery after the failure of treatment with the gamma knife. In these patients, the tumors adhere tightly to vital structures such as nerves, vessels, and the brainstem, making total removal very difficult and with greater risk. Gwak and associates[5] reported that, in cases of subtotal removal of a trigeminal schwannoma, the isolated residual tumor was stable after 5 years in 75% of patients, suggesting that, in cases of subtotal removal, it is worthwhile to wait and observe the residual until it grows. An important limit in the discussion of surgery versus radiosurgery series lies in the fact that most patients included in the surgery series are not suitable for radiosurgery because their lesions are too big to be irradiated. Because trigeminal schwannomas are benign, slow-growing lesions that mostly present in the third and fourth decades of life, we believe they must be treated surgically by experienced surgeons who persistently aim for total removal. Patients with a progressive tumor who are not surgical candidates, or who have residual or a recurrent tumor that cannot be removed, can be referred for radiosurgery, as current reports indicate that this modality induces good control of tumor growth and acceptable cranial nerve outcomes, but at a relatively short follow-up.

Stereotactic Radiosurgery for Trigeminal Schwannomas

Douglas Kondziolka, Hideyuki Kano, and L. Dade Lunsford

Case Presentation

The presented case is that of a 40-year-old with a history of facial pain and numbness, and the neurologic examination noted mild hypoesthesia and hypoalgesia in the second and third trigeminal divisions. The axial contrast-enhanced MRI

shows a mass in the right cavernous sinus extending along the course of the trigeminal nerve. It has a dumbbell shape that is typical of a trigeminal schwannoma.

The management of this patient includes both diagnosis and therapy, and the differential diagnosis for a lesion in this location could include a schwannoma, meningioma, lymphoma, metastasis, hemangioma, or nonneoplastic process such as granulomatous inflammation. The latter would be unusual in this case because of the extent of lesion outside the cavernous sinus. A metastasis would be less likely in a patient at this age and without a cancer history. The presentation and shape of the tumor are most consistent with a trigeminal schwannoma. We would therefore make that diagnosis without histology sampling and would manage the patient as such.

Therapeutic options include observation with serial imaging studies, microsurgical resection (complete or partial), SRS, fractionated radiotherapy, or combined approaches. Because this patient is symptomatic, we favor treatment over observation, and because the tumor is fairly small in volume, the patient is an ideal candidate for radiosurgery. In our experience, gamma knife radiosurgery is associated with a high rate of tumor response and regression and possible improvement in symptoms. This could be achieved without exposing the patient to the risks of craniotomy, or to a higher chance of impaired neurologic function or vascular injury.

Background

Trigeminal schwannomas are slow-growing, benign nerve sheath tumors that are uncommon compared with vestibular schwannomas.[21-25] They account for less than 1% of all intracranial tumors and 0.8 to 8% of all intracranial schwannomas.[7,21-27] Despite continued improvements in cranial-base surgical techniques, including endonasal surgery, a tumor's adherence to adjacent critical neurovascular structures makes complete removal difficult.[7,8,22-24] When such removal is attempted, new postoperative neurologic deficits are common.[7,13,18,23,27] The rate of new or worsened trigeminal function after tumor removal varies from 13 to 86%.[7,8,22,23,28]

There is increasing literature about the value of SRS for patients with trigeminal schwannomas.[4,29-34] In a recent review, we retrospectively assessed tumor control, clinical response, the risk of adverse radiation effects, and variables that affect treatment outcomes.[26]

Clinical Experience with Gamma Knife Radiosurgery

Over a 16-year interval before 2005, 33 patients with trigeminal schwannomas underwent SRS at the University of Pittsburgh with the gamma knife manufactured by Elekta Instruments (Norcross, GA) (**Table 6.2**). There were 17 males and 16 females with a median age of 49.5 years (range 15.1–82.5 years). Eleven patients (33%) had prior surgical resection and one patient was diagnosed through stereotactic biopsy. Twenty-two patients (67%) underwent SRS as primary management. As in the case presented, in our series the diagnosis was based on a combination of clinical symptoms or signs and confirmatory neuroimaging findings. All tumors extended along the course of the trigeminal nerve, had diffuse contrast enhancement identified by MRI, and had no dural tail. Six patients underwent SRS at the time of tumor recurrence identified by imaging. Tumor progression after initial management was defined as an increase in tumor volume delineated on MRI. The median duration between last surgical removal and progression was 22.1 months (range 9.4–76.5 months).

The classification of each lesion was based on the location of the tumor, and the tumors were classified into one of three types: root (tumor predominantly located in the posterior fossa); ganglion (tumor predominantly located in the middle fossa); and dumbbell (tumor involving both the middle and posterior fossa),[35] as in the case presented.

In our patients, the median tumor volume was 5.0 cm³ (range 0.5–18.0 cm³), similar to that of the presented case. A median of six isocenters (range 1–13) was used for dose planning. The median prescription dose delivered to the tumor margin was 15 Gy (range 12–22 Gy), and the prescription isodose was 50% in all cases. The maximum dose

Table 6.2 Characteristics of Patients (*n* = 33) in the University of Pittsburgh Series	
Median age (range)	49.5 (15.1–82.5)
Male	17
Female	16
Type: Root	6
Ganglion	17
Dumbbell	10
Solid	31
Cystic	2
Prior surgery	11
Mean/median target volume (cm³) (range)	5.0/4.2 (0.5–18.0)
Mean/median margin dose (Gy) (range)	15.0/15.0 (12–20)
Mean/median maximum dose (Gy) (range)	29.9/30.0 (24–40)

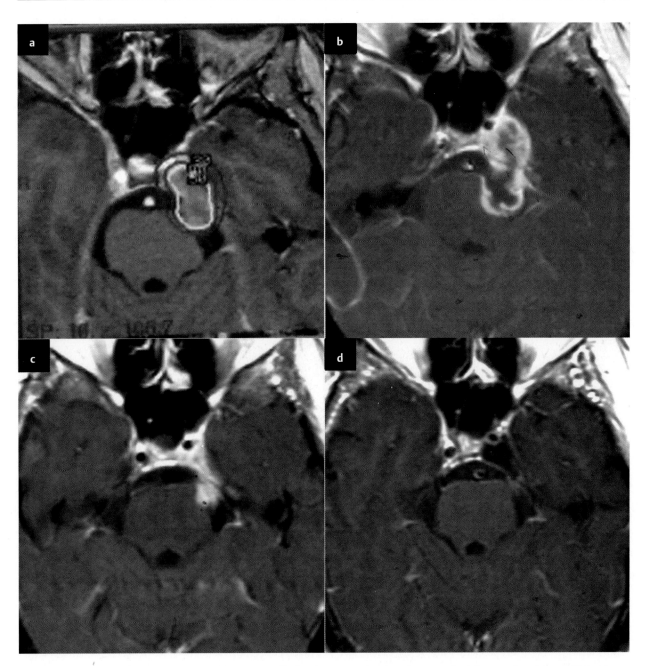

Fig. 6.8a–d **(a)** Axial MRI of a 44-year-old woman with facial numbness at the time of radiosurgery showing a dumbbell-shaped trigeminal schwannoma. **(b)** At 4 months, the MRI showed expansion of the tumor with central contrast loss. **(c)** However, at 8 months there was a marked decrease in volume. **(d)** The 7-year follow-up MRI showed complete resolution of the tumor without any cranial nerve deficit.

varied from 24 to 40 Gy (median 30 Gy). All patients had a minimum follow-up of 6 months (range 7.2–147.9 months), and 24 patients had a follow-up of 24 months or more. The mean follow-up time was 6 years.

Tumor Response After Radiosurgery

Follow-up imaging studies showed tumor control in 29 (87.9%) of 33 tumors after SRS. After radiosurgery, a complete resolution of volume was identified in two tumors (one ganglion and one dumbbell type) **(Fig. 6.8)**. A partial response was seen in 15 tumors (three root, eight ganglion, and four dumbbell). In 12 patients, the appearance of the tumor remained unchanged after radiosurgery (three root, seven ganglion, and two dumbbell). Delayed in-field tumor progression was seen in four cases (one ganglion and three dumbbell type), although two have required no further treatment. Two of four patients who had tumor progression underwent repeated SRS. One patient underwent repeated, staged SRS 5.5 years after the initial SRS. At the first stage, we treated the cerebellopontine angle component (tumor volume 8.5 cm³, margin dose 12 Gy). At the second

Table 6.3 Cranial Nerve Response to Radiosurgery (*n* = 33)

		Before SRS	After SRS		
			Improved	**No change**	**Worse**
Prior surgery (n = 11)					
Trochlear		0	0	0	0
Trigeminal	Neuropathy	7	0	6	1
	Pain	2	0	2	0
Abducens		2	1	1	0
Facial		0	0	0	0
Acoustic		1	0	1	0
No prior surgery (n = 22)					
Oculomotor		1	0	1	0
Trochlear		2	1	1	0
Trigeminal	Neuropathy	16	7	7	4
	Pain	6	2	3	2
Abducens		7	4	1	2
Facial		1	0	1	0
Acoustic		2	0	2	0

Abbreviation: SRS, stereotactic radiosurgery.

stage, 3 months later, the patient underwent SRS for the middle fossa component (tumor volume 17.5 cm³, margin dose 12 Gy). Two years after the second stage, the tumor was resected because of continued tumor growth and worsening facial sensory loss. Another patient underwent repeated SRS 26 months after the initial SRS. Six years later, both the tumor volume and symptoms remained unchanged. Two of four patients with slight tumor progression had no additional treatment. One patient with tumor growth (estimated volume increase of 300%) had no new symptoms 6 years after SRS. The progression-free survival after SRS was 97.0%, 88.3%, 82.0%, and 82.0% at 1, 3, 5, and 10 years after SRS, respectively.

A larger SRS target volume, male sex, and a dumbbell-type tumor were associated with worse progression-free survival. Other variables (age, neurofibromatosis type 2, cystic or solid tumor, margin dose, and prior surgical resection) were not significantly associated with better progression-free survival.

Tumor Configuration

In our series, six of 33 patients (18.2%) had root tumors, 17 (51.5%) had ganglion tumors, and 10 (30.3%) had dumbbell tumors. Four of the 33 patients (12.1%) showed progression in the SRS volume, but none of the six patients with root tumors showed progression after radiosurgery. One of 17 patients (5.9%) with a ganglion tumor exhibited progression within the SRS volume, whereas three of 10 patients (30%) with dumbbell tumors did so. With respect to tumor location, the 5-year progression-free survivals of patients with the root, ganglion, and dumbbell tumors were 100%, 91.7%,

and 56.3%, respectively. Patients with root and ganglion tumors had a 1-, 5-, and 10-year progression-free survival of 100%, 93.8%, and 93.8%, respectively. Those with dumbbell tumors had 1-, 5-, and 10-year progression-free survival of 90.0%, 56.3%, and 56.3%, respectively. The dumbbell tumors were associated with lower rates of control (*p* = 0.0314), although an excellent response occurred in some patients. Because tumor volume is always important, we found in this series that a volume of less than 8.0 mL was significantly associated with better tumor control (*p* = 0.0007).

Neurologic Deficits

As in the case presented, all patients in our series had neurologic symptoms related to their trigeminal schwannoma. After SRS, 11 of the 33 patients (33.3%) had clinical improvement in symptoms or signs at a median of 9.5 months (range 2.7–88.5 months). One of 11 patients (9.1%) who had prior surgical removal exhibited improvement in neurologic symptoms and signs, whereas 10 of 22 patients (45.5%) who had no prior surgical removal showed significantly better improvement in neurologic symptoms and signs (*p* = 0.0367). Eight of 11 improved patients (72.7%) also had a reduction in their tumor volume. We noted improvement in oculomotor nerve function in one of two patients and in trochlear nerve function in one of two patients. Seven of 23 patients (30.4%) with trigeminal neuropathy improved, as did two of eight patients (25%) with facial pain. Five of nine patients with abducens nerve palsies improved while three of 33 patients (9.1%) had progression of their neurologic deficits. Two patients developed new trigeminal deficits (facial sensory loss and pain) and both had tumor progression. Ten of 22 patients (45.5%) who underwent primary SRS (no prior surgery) exhibited improvement of their neurologic symptoms **(Table 6.3)**.

Radiosurgical Morbidity

After SRS, two patients (6.1%) in our series developed suspected adverse radiation effects. Two patients with root-type trigeminal schwannomas (who received 13 Gy and 15 Gy at the tumor margin) showed increased peritumoral T2 signal changes. Neither patient developed new symptoms, and both were successfully treated with oral corticosteroids.

Trigeminal schwannomas are typically managed with surgical resection, and newer generation skull-base approaches allow better tumor exposure and require less brain retraction. Nonetheless, the surgical removal of a trigeminal schwannoma is still associated with the development of new neurologic deficits in 13 to 86% of patients and persistent, high rates of cerebrospinal fluid leakage.[22,23,27,28,36,37] Although total surgical removal is a reasonable goal for trigeminal schwannomas, less morbid alternative strategies warrant further evaluation. In addition, minimally invasive methods are needed when tumors recur. Additional therapeutic options for trigeminal schwannomas include fractionated external beam radiotherapy and SRS.[15,18,38]

Other Series

Pollock and colleagues[39] reported outcomes after gamma knife radiosurgery in 24 patients with nonvestibular schwannoma; 10 of these patients had trigeminal schwannomas. They reported tumor control in nine of these 10 patients with trigeminal schwannomas. Three developed new or worsening trigeminal dysfunction after SRS. Pan and associates[17] treated 56 patients with trigeminal schwannomas using gamma knife radiosurgery and reported a 93% tumor control rate at a mean follow-up of 68 months. Hasegawa and coworkers[15] treated 37 patients with trigeminal schwannomas and reported actuarial 5- and 10-year tumor control rates of 84% at a mean follow-up of 54 months.

In their series, Hasegawa and coworkers noted that larger tumors greater than or equal to 15 cm³ were more likely to progress despite SRS. In our present series, the 3-year progression-free survival by tumor volume of less than 8.0 cm³ and 8.0 cm³ or more were 94.4% and 64.3%, respectively. A target volume of less than 8.0 cm³ was significantly associated with better progression-free survival ($p = 0.0007$). Hasegawa and coworkers emphasized the importance of location. In their experience, all but one tumor located predominantly in the middle fossa was successfully treated. Tumor control was achieved significantly less frequently in patients whose tumors compressed the fourth ventricle ($p = 0.01$). In our current series, dumbbell tumors had a higher rate of later tumor progression, which is likely related to increased tumor volume. We suspect that root and ganglion tumors are recognized at an earlier stage.

Symptomatic Relief

In their series, Pan and associates[17] noted that 25% of patients experienced complete relief of symptoms, 44% had improved symptoms, 14% had no change in symptoms, and 9% had slight worsening of symptoms. Hasegawa and colleagues[15] reported that 40% of their patients noted improvement in their symptoms. One third of our patients exhibited improvement in neurologic symptoms and 58% had no change. Three patients (9.1%) had delayed worsening of neurologic function and two of these developed facial anesthesia and facial pain due to tumor progression. Ten of 22 patients (45.5%) who underwent SRS for initial management had improvement in neurologic symptoms, whereas 10 who underwent initial surgical removal had no improvement in neurologic symptoms after SRS. Patients with no prior resection were more likely to improve. We noted that associated trochlear or abducens nerve dysfunction improved in approximately half of affected patients.

Conclusion

Patients who have smaller volume trigeminal schwannomas are ideal candidates for radiosurgery as an alternative to surgical resection. Larger dumbbell-shaped tumors may benefit from a combined approach of both resection and radiosurgery for any residual tumor. The majority of patients with trigeminal schwannomas can be expected to have a good neurologic outcome with the available treatment approaches.

Management of Trigeminal Schwannoma: Microsurgical Removal vs. Radiosurgery

Takeshi Kawase

The improvement in surgical techniques for removing trigeminal schwannomas may be one of the most prominent recent advancements in neurosurgery because it allows us to understand the microsurgical anatomy of the meninges of the parasellar compartment and the tumor location.[19,40] One characteristic of a trigeminal schwannoma is its extension into multiple fossae, namely the middle and posterior fossae through Meckel's cave.[8] It seldom extends into the cavernous sinus, however, and can be excised with a less invasive technique without exposing the temporal lobe and the cavernous sinus, as illustrated in Gragnaniello and Al-Mefty's section.

Even with its complicated location, the tumor is mostly separated from the cavernous sinus by a thickened inner layer, and any injury to ocular function can be prevented by careful preservation of the membrane. The trunk of the trigeminal nerve is preserved, leading to mild and acceptable postoperative facial hypesthesia.[3,8,41] Therefore, the gross total removal of a trigeminal schwannoma can be done less invasively than for acoustic tumors, which do not have such a membrane between the tumor and the cranial nerve VII–VIII complex. Complete surgical excision of a trigeminal schwannoma after radiosurgery, however, is more difficult because of the tumor's adhesion to the surrounding structures, as shown in one of our patients **(Fig. 6.9)**.

The golden standard of treatment for symptomatic benign tumors is total surgical removal, if it can be done with minimal neurologic deficit. This standard might not change even with the development of radiosurgery. Therefore, surgical removal should be the first choice, with radiosurgery reserved for cases of incomplete surgical removal or for elderly patients who do not have surgical indications. Asymptomatic or small tumors found incidentally can be observed without treatment.

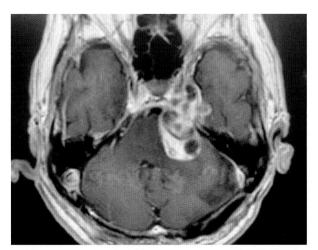
a

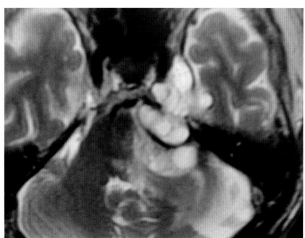
b

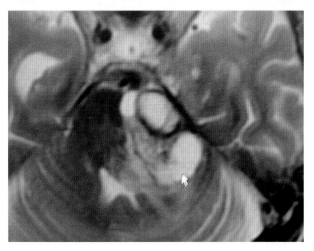
c

Fig. 6.9a–c **(a)** An example of a trigeminal schwannoma that regrew after treatment through surgery and with the gamma knife. The MRI with gadolinium enhancement shows a dumbbell-shaped tumor. The patient had undergone previous surgery through the pterional approach to remove the parasellar part, and the portion in the posterior fossa was treated with the gamma knife. **(b)** The T2-weighted MRI shows perifocal edema in the brainstem. **(c)** The postoperative MRI after the anterior petrosal approach. The portion in the middle fossa was removed, but the posterior fossa tumor (*white arrow*) could not be removed because of severe adhesion to the brainstem.

There are three surgical approaches to trigeminal schwannomas: Dolenc's approach, the anterior petrosal approach, and the zygomatic petrosal approach.[49] I must add a comment about the illustrative surgical technique to simplify the selection of the surgical approach.[51] Dolenc's approach might have an advantage for tumors having a major part in the middle fossa, or for dumbbell tumors having a wide opening of Meckel's cave, because tumor excision can take place through the widened Meckel's cave without incision of the tentorium (**Fig. 6.6**).[3] In contrast, the anterior petrosal approach has an advantage for hourglass-shaped tumors with minimal widening of Meckel's cave. Opening of the orbit and superior orbital fissure, therefore, might not be necessary if the tumor can be accessed more subtemporally with the anterior petrosal approach. Such a combined approach (the zygomatic petrosal approach) could be useful for a huge dumbbell tumor extending into three fossae, the middle, posterior, and infratemporal fossae.

References

1. Majoie CB, Hulsmans FJ, Castelijns JA, et al. Primary nerve-sheath tumours of the trigeminal nerve: clinical and MRI findings. Neuroradiology 1999;41:100–108

2. Al-Mefty O. Skull base: zygomatic approach. Neurosurgery 1986;19:674–675

3. Al-Mefty O, Ayoubi S, Gaber E. Trigeminal schwannomas: removal of dumbbell-shaped tumors through the expanded Meckel cave and outcomes of cranial nerve function. J Neurosurg 2002;96:453–463

4. Day JD, Fukushima T. The surgical management of trigeminal neuromas. Neurosurgery 1998;42:233–240, discussion 240–241

5. Gwak HS, Hwang SK, Paek SH, Kim DG, Jung HW. Long-term outcome of trigeminal neurinomas with modified classification focusing on petrous erosion. Surg Neurol 2003;60:39–48, discussion 48

6. Taha JM, Tew JM Jr, van Loveren HR, Keller JT, el-Kalliny M. Comparison of conventional and skull base surgical approaches for the excision of trigeminal neurinomas. J Neurosurg 1995;82:719–725

7. Samii M, Migliori MM, Tatagiba M, Babu R. Surgical treatment of trigeminal schwannomas. J Neurosurg 1995;82:711–718

8. Yoshida K, Kawase T. Trigeminal neurinomas extending into multiple fossae: surgical methods and review of the literature. J Neurosurg 1999;91:202–211

9. Dolenc VV. Frontotemporal epidural approach to trigeminal neurinomas. Acta Neurochir (Wien) 1994;130:55–65

10. Pamir MN, Peker S, Bayrakli F, Kiliç T, Ozek MM. Surgical treatment of trigeminal schwannomas. Neurosurg Rev 2007;30:329–337, discussion 337

11. Zhou LF, Mao Y, Zhang R. Surgical treatment of dumbbell-shaped neurinomas: report of an experience with 57 cases in a single hospital. Surg Neurol 2007;68:594–602

12. Moffat D, De R, Hardy D, Moumoulidis I. Surgical management of trigeminal neuromas: a report of eight cases. J Laryngol Otol 2006;120:631–637

13. Sarma S, Sekhar LN, Schessel DA. Nonvestibular schwannomas of the brain: a 7-year experience. Neurosurgery 2002;50:437–448, discussion 438–439

14. Mariniello G, Cappabianca P, Buonamassa S, de Divitiis E. Surgical treatment of intracavernous trigeminal schwannomas via a fronto-temporal epidural approach. Clin Neurol Neurosurg 2004;106:104–109

15. Hasegawa T, Kida Y, Yoshimoto M, Koike J. Trigeminal schwannomas: results of gamma knife surgery in 37 cases. J Neurosurg 2007;106:18–23

16. Phi JH, Paek SH, Chung HT, et al. Gamma knife surgery and trigeminal schwannoma: is it possible to preserve cranial nerve function? J Neurosurg 2007;107:727–732

17. Pan L, Wang EM, Zhang N, et al. Long-term results of Leksell gamma knife surgery for trigeminal schwannomas. J Neurosurg 2005;102(Suppl):220–224

18. Huang CF, Kondziolka D, Flickinger JC, Lunsford LD. Stereotactic radiosurgery for trigeminal schwannomas. Neurosurgery 1999;45:11–16, discussion 16

19. Nettel B, Niranjan A, Martin JJ, et al. Gamma knife radiosurgery for trigeminal schwannomas. Surg Neurol 2004;62:435–444, discussion 444–446

20. Morita A, Coffey RJ, Foote RL, Schiff D, Gorman D. Risk of injury to cranial nerves after gamma knife radiosurgery for skull base meningiomas: experience in 88 patients. J Neurosurg 1999;90:42–49

21. de Benedittis G, Bernasconi V, Ettorre G. Tumours of the fifth cranial nerve. Acta Neurochir (Wien) 1977;38:37–64

22. Goel A, Muzumdar D, Raman C. Trigeminal neuroma: analysis of surgical experience with 73 cases. Neurosurgery 2003;52:783–790, discussion 790

23. McCormick PC, Bello JA, Post KD. Trigeminal schwannoma. Surgical series of 14 cases with review of the literature. J Neurosurg 1988;69:850–860

24. Pollack IF, Sekhar LN, Jannetta PJ, Janecka IP. Neurilemomas of the trigeminal nerve. J Neurosurg 1989;70:737–745

25. Yasui T, Hakuba A, Kim SH, Nishimura S. Trigeminal neurinomas: operative approach in eight cases. J Neurosurg 1989;71:506–511

26. Kano H, Niranjan A, Kondziolka D, Flickinger JC, Dade Lunsford L. Stereotactic radiosurgery for trigeminal schwannoma: tumor control and functional preservation. Clinical article. J Neurosurg 2009;110:553–558

27. Taha JM, Tew JM Jr, van Loveren HR, Keller JT, el-Kalliny M. Comparison of conventional and skull base surgical approaches for the excision of trigeminal neurinomas. J Neurosurg 1995;82:719–725

28. Al-Mefty O, Ayoubi S, Gaber E. Trigeminal schwannomas: removal of dumbbell-shaped tumors through the expanded Meckel cave and outcomes of cranial nerve function. J Neurosurg 2002;96:453–463

29. Andrews DW, Suarez O, Goldman HW, et al. Stereotactic radiosurgery and fractionated stereotactic radiotherapy for the treatment of acoustic schwannomas: comparative observations of 125 patients treated at one institution. Int J Radiat Oncol Biol Phys 2001;50:1265–1278

30. Flickinger JC, Kondziolka D, Niranjan A, Lunsford LD. Results of acoustic neuroma radiosurgery: an analysis of 5 years' experience using current methods. J Neurosurg 2001;94:1–6; comment in J Neurosurg 2001;94:141–142

31. Flickinger JC, Kondziolka D, Pollock BE, Lunsford LD. Evolution in technique for vestibular schwannoma radiosurgery and

effect on outcome. Int J Radiat Oncol Biol Phys 1996;36:275–280

32. Niranjan A, Lunsford LD, Flickinger JC, Maitz A, Kondziolka D. Dose reduction improves hearing preservation rates after intra-canalicular acoustic tumor radiosurgery. Neurosurgery 1999;45:753–762, discussion 762–765

33. Régis J, Pellet W, Delsanti C, et al. Functional outcome after gamma knife surgery or microsurgery for vestibular schwannomas. J Neurosurg 2002;97:1091–1100

34. Suh JH, Barnett GH, Sohn JW, Kupelian PA, Cohen BH. Results of linear accelerator-based stereotactic radiosurgery for recurrent and newly diagnosed acoustic neuromas. Int J Cancer 2000;90:145–151

35. Lesoin F, Rousseaux M, Villette L, et al. Neurinomas of the trigeminal nerve. Acta Neurochir (Wien) 1986;82:118–122

36. Eisenberg MB, Al-Mefty O, DeMonte F, Burson GT. Benign non-meningeal tumors of the cavernous sinus. Neurosurgery 1999;44:949–954, discussion 954–955

37. Samii M, Babu RP, Tatagiba M, Sepehrnia A. Surgical treatment of jugular foramen schwannomas. J Neurosurg 1995;82:924–932

38. Zabel A, Debus J, Thilmann C, Schlegel W, Wannenmacher M. Management of benign cranial nonacoustic schwannomas by fractionated stereotactic radiotherapy. Int J Cancer 2001;96:356–362

39. Pollock BE, Foote RL, Stafford SL. Stereotactic radiosurgery: the preferred management for patients with nonvestibular schwannomas? Int J Radiat Oncol Biol Phys 2002;52:1002–1007

40. Kawase T, van Loveren H, Keller JT, Tew JM. Meningeal architecture of the cavernous sinus: clinical and surgical implications. Neurosurgery 1996;39:527–534, discussion 534–536

41. Muto J, Kawase T, Yoshida K. Meckel's cave tumors: relation to the meninges and minimally invasive approaches for surgery: anatomic and clinical studies. Neurosurgery 2010;67(3, Suppl Operative):ons291–ons298, discussion ons298–ons299

Chapter 7

Surgical Removal of a Pituitary Macroadenoma: Endoscopic vs. Microscopic

Case

A 45-year-old man presented with bitemporal hemianopsia and a nonsecreting pituitary tumor.

Participants

Is the Endoscope Useful for Pituitary Tumor Surgery?: Atul Goel

Endoscopic Removal of a Pituitary Macroadenoma: John A. Jane, Jr., Stephen J. Monteith, and Michael S. McKisic

The Endonasal Combined Microscopic Endoscopic with Free Head Navigation Technique to Remove Pituitary Adenomas: Ossama Al-Mefty, Mohamad Abolfotoh, and Cristian Gragnaniello

Moderator: Surgical Removal of a Pituitary Macroadenoma: Endoscopic vs. Microscopic: Mario Ammirati

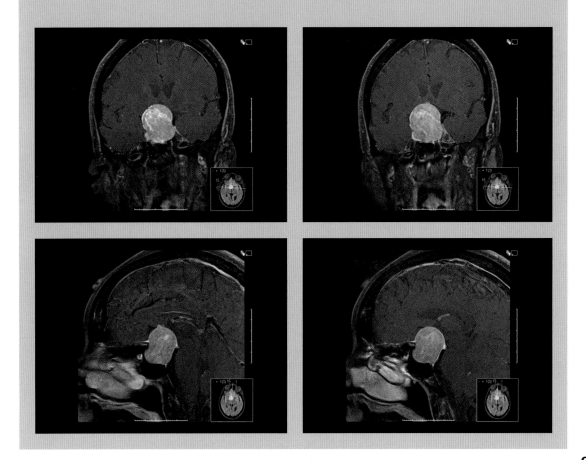

Is the Endoscope Useful for Pituitary Tumor Surgery?

Atul Goel

The introduction of the microscope drastically changed the entire visual aspect of pituitary tumor surgery. Good depth lighting and the ability to work with comfort and ease have made it possible for the surgeon to control the conduct of the entire operation. Thus, pituitary tumor surgery has become one of the most results-oriented neurosurgical procedures. After successful surgery, there can be a dramatic and immediate improvement in vision, a reversal of acromegaly and cushingoid features, and other similar results.

Giant pituitary tumors are among the most complex neurosurgical challenges. Despite their histologically benign nature, some of these tumors grow to a massive size. Because of the invasiveness and size of such tumors, surgical resection is difficult and, in some cases, dangerous.[1] But because the results of radiation therapy are inconsistent, surgery forms the mainstay of treatment.

The diagnosis of a pituitary tumor usually can be made on the basis of clinical features and their classic anatomic extensions seen on imaging.[2] Surgical biopsy for histological confirmation has no relevance. Small or partial resections can be dangerous, as bleeding from the residual tumor is frequent, an event defined earlier as "postoperative pituitary apoplexy."[1] Successful radical resection of the tumor can rapidly dispel symptoms and lead to an excellent long-term clinical outcome. After such resection, the recurrence rate of these tumors is low.

Anatomic Grading of Giant Pituitary Tumors[3,4]

Giant pituitary tumors have a maximum transverse dimension of at least 3 cm and can be divided into four grades:

Grade I tumors are located within the confines of the sella, remain underneath the superiorly elevated diaphragma sellae, and do not invade the cavernous sinus (**Fig. 7.1**). The diaphragma sellae is stretched superiorly, sometimes even beyond the corpus callosum, and it covers the entire superior dome of the pituitary tumor. Although the suprasellar extension of the tumor is intracranial, it is referred to as subdiaphragmatic.

Grade II pituitary tumors invade the cavernous sinus (**Fig. 7.2**). There is no exact anatomic or histological reason why some tumors extend into the cavernous sinus and some do not. Although several studies discuss the issue, the nature of the membranes that demarcate the cavernous sinus from the pituitary gland remains controversial.[5] Transgression of the lateral dural wall of the cavernous sinus has not been reported.

Grade III pituitary tumors elevate the roof of the cavernous sinus superiorly (**Fig. 7.3**).

Grade IV pituitary tumors transgress the boundary of the diaphragma sellae and enter the subarachnoid spaces of the brain (**Fig. 7.4**). These tumors encase the arteries of the circle of Willis and are considered aggressive because of their anatomic, clinical, and surgical behavior.

The Use of the Endoscope in Pituitary Tumor Surgery

In use for quite some time now, endoscopes are currently being recommended for several neurosurgical operations. The superiority of the endoscope in treating tumors of the

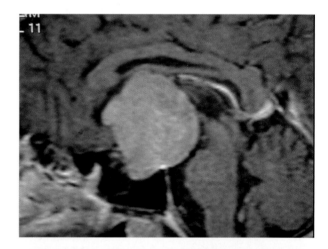

a

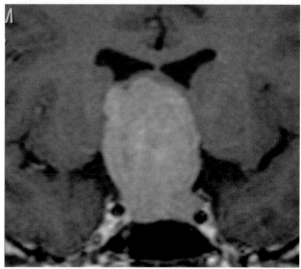

b

Fig. 7.1a,b **(a)** Contrast-enhanced sagittal magnetic resonance imaging (MRI) of a grade I pituitary tumor. The diaphragma sellae is elevated by the giant tumor. **(b)** Coronal image of the tumor.

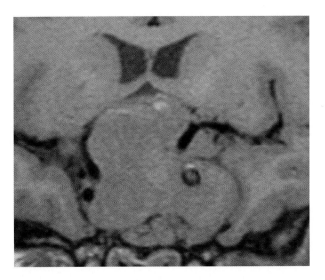

Fig. 7.2 Coronal MRI of a grade II tumor. The cavernous sinus is invaded by the tumor.

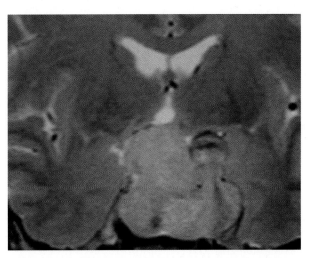

Fig. 7.3 Coronal MRI of a grade III pituitary tumor. The roof of the cavernous sinus is elevated by the tumor, which is also under the superiorly elevated diaphragma sellae.

paranasal sinus and clival regions and medial extradural cavernous sinus tumors is now accepted. The campaign in favor of the use of the endoscope has been quite intense. Even the general population has come to know this tool, and some patients even demand that their pituitary surgery be done with an endoscope. Several surgeons who are accustomed to using the microscope for pituitary tumor surgeries have acknowledged the value of the endoscope.

Personal Technique for the Presented Case

The tumor in the presented case is a large, but not giant, grade I pituitary tumor. The sella is large and ballooned, but

the tumor does not invade the cavernous sinus. The tumor appears to be of a standard consistency and vascularity.

My experience with pituitary tumor operations exceeds 1,700 cases over a 14-year period, and I prefer to do all pituitary tumor surgeries using the sublabial transseptal and transsphenoidal operative route with a microscope. I find the use of an endoscope, even as an assistant tool to the microscope, redundant and unnecessary.

Although the nostril is currently the route preferred by some surgeons, I do not like to do the operation through this route, as it limits the exposure and restricts the ability to open the speculum widely. Furthermore, damage to the hair follicles and the skin of the nostril can be quite painful for the patient. The sublabial approach is a cleaner avenue, is midline, and provides sufficient exposure to open the

a

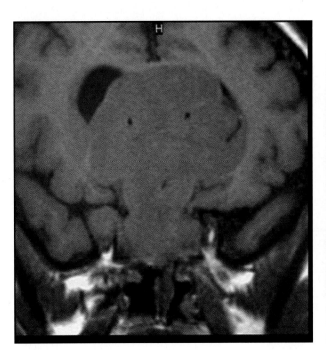

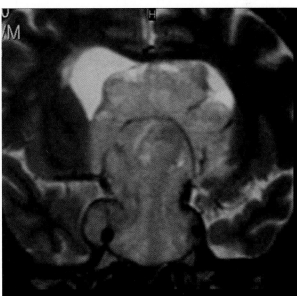

b

Fig. 7.4a,b **(a)** T1-weighted MRI of a grade IV tumor. Both anterior cerebral arteries are encased by the tumor. **(b)** T2-weighted image showing encasement of the anterior cerebral artery complex.

speculum widely. I do not use coagulation equipment on the operating table, and have found that coagulation can be entirely avoided in pituitary tumor surgery. Although this technique does create some bleeding in the operative field, it can easily be handled with the microscope. On the other hand, if one uses an endoscope, extensive mucosal coagulation may be necessary to provide a blood-free field, which prevents fogging of the endoscope lens.

I expose the anterior sellar wall and then resect it widely, initially using a chisel and then rongeurs. After the wall is open, I make a cruciate incision in the dura. The tumor is then progressively debulked. These tumors are usually soft, friable, and necrotic, which makes debulking safe and relatively quick. Despite the occasional high vascularity of these lesions, it is relatively easy to control bleeding with hemostats like Gelfoam and Surgicel, and intratumoral coagulation can be avoided.

Tumor resection is begun from the sella in the midline, and is followed by resection in the lateral aspect of the sella. It then continues superiorly. As resection continues, the tumor progressively falls and comes down into the operative field. The Valsalva maneuver is used during surgery to facilitate descent of the tumor mass, but to get the tumor into the field inferiorly requires experience and confidence. Frequently, the diaphragma sellae has to be retracted superiorly to expose the tumor within its folds. In my experience with pituitary tumors of grades I to III, the tumor under the diaphragma sellae can invariably be resected. Although some tumors are relatively firm and even fibrous and "elastic," they can always be progressively debulked, brought inferiorly into the operative field, and resected.

In our early experience, to resect the suprasellar component of the tumor, we preferred to remove the bone of the tuberculum sellae and planum sphenoidale. However, we have realized that removing this bone is necessary for only a minority of patients and can frequently be avoided even in patients with much larger tumors than that in the presented case. The use of the endoscope to view the suprasellar component is unnecessary, as the diaphragma sellae should be viewed anteriorly in the surgical field at the end of tumor resection. The use of curettes to resect the tumor in the lateral parts of the sella is generally satisfactory if the surgeon has sufficient experience in pituitary tumor surgery. The use of the endoscope for lateral visualization can be helpful but is not mandatory.

Some large tumors can be extensively vascular. In such cases, tumor resection has to be done during profuse bleeding. In such cases, it is much safer and more comfortable to use a microscope rather than an endoscope. On some occasions, there can be profuse bleeding from the cavernous sinus. With experience it may be possible to control such bleeding with an endoscope, but surgery under the microscope can be much more controlled in such a situation. Reconstruction of the region after surgery is rather straightforward when the conventional microneurosurgical approach is used, and the cerebrospinal fistula rate in most of the reported series is less than 2%.

Resecting the tumor within the confines of the cavernous sinus is a relatively complex technique. The anterior loop and the horizontal portion of the carotid artery can be exposed with a microscope and appropriate angulation of the speculum; however, working around the carotid artery depends mainly on the consistency of the tumor. In some cases, tumors that extend into the cavernous sinus are softer and more necrotic than those with no cavernous sinus extension. In these cases, the tumor can be resected safely and radically. However, whether to resect the section of tumor in the cavernous sinus in patients with nonfunctional pituitary tumors is controversial. Even in patients with a functioning pituitary tumor, whether to resect the cavernous sinus portion is controversial. In desperate situations in patients with functioning pituitary tumors, a lateral, basal, subtemporal extradural route can be used to resect this portion of the tumor. The advantages of using the endoscope to radically resect the portion of tumor within the cavernous sinus are yet to be evaluated and confirmed.

Apart from providing good images of the lateral aspect of the sella and optic nerves as well as the carotid artery bulge in the sphenoid sinus, there are no significant advantages in using an endoscope for pituitary tumor surgery. The need for extensive mucosal coagulation and the limitations in having to control bleeding can severely limit the ease of tumor resection with the endoscope.

Endoscopic Removal of Pituitary Macroadenoma

John A. Jane, Jr., Stephen J. Monteith, and Michael S. McKisic

Historical Perspectives on the Endoscopic Approach

The ancient Egyptians were the first to recognize the possibility of accessing the brain endonasally without dis-figurement. Computed tomography scans of mummies and archaeological findings confirm that the Egyptians used specialized instruments to perform the earliest transsphenoidal approaches, albeit postmortem.[6] It would be several thousand years before Schloffer, Von Eiselberg, and Kocher would carry out, in 1907, the earliest transsphenoidal surgeries to access a pathological lesion.[7] The sublabial transseptal approach was used by Cushing[8] in 1909 and was less traumatic than the endonasal and sublabial approaches introduced in 1910 by Hirsch and Halstead, respectively.[7] Cushing abandoned the approach, however, in part because of inadequate illumination, but in the late 1960s, Hardy overcame this obstacle by making use of the operating microscope. Since then, approaches have been modified with improved visualization for the surgeon and decreased postoperative discomfort for the patient.

The approaches done with the microscope essentially differ according to where the mucosal incision is made (sublabial, hemitransfixion, Killian, or direct sphenoidotomy) and the width of the sellar exposure each provides. Whereas the sublabial approach provides the widest exposure, it also requires the most soft tissue and mucoperichondrial dissection. By contrast, the direct endonasal sphenoidotomy requires no anterior septal dissection but has the narrowest exposure. The endonasal approaches decrease both the postoperative discomfort for the patient and the chances of anterior septal complications. However, the downsides of more direct approaches include diminished working room, a more limited sellar exposure, and an approach from an angled trajectory.[7]

Evolution of the Endoscopic Approach

The role of the endoscope has evolved over time. Initial reports describe the use of the endoscope as an adjunct to the standard approach with the microscope.[9,10] For example, the endoscope could be used for the anterior sphenoidotomy before introducing the microscope, or it could be simply introduced at the end of resection to inspect for residual tumor. The pure endoscopic transsphenoidal approach was introduced by Jho and Carrau[11] in the late 1990s, with modifications by Kassam and colleagues[12,13] that allowed the scope of the approach to expand to surgery for complex skull-base tumors. Other pioneers include Cappabianca and de Divitiis[14,15] in Italy, as well as Frank, Pasquini, Locatelli, and others who have made significant contributions to the development of endoscopic techniques and transsphenoidal surgery.[16–18]

Advantages of the Endoscopic Approach

The primary advantages of the endoscopic removal of adenomas lie in the panoramic field of view and the ability to attain an extreme close-up point of view. During the approach, the panoramic view allows superior visualization of the sphenoid anatomy. Unlike the approach with the microscope, in which a localization X-ray is necessary after speculum placement, image guidance is rarely needed during a standard endoscopic approach, which decreases the dose of radiation to both the patient and operator. Anatomic landmarks are clearly identifiable, even by the novice endoscopist, which increases the surgeon's confi-

dence and decreases the learning curve.[19] In the case of a repeated operation, distorted anatomy can be more clearly identified, and the existence of an operative corridor facilitates surgery with less risk of complications.[7,15] In addition, because there is no submucosal dissection, nasal packs are not routinely used, which improves overall patient satisfaction with the procedure.

Most significantly, the panoramic view allows a greater portion, if not all, of an adenoma to be removed under direct visualization. Tumor extensions toward the cavernous sinus walls and the suprasellar portions, which are often removed blindly by feel during an approach with the microscope, are instead removed with certainty. The magnification allows excellent visualization of the interface between the tumor and pituitary gland, potentially facilitating adenomectomy with minimal disruption of the surrounding tissues.[15] With the wide-angle lens view of the zero-degree endoscope and the use of angled endoscopes, the endoscopic surgeon can see around corners, which is not possible with the microscope.[16] This ability can be particularly helpful in patients with a macroadenoma that extends into the cavernous sinus or suprasellar space.[17] For tumors that invade the cavernous sinus, the endoscope affords a wider view when compared with the microscope and unrivaled maneuverability in the lateral compartment of the cavernous sinus.[17] Moreover, only the endoscope allows the surgeon to use the diving technique described by Locatelli and colleagues.[18] Intrasellar hydroscopy allows for more complete assessment of the surgical bed, during and after resection, with improved hemostasis. Blind curettage is therefore minimized and a larger extent of the tumor can be removed under direct visualization.

Disadvantages of the Endoscopic Approach and Strategies for Their Management

Despite its advantages, there are several disadvantages of the endoscopic approach, many of which can be overcome with training and experience. Neurosurgeons are comfortable using the operating microscope and the three-dimensional view it provides. When using the endoscope, a new skill set with a different type of hand–eye coordination must be learned and practiced. Some surgeons find the two-dimensional view on a monitor challenging, particularly with regard to depth perception.[19,20] This problem can be partly overcome with the help of a skilled endoscopist as the assistant. Such an assistant can help the surgeon with opportune in-and-out movements of the camera to create an artificial perception of depth. This notion of the endoscope as part of a "clock gear" mechanism was aptly described by Cavallo and associates.[21] Each part of the system depends on the others. If one part fails then the whole system fails. In addition, proprioception allows the surgeon to perceive the location of an instrument in one hand as it relates to the instrument in the other. Because of the current constraints with rigid endoscopes, there is a slight "barrel distortion" effect at the edges of the field of view. When the endoscope cannot be repositioned, an angled scope can overcome these distortive effects so that the surgeon can examine the edges and beyond the resection bed.

The endoscope does occupy space within the operative field and can obstruct the free movement of surgical instruments. Whereas the operative field during an adenomectomy done with the microscope is occupied by two instruments (suction and the dissector), the endoscopic technique requires the surgical field to be occupied by an additional instrument—the endoscope itself. Therefore, there is less room to maneuver instruments, and the sphenoidotomy must be larger to allow a similar range for instrument movement. Furthermore, the approach with the microscope is facilitated by the use of a nasal speculum, which is not typically used during an endoscopic approach because it occupies a significant amount of space and creates a rigid avenue that is not conducive to the approach. Without a speculum, the nasal mucosa is placed at risk of injury when instruments are introduced and the surgeon has greater difficulty freely introducing instruments and performing precise dissection during the removal of microadenomas.

Case Presentation and Relevance to the Described Technique

The case presented is that of a 45-year-old man with a nonfunctioning pituitary macroadenoma causing bitemporal hemianopsia. The representative magnetic resonance imaging (MRI) shows a large macroadenoma with a suprasellar extension (**Fig. 7.5**). Coronal images show likely cavernous sinus involvement bilaterally. Therefore, a complete resection is unlikely regardless of whether an endoscope or microscope is used. The primary goal of surgery is to decompress the optic chiasm. Secondary goals are to remove enough of the tumor to prevent recurrence and to preserve pituitary function. Because the patient is relatively young, these goals require as thorough a removal of tumor as possible.

Surgical Technique

An in-depth discussion of the endoscopic surgical technique is presented elsewhere,[7] but the key steps are described herein. The patient is placed in a lawn-chair position with approximately 20 degrees of back elevation, and the head is placed on a horseshoe headrest. We have found that this position improves venous drainage and decreases bleeding. Image guidance is not routinely used for first-time transsphenoidal approaches (although fiducials are present in this case) unless the patient has a presellar or conchal sphenoid anatomy. We use a three-handed approach with a wide anterior sphenoidotomy and posterior septectomy. Both middle turbinates are lateralized but not resected. We

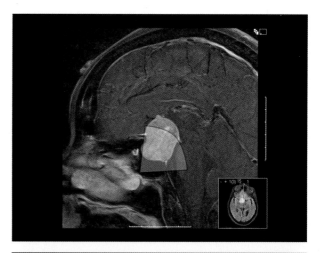

a

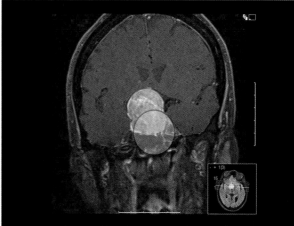

b

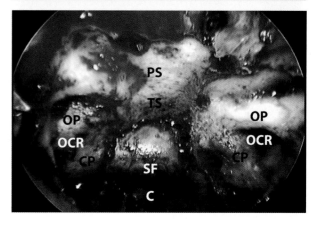

c

Fig. 7.5a–c **(a)** Sagittal view of the lesion with the endoscopic view superimposed in gray. **(b)** Coronal view of the lesion with the endoscopic view superimposed in gray. **(c)** Endoscopic photograph from within the sphenoid sinus of a different patient. C, clivus; CP, carotid protuberance; OCR, opticocarotid recess; OP, optic protuberance; PS, planum sphenoidale; SF, sellar floor; TS, tuberculum sellae.

would not advocate the placement of a lumbar drain in this patient because the tumor does not have an hourglass configuration. When the patient is at high risk of a cerebrospinal fluid leak (as in this case) and the sellar floor has been completely eroded by tumor (not likely in this case),

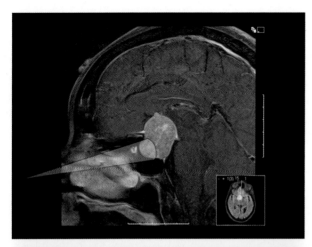

a

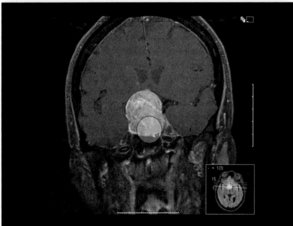

b

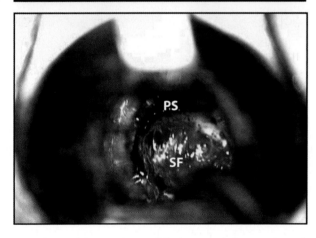

c

Fig. 7.6a–c **(a)** Sagittal view of the lesion with the view through the microscope superimposed in gray. **(b)** Coronal view of the lesion with the view through the microscope superimposed in gray. **(c)** Photograph through the microscope from within the sphenoid sinus of a different patient. PS, planum sphenoidale; SF, sellar floor.

landmarks with the pure microscopic approach **(Fig. 7.6)**, but with the endoscope, these landmarks are usually readily visible **(Fig. 7.5)**. In this patient, we would open the sellar floor to the limits of the cavernous sinus bilaterally. We would also remove the tuberculum and a small amount of the planum to facilitate visualization. The dura is opened with care so as not to disturb the underlying tumor capsule. For this access, a wide dural opening is essential; a narrow opening restricts the view into the sella and defeats the purpose of using the endoscope. Resection begins inferiorly, laterally, and then superiorly against the diaphragm. Care must be taken not to remove the superior portions of the tumor until the lateral portions against the cavernous sinus walls are resected. The endoscope is most helpful in this respect.[17]

On the preoperative MRI, the normal gland appears to be superior and along the right cavernous sinus wall **(Fig. 7.5a,b)**. The gland should be identified early during dissection and protected. Ideally with a soft tumor, the mass will come down into the operative field as resection progresses. The 30- and 45-degree scopes are also introduced to assess the completeness of resection along the cavernous sinus walls, diaphragm, and, in particular, along the junction of the cavernous sinus wall and diaphragm. The primary goal of surgery in this patient is chiasmatic decompression, which can be confirmed with confidence with the close-up view provided by the endoscope. If a cerebrospinal leak occurs, a fat graft is prepared and placed in the sella. This graft is tailored to the correct size and placed in the extradural plane, buttressed under any remaining sellar bone. A dural sealant is sprayed over the reconstruction with a powered sprayer and no packs are used. Patients are transferred to the ward (not to intensive care) with nasal decongestant sprays for 3 days, and given saline nasal sprays and sodium bicarbonate nasal rinses to be done at home for 6 weeks.

The main goal in this patient is to decompress the optic chiasm, preserve pituitary function, and prevent recurrence. Each of these goals can be accomplished with either the endoscope or the microscope. However, the panoramic view provided by the endoscope allows more of the tumor to be removed under direct visualization. Although a gross total resection may be possible, the size of the tumor and possible cavernous sinus involvement indicates that it is likely invasive. Therefore, the possibility of recurrence in this relatively young patient is real. Even with adequate visualization during surgery with the zero-degree and angled endoscopes, some residual cells are likely to remain even if the operative impression and immediate postoperative MRI indicate complete resection. Nevertheless, even if a gross total resection were accomplished, we would not move directly to gamma knife radiosurgery, particularly if the pituitary function had been preserved. If there is obvious cavernous sinus or bony invasion, however, and the patient had panhypopituitarism postoperatively, then we would have a lower threshold for early gamma knife treatment.

we prepare a nasoseptal flap for repairing the sella.[22] We would not raise a nasoseptal flap for this case.

We continue the sphenoidotomy until the key landmarks are identified and are clearly visible: the planum sphenoidale, optic protuberances, and opticocarotid recesses. We have often found it difficult to identify these

Future Directions

The technology of the endoscope has improved dramatically since its invention 200 years ago by Bozzini.[23] The size of the instruments and the associated degree of operative obstruction have decreased. In addition, high-definition endoscopes provide a very detailed, high-resolution image. Recently, with the introduction of three-dimensional endoscopes, we are poised for a new era in endoscopic pituitary surgery. Subjectively, improved depth perception and no increase in operative time have been reported by early adopters.[24] Although the quality of the images is not yet as high as the current technology allows, these endoscopes provide a three-dimensional (3D) view, which has been one of the major requests of experienced microscopic pituitary surgeons using the endoscopic approach. Whether the 3D endoscope improves patient outcomes remains to be determined.

Conclusion

The endoscopic approach provides an effective means to adequately resect a large macroadenoma like the one in this patient. The magnified, panoramic view of the surgical field minimizes blind curettage and maximizes the degree of tumor that is removed by direct sight. Technological advances will continue to push the endoscopic approach further. With regard to transsphenoidal pituitary surgery for macroadenomas, time will tell how long the microscopic-versus-endoscopic debate will continue.

The Endonasal Combined Microscopic Endoscopic with Free Head Navigation Technique to Remove Pituitary Adenomas

Ossama Al-Mefty, Mohamad Abolfotoh, and Cristian Gragnaniello

Pituitary surgery exemplifies the continuous refinement of surgical techniques. The transsphenoidal approach is the approach of choice to treat most pituitary adenomas, including the case presented here. The recent emphasis has been on minimally invasive surgery. The challenge in minimizing invasion lies in reducing postoperative complications and deficits, decreasing the length of hospital stays, and avoiding trauma to a healthy parenchyma while achieving the surgical goal. Continuous technical advancements have provided the means to overcome this challenge.[7,25–30]

Although endoscopic and microscopic techniques are presented in the literature as alternative and frequently competitive approaches, we believe they are complementary and that the use of both will improve our surgical technique to achieve the true meaning of minimal invasiveness. The combined use of both the endoscope and microscope in pituitary surgery was first described by Bushe and Halves[31] in 1978. The application of neuronavigation with free head movement enhances the benefits of these techniques, and has been described by Al-Mefty and colleagues.[32]

Description of the Technique

Patients should have a comprehensive preoperative clinical evaluation, including neurologic, neuro-ophthalmologic, and neuroendocrinologic evaluation. This should include measurement of the diluted prolactin level to avoid surgery in patients who can be treated medically. MRI accurately delineates the sellar region and surrounding structures, including the optic chiasm, the cavernous sinuses, and the carotid arteries. It shows the tumor extensions and can define the proper avenue for the transsphenoidal approach **(Fig. 7.7)**.

Computed tomography (CT) scans are obtained to define the anatomy and pneumatization of the sphenoid sinus along with its septation and keel, the shape of the sella, and the planum sphenoidale, and to evaluate the intercarotid distance. This anatomic imaging is especially advantageous during the procedure when the CT scans are merged with the MRI in the navigation system.

The patient is placed in the supine position and the patient's trunk is slightly elevated, with the head above the level of the heart to facilitate venous drainage. The patient's head is placed on a gel donut. Head fixation is not used, which allows the surgeon to move the patient's head intraoperatively to obtain the best angle and view. The head is positioned in a manner that best exposes the anatomy of the lesion; it is kept in a neutral position and slightly rotated to the surgeon's side. The nasal cavities, face, and nose are washed with Betadine, and a surgical sponge is placed in the retropharynx. The patient's abdomen is also prepared for fat harvesting if it is needed for closure.

Before the patient is draped in sterile fashion, the registration mask and its communication unit (Stryker, Kalamazoo, MI) are applied to the patient's face. This mask has an adhesive strip and leads on the surface, which allows a very simple and accurate registration phase when the system is

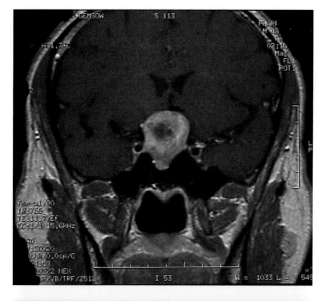

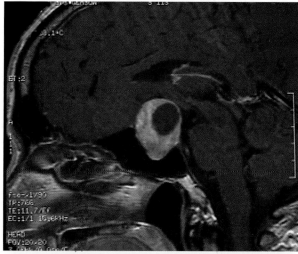

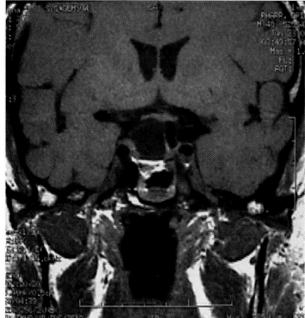

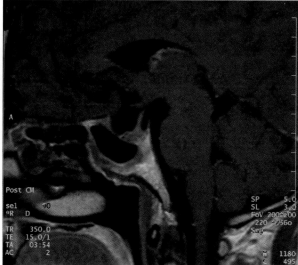

Fig. 7.7a–d Images of the illustrative case operated on with the combined technique. **(a,b)** Preoperative coronal and sagittal views depicting a large cystic pituitary adenoma with a suprasellar extension and compression of the optic chiasm and third ventricle. **(c,d)** Postoperative MRIs showing complete removal.

turned on **(Fig. 7.8)**. Once the patient is registered according to the MRI and the CT images, a tracker is mounted on the endoscope rod. The tip of the rod is used as a tool for navigation and reveals its exact position and projection on the screen. The microscope is then brought in and calibrated to make its focal point navigable **(Fig. 7.9)**.

Likewise, surgical instruments, dissectors, and curettes can be registered and calibrated, which ensures the surgeon's control over the position of the tools during surgery and, most importantly, tumor dissection. This system provides a major advantage for surgery because it avoids fluoroscopy, confirms the midline, gives positions in three planes, and shortens the anesthesia time. Neuronavigation is particularly useful for preventing injuries to eloquent structures, when there is a narrow distance between the carotid arteries, when the sphenoid sinus is poorly pneu-

matized, and in cases of recurrence or in patients who underwent previous nasal surgery, in whom the anatomy is distorted either by the lesion or scar tissue. The paramount advantage is the free head movement, which allows additional visualization by extension, flexion, or rotation to either side while maintaining accurate navigation.

The operation begins with a zero-degree endoscope advanced through the nostril to explore the narrow corridor between the middle turbinate and the septum with a close-up view. Under endoscopic visualization, the surgeon must note the available anatomic landmarks, especially in patients who have undergone previous surgery either for a pathological process of the septum or a recurrent tumor. The endoscope, whose position is confirmed by the navigation system, guides the surgeon in identifying the nasal anatomy when it has been distorted by previous surgery.

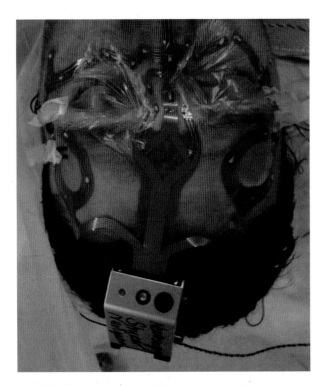

Fig. 7.8 The registration mask and its communication unit applied to the patient's prepared head, which is not fixed in the three-point holder.

The middle turbinate is recognized and followed until the anterior sphenoid wall is reached and the sphenoid ostium becomes visible as the camera moves upward. There is no attempt or need to resect the middle turbinate (**Fig. 7.10**).

A slim nasal speculum is placed to compress the middle turbinate laterally, the microscope is brought in, and a short incision divides the mucosa, which covers the junction of the bony septum and the rostrum. With a simple maneuver, the mucosa is dissected laterally and the septum is displaced to the other side to expose the whole rostrum, maintaining the integrity of the nasal cavity on the opposite side. This maneuver has the same effect as tunneling under the mucosa during the submucosal approach,

but with less dissection, less bleeding, and direct exposure. The rostrum is removed in one piece with a chisel so that it can be used for closure.

After the sinus is identified, the images are reviewed again to note the compartmentalization of the sinus and its pneumatization. Although the navigation system helps surgeons determine the best trajectory to the sellar floor, they must recognize anatomic landmarks in the sphenoid sinus, such as the carotid prominences, opticocarotid recesses, the clival indentation, the posterior and lateral walls of the sinus, and the floor of the sella. In particular, neuronavigation is of great help when addressing the septa of the sphenoid sinus, which, even if seen on the midline when the rostrum is removed, in most cases leads more laterally to an implant on the carotid prominence, with a consequent risk of injury to the artery.

The opening of the sella depends on its thickness. When it is thick, it can be approached with a chisel; when it is fine, it can be approached with a curette. Micro-Doppler is used before the dura is opened to ascertain the distance from the carotid and confirm the absence of an aneurysm. The dura is opened in an X shape. The approach to the dura is contingent on the type of lesion.

Removal of the lesion should progress with suction and microcurettes at the base and underside of the lesion, thus avoiding a cylinder coring of the tumor and allowing its downward delivery. Pituitary lesions almost always have a plane of dissection between them and the diaphragm. The endoscope with a 30-degree lens is then used to locate any lateral fragments.

Finally, closure depends on the size of the lesion and whether cerebrospinal fluid has been encountered during surgery. Closure might make use of fat harvested from the abdomen, which is then carefully placed into the sella and supported with fibrin glue. When cerebrospinal fluid has not been encountered, the fat is not necessary. As an additional precaution, fibrin glue can be used in the sella to stop microbleeding. The floor of the sella is reconstructed by using the rostrum that was removed during the opening. The speculum is removed, the rostrum is pushed into

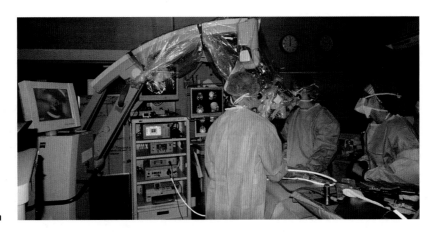

Fig. 7.9a,b **(a)** The setup of the operating room, with anesthesia equipment at the foot of the table facing the endoscopic navigation screen in relation to the position of the microscope.

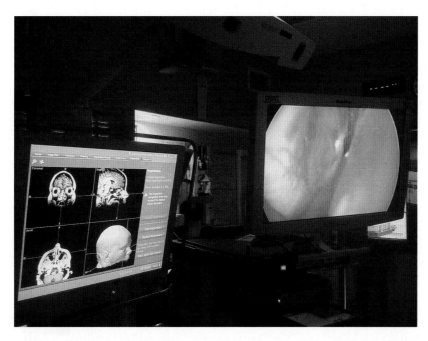

Fig. 7.9a,b (*continued*)   **(b)** The endoscope is advanced into the nasal cavity to identify the passage anatomically while confirming the location with navigation on a tracker-mounted endoscope.

the midline from the other nostril, and the small mucosal flap is reflected over the septum. The endoscope is placed once more to ensure that the mucosa is spread with no disruption of the normal anatomy; therefore, there is usually no need to pack the nasal cavity. Patients usually leave the hospital 1 or 2 days after surgery, depending on whether they need to be monitored for diabetes insipidus.

Conclusion

For many years, the transsphenoidal route has been the preferred approach to lesions of the sellar floor and upper clivus.[33,34] Several technical modifications have been introduced to minimize local complications, including the use of fluoroscopy, an endonasal route,[35] navigation, and en-

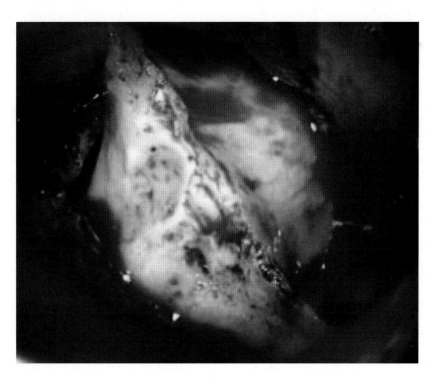

Fig. 7.10   The anterior wall of the sphenoid sinus is exposed with minimal disruption of the nasal mucosa by making a 1-cm flap at the keel and displacing the septum to the other side with its intact nostril mucosa.

doscopy.[9,26,28,31,36–42] The ongoing argument between supporters of the microscope and endoscope used alone most often overlook the fact that both scopes have undeniable advantages and disadvantages.[7,43] Our opinion is that a neurosurgeon must be a master of both techniques to choose the one most appropriate for a given phase of the operation.[36] A neurosurgeon must be ready at any moment to shift from binocular vision to that of the monitor. The endoscope grants surgeons a close-up view of the lesion and, with the use of angulated lenses, they can inspect areas away from the midline to identify fragments, which often sit in the cavernous sinus.[44] The visual plane, the "barrel effect" present at the margins of the image, and the difficulties of using the endoscope in the presence of sustained bleeding are still unsolved problems.[28,29,37]

The navigation system calibrates the focal point of the microscope, the tip of the endoscope, and the surgical instruments, thereby allowing the surgeon to know, in each instant of the procedure, the exact position of the instrument and its direction related to the structures at risk of injury, especially during the approach and tumor removal.[45] The registration mask is a great adjunct for navigating the facial skeleton because of its easy and intuitive use. Furthermore, the possibility of merging CT and MRI images is a significant advantage.

We believe the maneuver of overturning the mucosal flap with septal displacement adds significantly to the general outcome of the procedure.[39] It facilitates the opening and closing in a very short time, is limited to one side with minimal disruption of the normal anatomy, there is no need to resect the middle turbinate, and dissection of the mucosa can be limited. There is little need to pack the nose during the postoperative period, or for lengthy, local postoperative treatment of crusting and disturbed nasal mucosa.

Moderator
Surgical Removal of a Pituitary Macroadenoma: Endoscopic vs. Microscopic
Mario Ammirati

The case presented is that of a patient with a large nonsecreting pituitary macroadenoma with chiasmatic compression manifested by bitemporal hemianopsia. As this tumor has a straight suprasellar extension, a transsphenoidal approach is the approach of choice. The goal of surgery should be aggressive tumor removal leading to chiasmal decompression. In addition, surgery should be associated with a low complication rate, including maintaining pituitary function. The main determinant in achieving these goals is tumor consistency; clearly, a soft tumor can be removed much more easily than a fibrous one. Unfortunately, the tumor's consistency is difficult to ascertain preoperatively.[46]

The technical nuances used to reduce complications include fastidiously maintaining the surgery outside the arachnoidal membrane, avoiding aggressive pulling on the tumor, recognizing the normal pituitary, and being continuously aware of the position of the intracavernous carotid arteries.[47] Over the years, pituitary surgery done with the microscope has been shown to accomplish these goals with minimal complications across different practice settings, as Ciric and colleagues[48] showed in their survey of the late 1990s. Pituitary surgery with the microscope relies on three-dimensional visualization, and hence on the ability to operate in three-dimensional space.

Endoscopic pituitary surgery has been advocated for the surgical treatment of pituitary adenomas since the late 1990s. This recommendation is based on the improved visualization and the surgeon's ability to visualize around corners compared with surgery done with the microscope. Endoscopic surgery is also perceived as less invasive.[49] The main drawback is the monocular vision with a lack of a true three-dimensional view. It has also been argued, probably rightly so, that it is more invasive than its microscopic counterpart.[50]

Notwithstanding any of these considerations, over more than 20 years, endoscopic pituitary surgery has failed to show a better outcome than pituitary surgery that is done with the microscope.[51] This has been the case even in the hands of its very passionate proponents! It is also clear that, during the endoscopic learning period, one is faced with an increasing number of complications.[52] Although this number of complications and the resources needed to master and execute a new technique would be completely acceptable if the end result is a better outcome for the patient, they become difficult to justify when the outcome is, at best, similar.[53]

The popularity of endoscopic pituitary surgery in the absence of any consistent data to support its superiority demonstrates once more the need for a better system to evaluate the introduction of new surgical procedures if surgical innovation has to move from a marketing arena into a substantive, evidence-based arena. This need was addressed by the Balliol Colloquium held at the Balliol College in Oxford, United Kingdom, between 2007 and 2009. Participants included surgeons, methodologists, statisticians, and the evidence-based medical community; their recommendations were published in *Lancet* in 2009.[54] Aside from transformative innovations, such as tracheotomy for tracheal obstruction, that lead to "an advance that is clear and substantial and that cannot be explained by either chance or bias," the majority of surgical innovations are incremental and are "prone to overoptimistic assessments by their developers and, therefore, need controlled randomized studies, when possible."[54] The colloquium proposed a loose algorithm to evaluate surgical innovations—the IDEAL Recommendations.[53] According to this set of recommendations, the proposed surgical innovation should be tested through different stages of the IDEAL mnemonic:

> **Stage 1,** the *Idea* phase, should be a proof of a concept to address a clinical need. The innovation should be tested in few patients with careful, especially negative, outcome reporting.
>
> **Stage 2A,** the *Development* phase, relies on the deliberate use of the procedure in a small group of selected patients to garner outcomes on the safety of the procedure and on its technical and procedural success or lack thereof. Protocols are required, and they should be handled outside the surgeons' institution to ensure objectivity. Ethical approval and informed research consent should be obtained.
>
> **Stage 2B,** the *Exploration* phase, involves the exploration of the outcome of a rather well-defined procedure in a larger group of patients. Prospective rigorous trials to assess short-term outcomes (technical-clinical and patient-centered) must be used. Tight quality controls and ethical approval and informed research consent are mandatory.
>
> **Stage 3,** the *Assessment* phase, involves well-defined indications, a stable procedure executed by many surgeons, and the assessment of this procedure vis-à-vis the gold standard. This assessment may be accomplished through randomized clinical or other well-structured trials, such as parallel group nonrandomized studies, controlled interrupted-time series studies, tracker trials, or similar designs. Ethical approval and informed research consent are needed.
>
> **Stage 4,** the *Long-term study*, is a longitudinal surveillance phase through which the now-established procedure is evaluated for rare and long-term outcomes.

The use of these or similar guidelines is intended to minimize any evaluation bias and to maximize patients' safety. Clearly, not all proposed innovations will be as successful as their originators suggest; many of them will have their implementation altered and their indications refined while going through this or a similar process. This process of evaluating surgical innovations associated with a paradigm shift is possible, as shown by the consortium evaluating Natural Orifice Transluminal Endoscopic Surgery (NOTES) (www.noscar.org).

It is likely that a similar level of evidence will be mandated more and more in the future by third-party payers before they will cover the cost of a more expensive procedure. As neurosurgeons, we would better serve our patients and our field by proactively engaging and demanding this type of evidence before embracing unproven surgical innovations.

References

1. Goel A, Deogaonkar M, Desai K. Fatal postoperative "pituitary apoplexy": its cause and management. Br J Neurosurg 1995; 9:37–40

2. Goel A. Impact of arterial relationship on strategy for cavernous sinus tumour surgery. Neurol India 1998;46:94–101

3. Goel A, Nadkarni T, Muzumdar D, Desai K, Phalke U, Sharma P. Giant pituitary tumors: a study based on surgical treatment of 118 cases. Surg Neurol 2004;61:436–445, discussion 445–446

4. Goel A, Nadkarni T. Surgical management of giant pituitary tumours—a review of 30 cases. Acta Neurochir (Wien) 1996; 138:1042–1049

5. Goel A. Meningeal architecture of the cavernous sinus: clinical and surgical implications. Neurosurgery 1998;42:430–431 (Letter)

6. Cappabianca P, de Divitiis E. Back to the Egyptians: neurosurgery via the nose. A five thousand year history and the recent contribution of the endoscope. Neurosurg Rev 2007;30:1–7, discussion 7

7. Jane JA Jr, Han J, Prevedello DM, Jagannathan J, Dumont AS, Laws ER Jr. Perspectives on endoscopic transsphenoidal surgery. Neurosurg Focus 2005;19:E2

8. Cushing H. III. Partial hypophysectomy for acromegaly: with remarks on the function of the hypophysis. Ann Surg 1909; 50:1002–1017

9. Apuzzo MLJ, Heifetz MD, Weiss MH, Kurze T. Neurosurgical endoscopy using the side-viewing telescope. J Neurosurg 1977; 46:398–400

10. Halves E, Bushe KA. Transsphenoidal operation on craniopharyngiomas with extrasellar extensions. The advantage of the operating endoscope. [Proceedings] Acta Neurochir Suppl (Wien) 1979;28:362

11. Jho HD, Carrau RL. Endoscopic endonasal transsphenoidal surgery: experience with 50 patients. J Neurosurg 1997;87:44–51

12. Kassam A, Snyderman CH, Mintz A, Gardner P, Carrau RL. Expanded endonasal approach: the rostrocaudal axis. Part II. Posterior clinoids to the foramen magnum. Neurosurg Focus 2005;19:E4

13. Kassam A, Snyderman CH, Mintz A, Gardner P, Carrau RL. Expanded endonasal approach: the rostrocaudal axis. Part I. Crista galli to the sella turcica. Neurosurg Focus 2005;19:E3

14. Cappabianca P, de Divitiis E. Endoscopy and transsphenoidal surgery. Neurosurgery 2004;54:1043–1048, 1048–1050

15. Cappabianca P, Cavallo LM, de Divitiis O, Solari D, Esposito F, Colao A. Endoscopic pituitary surgery. Review. Pituitary 2008; 11:385–390

16. Har-El G. Endoscopic transnasal transsphenoidal pituitary surgery—comparison with the traditional sublabial transseptal approach. Otolaryngol Clin North Am 2005;38:723–735

17. Doglietto F, Lauretti L, Frank G, et al. Microscopic and endoscopic extracranial approaches to the cavernous sinus: anatomic study. Neurosurgery 2009;64(5, Suppl 2):413–421, discussion 421–422

18. Locatelli D, Canevari FR, Acchiardi I, Castelnuovo P. The endoscopic diving technique in pituitary and cranial base surgery: technical note. Neurosurgery 2010;66:E400–E401, discussion E401

19. de Divitiis E. Endoscopic transsphenoidal surgery: stone-in-the-pond effect. Neurosurgery 2006;59:512–520, discussion 512–520

20. Powell M. Microscope and endoscopic pituitary surgery. Acta Neurochir (Wien) 2009;151:723–728.

21. Cavallo LM, Dal Fabbro M, Jalalod'din H, et al. Endoscopic endonasal transsphenoidal surgery. Before scrubbing in: tips and tricks. Surg Neurol 2007;67:342–347

22. Kassam AB, Thomas A, Carrau RL, et al. Endoscopic reconstruction of the cranial base using a pedicled nasoseptal flap. Neurosurgery 2008;63(1, Suppl 1):ONS44–ONS52, discussion ONS52–ONS53

23. Doglietto F, Prevedello DM, Jane JA Jr, Han J, Laws ER Jr. Brief history of endoscopic transsphenoidal surgery—from Philipp Bozzini to the First World Congress of Endoscopic Skull Base Surgery. Neurosurg Focus 2005;19:E3

24. Tabaee A, Anand VK, Fraser JF, Brown SM, Singh A, Schwartz TH. Three-dimensional endoscopic pituitary surgery. Neurosurgery 2009;64(5, Suppl 2):288–293, discussion 294–295

25. Cushing H. Transsphenoidal methods of access. In: Cushing H, ed. The Pituitary Body and Its Disorders: Clinical States Produced by Disorders of the Hypophysis Cerebri. Philadelphia: JB Lippincott, 1912:296–303

26. Guiot G, Bouche J, Hertzog E, Vourc'H G, Hardy J. [Hypophysectomy by trans-sphenoidal route]. Ann Radiol (Paris) 1963;6: 187–192

27. Hardy J. [Excision of pituitary adenomas by trans-sphenoidal approach]. Union Med Can 1962;91:933–945

28. Jane JA Jr, Thapar K, Kaptain GJ, Maartens N, Laws ER Jr. Pituitary surgery: transsphenoidal approach. Neurosurgery 2002; 51:435–442, discussion 442–444

29. Jho HD. Endoscopic pituitary surgery. Pituitary 1999;2:139–154

30. Krisht AF. Transsphenoidal approach and its variants. In: Sekhar LN, Fessler RG, eds. Atlas of Neurosurgical Techniques: Brain. New York: Thieme, 2006:654–660

31. Bushe KA, Halves E. [Modified technique in transsphenoidal operations of pituitary adenomas. Technical note (author's transl)]. Acta Neurochir (Wien) 1978;41:163–175

32. Al-Mefty O, Pravdenkova S, Gragnaniello C. A technical note on endonasal combined microscopic endoscopic with free head navigation technique of removal of pituitary adenomas. Neurosurg Rev 2010;33:243–248, discussion 248–249

33. Sanai N, Quiñones-Hinojosa A, Narvid J, Kunwar S. Safety and efficacy of the direct endonasal transsphenoidal approach for challenging sellar tumors. J Neurooncol 2008;87:317–325

34. Sheehan MT, Atkinson JL, Kasperbauer JL, Erickson BJ, Nippoldt TB. Preliminary comparison of the endoscopic transnasal vs the sublabial transseptal approach for clinically nonfunctioning pituitary macroadenomas. Mayo Clin Proc 1999;74:661–670

35. Elias WJ, Laws ER Jr. Transsphenoidal approaches to lesions of the sella. In: Schmidek HH, Sweet WH, eds. Operative Neurosurgical Techniques: Indications, Methods and Results, 4th ed. Philadelphia: WB Saunders, 2000:373–384

36. Batay F, Vural E, Karasu A, Al-Mefty O. Comparison of the exposure obtained by endoscope and microscope in the extended trans-sphenoidal approach. Skull Base 2002;12:119–124

37. Cappabianca P, Cavallo LM, de Divitiis E. Endoscopic endonasal transsphenoidal surgery. Neurosurgery 2004;55:933–940, discussion 940–941

38. Fatemi N, Dusick JR, de Paiva Neto MA, Kelly DF. The endonasal microscopic approach for pituitary adenomas and other parasellar tumors: a 10-year experience. Neurosurgery 2008;63 (4, Suppl 2):244–256, discussion 256

39. Griffith HB, Veerapen R. A direct transnasal approach to the sphenoid sinus. Technical note. J Neurosurg 1987;66:140–142

40. Swearingen B. Transsphenoidal approach to pituitary tumors. In: Schmidek HH, Roberts DW, eds. Operative Neurosurgical Techniques: Indications, Methods, and Results, 5th ed. Philadelphia: WB Saunders, 2005:321–331

41. Wilson WR, Laws ER Jr. Transnasal septal displacement approach for secondary transsphenoidal pituitary surgery. Laryngoscope 1992;102:951–953

42. Snyderman C, Kassam A, Carrau R, Mintz A, Gardner P, Prevedello DM. Acquisition of surgical skills for endonasal skull base surgery: a training program. Laryngoscope 2007;117:699–705

43. Teo C, Nakaji P. Neuro-oncologic applications of endoscopy. Neurosurg Clin N Am 2004;15:89–103

44. Catapano D, Sloffer CA, Frank G, Pasquini E, D'Angelo VA, Lanzino G. Comparison between the microscope and endoscope in the direct endonasal extended transsphenoidal approach: anatomical study. J Neurosurg 2006;104:419–425

45. Barrow DL, Tindall GT. Loss of vision after transsphenoidal surgery. Neurosurgery 1990;27:60–68

46. Bahuleyan B, Raghuram L, Rajshekhar V, Chacko AG. To assess the ability of MRI to predict consistency of pituitary macroadenomas. Br J Neurosurg 2006;20:324–326

47. Ciric I, Rosenblatt S, Zhao JC. Transsphenoidal microsurgery. Neurosurgery 2002;51:161–169

48. Ciric I, Ragin A, Baumgartner C, Pierce D. Complications of transsphenoidal surgery: results of a national survey, review of the literature, and personal experience. Neurosurgery 1997; 40:225–236, discussion 236–237

49. Tabaee A, Anand VK, Barrón Y, et al. Endoscopic pituitary surgery: a systematic review and meta-analysis. J Neurosurg 2009;111:545–554

50. Oldfield EH. Editorial: Unresolved issues: radiosurgery versus radiation therapy; medical suppression of growth hormone production during radiosurgery; and endoscopic surgery versus microscopic surgery. Neurosurg Focus 2010;29:E16

51. Gondim JA, Almeida JP, de Albuquerque LA, Gomes E, Schops M, Ferraz T. Pure endoscopic transsphenoidal surgery for treatment of acromegaly: results of 67 cases treated in a pituitary center. Neurosurg Focus 2010;29:E7

52. Gondim JA, Almeida JP, Albuquerque LA, et al. Endoscopic endonasal approach for pituitary adenoma: surgical complications in 301 patients. Pituitary 2011;14:174–183

53. Ammirati M, Law I, Ciric I. Short term outcome of endoscopic versus micrscopic pituitary adenoma surgery: A systemic review and meta-analysis. J Neurol Neurosurg Psychiatry 12 Dec. 2012

54. McCulloch P, Altman DG, Campbell WB, et al; Balliol Collaboration. No surgical innovation without evaluation: the IDEAL recommendations. Lancet 2009;374:1105–1112

Surgical Approaches to Pituitary Macroadenomas with Cavernous Sinus Extensions: Transcranial vs. Transsphenoidal Approach

Case

A 50-year-old, right-handed man came to medical attention with decreased vision in his right eye and headache. On examination, he had a partial third nerve palsy. Vision in his right eye was 20/200. Neuro-endocrinologic tests showed a diluted prolactin level of approximately 40 IU and the patient had panhypopituitarism.

Participants

Cranial Approaches to Pituitary Adenomas with Cavernous Sinus Extensions: Gerardo Guinto and Roxana Contreras

The Endonasal Transsphenoidal Approach to Pituitary Macroadenomas with Cavernous Sinus Extensions: Ali Shirzadi, Doniel Drazin, and Wesley A. King

Moderators: Transcranial vs. Transsphenoidal Approach for Pituitary Macroadenomas with Cavernous Sinus Invasion: Nelson Oyesiku and Brandon A. Miller

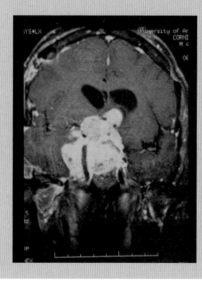 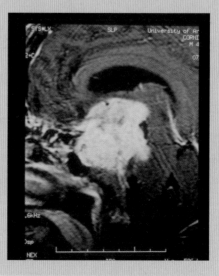

Cranial Approaches to Pituitary Adenomas with Cavernous Sinus Extensions

Gerardo Guinto and Roxana Contreras

Despite the current advances in neurosurgery, particularly the improved understanding of the microsurgical anatomy and further development of microsurgical instruments, the cavernous sinus remains one of the most complex areas to present a great challenge for skull-base surgeons.[1] In addition, the advent of radiosurgery has caused a controversy regarding the indications for removing lesions, particularly benign ones, affecting this region.

Throughout the years, the term *cavernous sinus* has been commonly used for this anatomic structure; however, it is well known that this term is a misnomer. The venous compartment is really formed by a complex network of capillaries rather than true dural sinuses. For this reason, this area should be referred to as a *lateral sellar compartment* or as a *parasellar region*.[2] Meningiomas are the lesions that most frequently invade the cavernous sinus. Pituitary adenomas are peculiar tumors that tend to respect the anatomic boundaries surrounding them and only rarely violate these frontiers and invade other areas. Another peculiarity of these tumors is that, even when they truly invade the sinus, patients only occasionally exhibit the classic signs and symptoms of oculomotor deficit, which is most common in patients with meningiomas.

There are many ways to access the cavernous sinus, but they can be divided into two approaches: transsphenoidal and transcranial. This section focuses on transcranial approaches.

Anatomy

The cavernous sinus (CS) is a paired tetrahedral structure located on both sides of the sella turcica. Because of its shape, it has four walls (anterior, posterior, lateral, and medial), a roof, and a floor, all composed of dura mater. The lateral wall is formed by two dural layers. The inner dural layer is continuous with the periosteum of the clivus, temporal bone, and sphenoid bone. In addition, this membrane is partially formed by the epineurium of the third, fourth, and fifth cranial nerves. The outer layer is thicker and is continuous with the dura of the middle fossa, tentorium, and the outer layer of the dura of the clivus. The clinoid segment of the internal carotid artery (ICA) has two rings, distal and proximal, that are fused medially but separated laterally by the anterior clinoid process. The distal ring is in contiguity with the outer layer of the lateral wall of the CS, whereas the proximal ring is continuous with the inner layer of this lateral wall and forms a part of the roof of the CS. Between the two layers of the lateral wall run the oculomotor nerves (III and IV) and the first (and sometimes second) branch of the fifth cranial nerve.[3]

The medial wall of the CS is contiguous with the dura mater of the floor of the sella turcica and the inner layer of the dura mater of the clivus. This wall is partially covered by a thin bony plate that forms the lateral wall of the sphenoid sinus. The anterior loop or bend of the ICA produces an impression in this bone known as the carotid prominence, an important anatomic landmark for medial approaches to the CS.

The ICA has a particular trajectory through the CS, and several different nomenclatures designate the anatomic portions of this vessel. Once it penetrates the skull through the carotid canal, the ICA curves forward and medially to traverse within the temporal bone in what is known as the petrous portion. Once it reaches the region of the foramen lacerum, it curves upward again, taking a vertical direction (the posterior vertical segment). This portion is covered by the trigeminal ganglion (gasserian), and is sometimes referred to as the trigeminal segment. In this region, the artery is surrounded by fibrous tissue known as the petrolingual ligament, which represents the true anatomic landmark between the petrous and the cavernous portion of the artery. Once inside the cavernous sinus, the ICA takes another curve to run horizontally and forward toward the superior orbital fissure. At the end of this horizontal portion, the artery takes one more bend, now in a superomedial direction, to take another vertical direction (the anterior vertical portion) and exits the CS to enter the subarachnoid space. In this area, the artery is covered by the aforementioned dural rings and the anterior clinoid process.[4]

The cavernous ICA has several collateral branches, but the most constant are two: the meningohypophyseal artery and the inferolateral trunk. The first branch has three divisions: the tentorial branch (Bernasconi-Cassinari), the dorsal meningeal artery, and the inferior hypophyseal artery. Another inconstant branch of the cavernous ICA is the capsular artery (McConnell), which irrigates the capsule of the pituitary gland. Finally, in 8 to 10% of patients, the ophthalmic artery has its origin in this cavernous portion of the ICA.

As mentioned, cranial nerves III, IV, V_1, and, occasionally, V_2 run between the two layers of the lateral wall of the CS and only the sixth nerve (abducens) and the sympathetic nerve fibers are really intracavernous, running in close contact with the ICA. The third cranial nerve enters the CS through the roof (oculomotor trigone), lateral to the posterior clinoid process, where it remains between the two layers of the lateral wall and travels toward the superior orbital fissure to enter the orbit. The fourth cranial nerve enters the tentorial edge to run toward the lateral wall of the CS, where it also travels between its layers, to reach the superior orbital fissure. The sixth nerve comes from the posterior fossa and penetrates Dorello's canal (formed by the clivus and the posterior petroclinoid ligament) to traverse the clivus. It then enters the CS, where it is in close contact with the lateral surface of the posterior vertical segment of the cavernous ICA. It then runs alongside this artery, attached to the inferolateral surface of its horizontal portion, and reaches the orbit through the superior orbital fissure. The ophthalmic branch of the trigeminal nerve (V_1) travels in almost its entire length in the lateral wall, between the layers, toward the superior orbital fissure.[5,6]

The cavernous venous plexus can be divided into four spaces—lateral, medial, posterior, and anterior—depending on their relationship with the ICA. Similarly, the CS has several extrinsic venous communications: the superior ophthalmic artery, the pterygoid plexus, the superior and inferior petrosal sinuses, and the sphenoparietal sinus. Finally, there are communications between both cavernous sinuses via the so-called anterior and posterior intercavernous sinuses found in the sella turcica, but mainly through the basilar venous plexus located between two folds of the dura mater of the clivus.

Surgical Indications

Considering the complexity of surgery in this region, the high rate of morbidity, and the availability of other treatment alternatives such as radiosurgery, there are precise indications for operating on patients with cavernous invasion by a pituitary adenoma.[7] The most important general indications are as follows: first, when there is a cavernous component of the tumor with dimensions greater than those acceptable for safe treatment with radiosurgery (2.5 cm); and second, when patients have an oculomotor deficit. For some patients with pituitary adenomas, there are alternatives for medical treatment. Prolactin-secreting tumors only rarely have to be operated on because even giant tumors usually respond positively to dopamine agonists such as bromocriptine and cabergoline.[8] Similarly, when growth hormone–producing tumors invade the CS, medical treatment with somatostatin analogues or dopamine agonists is preferred before attempting direct surgery. An adrenocorticotropic hormone (ACTH)-producing adenoma only rarely invades the CS; the majority of cases of Cushing's disease are related to microadenomas or intrasellar tumors. When there is cavernous invasion, initial management with ketoconazole may be indicated. Finally, some nonfunctioning pituitary adenomas may also show some response to dopamine agonists. This possibility has to be considered before making a decision to remove the intracavernous component of functioning tumors.

A final consideration for exposing and removing the intracavernous component of a pituitary adenoma is related to the tumor itself. If, during the resection of the extracavernous portion of the tumor, an experienced surgeon notes a favorable consistency, a weak adherence of the tumor to surrounding tissues, or a poor vascular supply, the surgeon may then decide to continue the tumor resection toward

the CS. For this reason, in most patients who have a pituitary adenoma with parasellar invasion, all the surgical steps for exposing the CS must be done during the approach so that the surgeon is prepared to access this region.

Preoperative Studies

Undoubtedly, magnetic resonance imaging (MRI) is the ideal and indispensable study to determine whether there is a real invasion of the tumor into the CS.[9,10] The most useful view is the T1-weighted, coronal projection with gadolinium enhancement. In this image, the medial wall appears as a hypointense line that separates the content of the sella turcica from the CS. This projection also provides valuable information regarding subcavernous tumor invasion into the lateral recess of the sphenoid sinus or, in rare cases, when there is invasion to the infratemporal fossa and parapharyngeal space.

The most important point is to analyze the behavior of the tumor in relation to the cavernous ICA. If this vessel is displaced laterally, if the tumor contacts it only in its medial surface, or if the artery is only partially surrounded, it is reasonable to rule out an invasion of the CS (**Fig. 8.1**). This tumor behavior is the most common in pituitary adenomas and it may be considered a displacement rather than a real invasion. On the other hand, if the artery is displaced medially or is completely surrounded by tumor with a reduction in its diameter, it is almost certain that there is a real invasion (**Fig. 8.2**). A T2-weighted image may provide information about the consistency of the tumor. If the tumor appears hyperintense in this phase, it likely has a favorable consistency, for which a more radical excision can be planned. In contrast, if the lesion remains

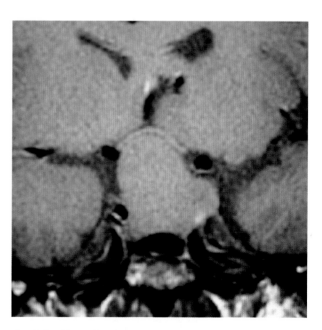

Fig. 8.1 T1-weighted magnetic resonance imaging (MRI), coronal view, showing a pituitary adenoma that is only displacing but not invading the left cavernous sinus.

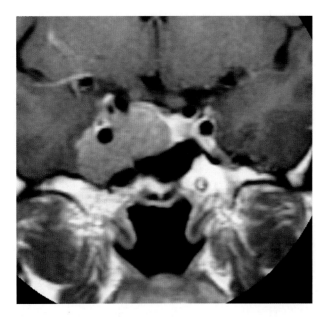

Fig. 8.2 T1-weighted MRI, coronal view with contrast enhancement, showing a pituitary adenoma with invasion of the cavernous sinus. The right internal carotid artery is completely surrounded by tumor.

hypointense or isointense in both phases (T1 and T2), it usually has a firmer consistency and, therefore, presents a greater degree of difficulty during removal. Axial cuts allow an adequate assessment of the growth pattern of the tumor to areas adjacent to the CS, particularly the orbit, the posterior fossa, and the anterior floor.[11,12]

Computed tomography (CT) provides only limited information compared with MRI. It is useful for assessing the anatomic characteristics of bone and the degree of erosion caused by the tumor, and for identifying the presence of calcifications (rare in pituitary adenomas). Angiography is usually unnecessary because, especially in cases of pituitary adenomas, the information provided by this study can be obtained through magnetic resonance (MR) angiography or CT angiography with lower risk for the patient. In addition, sacrificing the ICA or performing a bypass is almost never justified in patients with these types of tumors. For this reason, balloon test occlusion is not indicated.

In addition to standard preoperative studies, all patients must undergo an integral endocrine evaluation and a complete ophthalmologic examination, including visual field testing and evaluation of eye movements.

Surgery

Anesthesia

The patient is administered standard general anesthesia through endotracheal intubation. In general, muscle relaxants are used for most of the intracranial procedures. Commonly used medications for intracranial procedures are propofol, isoflurane, fentanyl, pancuronium, midazolam, and nitrous oxide, among others. To facilitate brain relax-

ation, it is preferable to use mild to moderate hyperventilation to maintain a $PaCO_2$ of 30 to 35 mm Hg, as well as administration of mannitol at doses of 0.5 to 1 g/kg. On rare occasions (particularly when resection is performed via an extended subfrontal approach), the placement of a lumbar subarachnoid catheter is indicated for releasing cerebrospinal fluid (CSF), which provides more brain relaxation. More intensive cerebral protection measures, such as hypothermia, hemodilution, and burst suppression in the electroencephalogram with barbiturates, are usually unnecessary. Finally, it is very important to ensure the venous return in the legs by using compression (preferably intermittent pneumatic) stockings.

Intraoperative Monitoring

Somatosensory evoked potentials are useful in detecting early changes in brain function, particularly when there is a carotid lesion that causes ischemia or to detect excessive brain retraction. The brainstem auditory evoked response is also very useful because it detects at an early stage any change in the conductivity of the brainstem caused by brain retraction, surgical manipulation, or the tumor itself. Finally, to help identify the oculomotor nerves within the CS, it is very useful to have neurostimulation equipment and electromyographic recording of the extraocular muscles. Similarly, electromyographic recording of the facial muscles may help identify the greater superficial petrosal nerve by its conduction toward the geniculate ganglion.

Surgical Approaches and Techniques

Cranial approaches to pituitary adenomas that invade the CS can be divided into two types: lateral and medial. The most widely used lateral approach is the orbitozygomatic, whereas the most commonly used medial approach is the extended subfrontal.

Orbitozygomatic Approach

For this approach, the patient is placed in the supine position with the head fixed in a three-pin head holder, rotated approximately 35 degrees contralaterally, and slightly extended so that the malar eminence is the highest point (**Fig. 8.3**). The patient has to be fixed securely to the operating table to allow for rotation on the long axis during the procedure. Similarly, the head elevation can be varied to promote venous return and increase brain relaxation.

A curvilinear incision is drawn in the skin in the frontotemporal region with a preauricular extension that reaches the ear lobe downward and is directed upward to the midline at the edge of the hairline. The incision can also be drawn as a question-mark shape with the same upper and lower limits to circumvent the bulk of the temporalis muscle, facilitating its elevation (**Fig. 8.4**). The incision and dissection is begun in the preauricular region, immediately in front of the tragus, to allow for early identification of the

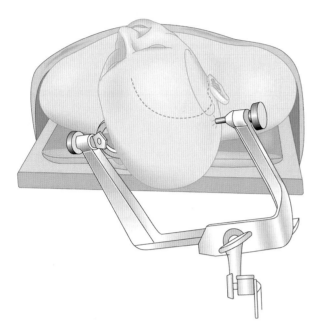

Fig. 8.3 The patient's position for the orbitozygomatic approach.

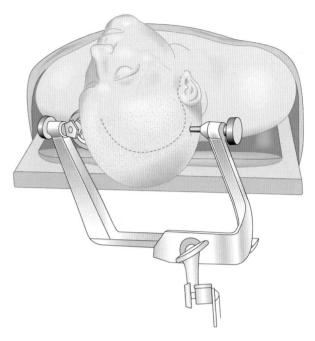

Fig. 8.4 Details of the skin incision for the orbitozygomatic approach. In this case, a question-mark–shaped incision is made.

superficial temporal artery and to improve the postoperative cosmetic result. Preserving this vessel is important for two reasons: to enable irrigation of the myocutaneous flap and to use it as a vascular trunk in rare cases when it is required to perform a bypass. The superficial temporal artery usually has a collateral branch that arises above the outer ear and that is directed dorsally. This branch must be coagulated and cut to displace the main trunk of the superficial temporal artery forward along with the skin flap.[13,14]

The pericranium is elevated preferably with the scalp and not with monopolar coagulation to prevent desiccation or damage. This dissection continues rostrally on the superficial temporal fascia up to the fat pad. This fat pad is usually found by drawing an imaginary line from the root of the zygomatic arch to the root of the external orbital process of the frontal bone. At this point, both layers of the superficial temporal fascia are cut in the same direction as this imaginary line to carry out an interfascial dissection, which allows preservation of the frontotemporal branch of the facial nerve that runs between the two layers of the superficial temporalis fascia.[15]

Blunt dissection continues on the fibers of the temporalis muscle, with the aim of maintaining the superficial temporal fascia attached to the skin flap until the orbit and superior border of the zygomatic arch are reached. Detachment is continued over the external surface of this arch until the malar bone is reached anteriorly, up to the level of the zygomatic-facial foramen and to the root of the zygomatic arch posteriorly. The glenoid cavity of the temporal bone (condylar fossa) can be included in this posterior dissection. With sharp dissection, the masseter is now removed from the inferior border of the zygomatic arch. The orbital rim is dissected up to the supraorbital notch, where

the supraorbital nerve is identified and protected. Dissection is continued on the lateral and superior walls of the orbit. The use of cottonoids during this dissection is very helpful because the periorbita can be protected. Likewise, the anesthesiologist should be notified at this stage because manipulation of the orbital contents may cause bradycardia, which occasionally may be marked. Dissection on the lateral wall of the orbit continues downward until the inferior orbital fissure is identified. Then the supraorbital nerve is skeletonized. In some cases, this nerve exits the cranium through a real orifice; therefore, skeletonizing becomes necessary to fracture the inferior osseous lip of this orifice with a high-speed drill or chisel. In most cases, however, there is no supraorbital orifice but there is a notch, so detaching the nerve is simple.

Surgery continues with the dis-insertion of the temporalis muscle with the periosteal elevator. This maneuver should be done in an ascending or retrograde direction, which better preserves the deep or periosteal temporal fascia, providing better cosmetic results. In this manner, the entire temporalis muscle is moved down and forward, exposing the pterional or frontotemporal region.[16]

Although there are descriptions of several ways of performing the frontotemporal craniotomy and the orbitozygomatic osteotomy in one piece,[17] the reality is that this is easier to do in two pieces. In this two-step maneuver, at least 2.5 cm of the superior and lateral walls of the orbit can be preserved and the condylar fossa can be included in the osteotomy. The cosmetic results are similar regardless of whether the craniotomy and orbitozygomatic osteotomy are done in one or two pieces. Other authors have described the use of three pieces.[18]

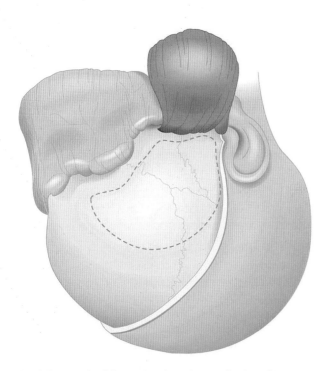

Fig. 8.5 Details of the pterional craniotomy for the orbitozygomatic approach.

The craniotomy is begun with the first bur hole made on the lateral facet of the frontal bone at its junction with the superior temporal line (the keyhole). Another, optional bur hole can be made just above the root of the zygomatic arch. Then, a standard frontotemporal craniotomy (pterional) 6 to 8 cm in diameter is done, centered on the pterion and with its medial limit on the supraorbital notch (**Fig. 8.5**). The cut that joins the two bur holes should be made in both directions (up/down), having as a center the sphenoid ridge (the greater wing of the sphenoid bone). The bone flap is elevated with the Penfield No. 1 to fracture the sphenoid ridge. This maneuver includes in the flap a wider part of the bone of the temporal region, which can be replaced at the end of the procedure.[19] The craniotomy should be expanded as closely as possible to the orbital rim and to the condylar fossa. The procedure continues with the removal of the remaining bone of the temporal region with rongeurs and Kerrisons and with the drilling of the sphenoid ridge until the superior orbital fissure is reached and then completely unroofed. The surgeon now prepares the surgical field for the orbitozygomatic osteotomy by detaching the frontal and temporal dura mater from the superior and lateral walls of the orbit as well as from the roof of the condylar fossa.

The orbitozygomatic osteotomy is done with a reciprocating saw, and the sequence of cuts varies according to the surgeon's preference. For the orbital osteotomy, cutting is begun on the roof of the orbit at the level of the supraorbital notch or slightly medial. From this point, the cut is directed backward over the orbital roof to a distance of 2.5 to 3 cm. At the posterior end of this cut, another perpendicular cut is started and directed laterally, now in the cor-

onal plane, from the orbital roof toward the lateral wall until it reaches the inferior orbital fissure. The next cut is made on the lateral wall of the orbit, facing the orbital surface. This cut begins on the inferior orbital fissure and runs toward the malar bone, without surpassing the site of the zygomatic-facial foramen to avoid entering the maxillary sinus. The cut in the malar bone is completed over the exocranial surface, in an inverted V shape, which facilitates replacement at the end of the procedure.

In almost all approaches to the CS, it is usually necessary to expose the petrous segment of the ICA. The main reasons for this are to obtain proximal control of this vessel and to determine its precise location, which may serve as an orientation reference during tumor removal. In these cases, it would be preferable to include the condylar fossa in the orbitozygomatic osteotomy because this maneuver notably increases the exposure on the petrous bone. To make this osteotomy, the surgeon begins with an extracapsular detachment of the joint, displacing it downward with the mandibular condyle. In the great majority of patients, the mouth is open because the operation takes place with orotracheal intubation. For this reason, the mandibular condyle is almost always found outside the condylar fossa and displaced forward. Once the condylar fossa is totally detached, a V-shaped osteotomy is then done (with the reciprocating saw) on its roof, with care being taken not to pass the level of the foramen spinosum medially; otherwise, there is a risk of injury to the petrous ICA. Similarly, care must be taken not to damage the cartilage and skin of the external ear conduct, which lies immediately behind the condylar fossa. In this way, an orbitozygomatic bar is obtained that includes 2.5 to 3 cm of the lateral and superior walls, two thirds of the roof of the condylar fossa, the zygomatic arch, and part of the malar bone (**Fig. 8.6**). This maneuver prevents the postoperative complications of pulsatile enophthalmos and chewing problems.

If it is not considered necessary to widely expose the petrous portion of the ICA but only to identify it, the surgeon does not need to include the condylar fossa in the exposure; therefore, the zygomatic osteotomy is done obliquely at the root of the arch. Once the craniotomy and orbitozygomatic osteotomy are finished, the temporalis muscle can be completely retracted and then the anterior and middle cranial floors are exposed.

The dura mater of the middle fossa is detached until the arcuate eminence is visualized, which is perpendicular to the longitudinal axis of the petrous bone. Then the middle meningeal artery, the foramen spinosum, V_3, and the foramen ovale are also identified and exposed. The floor of the middle fossa is drilled until V_3 and the middle meningeal artery are completely skeletonized. The artery is coagulated and cut to facilitate temporal retraction, and dissection is continued medially until the greater superficial petrosal nerve and its hiatus are identified. This nerve runs parallel to the petrous bone. To facilitate its identification, it can be stimulated during an electromyographic register of the muscles of the face. Sectioning of the greater superficial pe-

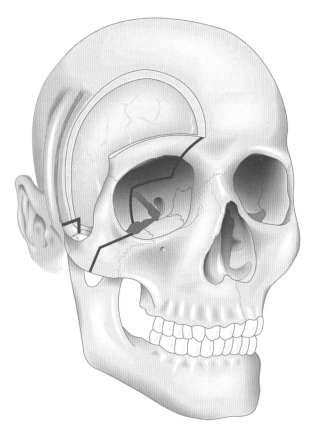

Fig. 8.6 The pterional craniotomy and orbitozygomatic osteotomy is done in two pieces. The orbitozygomatic bar includes 3 cm of the superior and lateral walls of the orbit and part of the malar bone. In this case, the osteotomy was extended to include two thirds of the condylar fossa.

trosal nerve is generally recommended to avoid excessive traction on the geniculate ganglion and subsequent postoperative hemifacial paralysis.

In many cases, the horizontal portion of the petrous ICA is only partially covered by bone, which facilitates its identification. When this is not the case, the artery can be localized just posterior and medial to V_3 and below the greater superficial petrosal nerve, where drilling is started. A diamond bur should be used to avoid damaging the ICA. The eustachian tube should not be damaged during drilling; otherwise, it has to be plugged with muscle and fibrin adhesive to avoid the risk of CSF leakage. The best reference for identifying the eustachian tube is the tensor tympani muscle, which lies immediately above it and in front of and below the petrous ICA. Both structures (muscle and eustachian tube) have the same direction as the petrous ICA. Drilling behind the carotid foramen must be avoided because this is the area where the basal turn of the cochlea is located.

The next step is to perform an anterior clinoidectomy, which is preferably done extradurally. When the anterior clinoid process is removed with the high-speed bur, extensive irrigation is necessary to prevent the heat generated by drilling that may damage the optic nerve. This bone removal

can also be done with rongeurs, with a gentle movement of the surgeon's wrist. The optic strut that represents the inferior wall of the optic canal can now be visualized and also removed with the drill or rongeur. To increase the exposure, the optic nerve can be completely unroofed, which allows its mobilization. This mobilization is facilitated by sectioning of the optic sheath. In some patients, the anterior clinoid process is very small; therefore, intradural extraction is preferred. When the approach is completed, all the bone between the CS and the surgeon is removed (**Fig. 8.7**).

Access to the Cavernous Sinus Through the Orbitozygomatic Approach

With the orbitozygomatic approach, two surgical routes are most commonly used to expose the CS in patients with pituitary adenomas: the inferolateral and the superior. These can be used in combination, depending on the growth pattern of the tumor. The inferolateral approach begins with extensive extradural work, which is started with the complete exposure of the three branches of the trigeminal nerve as follows. During the approach, the superior orbital fissure, and therefore the ophthalmic branch, is completely unroofed. The foramen ovale is also opened, exposing the mandibular nerve. Finally, all the bone located in the region of the foramen rotundum is removed to completely free the maxillary branch (**Fig. 8.8**).

Access to the CS begins with detaching or peeling of the dura of the middle fossa, separating it from the trigeminal branches and the gasserian ganglion. This maneuver completely exposes Meckel's cave. The peeling is extended backward and up toward the area of the third and fourth cranial nerves where, on occasion, it is preferable to leave a part of the dura mater intact, especially if it firmly adheres to these nerves. This makes it possible to preserve the nerve's blood supply and prevent an oculomotor deficit. However, considering that the majority of pituitary adenomas have a favorable consistency, in general an extensive peeling is not required, and it is sufficient to uncover the three branches of the trigeminal nerve and the gasserian ganglion. Usually, at the beginning of peeling, the tumor can be observed emerging between the trigeminal branches (**Fig. 8.9**). Removal is done with the aspirator, pituitary curettes, and biopsy forceps. In these tumors, it is usually sufficient to access the CS via the angle formed between V_2 and V_3 and between V_1 and V_2. The trigeminal branches are quite elastic and allow for some distraction to expand these spaces. On the other hand, extraction of the orbital rim (included in the orbitozygomatic osteotomy) enables the surgeon to vary the direction of the microscope, allowing entry at different angles.

When using this route, the main precaution during tumor removal is identifying the horizontal portion of the cavernous ICA. In complex and fibrous tumors, this vessel can be easily damaged during tumor removal. Intraoperative micro-Doppler can be very helpful for early and safe identification of the cavernous ICA.

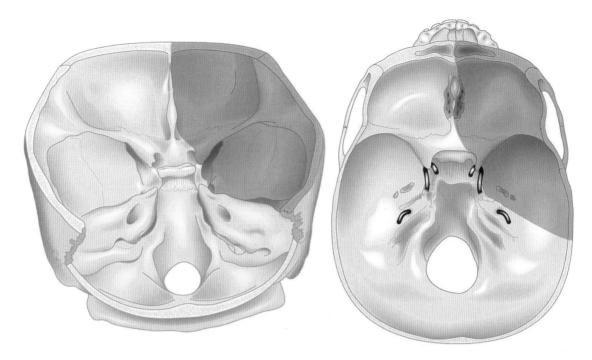

Fig. 8.7   Details of bone removal (craniotomy, osteotomy, and drilling) in the orbitozygomatic approach. The cavernous sinus is totally exposed from a lateral perspective.

Another anatomic reference to be kept in mind during this phase of surgery is the precise location of the abducens nerve. This cranial nerve may be damaged when the tumor is dissected from the lateral surface of the posterior vertical segment and from the inferolateral wall of the horizontal portion of the cavernous ICA. Finally, by complete drilling of the bone located between V_2 and V_3, access to the sphenoid sinus can be obtained, which is very useful in patients with these particular tumors because, in many cases, they invade this sinus in addition to the CS.

If this inferolateral access is insufficient, it becomes necessary to combine it with an intradural lateral approach. The dura mater is then opened with a C-shaped frontotemporal incision, and the dural flap is reflected over the orbital contents. Wide splitting of the sylvian fissure is required to continue the dural peeling intradurally up to the

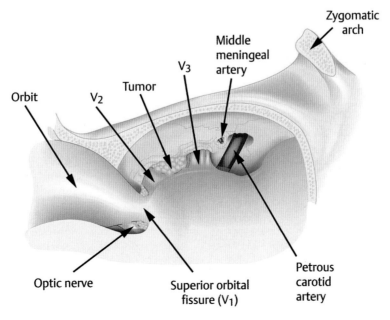

Fig. 8.8   The extradural exposure in the inferolateral approach to the right cavernous sinus (surgical position). V1, V2, V3, branches of the fifth cranial nerve.

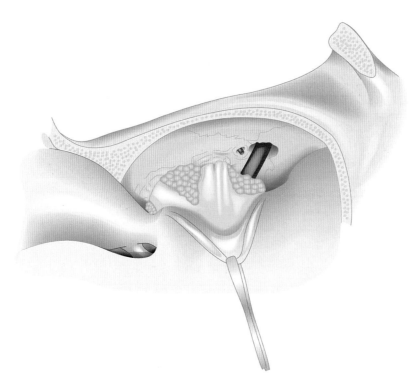

Fig. 8.9 Peeling of the middle fossa. The tumor is clearly seen between the trigeminal branches. The right cavernous sinus is in the surgical position.

exposure of the third and fourth cranial nerves. The CS is then accessed between nerves, preferably through Parkinson's triangle, which is formed by the fourth nerve and V_1.

The superior approach is preferred when the tumor is located above and medial to the horizontal portion of the cavernous ICA. This approach also adequately exposes the anterior vertical portion, the anterior loop, and the clinoid segment of the ICA, and likewise the third and fourth cranial nerves, but it is very difficult to expose the sixth nerve, V_1, V_2, and V_3. For this approach, the anterior clinoid process must be completely removed. A C-shaped dural opening is also made in the frontotemporal region and the dural flap is retracted over the orbital contents. Resection of the clinoid dura mater and sectioning of the optic nerve sheath are also mandatory to freely mobilize the nerve. Access to the CS is made by sectioning the dural rings of the ICA. In this manner, the CS is exposed from a superior perspective (**Fig. 8.10**).

The dural opening on the roof of the CS can be extended to reach the posterior clinoid process. However, this aperture must be made carefully because there is a risk of injury to the cavernous ICA, which is often found attached to the roof of the CS. The dura can also be opened along the course of the third nerve to facilitate its mobilization and to widen the exposure. This dural opening is recommended only for patients who have a preoperative oculomotor deficit to obtain maximum decompression of this nerve. The dissection can be continued around the pituitary gland into the sella turcica and even toward the contralateral CS.

Closure and reconstruction begin with suture of the dura mater as tightly as possible. When the sphenoid sinus has been opened, it must be packed with fat and fibrin adhesives to avoid the risk of CSF leakage. The orbitozygomatic bar is replaced and fixed with titanium miniplates. Considering that most of the orbital walls are replaced with this bar, reconstruction of the orbit is unnecessary. In fact, pulsatile enophthalmos is very rare when doing the orbitozygomatic osteotomy in this way. The temporalis muscle is replaced and sutured either to the surrounding fascia or to the adjacent bone through oblique holes made with the perforating drill. It is not necessary to fix or suture the masseter muscle to the zygomatic arch because it reinserts spontaneously. The bone flap is replaced and also fixed with miniplates or wire, and finally the fascia and skin are closed with running sutures.

Combination of the Orbitozygomatic Approach with Other Approaches

Tumors invading the CS can grow backward to the posterior fossa, particularly to petroclival region, or the cerebellopontine angle. This is very rare in patients with a pituitary adenoma and is most commonly seen in those with meningiomas. When invasion of these areas is small, it is sufficient to combine the orbitozygomatic approach with an anterior transpetrosal approach by the complete drilling of the petrous apex (Kawase's triangle). However, when the invasion is large, it becomes necessary to combine it with a posterior

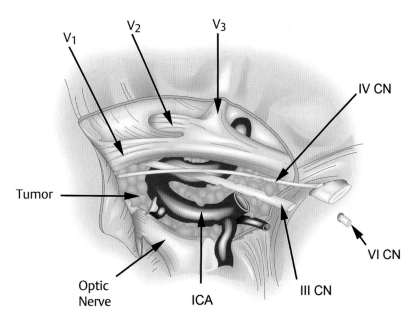

Fig. 8.10 Right cavernous sinus exposure (in the surgical position) for a superior intradural approach. CN, cranial nerve; ICA, internal carotid artery; V1, V2, V3, branches of the fifth cranial nerve.

transpetrosal approach.[20,21] To combine this with the or-bitozygomatic approach, another curvilinear skin incision must be made on the retro- and supra-auricular areas; this incision joins the previous incision at a right angle at its midpoint. A presigmoid retrolabyrinthine mastoidectomy is done along with a retrosigmoid craniectomy and posterior temporal craniotomy. The dural incision begins in the presigmoid region and goes upward to the superior petrosal sinus, which is ligated and cut. The dural cut is continued horizontally in the temporal region over the inferior temporal gyrus, forming a T when joining the presigmoid incision. Once the dura is opened, one retractor is placed to mobilize the cerebellum and sigmoid sinus backward; another retractor is placed in the subtemporal region for the gentle elevation of the temporal lobe. The tentorium is then exposed and cut up to its edge. Identifying and preserving the vein of Labbé is imperative to prevent postoperative edema of the temporal lobe. Once the tentorium is completely cut, the tumor in the petroclival region is widely exposed and can be removed.

Extended Subfrontal Approach

For the extended subfrontal approach, the patient is placed in the supine position with the head at 0 degrees and slightly extended **(Fig. 8.11)**. A bicoronal skin incision is made behind the hairline, starting immediately in front of the ear, from where it rises vertically to the other side. The skin flap is dissected and reflected rostrally, leaving the pericranium attached to bone. When the dissection reaches the orbital rims, the pericranium is then detached and elevated, with sectioning 3 to 4 cm behind the skin incision. This maneuver creates a longer pediculated pericranial flap

that will be used to reconstruct the anterior floor of the skull base. Bone dissection continues forward to fully expose the orbital rims, where the supraorbital nerves are skeletonized and freed. At the midline, dissection is extended downward to the frontonasal suture **(Fig. 8.12)**. Both periorbits are dissected from the superior, lateral, and medial walls of the orbit, at least 3 cm posterior to the supraorbital ridges. A bifrontal craniotomy is then done, as basal as possible, which entails the risk of opening the frontal sinuses.

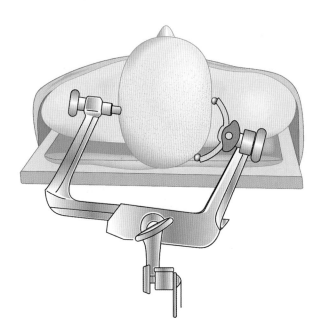

Fig. 8.11 The patient's position for the extended subfrontal approach.

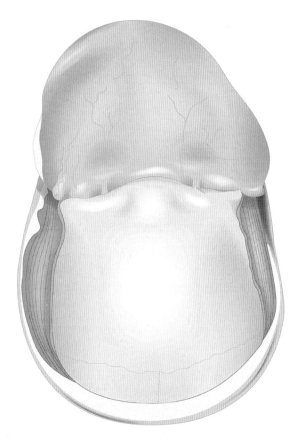

Fig. 8.12 After a bicoronal skin incision is made, the pericranium and the myocutaneous flap are reflected forward.

Sometimes the internal frontal crest is very prominent. In such cases, the bone in this region must be fractured during the craniotomy. The mucosa of the frontal sinuses is exenterated and the posterior wall of the sinuses is removed (cranialization).

Next, the dura mater of the crista galli is detached. A bilateral orbital osteotomy is then performed with three particular cuts. The first cut (anteroposterior) is made on each orbital roof beginning on the orbital rims just lateral to the supraorbital notch and ending 3 cm behind. The second, or coronal cut, is then made where the first cut ends (3 cm behind the orbital rim) and runs through the roof of both orbits, passing behind the cribriform plate of the ethmoid bone. The third, or axial, cut is made at the level of or just below the frontonasal suture and extends posteriorly to meet the coronal cut behind the cribriform plate. This cut risks injury to the ethmoidal arteries, which must be coagulated. Once the three cuts have been made, the bilateral fronto-orbito-ethmoid piece is removed (**Fig. 8.13**). Next, the frontal poles are gently retracted extradurally to expose the sleeves of the olfactory nerves (with the nerves inside), which are sectioned bilaterally. Dural detachment is continued to the planum sphenoidale. When all the dura of the anterior floor is detached, it is time to repair the dural defect created by the cut on the olfactory sleeves. Under the microscope, the rest of the ethmoid cells and planum sphenoidale are drilled. Both optic nerves are completely unroofed and the anterior wall of the sphenoid sinus is removed, thereby

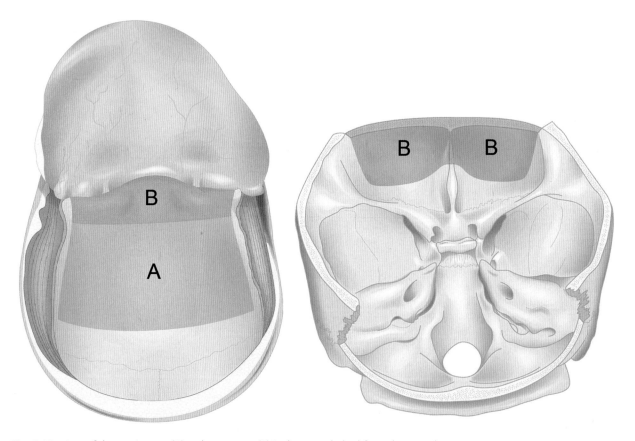

Fig. 8.13 Area of the craniotomy (A) and osteotomy (B) in the extended subfrontal approach.

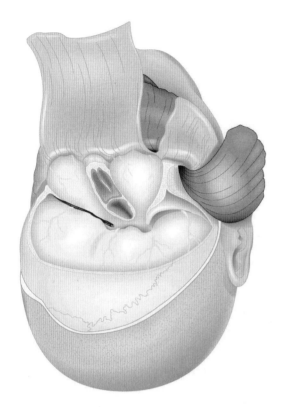

Fig. 8.14 The extradural exposure obtained through an extended subfrontal approach.

opening this sinus, which is often invaded by the tumor (**Fig. 8.14**). The floor of the sella turcica and the clivus are now identified. The sellar floor is drilled and tumor removal is continued into the sella turcica. With lateral movements of the microscope, it is possible to access both paraseellar regions where tumor removal is continued.[22,23]

The exposure of the cavernous sinus achieved with this approach is only partial. For this reason, this approach is recommended only for tumors with a favorable consistency. If the tumor is fibrous, it is very dangerous to attempt removal because of the high risk of injury to the cavernous ICA. Any injury to this artery is difficult to repair because of the lack of proximal control and the limited exposure of this vessel.

Reconstruction begins with placement of the pediculated pericranial flap, which is used to cover the defect created by drilling the anterior floor of the skull base. This flap must be split in its center to allow replacement of the orbital bar, which is fixed with miniplates. Finally, the bone flap is repositioned and the epicranial planes are closed in a standard manner.

Postoperative Care

After surgery, patients are routinely managed in the intensive care unit for the first 24 to 48 hours. They are extubated as soon as possible and undergo intensive neurologic and endocrinologic vigilance. After surgery, there is a high risk of electrolyte disequilibrium from manipulation of the hypothalamic-pituitary axis. Prophylactic antibiotics and anticonvulsant drugs are administered for 3 to 5 days. Steroids are given to reduce brain swelling and to replace any hormonal deficit as a result of manipulation of the sellar and suprasellar regions. Regardless of the patient's condition, a CT is done during the first 6 to 8 hours. Patients are usually discharged from the hospital 6 to 7 days postoperatively.

A control MRI is done after the first 4 to 6 weeks to assess the presence of residual tumor. External treatment of the patient should be done in conjunction with the endocrinology service to assess any need for definitive hormone replacement.

Complications

The possible complications of these approaches are the same as those of other, similar neurosurgical procedures and include infection, hematoma, seizures, and CSF leak. Other endocrinologic complications such as diabetes insipidus, hypothyroidism, hypocortisolism, or panhypopituitarism must be considered. There may be rare cases in which the brain manipulation damages the hypothalamic centers, leading to stupor and coma, thus endangering the patient's life.[24]

In any CS surgery, there is a high risk of deficit of the oculomotor nerves. In these cases, the patient should begin a physical therapy program or be referred to an oculoplasty service to evaluate the need for some type of reconstructive surgery for cases of permanent deficits. Finally, all these patients also have the potential risk of a serious complication generally associated with an ICA lesion.

Surgical Results

In general, when patients with a pituitary adenoma that invades the CS are appropriately selected, the results are surprising. Total resection of these tumors can often be achieved, unlike with meningiomas, with minimal functional deficits (**Figs. 8.15, 8.16, 8.17**). Moreover, because pituitary adenomas are benign tumors with a usually very low rate of proliferation, patients remain disease-free for longer periods.[25] However, achieving a real cure (as internationally accepted) of functioning tumors is virtually impossible when these lesions have invaded the CS.

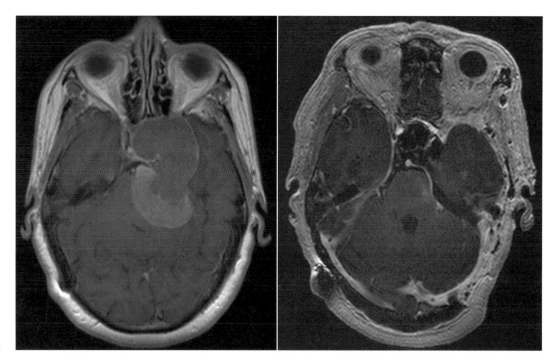

a

b

Fig. 8.15a,b T1-weighted MRI, axial view with contrast enhancement, of a 57-year-old woman with a pituitary adenoma invading the left cavernous sinus and petroclival region. The patient was operated on with a combination of the orbitozygomatic and posterior transpetrosal approaches. A total resection of the tumor was achieved in this patient with no neurologic deficit. **(a)** Preoperative image. **(b)** Postoperative image.

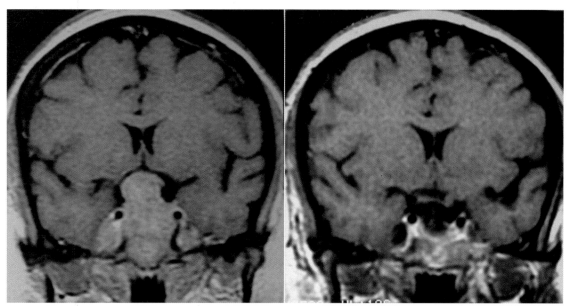

a

b

Fig. 8.16a,b T1-weighted MRI, coronal view with contrast enhancement, of a 51-year-old woman with a tumor invading the sellar and suprasellar regions as well as both cavernous sinuses. Through an extended subfrontal approach, the whole tumor (including the invasion into both cavernous sinuses) could be removed. **(a)** Preoperative image. **(b)** Postoperative image.

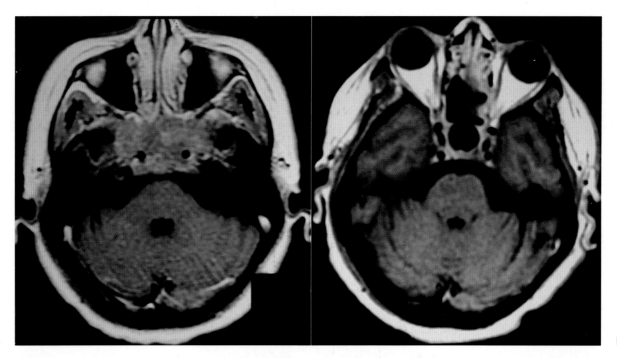

a   b

Fig. 8.17a,b T1-weighted MRI, axial view with contrast enhancement, of a 44-year-old man with bilateral invasion of the cavernous sinus by a pituitary adenoma. The tumor was completely removed through an extended subfrontal approach. **(a)** Preoperative image. **(b)** Postoperative image.

The Endonasal Transsphenoidal Approach to Pituitary Macroadenomas with Cavernous Sinus Extensions

Ali Shirzadi, Doniel Drazin, and Wesley A. King

Case Illustration

A 35-year-old woman presented for medical evaluation of decreased visual acuity and headache. No significant changes in her body habitus were noted. The physical examination was consistent with bilateral temporal hemianopsia; her visual acuity was 20/40 in the left eye and 20/70 in the right eye. MRI studies of the brain and sella revealed a large enhancing mass having characteristics most consistent with a nonfunctioning macroadenoma with a suprasellar extension and involvement of the bilateral cavernous sinuses, with a greater extension on the right **(Fig. 8.18)**. Judging by the marked enlargement and destruction of the sella turcica, the patient's tumor appeared most likely to be a nonsecreting pituitary adenoma. Based on the MRI findings, the probable diagnosis was a cavernous sinus extension, although this diagnosis could not be determined with certainty until the time of surgery. The patient's hormonal abnormalities were limited to a modest elevation in prolactin (55 ng/mL) attributed to compression of the pituitary stalk by the large tumor.

The patient underwent a transsphenoidal resection of the macroadenoma with the primary goal of decompressing the optic apparatus, with the hope of complete tumor removal. After surgery, she did well and had immediate improvement in her vision, and the postoperative image showed complete resection of her tumor **(Fig. 8.19)**. The patient was discharged from the hospital on postoperative day 2, with instructions to follow up with the endocrine and neurosurgery services.

Historical Review

The transsphenoidal approach has become a well-established method of resecting intrasellar and suprasellar pathologies. First proposed over a century ago,[26] the technique has progressed and improved with the introduction of the operative microscope, micro-instruments, and the endoscope.[27]

Giordano first proposed the transfacial approach for pituitary lesions in 1897, but it was Hemann Schloffer of

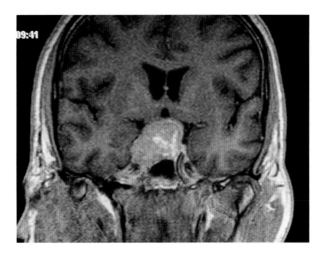

Fig. 8.18 A large enhancing mass with suprasellar and bilateral cavernous sinus extensions.

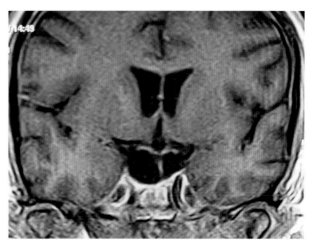

Fig. 8.19 Postoperative MRI showing complete resection of the tumor with decompression of the optic chiasm.

Austria who performed the first successful transsphenoidal resection of a pituitary tumor in 1907. Kocher and Hirsch modified the approach with multiple-stage resections of sellar tumors and the introduction of the nasal speculum.[28] Albert Halstead described the transsphenoidal sublabial approach in 1910, and Harvey Cushing redefined it in the 1920s. Dott, who studied under Cushing, continued using the transsphenoidal approach and trained Gerard Guiot, who introduced the use of radiofluoroscopy for trajectory confirmation in the 1950s and the use of the endoscope.[28,29] Hardy, a student of Guiot's, advanced the field with the incorporation of the operative microscope in the 1960s, dramatically changing the approach from just decompression to the inclusion of endocrinologic symptom relief.[28]

Although Guiot introduced the use of endoscopy, it was not until the 1970s that Apuzzo, Bushe, and Halves popularized the technique as an adjunct to microscopic resection of pituitary lesions.[29] In the 1990s, a collaboration of many neurologic and otolaryngological surgeons developed an endoscopic transsphenoidal approach to the sella. Jho and Carrau from the University of Pittsburgh became regarded as the leaders of pure endoscopic endonasal surgery for sellar tumors.[29] With continuing advances in radiology, navigation, and endoscopy, the field is continuing to improve, and reports describe decreased morbidity, better tumor resection, and the extension of the approach to suprasellar and third-ventricle pathologies.

Preoperative Evaluation

A careful and complete physical and neurologic examination of the patient is required before undertaking surgery of the cavernous sinus, regardless of the approach. Because of the risk of vascular and neural injury, patient selection is very important. In all cases, an MRI is done to delineate the extent of the lesion and assess any vascular involvement or abnormality. The MRI can depict a lesion's origin in the sella, clivus, or cavernous sinus, a critical distinction

in making a differential diagnosis and planning surgery. CT supplements the MRI by better defining bony expansion and destruction in selected cases. Usually, the MRI adequately demonstrates the relationship of the neoplasm to the ICA and documents patency of the artery and cavernous sinus, making a preoperative angiogram unnecessary. With pituitary adenomas, the caliber of the ICA is invariably normal, even when the artery is completely encased by the tumor. This phenomenon occurs because the tumor is soft and, unlike meningiomas, pituitary adenomas do not usually invade the arterial adventitia.

When an invasive pituitary tumor is suspected, preoperative blood studies, including hormonal levels, are essential. These studies may determine the course of treatment, for example, the use of a less aggressive surgical approach supplemented postoperatively by medical treatment (e.g., bromocriptine) or radiation therapy. The role of surgery in the treatment of prolactinomas remains controversial.[30] When surgery is undertaken on prolactinomas, we prefer to proceed with the operation and start bromocriptine treatment shortly thereafter, as this medication may promote fibrosis of the tumor and make surgical resection difficult. With surgery alone, the chances are small for a hormonal cure in a patient with a prolactinoma that has invaded the cavernous sinus, and therefore bromocriptine is usually required postoperatively. Overly aggressive surgery, with the undue risk of cranial nerve injury, is not indicated in this group of patients with pituitary tumors.

Surgery remains the first choice of treatment in patients with acromegaly, Cushing's disease, and hormonally inactive pituitary tumors.[31–35] In these patients, the surgeon must take a particularly aggressive stance, even if this means entering the cavernous sinus through a transsphenoidal approach. This is especially true with ACTH- and growth hormone–secreting tumors. When left untreated, these tumors have a significant associated morbidity, including malignancy in the case of acromegaly. An analogue of somatostatin, octreotide, has been introduced as a medical treatment modality for acromegaly.[32,34,36] Although it does not have the dramatic effect on tumor size that bromocriptine does with prolactinomas, octreotide has a high efficacy rate for lowering growth-hormone levels and will likely serve as a pre- and postoperative adjunct to surgery in patients with acromegaly.[32,34]

Growth Characteristics of Pituitary Adenomas

A relationship exists between the invasiveness of a pituitary tumor and its hormone-secretory status.[36] Specifically, hormonally active tumors tend to behave in a more invasive way than the hormonally silent adenomas. In general, previous studies have looked at the histological evidence of dural invasion by the tumor or the surgeon's observations at the time of surgery. MRI enables a preoperative assessment of the relationship of the tumor to cranial-base structures and a determination of the degree of invasiveness.[37–39] Cavernous sinus involvement is found in 6 to 10% of adenomas[37] with two distinct patterns of involvement. In the first pattern, adenomas can truly invade the sinus such that the venous spaces are obliterated and the ICA is partially or completely surrounded by the tumor. This behavior is frequently seen with nonfunctioning macroadenomas and is occasionally seen in growth hormone-secreting macroadenomas. In the second pattern, a tumor can compress the cavernous sinus without invading it. On MRI, the ICA may appear to have tumor partially surrounding it, but in no case is the artery completely encased. A fibrous dural layer is maintained between the tumor and the cavernous sinus.[37,38] This pattern is most typical for the nonsecreting or hormonally inactive tumors, with frank invasion of the cavernous sinus being rare. The involvement of the cavernous sinus remains a diagnosis made at the time of surgery. Finding an intact capsule adjacent to the cavernous sinus and ICA allows for easier tumor removal without significant intraoperative bleeding.[38]

Additionally, immunohistological studies with antiproliferating cell nuclear antigen (PCNA), an auxiliary protein of DNA polymerase, K_i-67, and methoxyisobutylisonitrile (MIBI), a novel anti–K_i-67 antibody, have been used to evaluate the growth rate and cavernous sinus invasion of pituitary adenomas.[40,41] Although these markers, especially MIBI, were correlated with a rapid growth of pituitary tumors, there was no correlation between cavernous sinus invasion and the growth rate of these tumors.[40] The reason for the differences in growth characteristics of these tumors remains unclear. Most likely, there are additional biochemical factors inherent to the invasive tumors that facilitate invasion of the cavernous sinus.

Patient Selection

We do not believe that cavernous sinus involvement should be a criterion for deciding to operate on a pituitary tumor transsphenoidally or transcranially. This decision should be based on the patient's age, health, and preoperative symptoms, and the direction of growth of the tumor. The surgeon's experience is also an important consideration. In our opinion, a craniotomy should be reserved for the patient who is otherwise in good health, whose tumor has grown either eccentrically under the temporal lobe or anteriorly under the frontal lobe. Posterior-superior growth can be treated satisfactorily through the transsphenoidal route. A craniotomy can be considered when a transsphenoidal procedure has not succeeded in achieving complete tumor removal.

Surgical Anatomy

Complete familiarity with and understanding of the inferomedial anatomy of the cavernous sinus is essential before undertaking surgery through the transsphenoidal approach. As with lateral and superior-medial approaches to the cavernous sinus, familiarity with the anatomy is best achieved through meticulous cadaveric dissection.[42–46] The dura of the medial wall of the cavernous sinus is thick, like that of the outer layer of the lateral wall, but unlike the lateral wall, an inner layer is absent. The dura of the pituitary fossa, which has two layers, is contiguous with that of the medial cavernous sinus. Interdural venous channels, in continuity with the cavernous sinus, can frequently be seen passing beneath the pituitary gland and can be the source of bleeding at the time of surgery. Many diagrammatic representations of the parasellar area show dura separating the gland from the ICA, but this is not always present.

The ICA lies close to the medial wall of the cavernous sinus and is usually separated from it by a thin medial venous space. Along the vertical segment of the ICA, there are usually no venous channels medial to the artery. All segments of the intracavernous portion of the ICA can be visualized through the transsphenoidal approach. The posterior vertical segment is found distal to the foramen lacerum. After the posterior bend, the artery runs anterior as the horizontal segment that ends at the anterior bend before leaving the cavernous sinus. To enter the subdural space, the artery must pierce the dural ring, which is tenaciously attached to the ICA. The dural ring actually consists of two fibrous rings that fuse medially where they are continuous with the dura of the diaphragma sellae. Laterally, the dural ring continues as the dura overlying the anterior clinoid. Several branches of the ICA can be visualized through the sphenoid sinus. The meningohypophyseal trunk and its branches can be seen rising from the convex portion of the posterior bend, and the artery of the inferior cavernous sinus is seen lateral to the ICA as it passes above the abducens nerve. Less frequently visualized arteries include the inferior hypophyseal and McConnell's capsular artery.

The neural relationships of the medial parasellar area are extraordinarily intricate. The optic nerve exits through the optic canal superior-medial to the cavernous sinus, with the ophthalmic artery applied to its inferior surface. The ophthalmic artery can occasionally arise from the horizontal segment of the ICA, in which case it enters the orbit through the superior orbital fissure. Cranial nerves III, IV, and VI can be visualized lateral to the ICA. The ophthalmic and maxillary branches of the trigeminal nerve can be exposed transsphenoidally and are rarely injured during surgery of the medial cavernous sinus. Sympathetic nerve fibers run along the ICA before joining the abducens nerve and ultimately supplying the intraorbital structures.

Surgical Procedure

Positioning of Patient and Equipment

For this approach, the nasotracheal tube is taped to the left lower portion of the patient's mouth immediately after a nasal decongestant is applied to the nasal mucosa with cottonoids. We use MRI with image guidance to evaluate soft tissue and the extension of tumor and its relationship to carotid arteries. The patient is turned 180 degrees from the anesthesiologist, with the surgeon standing on the right side of the patient and the technician standing on the other side of the bed. The navigation and endoscope monitors are placed at the head of the patient. This position frees the surgeon from any restriction and provides full access to the patient's nostrils with comfortable visualization of the monitors. The patient's head is secured with three-point fixation to reduce any movement and improve the accuracy of neuronavigation. The patient's head is turned to the right and the body is positioned on the right of the table with the back elevated and all pressure points padded.

Approach

We use a bilateral nasal access for better visualization, less crowding of instruments, and better control of hemorrhage in case of complications. The endoscope is introduced at the 12 o'clock position of the right nostril, with fracturing and mobilizing of the medial turbinate laterally. The ostium of the sphenoid sinus is identified and the mucosa surrounding it is coagulated with a suction Bovie instrument (**Fig. 8.20**). The ostium is widened with Kerrison rongeurs, a drill, or both. Damage to the sphenopalatine artery in the inferior-lateral aspect of the ostium should be avoided. The posterior septal mucosa covering the vomer is coagulated and the midline bone is removed, which provides access to the contralateral nostril (**Fig. 8.21**). These steps are repeated on the left nostril, creating a wide bilateral sphenoidotomy extending laterally to the medial pterygoid plates, superiorly to the planum sphenoidale, and inferiorly to the floor of the sphenoid sinus. The posterior septectomy is further extended with a back-biting instrument; care must be taken, however, to limit this resection to not more than the posterior third of the septum as further resection can cause postoperative whistling for the patient. For expanded endonasal approaches to the sella, an endonasal septal flap is created and placed inferiorly in the nasopharyngeal fossa, and the septal mucosa is

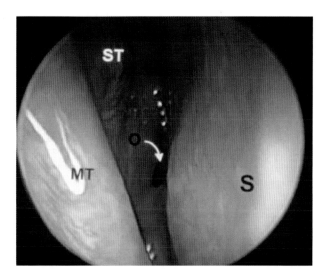

Fig. 8.20 Upon advancement of the endoscope, the septum (S) and medial turbinate (MT) can be identified medially and laterally, respectively. The ostia of the sphenoid sinus (O) is noted deep in the nostril.

not coagulated. This wide opening provides great access and enables the identification of key anatomic landmarks. At this point, the endoscope is secured on a holder, and binasal, bi-dextrous access to the sella is possible (**Fig. 8.22**).

The Sinus

After the sinus is entered and all of the mucosa within it is removed, several bony prominences are immediately visualized and should be noted before any bone within the sinus is removed. The carotid prominence, a bulge of the lateral wall of the sphenoid sinus, overlies the vertical and horizontal segment as well as the anterior bend of the ICA. Frequently, a bony prominence from the maxillary nerve can be identified. The location of the optic nerve can usu-

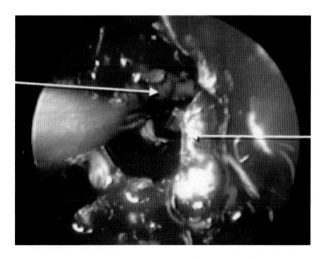

Fig. 8.21 By enlarging the ostia and removing the posterior septal wall and vomer (*bottom arrow*), bilateral access to the sella (*top arrow*) is facilitated.

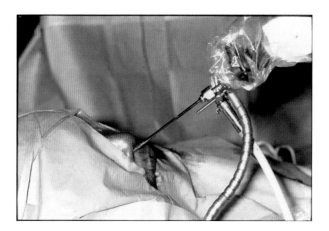

Fig. 8.22 By using an endoscope holder, the surgeon can free both hands and have bi-dextrous access to the sella.

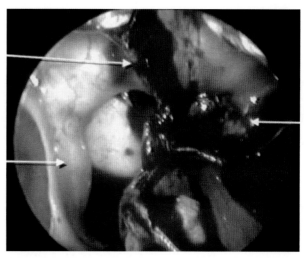

Fig. 8.23 When the sphenoid sinus is entered, the sella (*top arrow*) and bilateral (left, *middle arrow;* right, *bottom arrow*) internal cartid proturberances can be identified with the internal carotid arteries underneath them.

ally be identified along the superior-lateral aspect of the carotid prominence. The clivus and its recess are noted inferior to the sella, as the sella is mostly enlarged from the expanding tumor **(Fig. 8.23)**. In the case of a neoplasm, the sella or clivus can appear attenuated or distorted. Not infrequently, tumors extend into the sphenoid sinus.

Tumor Resection

The bone overlying the sella and medial sinus can be removed to expose the dura of the pituitary fossa and the ICA. Doppler ultrasonography is used to localize the carotid arteries before the dural opening, which is done with angled micro-feather blades. Any cavernous sinus bleeding should be controlled with an application of Gelfoam cottonoid pressure over the area. If bleeding is noted after micro-incision of the dura, it may be controlled by grasping both dural leaves with the bipolar cautery and coagulating them closed. Tumors involving the medial cavernous sinus typically obliterate the vascular space and can be removed in piecemeal fashion with ring curettes and microdissectors. These instruments can be passed gently around the ICA to remove tumor that has extended lateral to it. The endoscope may be introduced inside the sella to further visualize the extent of the mass, and further evaluation can be done with an angled scope. Tumors most often expand the sella, creating a corridor lateral to the carotid into the cavernous sinus, which can be easily followed with the endoscope. Significant venous bleeding is not usually a problem until the final stages of tumor removal as the patent part of the sinus is exposed. The adenoma can be further encouraged to collapse into the sinus through elevation of the subarachnoid fluid pressure with intermittent Valsalva maneuvers performed by the anesthesiologist or, alternatively, by injecting intrathecal saline through a lumbar subarachnoid catheter. Therefore, the tumor should be removed in a systematic manner, with bleeding controlled, and with absolute care taken to prevent injury to the optic nerves and carotid arteries.

Complications

Intraoperative complications of the transsphenoidal approach include CSF leakage, carotid laceration (rarely), and cranial nerve palsies. We reconstruct the sella with absorbable plates that are placed in the epidural space under the sellar bone. Most CSF leaks can be repaired with autologous abdominal fascia, or fascia lata, with fat and fibrin glue at the time of surgery. The postoperative diversion of CSF with a lumbar subarachnoid catheter, left in place for 3 to 5 days after surgery, helps to ensure good healing of the leak. In cases of carotid laceration, suture placement is impossible and pressure must be applied with cotton patties. An angiogram, if feasible, should be done immediately to evaluate the patency of the carotid and, if needed, a stent repair of the avulsed vessel should be done.

Discussion

The goal of pituitary surgery is surgical decompression of the neural structures, especially the optic apparatus, and complete removal of hormone-secreting tumors. We strongly believe that, as an initial procedure, the endoscopic transsphenoidal avenue should be used to approach this tumor. A craniotomy or, alternatively, radiotherapy can be undertaken as a second stage if the initial operation does not completely remove the lesion. The endoscopic approach provides great and wide visualization of the sella and skull base, which aids in complete removal of the entire tumor within the sphenoid sinus and immediate decompression of the optic nerves and brainstem with low associated morbidity. Pituitary tumors are typically soft and gelatinous and have a propensity to descend into the sphenoid sinus, thus making transsphenoidal resection feasible.

Although most pituitary tumors are avascular large adenomas, such as the tumor seen in this illustrative case, they can develop a blood supply and can be quite hemorrhagic. Concomitant with the increased vascularity is a tendency of the tumor to become fibrotic, firm, and multisegmented. Histologically, one does not always see the sheets of monotonous cells typical of pituitary adenomas, but rather one may see a nest of cells separated by a fibrovascular stroma. The result is that tumor extirpation is more difficult and may require sharp dissection to divide fibrous septation and to open tumor loculations. Further, the risk of CSF leakage in this setting is significantly higher than during surgery on more routine macroadenomas.

Advances in microsurgical techniques have allowed lesions of the cavernous sinus to be approached surgically.[47–49] One of the more challenging problems that has received considerable attention is when a pituitary tumor invades the medial cavernous sinus.[50,51] We believe that an endoscopic transsphenoidal approach provides for a safe and successful surgical resection of these tumors. It allows a panoramic view for magnified inspection of the resection cavity as well as wider and better identification of key anatomic structures.[52] With a two-handed microsurgical technique and an understanding of the two-dimensional depth perception of an endoscope, a surgeon can perform this microsurgical operation precisely with minimal brain manipulation and less frequent nasal packing.[52,53] Improvements in instruments have allowed the field of neurosurgery to advance and continue to expand the horizons of transsphenoidal surgery.

Moderators

Transcranial vs. Transsphenoidal Approach for Pituitary Macroadenomas with Cavernous Sinus Invasion

Nelson Oyesiku and Brandon A. Miller

In most centers, pituitary macroadenomas without invasion into the cavernous sinus are approached exclusively through transsphenoidal surgery. We almost exclusively use a transsphenoidal approach with three-dimensional endoscopy for the initial surgical treatment of all patients with pituitary adenomas. The utility of this approach, however, should not discourage familiarity with and a consideration of the transcranial approaches to the sella for tumors with a cavernous sinus extension. Although a transsphenoidal approach should be used for microadenomas and macroadenomas without extension outside the sella, tumors involving the cavernous sinus merit consideration of a broader range of surgical options. As described above, both endoscopic transsphenoidal and transcranial approaches can be used to approach pituitary tumors involving the cavernous sinus. The preceding authors' descriptions of both these approaches should serve as guides for neurosurgeons considering either approach. Here, we emphasize points we have learned through our experience in treating more than 2,000 patients with pituitary tumors, and we discuss the indications for a transcranial approach.

Preoperative Evaluation

Even with the widespread availability of CT and MRI, patients with pituitary macroadenomas often present with large invasive tumors, sometimes with invasion of the cavernous sinus. The slow-growing nature of these tumors and often subtle vision changes that accompany their growth frequently delay a patient's workup through visual testing or neuroimaging. This delay leads to the scenario of patients presenting with large or giant pituitary macroadenomas, often with cavernous sinus invasion.

Preoperatively, all patients should undergo MRI with and without contrast, formal visual fields testing, and endocrine evaluation. In the case of a prolactinoma causing significant mass effect, treatment with dopamine-agonist drugs may be indicated solely or in combination with surgery. Similarly, growth hormone–producing adenomas may respond to somatostatin analogues or dopamine agonists. In our multidisciplinary clinic, a neurosurgeon and endocrinologist evaluate all new patients at the same visit, which allows for the prompt initiation of medical management, if indicated, and the coordination of pre- and postoperative endocrine evaluations.

Surgery for a patient with an invasive macroadenoma causing vision loss must be considered most carefully. Although the goal of gross total resection, especially in younger patients, is admirable, it must be balanced against the potential risk of injury to neurologic and vascular structures. On the other hand, a large residual tumor is also less susceptible to radiosurgery and may predispose the patient to tumor progression.[54] Aspects of surgical morbidity such as hypopituitarism, injury to neurovascular structures, and the risk of a CSF leak must be considered. These factors should be discussed with the patient, and realistic expectations should be conveyed and analyzed. Preoperative counseling about such postoperative complications such as diabetes insipidus or a CSF leak will hasten their detection should they occur postoperatively.

Selecting the Approach

We approach all microadenomas and macroadenomas without cavernous sinus extension through a transsphenoidal route utilizing three-dimensional endoscopy. Tumors with a cavernous sinus extension present a more challenging situation. As Guinto describes, several cranial approaches may be used to resect large and irregularly shaped macroadenomas. All of these approaches involve a higher potential for neurovascular injury and postoperative cosmetic defects compared with transsphenoidal surgery. Additionally, there is the risk of postoperative hemorrhage and ischemia with transcranial approaches,[55,56] although this risk exists after transsphenoidal surgery as well.[55,57] The key advantages of cranial surgery for invasive pituitary adenomas are access to the lateral aspect of the cavernous sinus, which may be difficult to achieve via endoscopy, and the ability to safely control the ICA.[7]

The extended transsphenoidal approaches have improved the surgeon's ability to access the lateral cavernous sinus, and studies have shown the efficacy of this approach for adenomas invading the cavernous sinus.[58–60] Although limiting the surgeon's ability to achieve hemostasis in the case of large vessel injury, the endoscopic transsphenoidal approach has many advantages, especially with the recent advances in endoscopy, optics, and surgical instrumentation. The transsphenoidal route presents a more direct trajectory to pituitary tumors and eliminates the brain retraction that usually accompanies pterional and subfrontal exposures. Newer endoscopes, including systems that allow for three-dimensional visualization, include 30- and 45-degree lenses with illumination and magnification that give the surgeon an excellent view of the sellar and parasellar anatomy. Although working laterally toward and into the cavernous sinus is challenging, angled scopes and instruments allow for tumor resection at difficult angles. When there is venous bleeding from the sinus, Gelfoam, Floseal, or Surgifoam and pressure with cottonoids are quite effective for achieving hemostasis. We typically place a lumbar drain in patients with large tumors, which allows manipulation of the CSF volume during the case. Manipulating the CSF volume can help bring the tumor into the operative field or help unload the prolapsed diaphragma sella and arachnoid after tumor decompression to improve visualization within the tumor cavity. We typically leave lumbar drains in for 3 days after surgery for patients with an intraoperative CSF leak.

Although we favor the transsphenoidal approach whenever possible, several specific situations and tumor configurations complicate a transsphenoidal approach.[61] Tumors with a fibrous consistency often do not descend into the sella when resected from below, even after an extracapsular transsphenoidal approach, and may require subsequent resection through a transcranial approach.[7] As Guinto points out, a fibrous consistency may be predicted by a hypointense appearance on the T2-weighted MRI.[62] Adenomas extending over the planum sphenoidale often require an intracranial approach,[63] although they also can be approached via an extended transsphenoidal corridor through the anterior skull base with an angled lens.[1] Vascular considerations, such as "kissing" carotid arteries that critically constrict the sellar corridor or a coexisting cerebral aneurysm that is amenable to simultaneous clipping, indicate a transcranial approach.[63]

Furthermore, variations in the anatomy of the skull base, such as a lack of pneumatization of the sphenoid sinus, may restrict or even preclude transsphenoidal access. As King and colleagues state, an intracavernous extension of the tumor lateral to the carotid arteries may pose a challenge for transsphenoidal resection. Although it is possible to access the lateral cavernous sinus through an extended transsphenoidal approach, such as a transpterygoid approach, complete resection of these lesions can be difficult.[59] But this factor alone is rarely an indication for the transcranial versus the transsphenoidal route. With the availability of postoperative radiosurgery, it is quite reasonable to treat residual tumor in the lateral cavernous sinus after an endoscopic approach rather than use a transcranial approach purely to resect cavernous sinus disease, as long as the residual disease is minimal. Several studies of radiosurgery for pituitary adenomas have shown good results.[54,64,65] The most common reason we perform a craniotomy for pituitary adenoma is that any residual disease after a transsphenoidal operation is not amenable to radiotherapy. We approach these tumors first endoscopically, and then carry out a craniotomy for residual disease. Any residual tumor burden is treated with stereotactic radiosurgery or fractionated stereotactic radiotherapy, and patients undergo annual MRI and close neurosurgical, endocrinologic, and ophthalmologic follow-up. When the residual tumor left after a transsphenoidal approach is too large for effective radiosurgery, we perform a craniotomy on the right side unless the patient has severe vision loss on the left, in which case a left-sided approach has less chance of causing new visual deficits. In patients with large tumors and hydrocephalus, a ventriculostomy may be indicated before surgery. In select patients with large tumors, we have performed simultaneous transsphenoidal microscopic and transcranial approaches,[66] but this practice has fallen out of favor because of success with a staged endoscopic transsphenoidal-transcranial approach.

There are few data comparing the quality of different approaches for invasive pituitary adenomas. One recent review in the literature compared 66 patients undergoing endoscopic transsphenoidal resection with 106 patients undergoing transcranial surgery for giant adenomas.[57] The review found that, with the different surgical approaches used at different centers, including different surgeons with varying experience, retrospective analyses, nonrandomization, and missing data sets, appropriate and valid comparisons were impossible. The recent literature focusing on cavernous sinus disease has shown subtotal tumor resection but low morbidity after the transsphenoidal approach.[58–60,67,68] Although case series have shown a high rate of gross-total resection in transcranial approaches to the cavernous sinus,[56,69] there is a growing consensus that

the lower morbidity of the transsphenoidal approach combined with the effectiveness of postoperative radiosurgery makes it the more favorable avenue.[70–72] We advocate transsphenoidal resection followed by stereotactic radiosurgery or fractionated stereotactic radiotherapy for all but a select few patients with pituitary macroadenomas invading the cavernous sinus.

References

1. Youssef AS, Agazzi S, van Loveren HR. Transcranial surgery for pituitary adenomas. Neurosurgery 2005; 57(1, Suppl)168–175, discussion 168–175

2. Bogaev C, Sekhar LN. Cavernous sinus tumors. In: Sekhar LN, Fessler RG, eds. Atlas of Neurosurgical Techniques: Brain. New York: Thieme, 2006:633–653

3. Fukushima T, Diaz J. Surgical management of tumors invading the cavernous sinus. In: Schmidek HH, ed. Operative Neurosurgical Techniques. Indications, Methods and Results, 4th ed. Philadelphia: WB Saunders, 2000:351–369

4. Janjua RM, Al-Mefty O, Densler DW, Shields CB. Dural relationships of Meckel cave and lateral wall of the cavernous sinus. Neurosurg Focus 2008;25(6):E2

5. Isolan GR, Krayenbühl N, de Oliveira E, Al-Mefty O. Microsurgical anatomy of the cavernous sinus: measurements of the triangles in and around it. Skull Base 2007;17(6):357–367

6. Iaconetta G, de Notaris M, Cavallo LM, et al. The oculomotor nerve: microanatomical and endoscopic study. Neurosurgery 2010;66(3):593–601, discussion 601

7. Day JD. Surgical approaches to suprasellar and parasellar tumors. Neurosurg Clin N Am 2003;14(1):109–122

8. Wu ZB, Su ZP, Wu JS, Zheng WM, Zhuge QC, Zhong M. Five years follow-up of invasive prolactinomas with special reference to the control of cavernous sinus invasion. Pituitary 2008;11(1): 63–70

9. Knappe UJ, Jaursch-Hancke C, Schönmayr R, Lörcher U. Assessment of normal perisellar anatomy in 1.5 T T2-weighted MRI and comparison with the anatomic criteria defining cavernous sinus invasion of pituitary adenomas. Cent Eur Neurosurg 2009;70(3):130–136

10. Vieira JO Jr, Cukiert A, Liberman B. Evaluation of magnetic resonance imaging criteria for cavernous sinus invasion in patients with pituitary adenomas: logistic regression analysis and correlation with surgical findings. Surg Neurol 2006;65(2):130–135, discussion 135

11. Vieira JO Jr, Cukiert A, Liberman B. Magnetic resonance imaging of cavernous sinus invasion by pituitary adenoma diagnostic criteria and surgical findings. Arq Neuropsiquiatr 2004;62(2B): 437–443

12. Yamada S, Ohyama K, Taguchi M, et al. A study of the correlation between morphological findings and biological activities in clinically nonfunctioning pituitary adenomas. Neurosurgery 2007;61(3):580–584, discussion 584–585

13. Seçkin H, Avci E, Uluç K, Niemann D, Başkaya MK. The work horse of skull base surgery: orbitozygomatic approach. Technique, modifications, and applications. Neurosurg Focus 2008; 25(6):E4

14. Guinto G, Abello J, Félix I, González J, Oviedo A. Lesions confined to the sphenoid ridge: differential diagnosis and surgical treatment. Skull Base Surg 1997;7(3):115–121

15. Guinto G, Cohn F, Perez-de la Torre R, Gallardo M. Pituitary macroadenomas: transcranial approach. In: Sekhar LN, Fessler RG, ed. Atlas of Neurosurgical Techniques: Brain. New York: Thieme, 2006:661–669

16. Cheng CM, Chang CF, Ma HI, Chiang YH, McMenomey SO, Delashaw JB Jr. Modified orbitozygomatic craniotomy for large medial sphenoid wing meningiomas. J Clin Neurosci 2009; 16(9):1157–1160

17. Chang CW, Wang LC, Lee JS, Tai SH, Huang CY, Chen HH. Orbitozygomatic approach for excisions of orbital tumors with 1 piece of craniotomy bone flap: 2 case reports. Surg Neurol 2007; 68(Suppl 1):S56–S59, discussion S59

18. Campero A, Martins C, Socolovsky M, et al. Three-piece orbitozygomatic approach. Neurosurgery 2010; 66(3, Suppl Operative)E119–E120, discussion E120

19. Agazzi S, Youssef AS, van Loveren HR. The anterolateral approach for the transcranial resection of pituitary adenomas: technical note. Skull Base 2010;20(3):143–148

20. Klimo P Jr, Browd SR, Pravdenkova S, Couldwell WT, Walker ML, Al-Mefty O. The posterior petrosal approach: technique and applications in pediatric neurosurgery. J Neurosurg Pediatr 2009;4(4):353–362

21. Cho CW, Al-Mefty O. Combined petrosal approach to petroclival meningiomas. Neurosurgery 2002;51(3):708–716, discussion 716–718

22. Mortini P, Roberti F, Kalavakonda C, Nadel A, Sekhar LN. Endoscopic and microscopic extended subfrontal approach to the clivus: a comparative anatomical study. Skull Base 2003;13(3): 139–147

23. Ladziński P, Majchrzak H, Kaspera W, et al. Direct and remote outcome after treatment of tumours involving the central skull base with the extended subfrontal approach. Neurol Neurochir Pol 2009;43(1):22–35

24. Chang EF, Zada G, Kim S, et al. Long-term recurrence and mortality after surgery and adjuvant radiotherapy for nonfunctional pituitary adenomas. J Neurosurg 2008;108(4):736–745

25. Chang CZ, Huang YH, Howng SL. Follow-up of invasive pituitary macroadenoma in 56 patients within a duration of 5 years. Kaohsiung J Med Sci 2000;16(7):339–344

26. Liu JK, Das K, Weiss MH, Laws ER Jr, Couldwell WT. The history and evolution of transsphenoidal surgery. J Neurosurg 2001; 95(6):1083–1096

27. Dehdashti AR, Ganna A, Witterick I, Gentili F. Expanded endoscopic endonasal approach for anterior cranial base and suprasellar lesions: indications and limitations. Neurosurgery 2009; 64(4):677–687, discussion 687–689

28. Kanter AS, Dumont AS, Asthagiri AR, Oskouian RJ, Jane JA Jr, Laws ER Jr. The transsphenoidal approach. A historical perspective. Neurosurg Focus 2005;18(4):e6

29. Doglietto F, Prevedello DM, Jane JA Jr, Han J, Laws ER Jr. Brief history of endoscopic transsphenoidal surgery—from Philipp Bozzini to the First World Congress of Endoscopic Skull Base Surgery. Neurosurg Focus 2005;19(6):E3

30. Tyrrell JB, Lamborn KR, Hannegan LT, Applebury CB, Wilson CB. Transsphenoidal microsurgical therapy of prolactinomas: initial outcomes and long-term results. Neurosurgery 1999;44(2): 254–261, discussion 261–263

31. Boggan JE, Tyrrell JB, Wilson CB. Transsphenoidal microsurgical management of Cushing's disease. Report of 100 cases. J Neurosurg 1983;59(2):195–200

32. Carmichael JD, Bonert VS, Mirocha JM, Melmed S. The utility of oral glucose tolerance testing for diagnosis and assessment of treatment outcomes in 166 patients with acromegaly. J Clin Endocrinol Metab 2009;94(2):523–527

33. Ebersold MJ, Quast LM, Laws ER Jr, Scheithauer B, Randall RV. Long-term results in transsphenoidal removal of nonfunctioning pituitary adenomas. J Neurosurg 1986;64(5):713–719

34. Melmed S, Jackson I, Kleinberg D, Klibanski A. Current treatment guidelines for acromegaly. J Clin Endocrinol Metab 1998; 83(8):2646–2652

35. Saito K, Kuwayama A, Yamamoto N, Sugita K. The transsphenoidal removal of nonfunctioning pituitary adenomas with suprasellar extensions: the open sella method and intentionally staged operation. Neurosurgery 1995;36(4):668–675, discussion 675–676

36. Barkan AL, Kelch RP, Hopwood NJ, Beitins IZ. Treatment of acromegaly with the long-acting somatostatin analog SMS 201-995. J Clin Endocrinol Metab 1988;66(1):16–23

37. Cottier JP, Destrieux C, Brunereau L, et al. Cavernous sinus invasion by pituitary adenoma: MR imaging. Radiology 2000; 215(2):463–469

38. Knosp E, Steiner E, Kitz K, Matula C. Pituitary adenomas with invasion of the cavernous sinus space: a magnetic resonance imaging classification compared with surgical findings. Neurosurgery 1993;33(4):610–617, discussion 617–618

39. Lundin P, Nyman R, Burman P, Lundberg PO, Muhr C. MRI of pituitary macroadenomas with reference to hormonal activity. Neuroradiology 1992;34(1):43–51

40. Kawamoto H, Uozumi T, Kawamoto K, Arita K, Yano T, Hirohata T. Analysis of the growth rate and cavernous sinus invasion of pituitary adenomas. Acta Neurochir (Wien) 1995;136(1-2): 37–43

41. Landolt AM, Shibata T, Kleihues P. Growth rate of human pituitary adenomas. J Neurosurg 1987;67(6):803–806

42. Fujii K, Chambers SM, Rhoton AL Jr. Neurovascular relationships of the sphenoid sinus. A microsurgical study. J Neurosurg 1979;50(1):31–39

43. Inoue T, Rhoton AL Jr, Theele D, Barry ME. Surgical approaches to the cavernous sinus: a microsurgical study. Neurosurgery 1990;26(6):903–932

44. Rhoton AL Jr, Hardy DG, Chambers SM. Microsurgical anatomy and dissection of the sphenoid bone, cavernous sinus and sellar region. Surg Neurol 1979;12(1):63–104

45. Sekhar LN, Burgess J, Akin O. Anatomical study of the cavernous sinus emphasizing operative approaches and related vascular and neural reconstruction. Neurosurgery 1987;21(6):806–816

46. Sekhar LN, Sen CN, Jho HD, Janecka IP. Surgical treatment of intracavernous neoplasms: a four-year experience. Neurosurgery 1989;24(1):18–30

47. Dolenc V. Direct microsurgical repair of intracavernous vascular lesions. J Neurosurg 1983;58(6):824–831

48. Laws ER Jr, Onofrio BM, Pearson BW, McDonald TJ, Dirrenberger RA. Successful management of bilateral carotid-cavernous fistulae with a trans-sphenoidal approach. Neurosurgery 1979;4(2):162–167

49. Parkinson D. A surgical approach to the cavernous portion of the carotid artery. Anatomical studies and case report. J Neurosurg 1965;23(5):474–483

50. Hashimoto N, Kikuchi H. Transsphenoidal approach to infrasellar tumors involving the cavernous sinus. J Neurosurg 1990; 73(4):513–517

51. MacKay A, Hosobuchi Y. Treatment of intracavernous extensions of pituitary adenomas. Surg Neurol 1978;10(6):377–383

52. Jane JA Jr, Han J, Prevedello DM, Jagannathan J, Dumont AS, Laws ER Jr. Perspectives on endoscopic transsphenoidal surgery. Neurosurg Focus 2005;19(6):E2

53. Laws ER, Kanter AS, Jane JA Jr, Dumont AS. Extended transsphenoidal approach. J Neurosurg 2005;102(5):825–827, discussion 827–828

54. Gopalan R, Schlesinger D, Vance ML, Laws E, Sheehan J. Long-term outcomes after Gamma Knife radiosurgery for patients with a nonfunctioning pituitary adenoma. Neurosurgery 2011; 69(2):284–293

55. King WA, Rodts GE, Becker DP, Mc Bride DQ. Microsurgical management of giant pituitary tumors. Skull Base Surg 1996; 6(1):17–26

56. Spallone A, Gonzàlez-Gonzàlez JL, Mostes de Oca F, Verdial-Vidal R. [Pituitary adenomas invading the cavernous sinus. Transcranial transcavernous approach]. Neurocirugia (Astur) 2007; 18(4):294–300

57. Komotar RJ, Starke RM, Raper DM, Anand VK, Schwartz TH. Endoscopic endonasal compared with microscopic transsphenoidal and open transcranial resection of giant pituitary adenomas. Pituitary 2012;15(2):150–159

58. Ceylan S, Koc K, Anık I. Extended endoscopic transphenoidal approach for tuberculum sellae meningiomas. Acta Neurochir (Wien) 2011;153(1):1–9

59. Kitano M, Taneda M, Shimono T, Nakao Y. Extended transsphenoidal approach for surgical management of pituitary adenomas invading the cavernous sinus. J Neurosurg 2008;108(1): 26–36

60. Zhao B, Wei YK, Li GL, et al. Extended transsphenoidal approach for pituitary adenomas invading the anterior cranial base, cavernous sinus, and clivus: a single-center experience with 126 consecutive cases. J Neurosurg 2010;112(1):108–117

61. Zada G, Du R, Laws ER Jr. Defining the "edge of the envelope": patient selection in treating complex sellar-based neoplasms via transsphenoidal versus open craniotomy. J Neurosurg 2011; 114(2):286–300

62. Snow RB, Johnson CE, Morgello S, Lavyne MH, Patterson RH Jr. Is magnetic resonance imaging useful in guiding the operative approach to large pituitary tumors? Neurosurgery 1990;26(5): 801–803

63. Liu JK, Weiss MH, Couldwell WT. Surgical approaches to pituitary tumors. Neurosurg Clin N Am 2003;14(1):93–107

64. Loeffler JS, Shih HA. Radiation therapy in the management of pituitary adenomas. J Clin Endocrinol Metab 2011;96(7):1992–2003

65. Sheehan JP, Kondziolka D, Flickinger J, Lunsford LD. Radiosurgery for residual or recurrent nonfunctioning pituitary adenoma. J Neurosurg 2002; 97(5, Suppl)408–414

66. Alleyne CH Jr, Barrow DL, Oyesiku NM. Combined transsphenoidal and pterional craniotomy approach to giant pituitary tumors. Surg Neurol 2002;57(6):380–390, discussion 390

67. Di Maio S, Cavallo LM, Esposito F, Stagno V, Corriero OV, Cappabianca P. Extended endoscopic endonasal approach for selected pituitary adenomas: early experience. J Neurosurg 2011; 114(2):345–353

68. Frank G, Pasquini E. Endoscopic endonasal cavernous sinus surgery, with special reference to pituitary adenomas. Front Horm Res 2006;34:64–82

69. Dolenc VV. Transcranial epidural approach to pituitary tumors extending beyond the sella. Neurosurgery 1997;41(3):542–550, discussion 551–552

70. Agrawal A, Cincu R, Goel A. Current concepts and controversies in the management of non-functioning giant pituitary macroadenomas. Clin Neurol Neurosurg 2007;109(8):645–650

71. Murad MH, Fernández-Balsells MM, Barwise A, et al. Outcomes of surgical treatment for nonfunctioning pituitary adenomas: a systematic review and meta-analysis. Clin Endocrinol (Oxf) 2010;73(6):777–791

72. Musleh W, Sonabend AM, Lesniak MS. Role of craniotomy in the management of pituitary adenomas and sellar/parasellar tumors. Expert Rev Anticancer Ther 2006;6(Suppl 9):S79–S83

Treatment of Craniopharyngiomas: Total Removal vs. Subtotal Removal with Radiation

Case

A 14-year-old girl came to medical attention with diabetes insipidus and a visual field defect.

Participants

Subtotal Resection with Focal Irradiation for Craniopharyngiomas: Frederick A. Boop and Scott D. Wait

Radical Resection of Pediatric Craniopharyngiomas: Jeffrey H. Wiskoff and Robert E. Elliott

Moderators: Total Removal vs. Subtotal Removal with Radiation for Craniopharyngiomas: Edward R. Smith and R. Michael Scott

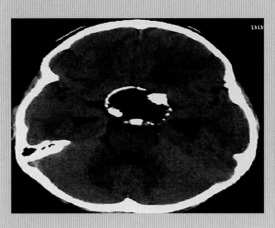
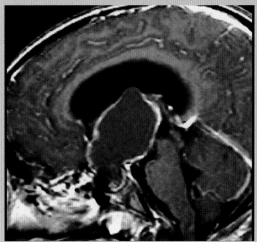

Subtotal Resection with Focal Irradiation for Craniopharyngiomas

Frederick A. Boop and Scott D. Wait

Here is a letter I recently received from the mother of a child with a craniopharyngioma:

> I have a 15-year-old son who was diagnosed at the age of 10 with a golf ball–sized craniopharyngioma. He had a gross total resection. ... He has all the usual complications: panhypopituitarism, diabetes insipidus, hyperphagia, hypothalamic obesity, and visual loss, plus he suffered a stroke when the surgeon "nicked" an artery. He also developed severe behavioral problems. He is extremely violent and self-abusive. One day, we noticed he didn't have any vision at all. We took him to his ophthalmologist and she recommended we take him to see his neurologist because she couldn't see anything wrong. We had appointments with endocrinology too so his neurologist worked him in. He was admitted and had an emergency MRI. It was found that a herpes virus had attacked his retina. His neurologist told us the MRI had shown a recurrence of the craniopharyngioma in the sella region. He gave us three options: (1) wait and see and re-scan in 3 months, (2) stereotactic radiosurgery, or (3) do nothing. The final option was given only because our son had developed other issues such as hypertension, spinal fusion due to idiopathic scoliosis, dystonia, two *Staph. aureus* infections, sleep apnea, diabetes, enlarged liver with elevated liver enzymes, lung depletion in the lower quadrants of his lungs, and depression. Right now we are planning on doing the radiation in the near future.

This letter is not to be misconstrued as an indictment of surgery for craniopharyngiomas but rather as an example of what is likely when a less experienced team cares for a child with a complicated craniopharyngioma. When one stops to consider that craniopharyngiomas represent only 1 to 2% of pediatric brain tumors, that the average children's hospital may see 30 to 40 pediatric tumors per year, and that there are generally two or more neurosurgeons on staff at a given hospital, then the average pediatric neurosurgeon might operate on only one craniopharyngioma every 2 to 3 years.[1] Thus, outside of major referral centers, it would be difficult for most neurosurgeons to gain enough experience with these tumors to consider themselves experts. More importantly, in interpreting the published literature on surgery for craniopharyngiomas, one cannot extrapolate the outcome or morbidity from a Wisoff, Yasargil, or Al-Mefty to one's own experience.[2] The care of children with these tumors is complex, requiring a well-organized multidisciplinary team willing to consider various treatment options for each individual patient. The team must provide a careful long-term follow-up to optimize functional recovery.

The treatment recommendations for the child cannot simply be "take it all out" versus "treat with focal irradiation." The reason that there are so many reported treatment options for this disease, such as observation, intracystic therapy, endoscopic drainage, stereotactic radiosurgery, conformal radiotherapy, proton beam therapy, and limited to complete resection, is that each of these treatments works well for some patients and none of these treatments works best for all patients. The treatment considerations for the child who presents with a headache, short stature, and normal vision with a small sellar lesion should be different from that for the child who presents with obtundation, panhypopituitarism, and acute hydrocephalus secondary to a giant craniopharyngioma[3] (**Figs. 9.1, 9.2**).

Preoperative Evaluation

The preoperative evaluation of each child is essentially the same. It includes high-definition magnetic resonance imaging (MRI), a formal visual evaluation, a detailed endocrinologic workup including stimulation testing, and psychosocial evaluation including developmental history, school performance, family stability, and available community support.[4] In the past quarter of a century, our microsurgical skills and training have allowed us to move from reporting morbidity and mortality throughout the 1970s to reporting basic functional outcome measures, such as the Glasgow Outcomes Scale at the end of the last century, and then to more detailed functional scales such as those of Karnofsky, Lansky, and others.

Treatment Strategies

In the current era, reporting of outcomes from craniopharyngioma treatment has moved to detailed neuropsychometric studies, quality-of-life measures, evaluations of school performance including attentional and processing problems in addition to visual acuity and fields, details of endocrinopathy and vasculopathy, and measures of progressive disease. Computed tomography (CT) and magnetic resonance angiography give us accurate assessments of postoperative pseudoaneurysms, moyamoya disease, and small-vessel arteritis. We also know that with each major intervention for craniopharyngiomas—surgery, radiotherapy, cyst catheter replacement, or shunt revision—the child will lose some measure of function. So when we review a series such as that reported by Hoffman, in which only 60% of children had a gross total resection of their tumor, and of those 15 to 20% recurred over time, the majority of these children will require a second craniotomy for recurrent disease, often followed by irradiation.[5] Under these circumstances, for the child who has had two or three major craniotomies with or without a shunt or shunt revision,

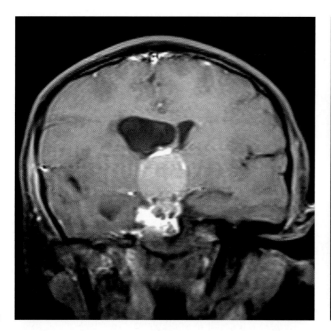

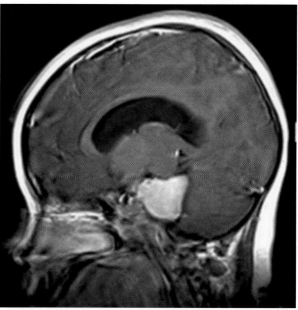

a

b

Fig. 9.1a,b **(a)** This is a T1-weighted gadolinium enhanced coronal image of an 8-year-old female presenting with headaches, normal visual exam, and normal endocrine status. Note the suprasellar tumor extending into the third ventricle and causing hydrocephalus. **(b)** A sagittal T1 gadolinium enhanced image of the same patient showing extension of the tumor into the posterior fossa nearly to the foramen magnum.

followed by medial forebrain irradiation, it is not realistic to expect the child to remain highly functional. Thus, minimizing the number of potential interventions is critical when designing a treatment strategy for these children.[6] A child with a small suprasellar craniopharyngioma should have an 80% chance for long-term cure with either complete resection of the tumor or with focal irradiation. The long-term recurrence risk after either treatment is approximately 20%. After focal irradiation, the child will likely eventually require a replacement of growth hormone, cortisol, and thyroid hormones, but is not likely to develop diabetes insipidus. The child having had surgical extirpation will likely require treatment for diabetes insipidus in addition to the other three hormones. Certainly, hormone replacement for diabetes insipidus is easier now that desmopressin is in a pill form, but in an unreliable social setting or for the family who cannot afford the medications, diabetes insipidus is life-threatening.[7]

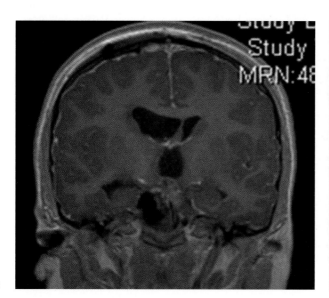

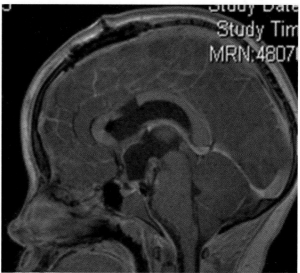

a

b

Fig. 9.2a,b The third ventricular portion in the same patient as in **Fig. 9.1** was resected through a transcallosal approach and the posterior fossa portion through a retrosigmoid approach, leaving tumor stuck to the hypothalamus. The patient then received focal conformal radiation to the small residual tumor. Two years following surgery, she is currently free of headaches with normal vision and requires only the replacement of growth hormone.

Regarding diabetes insipidus, many surgical articles have discussed the importance of preserving the pituitary stalk, even though most of the time the patient will develop diabetes insipidus after resection of the craniopharyngioma. In the case of larger craniopharyngiomas, diabetes insipidus may be secondary to hypothalamic injury, not just the pituitary stalk effect. Thus, if one considers diabetes insipidus as a dependent variable, children with this disease have an increased risk of obesity, attentional problems, and learning difficulties compared with those who do not have diabetes insipidus.[8] Given that diabetes insipidus is seen in association with radical resection of craniopharyngiomas in up to 90% of patients, whereas it is an uncommon consequence of treating a child with focal irradiation, one can understand that larger craniopharyngiomas with hypothalamic involvement would be better suited to partial resection and focal radiotherapy.

These data have led many neurosurgeons to propose grading systems for craniopharyngiomas in which treatment decisions are based on preoperative imaging characteristics. Puget and colleagues,[9] for example, have proposed a three-tier system in which children with a craniopharyngioma but no hypothalamic involvement undergo surgery with curative intent, whereas those with significant hypothalamic involvement undergo partial resection to decompress neurologic structures and reduce the treatment volume required for postoperative radiosurgery.

The optimal treatment of a child presenting with a craniopharyngioma is complex and should be based on a multidisciplinary evaluation when possible. Given the number of treatment options, the treatment should take into account the experience of the treating surgeon and radiation oncologist, the extent of involvement of neurovascular structures seen on imaging, and the resources available to the patient and family. Excellent long-term results can be obtained in the hands of experienced surgeons as long as neuroendocrine support and long-term follow-up are provided. Similar results can be obtained by less experienced teams with limited surgery and focal irradiation. In this group of children, progression-free survival rates of 80% or better can be expected at 10 and 20 years, with only a third of the patients requiring lifelong treatment for diabetes insipidus.[7] Using a paradigm of subtotal resection and irradiation should virtually eliminate surgical deaths. Thus, for the majority of pediatric neurosurgery centers and for children with a less reliable social milieu, this approach allows for a better outcome with less up-front risk.[10] For children with a recurrent craniopharyngioma or progression of disease after prior incomplete resection, it is best to consider referral to a specialty center for further treatment when possible. We are currently conducting a detailed prospective study to determine whether proton beam radiotherapy can improve the quality of life in children with this disease [A Phase II Trial of Limited Surgery and Proton Therapy for Craniopharyngioma and Observation for Craniopharyngioma After Radical Resection (NCT01419067); http://clinicaltrials.gov/ct2/show/NCT01419067.]

Management of Craniopharyngiomas

We published a monograph in 1996 on the management of craniopharyngiomas, in which we listed 10 recommendations.[2] Based on the improvements in care and in the understanding of this disease since that time, we have modified those 10 recommendations as follows:

1. The goal of treating craniopharyngiomas should be to control tumor growth while preserving the patient's cognitive, visual, and endocrine function.
2. Microsurgical decompression should be the initial treatment in any patient with rapid visual or neurologic decline or obstructive hydrocephalus. For hydrocephalus secondary to a large cystic craniopharyngioma, stereotactic or endoscopic placement of an Ommaya reservoir into the cyst, followed by aspiration and irradiation, has proven to be an effective alternative if the hydrocephalus is alleviated.
3. Microsurgical resection should be the initial consideration in children younger than 5 years of age in an effort to avoid the potential deleterious effects of radiation on the developing brain.
4. For patients with a large solid component to their tumor, both complete resection with curative intent and subtotal resection followed by focal irradiation appear to have equivalent control rates. Subtotal resection with focal irradiation affords better preservation of hypothalamic function.
5. Transsphenoidal resection should be considered the initial treatment for tumors located primarily within the sella turcica.
6. Surgical removal should be considered only for patients who have ready access to appropriate endocrinologic follow-up and replacement hormones, and for whom the family is capable of reliably providing for postoperative endocrinologic needs. Patients returning to underdeveloped countries or rural areas are at increased risk of death if these needs are not considered preoperatively. Compared with surgery, radiation therapy clearly reduces the likelihood of diabetes insipidus and the need for multiple hormone replacement.
7. For patients with primarily cystic tumors, intracystic therapy with the radioisotopes of phosphorus (^{32}P) or yttrium (^{90}Y) or with interferon appears to be efficacious, but its long-term ability to control the tumors has been called into question and many centers, including ours, have stopped using this modality in children.
8. Patients in whom a complete resection has been attempted by a skilled microneurosurgeon but has failed because of the tumor's adherence to vital structures may be closely followed with neuroimaging if progression is not likely to compromise visual or neurologic function. As two thirds of cases progress within 3 years of surgery, focused radiosurgery should be done at the time of clinical or radiographic progression. It should not be done for a fleck of residual calcification seen on a postoperative computed tomogram.

9. Patients presenting with solid or mixed tumor recurrence after what was initially believed to be a complete resection should undergo focal irradiation. Further surgery should be limited to decompression to improve the target volume for irradiation or restore loss of function. At present, there are no prospective data to say that one option is more effective than the other.

10. Stereotactic radiosurgery is best reserved for solid components of craniopharyngiomas that are small (less than 20 mm in diameter) and separated from the optic apparatus by 3 to 5 mm or more.

Radical Resection of Pediatric Craniopharyngiomas

Jeffrey H. Wisoff and Robert E. Elliott

Craniopharyngiomas comprise roughly 3% of all intracranial neoplasms[11,12] and are the most common nonglial brain tumor of childhood, constituting 6 to 8% of all pediatric brain tumors.[13,14] On a population scale, however, they are relatively rare lesions with an incidence of only 0.13 per 100,000 person years.[15] Fewer than 350 combined adult and pediatric craniopharyngiomas are diagnosed each year in the United States, and less than half of these occur in children.[15,16] Thought to arise from embryological remnants of the craniopharyngeal duct, these benign epithelial neoplasms with solid, cystic, and calcified components can arise anywhere along an axis from the third ventricle to the pituitary gland.[17-21]

The benign histology of craniopharyngiomas, however, belies their rather malignant clinical course in children. Described by Harvey Cushing[22] as "one of the most baffling problems to the neurosurgeon," their close proximity to the visual apparatus, circle of Willis, pituitary stalk, and hypothalamus predisposes these patients to severe adverse sequelae both at presentation and after treatment. Common findings include headache, vision loss, diabetes insipidus, panhypopituitarism, short stature, hypothalamic dysfunction with behavioral and memory disturbances, hyperphagia, and obesity.

Treatment Philosophy

Debate persists regarding the optimal treatment of patients with craniopharyngiomas. Regardless of the strategy selected, however, definitive tumor control or cure should be the goal of any treatment for pediatric craniopharyngiomas. Two critical factors for a potential cure are the extent of surgical excision and cranial irradiation. Some centers advocate radical resection for surgical cure, whereas others favor limited resection followed by radiation therapy to potentially limit injury to the hypothalamus. Both major paradigms provide similar rates of disease control and overall survival.[23-39] Although radical resection may have a higher potential for immediate perioperative morbidity,[9,23,29,40-44]

limited resection and radiation therapy causes more delayed morbidity including panhypopituitarism, visual deterioration, cognitive and attentional dysfunction, secondary central nervous system neoplasms, and cerebrovasculopathy, namely moyamoya disease.[31,45-53] Palliative procedures such as stereotactic cyst aspiration or Ommaya reservoir drainage may provide relief from the compression of neural and visual structures, but these effects are invariably transient. Progressive solid and cystic tumor recurrence and growth is inevitable. We believe such therapies should not be considered definitive or adequate treatment early in the course of disease.

The relative scarcity of craniopharyngiomas, the persistent lack of consensus regarding optimal treatment, and the potential morbidity of all forms of treatment combine to make it difficult, if not impossible, to determine the best management strategy. Given similar rates of disease control and survival with the two main treatment strategies, the focus of outcome assessment has shifted to quality-of-life metrics.[9,31,54-58] However, detailed quality-of-life outcomes from large series of uniformly treated patients are scarce. In this section of the chapter, we describe our preferred treatment paradigm for craniopharyngiomas in children: radical resection with the aim of surgical cure.

Preoperative Evaluation

Depending on the patient's age and the clinical status before surgery, we prefer a complete evaluation by various specialists that includes ophthalmologic, endocrinologic, and neuropsychological testing. Parents and families are counseled as to the expected short- and long-term postoperative course.

Our preoperative imaging protocol consists of MRI with frameless stereotactic image acquisition and CT. CT provides detailed information about the extent and location of tumoral calcification. Careful evaluation of multiplanar MRI scans is essential to understand the often complex relationship that craniopharyngiomas have to the visual apparatus, hypothalamus, and surrounding vasculature, and will lead to improved outcomes.

First, the location of the tumor in relation to the optic apparatus must be determined. Tumors can be entirely subchiasmatic primarily within the sella, prechiasmatic with or without a subfrontal extension, retrochiasmatic involving the floor of the third ventricle and the hypothalamus, or have a complex relationship to the chiasm with both prechiasmatic and retrochiasmatic components. Second, attention must be paid to the relationship of the dorsal aspect of the tumor and the hypothalamus. An increased involvement and deformation of the hypothalamus has been shown to predict the level of preoperative hypothalamic dysfunction as well as the operative morbidity of resection. Third, as craniopharyngiomas enlarge, they can form multilobulated cysts that extend along the pathways of least resistance and invade nearby anatomic spaces in the anterior, middle, and posterior fossae. These extensions must be recognized to optimize the surgical approach and minimize any retraction injury to normal brain parenchyma.

Surgical Approaches

Given the variability of the precise location and size of craniopharyngiomas, a variety of approaches have been described by different surgeons. These include the subfrontal,[5,13,59–62] pterional,[23,26,44,63,64] combined,[9,24,37,39,41] bifrontal interhemispheric,[65,66] transcallosal,[67] subtemporal,[68] transpetrosal,[69] and transsphenoidal approaches.[70–73]

We prefer a modified pterional exposure that includes removal of the supraorbital rim, anterior orbital roof, and the zygomatic process of the frontal bone. This approach provides the shortest, most direct route to the suprasellar region. It minimizes frontal and temporal lobe retraction with wide splitting of the sylvian fissure, allows early release of cerebrospinal fluid from the sylvian and carotid cisterns to aid brain relaxation, and facilitates early visualization of the carotid arteries and optic apparatus. Tumors extending from the pontomedullary junction to above the foramen of Monro can be successfully and safely removed through this approach without the need for corticectomy or sacrifice of the olfactory nerve, or potential cognitive dysfunction from the retraction of both frontal lobes.

Surgical adjuncts include the Cavitron Ultrasonic Surgical Aspirator (CUSA; Tyco Healthcare Radionics, Burlington, MA), frameless stereotaxy, and rigid and flexible endoscopes, and these should all be used when appropriate. Recently, we have found that endoscopic visualization during dissection of the tumor from the ventral surface of the chiasm and floor of the third ventricle greatly enhances the safety of tumor removal in this critical region and enables the complete removal of small fragments of tumor, calcium deposits, or both, that may or may not contain viable tumor cells. The endoscope is also useful for intraventricular visualization and the potential resection of tumor that lies within the third or lateral ventricles and is not accessible through the transsylvian approach. We reserve the transsphenoidal approach for tumors that are primarily or completely within the sella turcica.

Operative Technique

After intubation and the induction of anesthesia, the patient is positioned and stereotaxy is registered. Then dexamethasone (0.1 mg/kg), phenytoin (15 mg/kg), and cephalexin (25 mg/kg) are administered. Mannitol (0.25 g/kg) is given at the time of skin incision to aid brain relaxation. The diuretic effect is maximal within 1 hour of infusion and, ideally, at the time of brain and tumor manipulation. Hyperventilation and the progressive drainage of cerebrospinal fluid from the sylvian and basal cisterns usually provide excellent brain relaxation, even in the presence of hydrocephalus. Ventricular drainage is reserved for cases refractory to these maneuvers or in patients with severe, increased intracranial pressure unresponsive to medical management. However, if severe hydrocephalus is present or if there is a significant solid tumor component superiorly within the third ventricle, a 4-mm endoscope is placed into the lateral ventricle and held in place with a rigid retractor. This maneuver allows the surgeon to alternate visualization and the dissection of tumor from the endoscopic, intraventricular, or microscopic transsylvian routes.

A Z-plasty skin incision posterior to the hairline is made from the tragus to just beyond the midline. The temporalis fascia and muscle are sharply incised with a No. 15 blade and bluntly dissected from the underlying calvaria with a periosteal elevator to allow for excellent reapproximation at the end of the procedure and to minimize atrophy of the temporalis muscle. A one-piece, modified pterional craniotomy with removal of the anterior orbital roof, supraorbital rim, and zygomatic process of the frontal bone is then performed with the craniotome and a chisel and mallet. A brain retractor is used to prevent injury to the orbital contents or laceration of the periorbita during the orbital and supraorbital osteotomies. The dura is dissected from the sphenoid bone, which is removed with rongeurs down to the supraorbital fissure.

The dura is then elevated with a dural hook and incised in a C-shaped fashion. Especially for large tumors that distort the anatomy of or extend beyond the suprasellar cisterns, identifying the vascular anatomy provides critical internal landmarks for safe navigation. Laterally, the sylvian fissure is widely split and the branches of the middle cerebral artery are identified. Arachnoidal dissection of the fissure proceeds medially to the bifurcation of the internal cerebral artery. Once the carotid artery comes into view, the anterior cerebral artery and optic nerve, chiasm, and tracts are carefully inspected to reveal the relationship of these structures to the tumor (**Figs. 9.3, 9.4**).

We caution against early decompression of the cystic portion of the tumor, as this can result in redundancy of the tumor capsule and the overlying attenuated arachnoid. This loss of turgor can obscure the planes of dissection. The

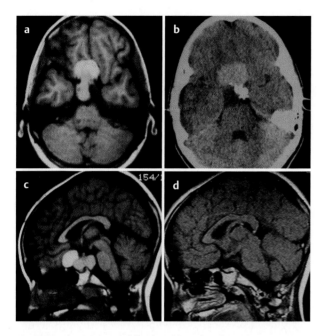

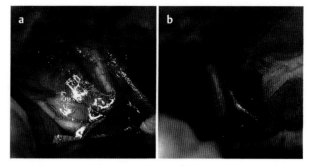

Fig. 9.4a,b **(a)** This intraoperative photograph taken after splitting of the right sylvian fissure confirmed the prechiasmatic nature of the craniopharyngioma seen in **Fig. 9.3.** The left optic nerve is elevated by the tumor, rotated into view, and exhibits pallor. **(b)** After gross total resection of the tumor, the optic nerves were decompressed and vasospasm was evident in the right internal carotid artery and the A1 segment of the anterior cerebral artery.

Fig. 9.3a–d A 9-year-old girl presented with a severe, progressive headache. On examination, she was found to have partial palsy of the third cranial nerve on the left and 20/40 visual acuity on the left. **(a,c)** Magnetic resonance imaging (MRI) scans after gadolinium enhancement revealed a 4-cm mixed cystic and solid tumor with a post-fixed chiasm. **(b)** Solid calcification in the left suprasellar region was apparent on the computed tomography (CT) scan. **(d)** Through a right pterional craniotomy, the patient underwent gross total resection of the adamantinomatous craniopharyngioma with transient worsening but eventual improvement in her cranial nerve palsy. Her visual acuity improved to 20/25 after surgery. Although the pituitary stalk was preserved, she developed diabetes insipidus and requires desmopressin. She is now 18 years past surgery, has been without disease recurrence, and completed graduate school after attending college.

overarching strategy for craniopharyngioma resection is to develop an arachnoid plane circumferentially around the tumor within the suprasellar cisterns followed by inspection and possible sectioning of the stalk. The last and most critical step is manipulation and excision of the dorsal portion of the tumor involving the hypothalamus.

Working in the opticocarotid, prechiasmatic, and carotidotentorial triangles, an arachnoidal plane is developed between the tumor capsule and the arteries of the circle of Willis. Careful attention must be paid to ensure preservation of the basal perforators. This plane is developed in a posterior direction until the basilar artery is identified through the usually intact membrane of Liliequist. This extracapsular dissection is usually facilitated by well-demarcated and preserved arachnoidal planes. In patients with recurrent tumors, these planes can be heavily scarred and may require an increased use of sharp microdissection.

After the cerebral vasculature is separated from the tumor capsule, the cyst can be aspirated and the solid components debulked. All attempts should be made to preserve the capsule of the tumor to allow gentle traction for even-

tual dissection of the tumor from its remaining attachments, especially the floor of the hypothalamus. With continuing respect for the arachnoidal planes, the surgeon then dissects the tumor free from the optic chiasm and the contralateral carotid artery and its branches. Although an attempt is always made to identify and preserve the pituitary stalk, we have found this successful in only 30% of patients. We recommend sectioning the stalk as distal as possible, without compromising negative margins, to potentially limit the severity of diabetes insipidus. After the tumor is separated from the entire circle of Willis and the pituitary stalk and optic apparatus, the capsule is grasped, and, with a combination of gentle traction and blunt dissection, a gliotic plane is developed between the dorsal aspect of the tumor and the floor of the third ventricle and hypothalamus in the region of the tuber cinereum. After the tumor is removed, the entire tumor bed must be inspected for residual disease with either a micro-mirror or an angled endoscope. Papaverine-soaked Gelfoam pledgets are then placed around the arteries of the circle of Willis to help ameliorate vasospasm **(Fig. 9.4)** and are removed before dural closure.

If the tumor has a significant retrochiasmatic or intraventricular component, the lamina terminalis must be fenestrated **(Fig. 9.5)**. The lamina terminalis is distinguished from the chiasm by its pale, avascular appearance and is often distended and attenuated by the underlying tumor. Tumor within the third ventricle can be simultaneously delivered through both the lamina terminalis and from below the chiasm. We find the use of a 4-mm endoscope inserted into the third or lateral ventricle to be extremely helpful to assist in the delivery of the intraventricular component of the tumor, obviating the need for a transcallosal approach to achieve complete resection. For tumors with a significant extension into the sella turcica, removal of the tuberculum sellae and posterior planum sphenoidale may be necessary to gain adequate exposure of the intrasellar

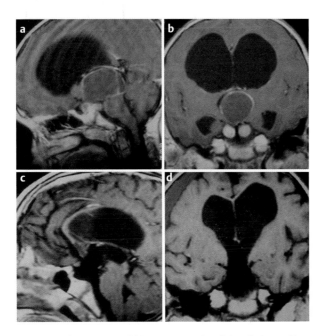

Fig. 9.5a–d A 7-year-old boy presented with headache and behavioral outbursts. **(a,b)** MRI scans revealed a 5-cm retrochiasmatic tumor with significant extension into the third ventricle, causing obstructive hydrocephalus. **(c,d)** After gross total resection of his adamantinomatous craniopharyngioma through a right pterional approach and fenestration of the lamina terminalis, he remained neurologically, visually, and hormonally intact, and his hydrocephalus resolved after the tumor was removed. He did, however, experience slight worsening of his short-term memory but was able to do well in school and currently attends college. He remains free of disease 14 years after resection.

space. After tumor removal, all bony defects in the sinuses must be repaired to prevent cerebrospinal fluid fistulas.

Postoperative Care

Following surgery and neurologic examination, all children are transferred immediately to the pediatric intensive care unit. A multidisciplinary team of pediatric endocrinologists, neuro-oncologists, and intensivists collaborate in the postoperative care. Frequent urine and electrolyte analyses are done to monitor for and aggressively treat electrolyte disturbances, namely diabetes insipidus. Dexamethasone is tapered over the course of 1 week, and phenytoin is continued for 3 weeks after surgery. The phenytoin is further continued for extended periods only in patients with seizures that cannot be attributed to electrolyte disturbances.

Postoperative MRI and CT scans are done within 48 hours after surgery to ensure complete resection. Surveillance MRI scans and clinical follow-up occur every 3 months during the first year, every 4 months during the second year, every 6 months for the next 3 years, and every year for the next 5 years. Frequent imaging allows for the early detection of recurrence while tumors are small and preferably asymptomatic. However, long-term imaging and follow-up are important, as late recurrences have been

reported. Regular evaluations by dedicated pediatric endocrinologists, ophthalmologists, and neuro-oncologists are essential in managing these cases long-term.

Outcomes and Complications

In the era of MRI, radiographically confirmed complete resection is possible in 80 to 100% of patients. Perioperative mortality after aggressive surgery has also declined substantially over the past two decades secondary to advances in neuroimaging and microsurgical techniques, from more than 10% to 0 to 4% in most current series.[5,9,13,23–26,29,30,32,39,40,45,63,64,74–80] Multiple authors report that the surgeon's experience with craniopharyngiomas has a significant impact on the likelihood of achieving complete resection and good functional outcomes.[9,35] Surgeons performing more than two operations per year for radical resection had good outcomes in 87% of children compared with only 52% in those performing fewer operations.[35]

Numerous centers have reported excellent rates of disease control and functional outcomes with the strategy of radical resection. In a large series by Zuccaro,[39] complete resection was achieved in 69% of 153 children. All children who underwent complete resection were in school and no more than 1 year behind in grade level, in contrast to only 62% of children who had limited resection and radiation. Di Rocco and colleagues[25] reported complete resection in 78% of 54 children treated with curative surgical intent. In their series, overall improvement in the patients' intelligence quotient (IQ) occurred after resection with a mean postoperative IQ of 112 (range 95–130). All but two of 50 surviving patients enjoyed normal social interactions. In a series by Hoffman and associates,[5] 26 of 27 children who underwent aggressive resection had IQ scores at or above average levels. Although 16 children had memory deficits, 14 of them attended regular schools. These authors contend that "memory impairment did not interfere with school progress if intelligence was adequate." Yaşargil and colleagues[44] reported good outcomes in 72.5% of children after initial surgery, and Fahlbusch and associates[63] reported functional independence in 78% of adult and pediatric patients after radical resection.

In our series of 86 children who underwent radical resection of a craniopharyngioma, gross total resection was accomplished in all 57 patients with primary tumors (100%) and in 18 of 29 (62%) with recurrent tumors with acceptably low morbidity **(Table 9.1)**. In contrast to the findings of other centers of increased morbidity, mortality, and worse functional outcomes at reoperation,[23,29,30,44,63,81–85] we found no such differences in our series. Good to excellent functional outcomes were achieved in 80% of children, and more than 60% of college-aged patients either attended or graduated from college—a clear indication of the high functionality of the majority of these children. New hypothalamic morbidity occurred in 25% of children and was mild or moderate in all but one case. Fewer than 20% of our patients developed obesity, and only two patients de-

Table 9.1 Morbidity and Mortality in 86 Children after Radical Resection of Craniopharyngiomas

	No. of Patients (%)	
	Primary	**Recurrent**
Perioperative mortality	2 (3.5%)	1 (3.4%)
Neurologic morbidity*		
Stroke	2 (4%)	2 (9%)
Mild hemiparesis	1 (2%)	0 (0%)
Transient cranial nerve palsy	8 (16%)	1 (4%)
Permanent cranial nerve palsy	1 (2%)	1 (4%)
Lethargy/abulia	2 (4%)	1 (4%)
Visual acuity		
Preoperative deficit	14 (27%)	15 (60%)
Improved	10 (19%)	3 (12%)
Stable	35 (67%)	17 (68%)
Worse	7 (13%)	5 (20%)
Visual fields		
Preoperative deficit	23 (43%)	22 (85%)
Improved	13 (25.5%)	7 (27%)
Stable	25 (49%)	12 (46%)
Worse	13 (25.5%)	7 (27%)
Diabetes insipidus		
Preoperative	6 (12%)	19 (73%)
Postoperative, new	33 (73%)	6 (67%)
Postoperative, total	39 (78%)	25 (89%)
Anterior pituitary dysfunction: mean number of hormones required ± SD	2.5 ± 1.1	2.1 ± 0.9

Abbreviations: SD, standard deviation.

*There were no significant differences between operative mortality and neurologic, visual, or endocrinologic morbidity between patients with primary and recurrent tumors ($p > 0.05$).

veloped severe or morbid obesity. These results contrast greatly with those from a German multicenter study that reported severe obesity in 44% of 185 children treated for craniopharyngiomas using various treatment modalities.[56] Although some centers contend that an increasing tumor size limits the extent of resection and local disease control,[38,40,63,86–92] we agree with other authors that size has no impact on the ability to achieve gross-total resection, at least for the initial tumors.[39,60,64,93] Nevertheless, given the large size and multicompartmental nature of giant craniopharyngiomas, a flexible and at times staged approach may be required for successful and safe extirpation of these tumors (**Fig. 9.6**).

Although our data did corroborate prior studies reporting worse overall survival for children with recurrent tumors,[34,38,44,63,81,94] subgroup analysis revealed excellent survival for children with nonirradiated recurrent tumors

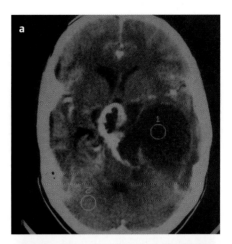
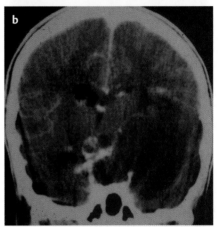
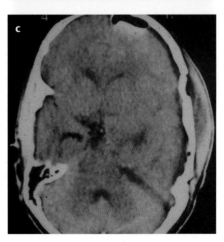

Fig. 9.6a–c **(a,b)** A 12-year-old boy presented with headache and was found on CT to have a giant, mixed cystic and solid tumor with extensive calcification in the suprasellar region and cystic extension into the left middle fossa. **(c)** After gross total removal of this adamantinomatous craniopharyngioma, he experienced a stroke that left him with a mild right hemiparesis, which improved over time. He did not develop diabetes insipidus but was left with a new right superior quadrantanopsia, likely from retraction of the left side of the optic chiasm during tumor removal. He experienced a 2-cm recurrence that was also removed 5 months after his initial surgery. He received passing grades at appropriate levels in school, required no adjuvant therapy, and has been free of disease for 23 years since his last surgery.

and those of smaller size at reoperation. Thus, prior failed radiation therapy and a large size at recurrence significantly limited our ability to achieve complete resection, the only remaining option for potential cure for these patients, and resulted in worse overall survival. In contrast, prior radical resection per se did not diminish the chance of achieving complete resection at reoperation, leading to improved disease control and survival. Fourteen children experienced a total of 15 recurrences after gross total resection at our hospital. All underwent reoperation at the time of recurrence, except one child who had radiosurgery because of fusiform dilation of the internal carotid artery. Gross total resection was achieved in 79% with no surgical morbidity or mortality. One patient had slight deterioration in vision but none of the children experienced hypothalamic or memory dysfunction. Overall survival for this cohort was 92% at a mean follow-up of 8 years, markedly higher than the rate of survival in patients with recurrent tumors reported in the literature.

Recurrence is one of the most common complications of craniopharyngiomas and usually occurs within the first 3 to 4 years after treatment.[5,21,24,26,30,39,41-44,63,64,76,80,85,95] In modern series, it occurs in roughly 20% of patients after imaging-confirmed complete resection and in 20 to 30% of patients after radiation therapy.[5,13,21,23,24,26,29,30,32,39,44,63,64,74,80,83,84,95] These facts must be considered when assessing the efficacy and safety of any treatment algorithm. Thus, in addition to the commonly reported morbidity, one must consider the potentially deleterious effects of early irradiation on the safety and efficacy of subsequent treatments, which prove necessary in up to one third of children. In experienced hands, radical resection alone may afford a greater chance of up-front disease control and potential cure compared with planned limited resection plus radiation, and provide more effective and safer treatment options should recurrence arise.

Craniopharyngiomas in Very Young Children

The aforementioned risks of radiation therapy are even more common and potentially detrimental in very young children (ages 5 and under).[31,50] Multiple centers have reported worse functional outcomes, higher rates of tumor recurrence, and decreased overall survival in younger children.[26,31,33,39,40,76,83,96-98] Importantly, one of the main treatment modalities after subtotal resection or recurrence—radiation therapy—is usually withheld in very young patients given the age-dependent cognitive morbidity, risk of secondary malignancy, visual deterioration, hypothalamic-pituitary axis dysfunction, and cerebrovasculopathy, namely, moyamoya disease.[31,45-53] In accordance with other centers, we strongly advocate radical resection as the optimal treatment in very young children with craniopharyngiomas.[35,83,85,98]

A retrospective review of our entire series of 86 children identified 19 children who were age 5 or younger at the time of surgery. Gross total resection was achieved in all but one child—a child who had undergone numerous prior resections, radiation therapy, and cyst aspirations before referral to the senior author for salvage therapy. The other 18 patients (95%) were alive at a mean follow-up of 9.4 years. Six patients experienced a total of seven recurrences. Six of these were successfully cured with a repeated resection, and the seventh child had radiosurgery because of fusiform dilation of the internal carotid artery. Four patients had transient cranial nerve palsies, but no permanent neurologic deficits occurred. New diabetes insipidus occurred in 50% of these children, and only one child (6%) experienced visual deterioration. The mean body mass index after resection was +1.4 standard deviations and within normal limits. New hypothalamic morbidity occurred in two children (short-term memory impairment and obesity, respectively), and two patients had worsening of their severe hypothalamic disturbance that was present preoperatively. Only one of 15 children (6.7%) with a normal body mass index before surgery experienced obesity, and a single patient experienced cognitive deterioration after radical resection. We found no differences in the rate of recurrence, recurrence-free, or overall survival between children ages 5 and younger and those who were older at the time of surgery. None of the children required conventional fractionated radiotherapy.

Given the increased risks of radiation therapy in young children, we agree with other centers[35,83,85,98] and strongly advocate radical resection as the optimal treatment in very young children with craniopharyngiomas. As our results demonstrate, in experienced hands, excellent oncological and functional outcomes can be obtained in this population with minimal morbidity, sparing this vulnerable population the inherent risks of cranial irradiation.

Impact of the Surgeon's Experience

Preliminary data have suggested that the surgeon's experience has an impact on the extent of resection and functional outcomes.[9,35] However, other large studies have yet to support this finding. We performed a detailed review of our data that supports the notion of increasing surgeon experience correlating with improved outcomes. From 1986 to 2011, our surgeons have performed a total of 116 resective operations for craniopharyngiomas in 99 children. Complete resection was the goal in all cases. The functional status of the children was scored using a four-tiered Craniopharyngioma Clinical Status Scale (CCSS) before surgery and at final follow-up. The CCSS assesses five major domains: neurologic, visual, hypothalamic, pituitary, and educational-occupational functioning.[99] The scoring of deficits is as follows: 1, normal; 2, mild; 3, moderate; and 4, severe. Perioperative death was scored as 5 across all domains for purposes of statistical analysis. All 116 surgeries were treated as discrete events and divided into quintiles of 23 cases for analysis; the final group comprised 24 cases.

Gross total resection was achieved in 96 surgeries (82.8%). A significantly larger proportion of complete resection was obtained in primary tumors (65 of 65 [100%]) compared with recurrent craniopharyngiomas (31 of 51 [60.8%]; $p < 0.0001$). There was no difference in the proportion of gross total resection among the quintile groups, indicating that the surgeon's experience had no observable impact on the extent of resection. Multivariate ordinal regression analysis showed that the preoperative CCSS score was the most significant predictor of the CCSS score for each domain at the time of final follow-up. The surgeon's increased surgical experience was a significant predictor of better postoperative CCSS scores for neurologic ($p = 0.04$) and cognitive (educational-occupational; $p = 0.03$) outcomes and was marginally associated with improved hypothalamic outcomes ($p = 0.08$). There was no observable impact of experience on visual or pituitary outcomes.

We believe these data support the practice of early referral to centers of experience with craniopharyngiomas. We are confident outcomes can be improved if patients are treated by tertiary referral centers and argue that this benefit is likely realized regardless of the treatment paradigm (subtotal resection with radiation versus radical resection).

Case Example

A 14-year-old girl presents with diabetes insipidus and a visual field deficit. In our series, postoperative diabetes insipidus was common with aggressive resection, and the resolution of preoperative diabetes insipidus was rare. The patient's visual status tended to improve or remain stable with radical resection. Transient contralateral hemianopia from manipulation of the optic tract was not uncommon but resolved or significantly improved with time. In this clinical scenario, we recommend aggressive surgical extirpation with an attempt to cure this adolescent girl and spare her the potential adverse effects of cranial irradiation.

Conclusion

We continue to believe that children with craniopharyngiomas should be treated with curative intent at presentation, whether through radical surgery or limited surgery plus irradiation. In accordance with other authors,[23,39,41,82,85,100] however, we believe that, in experienced hands, the radical resection of a craniopharyngioma at both presentation and recurrence offers the best chance of durable disease control and potential cure in pediatric patients. Given that most recurrences happen in the first few years after resection and the morbidity of reoperation is lower in smaller tumors,[100] frequent surveillance imaging in the early postoperative period is necessary to identify and treat recurrence early. Late recurrences, however, do occur and require continued long-term follow-up and imaging.

Nevertheless, the conclusions drawn from our experience may not be generalizable to all practices and patients. The success and safety of radical resection depend on the surgeon's expertise,[9,35] postoperative endocrinologic support, and the familial and societal resources available for the patient to cope with postoperative care and endocrine and hypothalamic deficits.[101] Educational assistance or tutoring may be required to maintain the child's schooling at the appropriate grade level. If the family structure and socioeconomic conditions of an individual patient do not provide appropriate support, the potential morbidity of radical resection may overshadow the merits of curative resection.[102]

Moderators

Total Removal vs. Subtotal Removal with Radiation for Craniopharyngiomas

Edward R. Smith and R. Michael Scott

The above sections describe alternative approaches to the management of craniopharyngiomas, with Wisoff and Elliott advocating total resection and Boop and Wait promoting subtotal removal coupled with the application of radiotherapy. The authors are all experienced, well-published leaders in the field of pediatric neurosurgery and make their cases persuasively by drawing on both personal experience and evidence from the literature.

The relative rarity of this tumor, coupled with the remarkably varied range of presentations, treatment strategies, and general paucity of published long-term outcomes, makes it impossible to render a definitive statement on the single best possible treatment. Underscoring these issues are the difficulties unique to treating a pediatric population. Attempts to measure outcomes are challenging enough when the goal is a return to baseline before the onset of illness. The ability to compare outcomes between different treatments is substantially more complicated when the baseline is dynamically changing in the setting of a developing child—in essence, moving the finish line while running the race. The inability of younger children to adequately articulate the effects of illness or the changes resulting from interventions adds a remarkable amount of complexity to the already difficult task of assessing the burden of disease or the efficacy of treatment. Paradoxically, the remarkable plasticity of the childhood nervous system may obscure the treatment effects. It may be unclear if a recovery is primarily the result of a specific intervention (or lack thereof) or predominantly due to the inherent regenerative capacity of a child's brain. Long-term follow-up to adequately assess the delayed effects on development, late-term recurrence, and unforeseen complications is of paramount importance in pediatric patients with a craniopharyngioma.

However, it is striking to note the number of similar, and even identical, principles of care supported by the seemingly opposing viewpoints. Both teams of authors cite the need to evaluate patients in centers experienced in the care of pediatric craniopharyngioma patients, with the input of multidisciplinary teams when formulating treatment plans. The authors make very clear the importance of curative intent at the time of initial diagnosis and treatment, given the reduced likelihood of success with each recurrence. Lastly, they acknowledge the intrinsic difficulty of treating this particular tumor, with the near-unique need for long-term follow-up to appropriately categorize treatment successes and failures.

As moderators, our objective is not to name a winner or a loser, as in a sporting match, but rather to emphasize the common practices in the two approaches, highlight relevant evidence-based points that can be cited in direct decision making, and offer an example of a practice that incorporates some elements of both approaches.

Common Practices

All pediatric patients with a craniopharyngioma should undergo an initial evaluation that incorporates imaging, endocrinologic studies, and visual field testing. Although some centers include psychosocial testing, which is likely helpful, such testing is variable in its methodology and not universally employed. In the United States, the use of MRI is the mainstay of anatomic evaluation. Multiplanar reconstructions and thin cuts through the region of the sella and infundibulum may help to reveal subcentimeter masses. MRI is particularly useful to identify tumors and delineate the relationship of the tumor to surrounding neurovascular structures, including the carotid arteries and their branches, the optic apparatus, the pituitary gland and stalk, and the hypothalamus and ventricular system. The tumor may appear heterogeneous, with bright cystic components on T1- and T2-weighted images, with solid portions of the tumor exhibiting variable enhancement after the administration of contrast. Obtaining MRI scans in axial, sagittal, and coronal planes with and without contrast is critical to preoperative planning and postoperative follow-up. Increasingly, magnetic resonance angiography is helpful in delineating the vascular anatomy for these same reasons.

Computed tomography is important in the diagnosis and surgical planning for craniopharyngiomas. A distinguishing feature of these tumors is the presence of calcium, which may be difficult to detect on MRI **(Fig. 9.7)**. Regions of calcification are present in the majority of these tumors in pediatric patients (up to 90%) and more than half of lesions in adults.[65,103,104] The preoperative radiographic visualization of solid calcium deposits (when present) is invaluable to the surgeon in determining the feasibility of specific operative approaches. Moreover, CT is helpful in ascertaining the degree of pneumatization of the sphenoid, ethmoid, and frontal sinuses, information relevant to the transsphenoidal approaches to sellar tumors (sphenoid), drilling down the planum sphenoidale for frontal approaches (sphenoid/ethmoids), and bifrontal approaches for suprasellar tumors (frontal).

Patients should also undergo preoperative endocrinologic assessment.[83,105,106] It is common to consult the endocrinology service before planning surgery and to obtain a panel of laboratory studies to evaluate pituitary function **(Table 9.2)**. Deficient hormones should be replaced

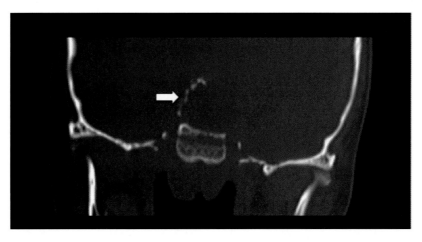

Fig. 9.7   Coronal reconstruction of noncontrast CT scan showing calcification along the lateral wall of a craniopharyngioma (*arrow*).

Table 9.2 Laboratory Tests for Endocrinology Evaluation

Prolactin

Thyroxine (T$_4$), thyroid hormone binding ratio (THBR), thyroid-stimulating hormone (TSH), free T$_4$

Insulin-like growth factor-1 (IGF-1), insulin-like growth factor binding protein-3 (IGFBP-3)

Cortisol (if not receiving steroids)

Dehydroepiandrosterone (DHEA) sulfate for patients older than 6 years (if not receiving steroids)

Follicle-stimulating hormone (FSH), luteinizing hormone (LH)

Estradiol (if female)

Testosterone (if male)

Electrolytes, blood urea nitrogen (BUN), creatinine, and serum osmolality

Bone age (if growth delay is possible)

as needed, with particular attention paid to a cortisol deficiency; patients with a craniopharyngioma should be considered to be in need of supplemental stress-dose steroids perioperatively.

When possible, a formal assessment of visual fields and an ophthalmologic examination should be done before surgery.[105,107] This not only establishes a baseline, but also may help guide the surgical approach if one optic nerve is substantially impaired and the other has retained function. Although often not practical in the setting of an acutely ill patient, those who present in a more elective fashion may be candidates for detailed neuropsychological evaluation, allowing caregivers and families to more effectively follow changes over the course of treatment and develop more tailored coping strategies.[108,109]

Once these data have been collected, the surgeon, associated caregivers, and family can then more effectively interpret the published evidence to drive informed decision making when formulating a treatment plan.

Evidence Relevant to Selecting the Treatment Approach

The two author teams in this chapter agree that surgical intervention of some sort is an established method for treating craniopharyngiomas in pediatric patients. Before undertaking an operation, it is critical to define the goals of surgery. Whether the objective is a complete resection or a planned subtotal debulking, a common theme is the need to have these complex patients assessed and treated at experienced centers that offer multimodality treatments.[1,5,8,21,83,105,110–112] If surgery is to be done, the data support the idea that the initial surgery is most important, as each relapse and subsequent intervention increases the risk of cumulative impairment.[6,109] Thus, another important decision for the caregiver is to objectively assess how likely

it is that the proposed treatment will definitively cure the craniopharyngioma.[1,105,112] Although it is impossible to predict any outcome with certainty, the accuracy of treatment increases when surgery is done by those with extensive experience and when surgeons honestly assess their capabilities.[1] Data suggest that many smaller craniopharyngiomas that do not involve the hypothalamus are more likely to be totally excised with lower morbidity, making this subgroup of tumors one that can likely be treated with an operative intent of total resection, an approach likely to be endorsed by the two author teams.[9,105,111]

Lastly, it is clear that larger tumors (> 5 cm), especially those that are suprasellar, heavily calcified, associated with hydrocephalus, or extensively involve the hypothalamus, provide substantially greater risk of perioperative morbidity (and, in some studies, mortality).[1,9,112,113] These risks, including loss of pituitary function (especially diabetes insipidus), hypothalamic obesity, cognitive loss, and vascular injury (stroke, arterial injury, etc.), need to be recognized and frankly addressed in the formulation of the treatment plan. It is this subset of craniopharyngiomas that most starkly highlights the variation in treatment algorithms among institutions. The same data are presented, convincingly, in different ways by both teams of authors—namely, that, within this group, subtotal resection with radiation offers a lower up-front morbidity (especially if done by less experienced surgeons) with a probable benefit of lower rates of diabetes insipidus. These benefits are contrasted to the probable, slightly higher, long-term "cure" rates (with cure placed in quotation marks because of the variable definition of what constitutes long term) offered through radical resection, coupled with the uncertainty of delayed secondary effects from radiation (at least as compared with the decades of experience with surgery). Both approaches lose efficacy when performed by less experienced physicians, but if the goal is radical resection, the surgeon's experience is paramount in minimizing complication rates.[9,112]

Practice Example

It is the practice at Boston Children's Hospital to incorporate aspects of both approaches—radical resection and subtotal resection with radiation—in the treatment of pediatric patients with a craniopharyngioma. It is a high-volume center, with the former chairman, R. Michael Scott, having treated nearly 100 such patients since 1988.[105] The general principle is to attempt radical resection, with the caveat of offering subtotal resection for patients with tumors that markedly involve the hypothalamus or those with bulk areas of calcification, especially in the regions of the hypothalamus, enwrapping the major arterial branches, or invading the optic apparatus. If the tumor is predominantly in the third ventricle, with limited access through an inferior approach, subtotal resection may be planned through a transcallosal approach, with the goals of opening cerebro-

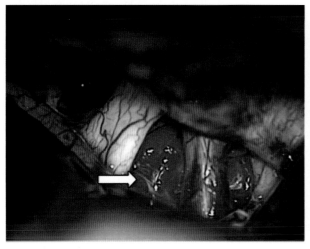
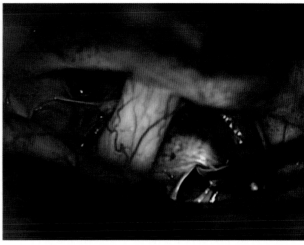

a

b

Fig. 9.8a,b Preoperative (**a**) and postoperative (**b**) images of a craniopharyngioma showing the radical resection of the tumor below the third ventricle. Note the tumor splaying the optic nerve and carotid artery (*arrow* in **a,** viewed through the pterional ap- proach) and subsequent resection with a view into the prepontine cistern through the arachnoid membrane (**b,** with instrument in the cistern).

spinal fluid pathways (to promote shunt independence) and debulking to reduce the size of the target for radiation. If at any point during an operation blind dissection on the walls of the third ventricle becomes the only means by which to proceed, it is likely that further resection will be abandoned.

Collectively, this general approach is geared toward radical resection as a primary treatment for pediatric patients with a craniopharyngioma, but is distinguished by outlining specific criteria for subtotal resection based on preoperative imaging, and defines critical intraoperative findings that would prompt aborting further tumor removal. Using this algorithm, recurrence rates range from 15 to 22% over 10 years, with no intraoperative deaths.[105,114] As with other reports, the most important criterion for reducing the likelihood of recurrence was definitive treatment at the time of initial diagnosis—whether radical resection or subtotal removal with radiation—and not leaving untreated bulk residual disease[114] (**Fig. 9.8**).

Conclusion

Craniopharyngiomas remain among the most challenging of all tumors in the pediatric population. Affected children should be referred to high-volume centers, given that the first attempt at treatment offers the best chance for long-term tumor control. Treatment plans should be formulated after detailed preoperative assessment (including imaging, endocrine studies, and assessment of visual fields) and in collaboration with associated nonsurgical care teams. Both radical resection and subtotal resection with radiation can provide high rates of disease-free survival, with slightly higher rates of long-term control after radical resection (when done by experienced surgeons), but at a potential cost of an increased risk of endocrinopathy and hypothalamic injury. Surgeons should clearly outline their rationale for operative intervention, along with criteria for aborting a procedure, with defined surgical goals to achieve optimal outcomes.

References

1. Sanford RA. Craniopharyngioma: results of survey of the American Society of Pediatric Neurosurgery. Pediatr Neurosurg 1994;21(Suppl 1):39–43
2. Boop FA. Conservative vs. aggressive treatment of craniopharyngiomas. In: Al-Mefty O, Origitano TC, Harkey HL, eds. Controversies in Neurosurgery. New York: Thieme, 1996:27–28
3. Wisoff JH, Elliott RE, Boop FA, Yam DA, Merchant TE. Craniopharyngioma. In: Jallo GI, Kothbauer K, Pradilla G, eds. Controversies in Pediatric Neurosurgery. New York: Thieme, 2010
4. Wisoff JH, Elliott RE. Radical resection. In: Jallo GI, Kothbauer K, Pradilla G, eds. Controversies in Pediatric Neurosurgery. New York: Thieme, 2010:63–70

5. Hoffman HJ, De Silva M, Humphreys RP, Drake JM, Smith ML, Blaser SI. Aggressive surgical management of craniopharyngiomas in children. J Neurosurg 1992;76:47–52
6. Merchant TE, Kiehna EN, Kun LE, et al. Phase II trial of conformal radiation therapy for pediatric patients with craniopharyngioma and correlation of surgical factors and radiation dosimetry with change in cognitive function. J Neurosurg 2006;104(2, Suppl):94–102
7. Boop FA, Yam DA, Merchant TE. Subtotal resection with adjuvant therapy. In: Jallo GI, Kothbauer K, Pradilla G, eds. Controversies in Pediatric Neurosurgery. New York: Thieme, 2010: 70–79

8. Merchant TE, Kiehna EN, Sanford RA, et al. Craniopharyngioma: the St. Jude Children's Research Hospital experience 1984-2001. Int J Radiat Oncol Biol Phys 2002;53:533–542

9. Puget S, Garnett M, Wray A, et al. Pediatric craniopharyngiomas: classification and treatment according to the degree of hypothalamic involvement. J Neurosurg 2007;106(1, Suppl):3–12

10. Clark A, Aranda D, Parsa AT, Auguste KI, Gupta N. A systematic review examining treatment-related morbidity for pediatric craniopharyngioma. J Neurosurg Pediatr 2012; in press

11. Burger PC, Scheithauer BW, Vogel FS. Surgical Pathology of the Nervous System and Its Coverings, 3rd ed. Oxford, England: Churchill Livingstone, 1990

12. Russell D, Rubinstein L. Pathology of Tumors of the Nervous System, 5th ed. Baltimore: Williams & Wilkins, 1989

13. Baskin DS, Wilson CB. Surgical management of craniopharyngiomas. A review of 74 cases. J Neurosurg 1986;65:22–27

14. Carmel PW, Antunes JL, Chang CH. Craniopharyngiomas in children. Neurosurgery 1982;11:382–389

15. Bunin GR, Surawicz TS, Witman PA, Preston-Martin S, Davis F, Bruner JM. The descriptive epidemiology of craniopharyngioma. J Neurosurg 1998;89:547–551

16. Weiner HL, Wisoff JH, Rosenberg ME, et al. Craniopharyngiomas: a clinicopathological analysis of factors predictive of recurrence and functional outcome. Neurosurgery 1994;35:1001–1010, discussion 1010–1011

17. Mollá E, Martí-Bonmatí L, Revert A, et al. Craniopharyngiomas: identification of different semiological patterns with MRI. Eur Radiol 2002;12:1829–1836

18. Prabhu VC, Brown HG. The pathogenesis of craniopharyngiomas. Childs Nerv Syst 2005;21:622–627

19. Pusey E, Kortman KE, Flannigan BD, Tsuruda J, Bradley WG. MR of craniopharyngiomas: tumor delineation and characterization. AJR Am J Roentgenol 1987;149:383–388

20. Wang KC, Hong SH, Kim SK, Cho BK. Origin of craniopharyngiomas: implication on the growth pattern. Childs Nerv Syst 2005;21:628–634

21. Wisoff JH. Surgical management of recurrent craniopharyngiomas. Pediatr Neurosurg 1994;21(Suppl 1):108–113

22. Cushing H. The craniopharyngiomas. In: Intracranial Tumors: Notes Upon a Series of Two Thousand Verified Cases with Surgical-Mortality Percentages Pertaining Thereto. Springfield, IL: Charles C. Thomas, 1932

23. Caldarelli M, Massimi L, Tamburrini G, Cappa M, Di Rocco C. Long-term results of the surgical treatment of craniopharyngioma: the experience at the Policlinico Gemelli, Catholic University, Rome. Childs Nerv Syst 2005;21:747–757

24. Dhellemmes P, Vinchon M. Radical resection for craniopharyngiomas in children: surgical technique and clinical results. J Pediatr Endocrinol Metab 2006;19(Suppl 1):329–335

25. Di Rocco C, Caldarelli M, Tamburrini G, Massimi L. Surgical management of craniopharyngiomas—experience with a pediatric series. J Pediatr Endocrinol Metab 2006;19(Suppl 1):355–366

26. Erşahin Y, Yurtseven T, Ozgiray E, Mutluer S. Craniopharyngiomas in children: Turkey experience. Childs Nerv Syst 2005;21:766–772

27. Habrand JL, Ganry O, Couanet D, et al. The role of radiation therapy in the management of craniopharyngioma: a 25-year experience and review of the literature. Int J Radiat Oncol Biol Phys 1999;44:255–263

28. Hetelekidis S, Barnes PD, Tao ML, et al. 20-year experience in childhood craniopharyngioma. Int J Radiat Oncol Biol Phys 1993;27:189–195

29. Kalapurakal JA, Goldman S, Hsieh YC, Tomita T, Marymont MH. Clinical outcome in children with craniopharyngioma treated with primary surgery and radiotherapy deferred until relapse. Med Pediatr Oncol 2003;40:214–218

30. Karavitaki N, Brufani C, Warner JT, et al. Craniopharyngiomas in children and adults: systematic analysis of 121 cases with long-term follow-up. Clin Endocrinol (Oxf) 2005;62:397–409

31. Merchant TE, Kiehna EN, Kun LE, et al. Phase II trial of conformal radiation therapy for pediatric patients with craniopharyngioma and correlation of surgical factors and radiation dosimetry with change in cognitive function. J Neurosurg 2006;104(2, Suppl):94–102

32. Merchant TE, Kiehna EN, Sanford RA, et al. Craniopharyngioma: the St. Jude Children's Research Hospital experience 1984–2001. Int J Radiat Oncol Biol Phys 2002;53:533–542

33. Rajan B, Ashley S, Gorman C, et al. Craniopharyngioma—a long-term results following limited surgery and radiotherapy. Radiother Oncol 1993;26:1–10

34. Regine WF, Kramer S. Pediatric craniopharyngiomas: long term results of combined treatment with surgery and radiation. Int J Radiat Oncol Biol Phys 1992;24:611–617

35. Sanford RA. Craniopharyngioma: results of survey of the American Society of Pediatric Neurosurgery. Pediatr Neurosurg 1994;21(Suppl 1):39–43

36. Scott RM, Hetelekidis S, Barnes PD, Goumnerova L, Tarbell NJ. Surgery, radiation, and combination therapy in the treatment of childhood craniopharyngioma—a 20-year experience. Pediatr Neurosurg 1994;21(Suppl 1):75–81

37. Tomita T. Management of craniopharyngiomas in children. Pediatr Neurosci 1988;14:204–211

38. Wen BC, Hussey DH, Staples J, et al. A comparison of the roles of surgery and radiation therapy in the management of craniopharyngiomas. Int J Radiat Oncol Biol Phys 1989;16:17–24

39. Zuccaro G. Radical resection of craniopharyngioma. Childs Nerv Syst 2005;21:679–690

40. De Vile CJ, Grant DB, Kendall BE, et al. Management of childhood craniopharyngioma: can the morbidity of radical surgery be predicted? J Neurosurg 1996;85:73–81

41. Kim SK, Wang KC, Shin SH, Choe G, Chi JG, Cho BK. Radical excision of pediatric craniopharyngioma: recurrence pattern and prognostic factors. Childs Nerv Syst 2001;17:531–536, discussion 537

42. Lena G, Paz Paredes A, Scavarda D, Giusiano B. Craniopharyngioma in children: Marseille experience. Childs Nerv Syst 2005;21:778–784

43. Sosa IJ, Krieger MD, McComb JG. Craniopharyngiomas of childhood: the CHLA experience. Childs Nerv Syst 2005;21:785–789

44. Yaşargil MG, Curcic M, Kis M, Siegenthaler G, Teddy PJ, Roth P. Total removal of craniopharyngiomas. Approaches and long-term results in 144 patients. J Neurosurg 1990;73:3–11

45. Anderson V, Godber T, Smibert E, Ekert H. Neurobehavioural sequelae following cranial irradiation and chemotherapy in children: an analysis of risk factors. Pediatr Rehabil 1997;1:63–76

46. Anderson VA, Godber T, Smibert E, Weiskop S, Ekert H. Cognitive and academic outcome following cranial irradiation and chemotherapy in children: a longitudinal study. Br J Cancer 2000;82:255–262

47. Keene DL, Johnston DL, Grimard L, Michaud J, Vassilyadi M, Ventureyra E. Vascular complications of cranial radiation. Childs Nerv Syst 2006;22:547–555

48. Mabbott DJ, Spiegler BJ, Greenberg ML, Rutka JT, Hyder DJ, Bouffet E. Serial evaluation of academic and behavioral outcome after treatment with cranial radiation in childhood. J Clin Oncol 2005;23:2256–2263

49. Mulhern RK, Merchant TE, Gajjar A, Reddick WE, Kun LE. Late neurocognitive sequelae in survivors of brain tumours in childhood. Lancet Oncol 2004;5:399–408

50. Neglia JP, Robison LL, Stovall M, et al. New primary neoplasms of the central nervous system in survivors of childhood cancer: a report from the Childhood Cancer Survivor Study. J Natl Cancer Inst 2006;98:1528–1537

51. Ron E, Modan B, Boice JD Jr, et al. Tumors of the brain and nervous system after radiotherapy in childhood. N Engl J Med 1988;319:1033–1039

52. Schmiegelow M, Feldt-Rasmussen U, Rasmussen AK, Lange M, Poulsen HS, Müller J. Assessment of the hypothalamo-pituitary-adrenal axis in patients treated with radiotherapy and chemotherapy for childhood brain tumor. J Clin Endocrinol Metab 2003;88:3149–3154

53. Spiegler BJ, Bouffet E, Greenberg ML, Rutka JT, Mabbott DJ. Change in neurocognitive functioning after treatment with cranial radiation in childhood. J Clin Oncol 2004;22:706–713

54. Carpentieri SC, Waber DP, Scott RM, et al. Memory deficits among children with craniopharyngiomas. Neurosurgery 2001; 49:1053–1057, discussion 1057–1058

55. Cavazzuti V, Fischer EG, Welch K, Belli JA, Winston KR. Neurological and psychophysiological sequelae following different treatments of craniopharyngioma in children. J Neurosurg 1983;59:409–417

56. Müller HL, Bueb K, Bartels U, et al. Obesity after childhood craniopharyngioma—German multicenter study on pre-operative risk factors and quality of life. Klin Padiatr 2001;213:244–249

57. Riva D, Pantaleoni C, Devoti M, Saletti V, Nichelli F, Giorgi C. Late neuropsychological and behavioural outcome of children surgically treated for craniopharyngioma. Childs Nerv Syst 1998;14:179–184

58. Sands SA, Milner JS, Goldberg J, et al. Quality of life and behavioral follow-up study of pediatric survivors of craniopharyngioma. J Neurosurg 2005;103(4, Suppl):302–311

59. Matson DD, Crigler JF Jr. Radical treatment of craniopharyngioma. Ann Surg 1960;152:699–704

60. Al-Mefty O, Hassounah M, Weaver P, Sakati N, Jinkins JR, Fox JL. Microsurgery for giant craniopharyngiomas in children. Neurosurgery 1985;17:585–595

61. Colangelo M, Ambrosio A, Ambrosio C. Neurological and behavioral sequelae following different approaches to craniopharyngioma. Long-term follow-up review and therapeutic guidelines. Childs Nerv Syst 1990;6:379–382

62. Sweet WH. Radical surgical treatment of craniopharyngioma. Clin Neurosurg 1976;23:52–79

63. Fahlbusch R, Honegger J, Paulus W, Huk W, Buchfelder M. Surgical treatment of craniopharyngiomas: experience with 168 patients. J Neurosurg 1999;90:237–250

64. Van Effenterre R, Boch AL. Craniopharyngioma in adults and children: a study of 122 surgical cases. J Neurosurg 2002;97:3–11

65. Samii M, Bini W. Surgical treatment of craniopharyngiomas. Zentralbl Neurochir 1991;52:17–23

66. Shibuya M, Takayasu M, Suzuki Y, Saito K, Sugita K. Bifrontal basal interhemispheric approach to craniopharyngioma resection with or without division of the anterior communicating artery. J Neurosurg 1996;84:951–956

67. Zhang YQ, Ma ZY, Wu ZB, Luo SQ, Wang ZC. Radical resection of 202 pediatric craniopharyngiomas with special reference to the surgical approaches and hypothalamic protection. Pediatr Neurosurg 2008;44:435–443

68. Symon L, Sprich W. Radical excision of craniopharyngioma. Results in 20 patients. J Neurosurg 1985;62:174–181

69. Al-Mefty O, Ayoubi S, Kadri PA. The petrosal approach for the resection of retrochiasmatic craniopharyngiomas. Neurosurgery 2008;62(5, Suppl 2):ONS331–ONS335, discussion ONS335–ONS336

70. Chakrabarti I, Amar AP, Couldwell W, Weiss MH. Long-term neurological, visual, and endocrine outcomes following transnasal resection of craniopharyngioma. J Neurosurg 2005;102: 650–657

71. Gardner PA, Kassam AB, Snyderman CH, et al. Outcomes following endoscopic, expanded endonasal resection of suprasellar craniopharyngiomas: a case series. J Neurosurg 2008;109:6–16

72. Laws ER Jr. Transsphenoidal removal of craniopharyngioma. Pediatr Neurosurg 1994;21(Suppl 1):57–63

73. Maira G, Anile C, Albanese A, Cabezas D, Pardi F, Vignati A. The role of transsphenoidal surgery in the treatment of craniopharyngiomas. J Neurosurg 2004;100:445–451

74. Albright AL, Hadjipanayis CG, Lunsford LD, Kondziolka D, Pollack IF, Adelson PD. Individualized treatment of pediatric craniopharyngiomas. Childs Nerv Syst 2005;21:649–654

75. Fischer EG, Welch K, Shillito J Jr, Winston KR, Tarbell NJ. Craniopharyngiomas in children. Long-term effects of conservative surgical procedures combined with radiation therapy. J Neurosurg 1990;73:534–540

76. Fisher PG, Jenab J, Gopldthwaite PT, et al. Outcomes and failure patterns in childhood craniopharyngiomas. Childs Nerv Syst 1998;14:558–563

77. Mottolese C, Szathmari A, Berlier P, Hermier M. Craniopharyngiomas: our experience in Lyon. Childs Nerv Syst 2005;21:790–798

78. Ohmori K, Collins J, Fukushima T. Craniopharyngiomas in children. Pediatr Neurosurg 2007;43:265–278

79. Stripp DC, Maity A, Janss AJ, et al. Surgery with or without radiation therapy in the management of craniopharyngiomas in children and young adults. Int J Radiat Oncol Biol Phys 2004;58:714–720

80. Tomita T, Bowman RM. Craniopharyngiomas in children: surgical experience at Children's Memorial Hospital. Childs Nerv Syst 2005;21:729–746

81. Barua KK, Ehara K, Kohmura E, Tamaki N. Treatment of recurrent craniopharyngiomas. Kobe J Med Sci 2003;49:123–132

82. Caldarelli M, di Rocco C, Papacci F, Colosimo C Jr. Management of recurrent craniopharyngioma. Acta Neurochir (Wien) 1998;140:447–454

83. [Craniopharyngioma in Children. 41st Annual Congress of the French Society of Neurosurgery. Lisbon, Portugal, June 4–7, 1991]. Neurochirurgie 1991;37(Suppl 1):1–174

84. Duff J, Meyer FB, Ilstrup DM, Laws ER Jr, Schleck CD, Scheithauer BW. Long-term outcomes for surgically resected craniopharyngiomas. Neurosurgery 2000;46:291–302, discussion 302–305

85. Vinchon M, Dhellemmes P. Craniopharyngiomas in children: recurrence, reoperation and outcome. Childs Nerv Syst 2008; 24:211–217

86. Djordjević M, Djordjević Z, Janićijević M, Nestorović B, Stefanović B, Ivkov M. Surgical treatment of craniopharyngio-

mas in children. Acta Neurochir Suppl (Wien) 1979;28:344–347

87. Gordy PD, Peet MM, Kahn EA. The surgery of the craniopharyngiomas. J Neurosurg 1949;6:503–517

88. Guidetti B, Fraioli B. Craniopharyngiomas. Results of surgical treatment. Acta Neurochir Suppl (Wien) 1979;28:349–351

89. Kahn EA, Gosch HH, Seeger JF, Hicks SP. Forty-five years' experience with the craniopharyngiomas. Surg Neurol 1973;1:5–12

90. Rougerie J. What can be expected from the surgical treatment of craniopharyngiomas in children. Report of 92 cases. Childs Brain 1979;5:433–449

91. Shapiro K, Till K, Grant DN. Craniopharyngiomas in childhood. A rational approach to treatment. J Neurosurg 1979;50:617–623

92. Trippi AC, Garner JT, Kassabian JT, Shelden CH. A new approach to inoperable craniopharyngiomas. Am J Surg 1969;118:307–310

93. Ammirati M, Samii M, Sephernia A. Surgery of large retrochiasmatic craniopharyngiomas in children. Childs Nerv Syst 1990;6:13–17

94. Katz EL. Late results of radical excision of craniopharyngiomas in children. J Neurosurg 1975;42:86–93

95. Tomita T, McLone DG. Radical resections of childhood craniopharyngiomas. Pediatr Neurosurg 1993;19:6–14

96. Hayward R. The present and future management of childhood craniopharyngioma. Childs Nerv Syst 1999;15:764–769

97. Poretti A, Grotzer MA, Ribi K, Schönle E, Boltshauser E. Outcome of craniopharyngioma in children: long-term complications and quality of life. Dev Med Child Neurol 2004;46:220–229

98. Thompson D, Phipps K, Hayward R. Craniopharyngioma in childhood: our evidence-based approach to management. Childs Nerv Syst 2005;21:660–668

99. Elliott RE, Sands SA, Strom RG, Wisoff JH. Craniopharyngioma Clinical Status Scale: a standardized metric of preoperative function and posttreatment outcome. Neurosurg Focus 2010;28:E2

100. Minamida Y, Mikami T, Hashi K, Houkin K. Surgical management of the recurrence and regrowth of craniopharyngiomas. J Neurosurg 2005;103:224–232

101. Shiminski-Maher T, Rosenberg M. Late effects associated with treatment of craniopharyngiomas in childhood. J Neurosci Nurs 1990;22:220–226

102. Wisoff JH, Donahue BR. Craniopharyngiomas. In: Albright AL, Pollack IF, Adelson PD, eds. Principles and Practice of Pediatric Neurosurgery, 2nd ed. Stuttgart: Thieme, 2007:560–578

103. Samii M, Tatagiba M. Surgical management of craniopharyngiomas: a review. Neurol Med Chir (Tokyo) 1997;37:141–149

104. Zada G, Lin N, Ojerholm E, Ramkissoon S, Laws ER. Craniopharyngioma and other cystic epithelial lesions of the sellar region: a review of clinical, imaging, and histopathological relationships. Neurosurg Focus 2010;28:E4

105. Scott RM. Craniopharyngioma: a personal (Boston) experience. Childs Nerv Syst 2005;21:773–777

106. Curtis J, Daneman D, Hoffman HJ, Ehrlich RM. The endocrine outcome after surgical removal of craniopharyngiomas. Pediatr Neurosurg 1994;21(Suppl 1):24–27

107. Feletti A, Marton E, Mazzucco GM, Fang S, Longatti P. Amaurosis in infancy due to craniopharyngioma: a not-exceptional but often misdiagnosed symptom. Neurosurg Focus 2010;28:E7

108. Waber DP, Pomeroy SL, Chiverton AM, et al. Everyday cognitive function after craniopharyngioma in childhood. Pediatr Neurol 2006;34:13–19

109. Müller HL, Bruhnken G, Emser A, et al. Longitudinal study on quality of life in 102 survivors of childhood craniopharyngioma. Childs Nerv Syst 2005;21:975–980

110. Jane JA Jr, Laws ER. Craniopharyngioma. Pituitary 2006;9:323–326

111. Wisoff JH. Craniopharyngioma. J Neurosurg Pediatr 2008;1:124–125, discussion 125

112. Elliott RE, Hsieh K, Hochm T, Belitskaya-Levy I, Wisoff J, Wisoff JH. Efficacy and safety of radical resection of primary and recurrent craniopharyngiomas in 86 children. J Neurosurg Pediatr 2010;5:30–48

113. Hoffman HJ. Surgical management of craniopharyngioma. Pediatr Neurosurg 1994;21(Suppl 1):44–49

114. Winkfield KM, Tsai HK, Yao X, et al. Long-term clinical outcomes following treatment of childhood craniopharyngioma. Pediatr Blood Cancer 2011;56:1120–1126

Chapter 10

Surgical Approaches to Retrochiasmatic Craniopharyngiomas

Case

An 18-year-old male presented to his pediatrician with the chief complaints of progressive visual loss, frequent urination, and marked obesity over the past several months. A magnetic resonance imaging study was done and the patient was referred to neurosurgeons.

Participants

Endoscopic Surgical Resection of Craniopharyngiomas: Edward R. Laws and Garni Barkhoudarian

The Petrosal Approach to Retrochiasmatic Craniopharyngiomas: Paulo Kadri and Ossama Al-Mefty

The Combined Approach for Craniopharyngiomas (Anterior Interhemispheric Transcallosal and Pterional-Transsylvian Routes): Uğur Türe and Ahmet Hilmi Kaya

The Translaminar Approach to Craniopharyngiomas: Edward R. Smith and R. Michael Scott

Moderators: Craniopharyngioma: Choosing the Optimal Neurosurgical Approach: James T. Rutka and Osaama H. Khan

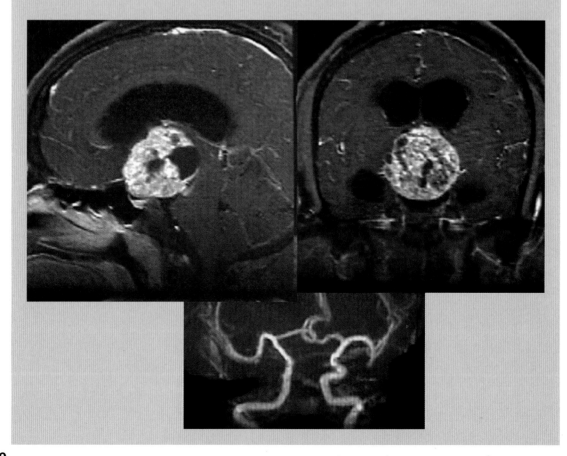

Endoscopic Surgical Resection of Craniopharyngiomas

Edward R. Laws and Garni Barkhoudarian

The patient was found to have a large suprasellar tumor and diabetes insipidus along with the symptoms he reported to his doctor. Further details of the endocrine evaluation are not available. Clearly, this tumor compresses the optic nerves and optic chiasm, and causes hypothalamic dysfunction (see the figure accompanying the case).

The imaging evaluation shows a lesion with an epicenter in the suprasellar region, almost certainly affecting the pituitary stalk. The lesion is primarily solid, but has some cystic components. A computed tomography (CT) scan would help in assessing the nature and degree of any calcification, but none is available. There is evidence of obstructive hydrocephalus from occlusion of the foramen of Monro.

There is no argument to be made for conservative treatment in this patient, as the tumor, almost certainly a craniopharyngioma, and the symptoms and signs it produces are progressive. Likewise, it would be our opinion that, at this point, neither radiation therapy nor chemotherapy would be effective treatment options. The best opportunity for a good outcome and prolonged control of disease is with surgical treatment.[1]

For a neurosurgeon, resecting a craniopharyngioma is a great challenge, both technically and philosophically. Significant controversy exists as to whether these lesions should be removed totally or whether, in some cases, a palliative resection followed by adjunctive therapy (usually radiation) is the wiser treatment option.[2] The only chance for a true cure lies with complete surgical resection.[3–6] Unfortunately, complete resection occasionally produces new damage to the visual system and the hypothalamus, making the outcome less than ideal.[5]

We will further discuss this case assuming that the optimal goal is complete surgical removal of the tumor. We will not further discuss palliative or temporizing measures such as cerebrospinal fluid (CSF) shunting, cyst aspiration, the installing of substances such as radioisotopes, or the use of bleomycin or interferon.

If resective surgery is the major goal, then there are two primary options: craniotomy or the transsphenoidal approach. Several anatomic and pathological considerations help the surgeon choose which of these two valid approaches is preferable. The answers to the following questions provide critical information in making the surgical choice:

1. *What is the epicenter of the tumor?* In this patient, the epicenter of the tumor is in the immediate suprasellar area and is retrochiasmatic. The expansion of the tumor from this epicenter has produced hydrocephalus, and has distorted the anatomy of the skull base in the region of the tuberculum sellae, with complete erosion of the posterior clinoids.
2. *What is the consistency of the tumor?* Does it have a major cystic component? Are there significant areas of

calcification? In this patient, it is evident that we are dealing with a primarily solid tumor. There is no major cystic component. We are uncertain about the presence of calcifications but do not believe that there is a large solid calcification in the lesion.

3. *What is the skull-base anatomy as related to the approach?* Is the sella enlarged or expanded? Is the sphenoid sinus well aerated? What is the relationship of the tumor to the vessels of the circle of Willis and carotid arteries in the cavernous sinus? In this case, the sphenoid sinus is well aerated, the sella is enlarged, the cavernous carotids are somewhat laterally displaced, particularly on the right, and the posterior clinoids are absent. The tumor, even though quite large, lies between the supraclinoid carotid arteries.
4. *What is the relationship of the tumor to the optic nerves, optic chiasm, and optic tracts?* In this patient the tumor is retrochiasmatic, and it has elevated the chiasm and separated the optic nerves and the optic tracts.
5. *Is there evidence of hydrocephalus and increased intracranial pressure?* In this patient there is clear evidence of obstructive hydrocephalus with ventricular enlargement. There is also significant mass effect from the tumor, and one can imply the presence of increased intracranial pressure from the erosion of the clinoid processes.
6. *Has there been prior therapy?* Prior surgery increases the difficulty and the risk of complications related to a subsequent surgical procedure. Radiation therapy or radiosurgery may also produce changes that make subsequent surgery more difficult. It is our understanding that there has been no prior therapy administered to this patient, making an initial surgical approach more advantageous.
7. *What is the nature and extent of endocrine malfunction?* The presence of preoperative diabetes insipidus in this patient implies that it will be permanent even after successful surgery. The nuances of preoperative endocrine preparation of the patient for surgery and proper management of endocrine deficiencies afterward portend an excellent outcome.[7,8]

An important consideration when surgery has been recommended lies with the nuances of craniotomy techniques versus the various transsphenoidal approaches.

Craniotomy Approaches

The following craniotomy approaches must be considered[9–11]:

1. The nondominant subfrontal approach, which is most commonly used in children and in patients with a postfixed optic chiasm[12]

2. The standard pterional approach, splitting the sylvian fissure, and working through the opticocarotid triangle, the lamina terminalis, or both[2,6,12–14]

3. The cranio-orbital approach, in which the superior rim of the orbit is resected to provide a lower trajectory of approach. The cranio-orbitozygomatic variant allows a broader exposure and improved mobilization of the temporal lobe when that is necessary[15]

4. The bifrontal interhemispheric approach, which is rarely used currently, although it enjoyed a brief period of popularity[16]

5. The transcallosal approach, which may be useful for tumors that are primarily intraventricular, and can be combined with additional approaches[13,17]

6. The subtemporal approach, which can be used for primarily retrochiasmatic tumors[18]

7. The transpetrosal approach, which is particularly suited to tumors that extend into the posterior fossa[19,20]

Transsphenoidal Approaches

We favor a transsphenoidal approach for this patient. The transsphenoidal approaches are variations and extensions of the traditional transsphenoidal route to the sella using the microscope. They can be considered minimally invasive when compared with craniotomy, but this is not always the case. The basic approaches are as follows:

1. The sublabial transsphenoidal microscope approach to the sella, which is primarily suitable for children and patients with intrasellar craniopharyngiomas[1,21]

2. The endonasal transsphenoidal microscope approach to the sella[14,21,22]

3. Endoscope-assisted variants of the prior two approaches[23,24]

4. Extended transsphenoidal anterior skull-base approaches, which can include microscope, endoscope-assisted, and purely endoscopic techniques[25–29]

In this patient, it will be difficult to carry out a safe total resection of this lesion with any given approach. In our experience, thorough resection can be achieved with the endoscopic approach (**Fig. 10.1**). We therefore advocate the endoscopic extended transsphenoidal skull-base approach to this very difficult lesion.

Endoscopic Extended Transsphenoidal Approach

This approach takes advantage of the surgical anatomy of the patient and the lesion. The sphenoid sinus is well aerated. Resecting the base of the sella, the tuberculum sellae, and the planum sphenoidale is straightforward and allows for excellent access along the long axis of the tumor, recognizing that it is retrochiasmatic and intimately associated with the hypothalamus.

The first surgical step is to expose the dura of the anterior fossa and the dural envelope of the sella. The superior circular sinus is often a robust structure and can be a bar-

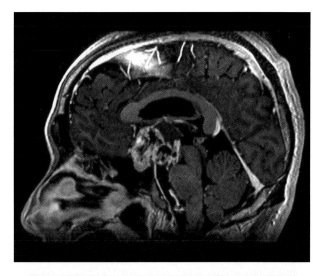

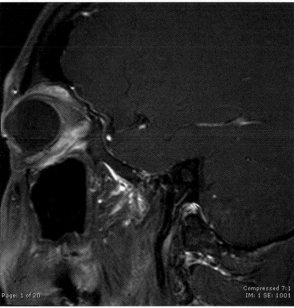

Fig. 10.1a,b **(a)** Preoperative sagittal magnetic resonance imaging (MRI) with contrast of a patient who underwent endoscopic transsphenoidal resection of a craniopharyngioma. **(b)** Postoperative sagittal postcontrast image showing gross total resection of the tumor. The fat graft is seen with a hyperintense signal on the T1-weighted image.

rier to good exposure. Before its division, the circular sinus must be controlled with electrocautery, hemostatic agents, or occasionally with clips. It is opened like a book and provides excellent exposure of the arachnoid membrane above the floor of the frontal fossa and above the diaphragm.

The initial exposure enables dissection and mobilization of the residual pituitary gland in the floor of the sella. In this case, particularly because the patient has preoperative diabetes insipidus, our initial strategy would be to dissect across the superior aspect of the pituitary gland back to the insertion of the stalk, and to section sharply the pituitary stalk, liberating the inferior aspect of the tumor from its attachments to the sella. Subsequent to this, the remnant of the diaphragm of the sella must be detached from its attachments to the tuberculum anteriorly and to the dorsum sellae and posterior clinoids posteriorly. In tumors that arise within the sella, the diaphragm acts as a barrier between the superior aspect of the tumor and the optic chiasm and hypothalamus, and helps in obtaining complete removal. In this case, although the diaphragm may be partially intact, the tumor lies primarily above the diaphragm and is in intimate contact with the arachnoid beneath and behind the optic chiasm and with the hypothalamus posteriorly and superiorly.

The arachnoid is carefully opened to expose the anterior face of the tumor, and maintaining the arachnoid plane is the initial goal. After some debulking of the lesion, the surgeon must separate the tumor from the inferior aspect of the optic chiasm, preserving the microvasculature intact. Once this is accomplished, further debulking of the lesion ultimately enables the inferolateral aspects of the tumor to be mobilized and its careful mobilization from the vessels of the circle of Willis, and ultimately from its attachments to the hypothalamus. These manipulations are accomplished with the operating endoscope and appropriate instruments, such as various-sized suctions and micro-instruments, including cupped forceps and dissectors.[30] Angled endoscopes are often useful, as are malleable instruments that can follow the visual path afforded by the endoscopic view. Long, fine bipolar instruments are essential for coagulating capsular vessels, which must be controlled in a methodical and progressive fashion to prevent bleeding from the dorsal aspect of the tumor.

The most difficult choice for the surgeon relates to the dissection of tumor from the hypothalamus. Frequently, a gliotic border can be identified and carefully separated from the capsule of the tumor. Unfortunately, the tumor itself often invades the brain in this area, and overly aggressive resection can cause devastating damage to the hypothalamus, producing both memory loss and obesity. For this reason, it is sometimes necessary to leave tumor remnants attached to the hypothalamus, which are then treated with adjunctive radiosurgery or radiotherapy.

Once the tumor is removed to the greatest extent possible, closure becomes a major challenge. Initial attempts with the extended transsphenoidal approach had rather high postoperative rates of CSF leaks. Several solutions have been proposed with various methods to reconstruct the skull base, and each has a certain advantage. The advent of nasal septal flap repair of the face of the sella has revolutionized this aspect of the operation, and subsequent CSF leakage has become a much less significant problem.[31,32]

Discussion

Since the introduction of endoscopy to neurosurgery, its advantages and disadvantages have been extensively debated. In certain situations, endoscopic approaches offer significant benefits in visualization and access to the lesion without significant brain retraction. However, disadvantages such as decreased working space and loss of stereoscopy favor the traditional microscope approaches. Ultimately, the surgeon's training, experience, and skill lead to improved outcomes with both technologies, and subgroups of craniopharyngioma patients show a difference in clinical outcomes with each technique.[2,7,14] In several studies, patients with completely or predominantly intrasellar craniopharyngiomas showed a higher likelihood of gross total resection with the endoscopic endonasal approach.[33,34]

A meta-analysis of the literature shows that patients who underwent the transsphenoidal approach had better gross total resection.[35] The use of endoscopy improved visual outcomes but with increased pituitary dysfunction, including diabetes insipidus. Inherent to the transsphenoidal approach is an increased incidence of CSF leaks (9–18%). Conversely, inherent to the transcranial approach is an increased rate of postoperative seizures (8.5%). A selection bias plays an important role in these reported outcomes.

Gross total resection, the ultimate goal of craniopharyngioma surgery, has been reported in upward of 80% of patients. Patients with no previous resection have even higher rates of resection (90%).[29] Compared with subtotal resection, there is a significant decrease in early and delayed recurrence rates. Duff and associates[5] found a 58.7% recurrence rate with subtotal resection compared to 19% with gross total resection at 10 years. Postoperative radiation decreases these rates to 9.6% and less than 1%, respectively.

Overall visual function is more likely to improve with the transsphenoidal approach. In their series, Yamada and colleagues[29] have observed some visual improvement in 90% of their patients, with a low incidence of new visual deterioration (3.4%). Other studies have similar findings.[7,33]

These differential outcomes are due, in part, to the characteristics of the tumor, which dictate the surgical approach. Intuitively, lesions that are primarily intraventricular or lateral to the midline are not amenable to the transsphenoidal approach. Consequently, the decision algorithm mentioned here can appropriately direct the surgical approach. Safe, gross total resection is therefore achievable with good long-term outcomes for this subset of patients. Experience, skill, and surgical judgment are always necessary to deal with this difficult neurosurgical challenge.

The Petrosal Approach to Retrochiasmatic Craniopharyngiomas

Paulo Kadri and Ossama Al-Mefty

This chapter's case is an 18-year-old who presented with visual loss, diabetes insipidus, and obesity secondary to an extra-axial, solid, cystic tumor occupying the suprasellar cistern. The tumor extends into and distorts the floor and fills the cavity of the third ventricle, and the interpeduncular and prepontine cisterns, and also blocks the drainage of CSF, creating secondary hydrocephalus. Compression and distortion of the optic chiasm, the pituitary stalk, and the hypothalamic nuclei in the anterior portion of the third ventricle explain the patient's clinical features. With information from the clinical examination and magnetic resonance imaging (MRI), the preoperative diagnosis is most likely a craniopharyngioma.

Craniopharyngiomas are epithelial neoplasms that arise from embryological remnants of squamous epithelium of the craniopharyngeal duct. Mainly tumors of childhood, craniopharyngiomas are benign lesions and the most common nonglial tumor in children. The optimal treatment is total removal with preservation of neural and endocrinologic function.

The tumor's precise site of origin in relation to the diaphragma sellae determines its relationship to the surrounding sellar structures and impinges on the favored route of tumor extension. The site of origin and the extension of a craniopharyngioma affect the clinical presentation, choice of surgical approach, and outcome of the patients. With respect to the optic chiasm, a tumor with a subdiaphragmatic origin is more likely to have an infra- or prechiasmatic extension, whereas tumors with a supradiaphragmatic site of origin are more likely to have a retrochiasmatic extension.

Recognizing a retrochiasmatic extension of the tumor is of paramount importance because of the difficult exposure of these tumors and their association with high surgical morbidity, a failure of total removal, increased surgical complications (primarily hypothalamic dysfunction), and higher recurrence rates. The various views provided by high-quality MRI precisely pinpoint the anatomic relation of the tumor and its usual extension downward toward the posterior fossa and upward into the third ventricle, displacing the midbrain posteriorly and the optic chiasm anteriorly. Visualizing the anterior cerebral–anterior communicating artery complex on magnetic resonance (MR) angiography or digital subtraction angiograms is of supreme relevance to distinguish between pre- and retrochiasmatic lesions. In patients with retrochiasmatic lesions, like the patient described in this chapter, the anterior cerebral arterial complex is not displaced upward as it is usually in patients with prechiasmatic lesions. CT adds information about the type and extension of calcification.

Hidden behind the optic chiasm and extending into the third ventricle and interpeduncular or even prepontine cisterns, the retrochiasmatic craniopharyngioma is a challenge to approach and expose through conventional routes, which are usually unsatisfactory. Several conventional routes approach these tumors from an anterior direction, risking injury to the anterior perforating arteries, the main blood supply to the hypothalamus and chiasm, magnifying the damage to these vital structures. But a wide exposure under direct view is achieved through the petrosal approach. Because it requires mobilizing the sinus medially, the petrosal approach provides an upward avenue to the tumor, which then presents itself, facilitating dissection from below and behind and preserving the hypothalamus and optic pathways.

The petrosal approach is indicated for patients with a large retrochiasmatic craniopharyngioma, such as in the patient presented for discussion, and even in younger pediatric patients, who do not have fully developed mastoid air cells to perform a mastoidectomy. In this section, we discuss the operative nuances of this approach.

Surgical Technique

Patient Positioning

For the petrosal approach, the patient is placed in the supine position on the operating table, with the trunk and head elevated approximately 20 degrees. The ipsilateral shoulder is slightly elevated with a roll. The head is turned and tilted to the contralateral side, inclined toward the floor, and then fixed in the three-point headrest. Compression of the contralateral jugular vein is prevented during head positioning.

Intraoperative Monitoring

Electromyographic activities of the third, sixth, and seventh cranial nerves are routinely recorded. Brainstem auditory evoked potentials and median nerve somatosensory-evoked potentials are recorded continuously. Other cranial nerves are monitored as required.

Skin Flap

The skin incision begins at the zygoma in front of the tragus, turning 2 to 3 cm above the ear, and then circling to descend approximately 4 cm medial to the mastoid process. The superficial temporal artery is preserved over the superficial temporal muscle fascia to preserve the blood supply of the temporal muscle. The skin incision is then raised sharply to the level of the external auditory meatus. The temporal fascia is incised and separated from the muscle along the anterior, superior, and inferior borders of the skin incision, and elevated posteriorly in continuity with the sternocleidomastoid muscle to produce a well-vascularized muscle–fascial flap for reconstruction. The posterior portion of the temporal muscle is detached sharply from the bone in an inferior-to-superior maneuver, preserving its deep fascia and thereby the remaining blood supply and its main innervations. The bony surfaces of the temporal fossa, mastoid, and lateral posterior fossa are thus exposed.

Craniotomy

The bone flap combines a supra-infratentorial craniotomy through four bur holes crossing the transverse-sigmoid sinus junction and the transverse sinus. The asterion, located at the junction of the lambdoidal, occipitomastoidal, and parietomastoidal sutures, is the key landmark, which guides placement of the first bur hole located medial and inferior to it, opening into the posterior fossa below the transverse-sigmoid sinus junction. A second hole, located at the squamomastoid junction of the temporal bone along the projection of the superior temporal line, opens into the supratentorial compartment, exposing the dura mater covering the posterior portion of the temporal lobe. These two bur holes flank the junction of the sigmoid and transverse sinuses. The other two holes are placed medial to the first two, on each side of the transverse sinus projection delineated by a line that follows along the zygomatic arch posteriorly.

The temporal and occipital bones are incised between the bur holes, supra- and infratentorially, with the foot attachment of the high-speed drill. For a retrochiasmatic craniopharyngioma, the occipital part of the craniotomy is somewhat smaller than the flap used for petroclival lesions. The tight adhesion of the sinus, which usually forms a high-domed bony impression on the inner surface of the skull, precludes the use of the foot attachment to connect the holes crossing it. Instead, a small drill is used to carefully expose the sinus between each of the flanking bur holes. The single bone flap is then dissected and carefully elevated from the sinus and dura mater.

Mastoidectomy

For the mastoidectomy, a small bone flap comprising the cortices of the mastoid is elevated in one piece. This flap is used at the end of the procedure to reconstruct the mastoid area. A complete mastoidectomy is done with the high-speed drill. The superficial and retrofacial air cells of the mastoid are drilled out, identifying the solid angles of the semicircular and facial canals, which are kept intact to preserve hearing. The sigmoid sinus is skeletonized down to the jugular bulb, exposing the dura on both sides of the sinus. The dura anterior to the sigmoid sinus is exposed only enough to open and close the dura. The sinodural angle is exposed to skeletonize the superior petrosal sinus, and the drilling is performed along the pyramid to thin the petrous bone toward its apex.

Dural Opening

The temporal dura is opened along the floor of the middle fossa and the incision extends posteriorly, parallel to the transverse sinus. A vertical incision is made in the presigmoid posterior fossa dura and extended toward the supratentorial incision. The exposed temporal lobe is inspected to define the point where the superior petrosal sinus will be coagulated and divided, preserving the insertions of the vein of Labbé complex and the posterior temporal veins.

Sectioning the Tentorium and Opening the Arachnoid

The tentorium is sectioned parallel to the drilled pyramid, all the way through to the incisura. Before the free edge of the tentorium is severed, the fourth cranial nerve is identified, preventing its injury, and the final cut is completed posterior to its entry point in the tentorial edge. This maneuver renders the sigmoid sinus free for posterior mobilization while the posterior leaf, together with the temporal lobe, is supported with a brain spatula. The arachnoid membrane of the crural, ambient, and cerebellomedullary cisterns are opened to release CSF and relax the brain. The third and fourth cranial nerves, the posterior cerebral artery, and the superior cerebellar artery at the incisura are identified. At this juncture, the tumor is widely exposed under the chiasm and the hypothalamus, as well as at the retrosellar area, in front of the midbrain and atop the basilar artery.

Exposing and Debulking the Tumor

The tumor is identified anterior to the midbrain in the retrosellar area. The cystic portion is aspirated, and cottonoids are placed around the area to prevent spillage of the contents. A specimen is taken for immediate histological confirmation, the tumor capsule is entered, and the tumor is debulked internally. Solid calcifications might require the use of ultrasonic aspiration.

Dissecting the Tumor

After the capsule is debulked, it can be freed from the surrounding structures, including the third and fourth nerves and the basilar artery and its perforators. The capsule in the interpeduncular fossa is separated from the anterior aspect of the brainstem, and the dissection progresses anteriorly toward the dorsum sella while the tumor descends free from the third ventricle, giving way to a gliotic plane of dissection between the tumor capsule and the hypothalamic floor. The tumor is dissected off the inferior surface of the hypothalamus, and a change in the appearance of the tissue is seen between the tumor and hypothalamus. The hypothalamus, with its feeding perforators, remains intact. As dissection progresses anteriorly, the tumor is dissected from the carotid artery and the posterior communicating artery. The pituitary stalk is identified, preserved, and followed into the sella, where the intrasellar portion of the tumor is dissected, preserving the gland itself. The gland is usually compressed but identifiable by its color and texture.

The tumor that lies beneath the optic nerves is dissected with care to avoid injuring the nerves. As the capsule of the tumor extending to the contralateral side is dissected, the contralateral third cranial nerve and posterior cerebral artery are identified. If the tumor extends into the third ventricle, it will descend as removal continues. This part of the tumor is removed in piecemeal fashion. The third ventricle is entered superior to the pituitary stalk and anterior to the mamillary bodies. When the tumor extends into the posterior fossa, it is dissected off the clivus; the dorsum sella; the fifth, seventh, and eighth cranial nerves; the lower cranial nerves; and the jugular foramen.

Closure

The temporal dura mater is resutured. The presigmoid dura usually shrinks, and a pericranial graft is used, if necessary, to achieve a watertight closure. The drilled mastoid cavity is filled with fat taken from the patient's abdomen. The temporal muscle is rotated over the defect and sutured to the sternocleidomastoid muscle, and the temporal fascia is sutured back to the temporal muscle. The soft tissue and skin are then closed in layers.

Managing Complications

Cerebrospinal Fluid Leak

After the petrosal approach, a CSF leak can occur from the skin or, more often, in the form of rhinorrhea through the mastoid air cells. Meticulous closure is critical in preventing such a leak. If fluid does leak, a CT scan is obtained to rule out hydrocephalus; if hydrocephalus is present, a shunt is placed. In the absence of hydrocephalus, a spinal drain is used for 72 hours and the CSF is tested for any evidence of chemical meningitis. If the leak continues, the wound is reexplored. If bacterial meningitis occurs as a result of a CSF leak, it is treated with antibiotics and spinal drainage.

Diabetes Insipidus

The patient's hourly fluid intake and output and specific gravity are monitored during and after surgery. Serum electrolytes and osmolarity are measured every 6 hours during the first postoperative day. In the first 24 hours, fluids are given to equalize intake with output on an hourly basis. If diabetes insipidus is diagnosed, treatment with 1-deamino-8-D-arginine vasopressin (DDAVP) is initiated, and sodium and electrolytes are closely monitored. If the patient's sodium concentration is low, DDAVP treatment is withheld until fluid overload is ruled out as the cause of polyuria. This is done through close and frequent monitoring of the patient's sodium level and urine output. If diabetes insipidus persists, DDAVP is given in scheduled doses.

Discussion

Retrochiasmatic craniopharyngiomas, especially the giant ones, are a formidable challenge for treatment. Increased surgical mortality, morbidity with poor neurologic and endocrinologic outcomes, a failure of total resection, and high recurrence rates are thoroughly reported in the literature, portending a rather malignant behavior despite their benign histological appearance. The literature describes treatments including partial removal with close surveillance, simple cyst aspiration, intracystic placement of a drainage catheter followed by different types of radiation therapy and chemotherapy, and even conservative treatments. The side effects of radiation and future complications of radiation therapy, regardless of the form used (conformational, radiosurgery, or brachytherapy), are clearly underestimated. Visual, cognitive, neurologic, and endocrine side effects, along with potentially radiation-induced tumors, are serious, life-threatening complications and occur frequently. The intracystic use of bleomycin and interferon has yet to be proved as a consistent form of treatment.

Craniopharyngiomas are benign lesions; their total surgical removal with preservation of the neuroendocrinologic structures ensures cure with a good quality of life for patients. Several approaches have been proposed to remove retrochiasmatic craniopharyngiomas. Most of them, including the pterional, frontopterional, cranio-orbitozygomatic, subfrontopterional, bifrontal interhemispheric, zygomatic, and the basal interhemispheric supra- or infrachiasmatic approaches, use a translamina terminalis route. Transsphenoidal and endoscopic procedures also have been proposed. The pterional approach provides a narrow surgical corridor, with the perforating arteries obstructing the lateral view through the optic carotid triangle. The mobilization of perforating arteries and the anterior cerebral arteries, manipulation close to the chiasm, and the inaccessibility of the upward extension into the third ventricle magnify the risk and failure of total resection through the horizontally projected approaches through the lamina terminalis. Apart from that, any draining vein from the frontal lobe to the sinus, which might be cut if the interhemispheric corridor is used to gain access to the lamina terminalis, may lead to subcortical hemorrhaging or a reduction in blood flow. The lateral-horizontal projected zygomatic approach is obstructed by the posterior cerebral arteries and optic tract, and gives only limited access to the upward extension of the tumor. The transsphenoidal approach, particularly for large lesions, is likely to provide even less of a chance of total removal, even with the addition of endoscopic techniques. These limitations lead to subtotal removal, resulting in higher recurrence rates. A second surgery for recurrent tumors is associated with high rates of complications.

Despite our emphasis on and commitment to total removal, this is not always possible. The risks posed to critical structures might derail this intention, but a direct view, unobstructed by any vital structure, blood vessels, or perforating vessels, can be achieved with the petrosal approach. This approach allows direct visualization with preservation of the hypothalamus, the walls of the third ventricle, and the inferior surface of the optic chiasm. Even in pediatric patients, who have typically small and poorly aerated mastoid cells that could hinder application, the advantages of the petrosal approach remain.

Conclusion

The surgical avenue (posterior-anteriorly and inferior-superiorly) provided by the petrosal approach is superb for exposure, particularly of the upper pole of retrochiasmatic craniopharyngiomas. It provides a direct and unobstructed view of the tumor and minimizes manipulation of the chiasm, optic nerve, major vessels, and perforators. Vascularization and the function of the hypothalamus are thus preserved.

The Combined Approach for Craniopharyngiomas (Anterior Interhemispheric Transcallosal and Pterional-Transsylvian Routes)

Uğur Türe and Ahmet Hilmi Kaya

This chapter's case is an 18-year-old who presented with visual loss, diabetes insipidus, obesity, an inhomogeneously enhancing parasellar mass involving the sella and third ventricle, hydrocephalus, and some cystic areas seen on radiological examinations. This combination of facts coheres to suggest to the neurosurgeon that the diagnosis is most probably a craniopharyngioma.

Pathology

Craniopharyngiomas are benign tumors histopathologically, and they originate from squamous rests located along the pituitary stalk. Their "malignancy" comes from their location and the difficulty of their radical resection. Visual pathways, the hypothalamus, the pituitary stalk and gland, major arterial structures with their perforators (internal carotid, anterior cerebral, and basilar arteries), and the surface of the third ventricle may all have an intimate relationship with the tumor, as in the case described here. The disease has a bimodal distribution by age, with peak incidence rates in children (5–14 years) and among older adults (45–60 years). The clinical findings of the disease relate to mass effects on these different structures: compression of the pituitary gland or stalk may cause endocrinologic problems, hypothalamic compression may cause diencephalic syndrome, optic pathway compression causes visual loss, and ventricular compression may cause hydrocephalus.[9,11,12,36–48]

In this patient, we would aim for total resection in the same sitting with a combined approach, that is, the combination of the pterional-transsylvian parachiasmatic and anterior interhemispheric transcallosal-transforaminal approaches, which has been described by Yaşargil.[11,46,47] In this section of the chapter, we discuss our treatment strategy.

The Rationale for Surgery

The appropriate treatment for patients with a craniopharyngioma is controversial. Some authors have determined that either gross total resection or subtotal resection combined with radiotherapy offers the same progression-free survival at follow-up periods of 5 to 10 years.[49–53] This conclusion implies that radiotherapy substitutes for the effort of total resection, thereby limiting serious complications such as hypothalamic injury. These conclusions are based on several choices of fractionated or stereotactic radiotherapy. These fractionated and precisely localized radiotherapies are also said to decrease side effects, such as panhypopituitarism, cognitive difficulties, and optic pathway injury.[54–59]

On the other hand, large surgical series present the results of microneurosurgical resection of this benign lesion and show definitive cure.[2,9,11,12,36,46,60,61] Several recent series especially emphasize that radical resection offers the best chance to control disease with potential cure and acceptable morbidity, and that the disease can be altered from lethal to survivable in children, who might then have a functional adult life.[44,48,62,63] In our opinion, understanding the difference in meaning between "chance of cure" and "progression-free survival" is crucial to wading through this controversy. A chance of cure in such patients denotes no tumoral tissue seen radiologically during the 5- to 10-year follow-up period, and this chance still predominates convincingly even though late recurrence is seen. But progression-free survival denotes irradiated residual tumor tissue with the same appearance on serial radiological examinations during the 5- to 10-year follow-up period. However, the expectation of cure in such a situation is definitely an overestimation.

Because craniopharyngiomas have a bimodal distribution by age, and a follow-up period of 10 years is very limited for children, an even longer progression-free survival is still not enough to compare these treatment strategies. we believe that totally removing the tumor always harbors a chance of cure, and we prefer this to irradiated residual tumoral tissue.

Today, with a better understanding of microneurosurgical anatomy and techniques that employ modern radiological tools, the surgery of craniopharyngiomas can be successful, with no damage to critical structures, including the perforating branches of the carotid, basilar, and anterior cerebral arteries; the optic nerve, chiasm, and tract; and the hypothalamus with its ventricular surfaces. Nonetheless, the hypophyseal stalk may need to be resected to achieve complete removal because the tumor may arise diffusely from the stalk and dissection may not be possible. Thus, panhypopituitarism may be inevitable, but good replacement therapy with good endocrinologic follow-up can be satisfactory.

The Rationale for Choosing the Approach

For the successful removal of a craniopharyngioma, the surgeon must carry out fine microsurgical excision of the tumor under direct microscopic visualization while respecting neighboring tissue. Such effort is crucial to prevent complications and achieve total resection. The location of the craniopharyngioma may vary according to the origin of the tumor.[11,38,42,45,46] A more inferior origin from the stalk may lead to a sellar location, whereas a more superior origin may result in tumor in the third ventricle. Thus, craniopharyngiomas can appear in sellar, suprasellar, and intraventricular locations, but a combination is also common. Different classification systems have been proposed for such panoramic locations.[11,37–42,46]

Several avenues of approach have been used for craniopharyngiomas, primarily the superior (anterior interhemispheric-transcallosal) and basal (frontobasal, pterional, cranio-orbitozygomatic, petrosal, and transsphenoidal) approaches.[3,9,11,12,19,36,39–44,46,48,64–67] The superior approaches mainly unveil the intraventricular and suprachiasmatic area, whereas the basal avenues open the intrasellar and parasellar areas.

Our preference is to approach a pure sellar location via the transsphenoidal route, but the suprasellar location is best visualized bilaterally via the pterional-transsylvian parachiasmatic approach. We understand the pterional approach to be a combined skull-base approach that unveils either the anterior and lateral base of the skull or the whole parasellar area, including the chiasmatic, carotid, and interpeduncular cisterns, which can be well visualized microsurgically. For tumors that dominate the ventricular location, we prefer the anterior interhemispheric transcallosal-transforaminal approach because the superior sightline allows the surgeon to see the whole border of the tumor with its third ventricular surface and, most importantly, the hypo-

thalamus. In particular, the presence of unilateral or bilateral hydrocephalus in patients with tumor in the third ventricle indicates an intimate relationship between the tumor and the foramen of Monro. In such situations, the superior view allows inspection of the most posterosuperior part of the tumor (third ventricular roof), which could cause inadvertent choroidal hemorrhage during surgery.

The translamina terminalis is also a natural corridor to the third ventricle during the pterional approach, but either the ipsilateral or the superior part of the ventricle cannot be well visualized even when the tumor is more anterolaterally oriented above the supraorbital trajectory. Still, this approach can be used for craniopharyngiomas involving the anterior part of the third ventricle if it is feasible. The translamina terminalis route requires more retraction of the peritumoral third ventricular walls, so we hesitate to use this avenue routinely. With respect to every surgeon's choice of approach, which is often guided by the surgeon's training, experience, and preferences, for tumors that dominate the ventricle and also the suprasellar location, as in the presented case, we prefer a combined approach consisting of superior (anterior interhemispheric transcallosal-transforaminal) and lateral (pterional-transsylvian parachiasmatic) approaches in the same sitting **(Fig. 10.2)**.

The Combined Approach for Craniopharyngiomas

The first and most crucial steps to successfully removing these lesions are detailed preoperative evaluation and planning the surgical strategy accordingly before entering the operating room. Nevertheless, one should be ready for surprises when dealing with a craniopharyngioma. Unfortunately, no radiological imaging system is yet available to help the surgeon determine how much the tumor adheres to its surroundings; therefore, evaluating this feature is possible only during surgery. The practical advantage of the combined approach mainly arises from its flexibility when it comes to dealing with surprises. For example, let's consider a scenario in which the craniopharyngioma is located mostly in the third ventricle. If dissecting the inferior part of tumor adhering to the surrounding tissue is difficult through the anterior interhemispheric transcallosal-transforaminal approach, switching to the pterional approach is the key to gross total excision. Or if dissecting the upper part of a prechiasmatic craniopharyngioma is not possible through the pterional approach, the surgeon can employ the anterior interhemispheric transcallosal-transforaminal approach. The surgeon's only requirement is to be ready to switch between the two approaches.

The surprises presented by a craniopharyngioma are not always negative. A lesion that appears frightening on MRI scans can sometimes be easily dissected and removed through one approach. Although this situation is rare, when it does happen the surgeon might regret making a large incision for a combined approach. To overcome this problem,

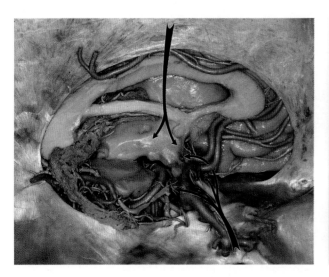

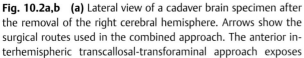

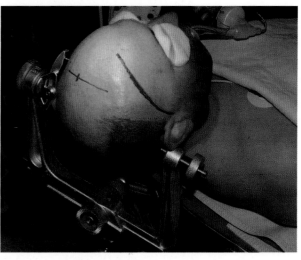

a

b

Fig. 10.2a,b **(a)** Lateral view of a cadaver brain specimen after the removal of the right cerebral hemisphere. Arrows show the surgical routes used in the combined approach. The anterior interhemispheric transcallosal-transforaminal approach exposes the most superior and posterior part of the tumor, whereas the pterional-transsylvian parachiasmatic approach exposes the parasellar part of the tumor. **(b)** Two separate incisions are used to avoid creating a huge skin flap.

in recent years, we have preferred to make two small incisions rather than one large incision for the combined approach. We draw two incision lines but begin with the most suitable approach according to the location and extension of the tumor. We make the second incision only when the second approach is necessary **(Fig. 10.2b)**.

When a craniopharyngioma is large enough to force the surgeon to consider a combined approach, choosing the initial approach depends on an evaluation of the parasellar part of the tumor. If this part is small and the majority of the tumor is located in the third ventricle, which opens the possibility of removal through one craniotomy, then the initial avenue should be the anterior interhemispheric transcallosal-transforaminal approach. Otherwise, if the tumor has a bulky parasellar portion, surgery should begin with the pterional-transsylvian approach.

In the following sections we describe the technique of each approach and the case of a patient with a tumor similar to that presented here who was operated on via this combined approach **(Fig. 10.3)**.

The Pterional-Transsylvian Parachiasmatic Approach

We generally prefer to make a right-sided pterional craniotomy. However, if the tumor extends mostly to the left side and vision in the left eye has severely deteriorated, we prefer to use a left-sided pterional craniotomy to protect the healthier right-side vision from potential risks. Positioning the patient's head correctly is a major step in the success of the combined approach. The fixation system must be applied wisely to allow the surgeon to change the position of the head during the operation, to switch from the pterional approach to the anterior interhemispheric transcallosal-transforaminal approach.

The patient is placed in the supine position, the back section of the operating table is elevated approximately 15 degrees, and the seat section is positioned parallel to the ground. The single pin of the three-point rigid cranial fixation system (Mayfield Modified Skull Clamp, Plainsboro, NJ) is applied to the ipsilateral mastoid process and the other two pins are applied to the contralateral parietal bone. The head is then fixed with 30 degrees of rotation to the opposite side and the neck is moderately extended. After positioning, the scalp is prepared for two small incisions.

The pterional-transsylvian approach has been described in detail by Yaşargil, and only an outline is given here. The pterional craniotomy is designed to take advantage of natural anatomic planes and space intervals between structures, and to expose the base of the brain using minimal or no retraction. The sphenoid ridge, with its pyramid shape, separates the frontal and temporal lobes. In the pterional approach, adequate bone drilling is crucial to sufficiently expose the anterior cranial base. To avoid entering the sinus, the surgeon should encounter the extension of the frontal sinus before the craniotomy. The base of the sphenoid ridge should be drilled away with a high-speed drill. We also remove the anterior clinoid process to gain more space and the ability to mobilize the internal carotid artery during tumor removal. The dura is opened in a semicircular fashion around the sylvian fissure, arching toward the sphenoid ridge, and is reflected.

A wide opening of the proximal part of the sylvian fissure is crucial to expose and remove the tumor. The tumor's relationship to the M1 segment of the middle cerebral artery, the A1 segments of the anterior cerebral arteries on the right and left sides, and the anterior communicating, anterior choroidal, and posterior communicating arteries is explored, as is the relationship to the optic nerves and chiasm and the oculomotor nerves. Of course, this exploration has limita-

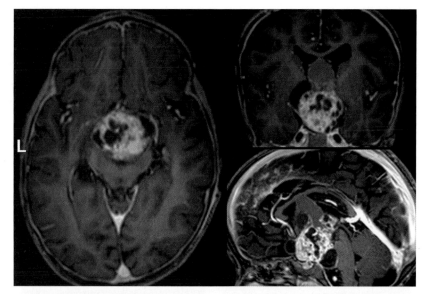

a

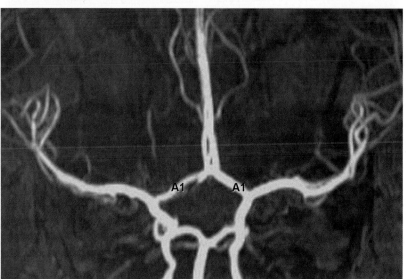

A1   A1

b

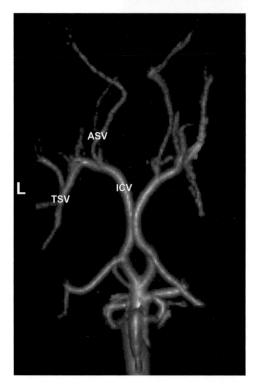

ASV

L   ICV

TSV

c

Fig. 10.3a–g A 5-year-old boy with an intra- and extraventricular cranio-pharyngioma. **(a)** The preoperative T1-weighted axial, coronal, and sagittal MRI scans with contrast enhancement demonstrate a giant craniopharyngioma extending from the parasellar region to the corpus callosum through the third ventricle. Because of hydrocephalus, the patient had a ventriculoperitoneal shunt placed by surgeons at another institution. **(b)** Preoperative MR angiography shows slightly elevated A1 segments of the anterior cerebral arteries, evidence of the retrochiasmatic location of the tumor. **(c)** MR venography of the sub-ependymal venous system shows the anterior septal veins (ASV) separated from each other by the tumor. The slightly posterior location of the junction of the right-sided thalamostriate vein (TSV) and ASV delineates the possibility of enlarging the right foramen of Monro via the anterior interhemispheric transcallosal-transforaminal approach. ICV, internal cerebral vein; L, left.

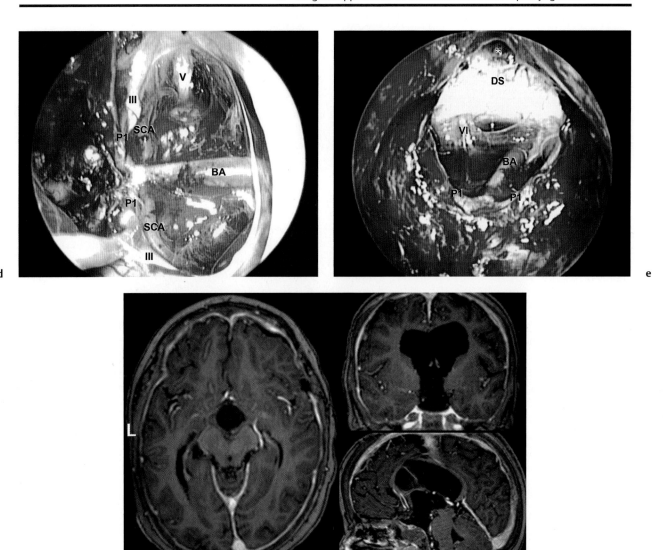

d

e

f

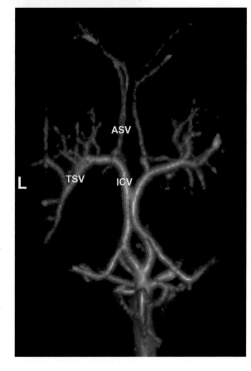

g

Fig. 10.3a–g (*continued*)   Intraoperative endoscopic pictures via the pterional-transsylvian **(d)** and transcallosal-transforaminal **(e)** routes show total removal of the tumor with the pituitary stalk. The asterisk indicates the base of the pituitary stalk. III, third nerve; V, fifth nerve; VI, sixth nerve; BA, basilar artery; DS, dorsum sella; P1, first segment of the posterior cerebral artery; SCA, superior cerebellar artery. **(f)** Postoperative T1-weighted axial, coronal, and sagittal MRI scans with contrast enhancement show total resection of the tumor through the combined approach (anterior interhemispheric transcallosal-transforaminal and pterional-transsylvian parachiasmatic). **(g)** Postoperative MR venography shows both anterior septal veins (ASV) approximated to each other, and the venous complex is preserved intact. TSV, thalamostriate vein; ICV, internal cerebral vein.

tions depending on the size and extension of the tumor. The surgeon also explores the subchiasmatic portion of the tumor through the narrow space intervals, the so-called prechiasmatic, opticocarotid, carotid-tentorial, and supracarotid triangles, and finally through an opening in the lamina terminalis (**Fig. 10.2a**). The surgeon should first aspirate the cystic component of the tumor, if it exists. After piecemeal removal of the solid parts to achieve central decompression, the peripheral surfaces of the tumor can be explored in the arachnoidal cleavage plane for complete removal.

Because of vital neurovascular structures, such as the basilar artery, basilar bifurcation, and the P1 segments of the posterior cerebral arteries and their perforating branches accommodating the interpeduncular fossa and the retro-clival-prepontine area, the basal part of the tumor in these locations must be dissected with utmost care. It may be difficult to differentiate small tumoral arteries from the perforators of the chiasm. Therefore, we should avoid the excessive coagulation of arteries. Oozing from small veins can be controlled through the application of small pieces of gelatin sponge (Spongostan, Ethicon, Inc., Somerville, NJ) and gentle compression with a moist cottonoid. The excessive use of bipolar coagulation near mesencephalic structures should be avoided.

The hidden parts of the tumor in the midline under the chiasm are explored through a window made into the lamina terminalis, which is already expanded by the tumor. Attention is focused on identifying the pituitary stalk. When a craniopharyngioma originates from the stalk with a broad base, dissection is almost impossible. In this situation, the stalk is resected together with the tumor to achieve complete removal. Postoperative endocrine substitution therapy is preferred rather than the risk of tumor recurrence and a second operation.

Furthermore, the pterional-transsylvian approach allows exploration of the sella, parasellar area, and anterior and middle fossae, which may also be invaded by tumor. Some of the tumor extending to the third ventricle may not be accessible through the pterional-transsylvian parachiasmatic approach, however, and switching to the anterior interhemispheric transcallosal-transforaminal approach becomes necessary.

The Anterior Interhemispheric Transcallosal-Transforaminal Approach

When using the anterior interhemispheric transcallosal-transforaminal approach after the pterional approach, the position of the patient's head must be readjusted. The head is brought to the neutral position and then fixed without rotation but with an optimal degree of elevation after the fixation system is released. Correct positioning should make visualization of the tumor possible from above vertically through the anterior interhemispheric fissure and incised corpus callosum, revealing the foramen of Monro, and as far as the infundibular areas, directly in one plane.

Before beginning the right-sided posterior frontal-para-sagittal craniotomy, the surgeon must carefully analyze the preoperative venogram or MR venography to determine the number and course of the frontal ascending veins, the size and variation of the superior sagittal sinus, and the possible presence of paramedian venous lacunae. Precise placement of the bone flap relative to the venous pattern in this area is thus ensured. It is important to recognize the position of the coronal suture, which in most instances lies vertical to the foramen of Monro. Sagittal MRI studies are an effective resource to guide the surgeon in targeting the foramen of Monro.

Exploring the anterior interhemispheric fissure, especially in pediatric patients, may be uncomplicated because multiple and wide corridors often exist between cortical veins draining into the sinus. However, in some cases, advancing through the interhemispheric fissure can be challenging when these corridors are narrower or the arachnoid bands tethering these veins are thicker than usual. With sharp dissection of the arachnoid bands, the draining veins are mobilized and, if at all possible, none of them are sacrificed. Moist cottonoids of increasing size are placed at the anterior and posterior points of dissection to provide a sufficient opening in the fissure and therefore avoid the need for a self-retaining retractor. Occasionally, the falx may be short or it may have fenestrations and compact arachnoidal adhesions among bilateral medial, frontal, or bilateral cingulate gyri across the midline. In some cases, pericallosal arteries provide small branches to the falx. To prevent their inadvertent avulsion, these branches are coagulated and severed.

Upon reaching the body of the corpus callosum, the surgeon must be aware that one, two, or even three pericallosal arteries may be present. The surgeon should carefully study the arterial pattern in this region on preoperative MR angiography and correlate this information with the surgical anatomy. Generally, the corpus callosum is incised approximately 5 to 10 mm in length between two pericallosal arteries. An incision into the corpus callosum initiates the free flow of CSF and decompression of the right lateral ventricle. Unless there are tiny natural vents in the septum pellucidum, CSF from the left lateral ventricle will not drain and the septum pellucidum will bulge to the right, obscuring the surgeon's view. A 5- to 10-mm fenestrating incision into the septum pellucidum allows drainage of the left lateral ventricle, giving the surgeon adequate access to both lateral ventricles as well as both foramina of Monro, regardless of the size of the ventricles.

Both foramina of Monro and the course of the veins joining the internal cerebral vein, in particular the anterior septal and thalamostriate veins, are inspected. In the classic definition, these veins are described as converging at the posterior margin of the foramen of Monro and are covered by the choroid plexus. In the majority of patients, however, the location of the junction between the anterior septal and internal cerebral veins is found beyond the posterior margin of the foramen of Monro, within the velum interpositum, mainly unilaterally but occasionally bilaterally. The drainage patterns of the anterior septal, thalamostriate, and internal cerebral veins, which are intimately associated with the surgical exposure of the third ventricle, can be studied preoperatively on MR venography[68] (**Fig. 10.3c**). In patients with a large tumor, one or both foramina of Monro are often grossly enlarged, and in such situations it has not been found necessary to mobilize the choroid plexus and tela choroidea. In patients with a small foramen of Monro bilaterally, we recommend defining the location of the junction of the anterior septal and internal cerebral veins and, in the case of a posteriorly located junction, we advocate opening the choroidal fissure as far as the junction to enlarge the ipsilateral foramen of Monro posteriorly. This technique allows adequate access to the entire third ventricle without injuring vital paraforaminal neural and vascular structures.[68]

In patients with a cystic tumor, the cyst is punctured and the contents aspirated, which facilitates dissection of the collapsed tumor from the wall of the third ventricle. In the absence of a cystic component, the lesion is debulked piecemeal using bipolar forceps, a rongeur, and suction, until an optimal central decompression has been achieved. Thereafter, the peripheral surface of the tumor around both foramina of Monro and in the posterosuperior aspect of the third ventricle can be dissected, especially from the choroid plexus. This is the main advantage of the combined approach, which facilitates dissection of the superior portion of the tumor under direct visual control instead of pulling the tumor down blindly, as is done in the pterional or other lateral approaches. The displaced massa intermedia and the entrance to the aqueduct are identified. Fortunately, in the majority of patients, a relatively well-defined cleavage exists between the ventricular wall and the tumor surface, and it is essential to keep track of this cleavage pattern. During dissection in the laterobasal areas of the third ventricle, the course of the optic tract must be taken into account. Deeper exploration exposes the chiasm, infundib-

ulum, mamillary bodies, and basilar bifurcation within the interpeduncular fossa.

After the tumor is removed, the explored areas are inspected to secure hemostasis. Pterional exploration continues to ensure that no residual tumor remains and that hemostasis is absolute. The surgical field of both craniotomies is reinspected with a 0-degree and a 30-degree endoscope to visualize any residual tumor in the retrochiasmatic and interpeduncular compartments, the posterior and superior walls of the third ventricle, and the intrasellar compartment, especially on the blind side of the sella where the craniotomy is established (**Fig. 10.3d,e**). Once total resection is achieved, hemostasis is established and watertight closure is ensured.

Conclusion

This combined approach provides an effective surgical method, under direct and full visual control, to explore and completely remove intra- and extraventricular types of craniopharyngiomas extending superiorly into the third ventricle up to the foramen of Monro. This approach is especially suitable when the tumor causes unilateral or bilateral hydrocephalus. The anatomic relationship of the inferior part of the tumor in subchiasmatic, interpeduncular, and prepontine areas, as well as the parasellar tumor extensions, can be identified and precisely dissected through a pterional-transsylvian parachiasmatic approach. The posterosuperior part of the tumor and its relation to structures in the foramen of Monro and third ventricle, especially adhesions to the choroid plexus and tela choroidea, can be explored and identified through the anterior interhemispheric transcallosal-transforaminal approach.

Separate small, free pterional and posterior frontal parasagittal bone flaps can be made with separate skin incisions. The combination of these two approaches unites the advantages of each and allows for safe and complete removal of these formidable lesions.

The Translaminar Approach to Craniopharyngiomas

Edward R. Smith and R. Michael Scott

Craniopharyngiomas are tumors usually found in the region of the infundibulum, although they can develop anywhere along an axis from the nasopharynx to the third ventricle. They comprise approximately 5 to 10% of pediatric brain tumors and present with signs and symptoms referable to their location, including visual loss, hormonal disturbances, hydrocephalus, and headache. The broad spectrum of strategies used to treat these tumors, in-

cluding surgical resection, radiation, and the intratumoral delivery of chemotherapeutic agents or radioisotopes, underscores the difficulty of achieving successful cures with acceptable morbidity, and has fostered considerable controversy among physicians involved in the care of children with these lesions. Among the most challenging of these lesions are those situated entirely within the third ventricle. This section provides a case-based review of one surgical technique to access tumors in this location by creating an opening in the lamina terminalis: the translaminar approach.

Presentation of the Case

An 18-year-old male presented to his pediatrician with the chief complaints of progressive visual loss, frequent urination, and marked obesity over the past several months. An MRI study was obtained (see case figure) with subsequent referral to neurosurgery.

Initial Steps

Diagnostic Evaluation

The patient's history and imaging support the presumptive diagnosis of a craniopharyngioma. These lesions originate from cells derived from the development of the adenohypophysis and tend to arise primarily from the region of the infundibulum.[69,70] Craniopharyngiomas are composed of two distinct subtypes, adamantinomatous and papillary, which differ pathologically. Adamantinomatous craniopharyngiomas are most common in children, have a tendency to produce calcified deposits intratumorally, and have a keratinized squamous layer that flakes off and degenerates into a characteristic cholesterol-rich "crankcase oil" fluid.[71-73] In contrast, the papillary subtype (also called squamous papillary) is found nearly exclusively in adults (albeit still less frequently than adamantinomatous tumors) and is characterized by stratified squamous epithelium that does not usually exhibit the calcification or cystic degeneration evident in the adamantinomatous tumors.[71-74]

Clinical Evaluation

Although craniopharyngiomas can be discovered in the asymptomatic patient, the vast majority of cases are identified with the onset of characteristic signs and symptoms.[75] The most common clinical findings include sequelae of increased intracranial pressure from mass effect and hydrocephalus (especially headache, nausea, and vomiting), particularly visual loss, or endocrinologic dysfunction, or both.[69,75,76] In the published series from Children's Hospital in Boston, symptoms resulting from increased intracranial pressure were the most common causes, leading to discovery of the tumor in 44% of patients.[75] Nearly 25% of patients with a craniopharyngioma have hydrocephalus at presentation—a finding in the patient presented here—secondary to obstruction of the third ventricle by the tumor.[76]

As in this patient, visual deterioration can be quite severe before it is detected by family or clinicians and may be asymmetric depending on the growth pattern of the tumor.[75,77] Similarly insidious is the development of endocrinologic dysfunction, which may remain unnoticed for long periods of time because of the often subtle onset of symptoms such as growth delay. Although a deficiency of growth hormone is the most common endocrinologic problem found in the setting of a craniopharyngioma (followed by hypothyroidism and diabetes insipidus—the cause of the frequent urination in the patient presented here), abnormalities of any and all of the pituitary hormones may be manifest, and a careful retrospective analysis of patients reveals some form of endocrine dysfunction in 60 to 90% of patients at diagnosis.[75,78] Hormonal symptoms can be compounded by effects resulting from hypothalamic injury, particularly common in patients with tumors filling the third ventricle. These findings include temperature intolerance or dysregulation, behavioral disturbances, and, as in the reviewed patient, weight gain.

For this patient, a formal assessment of visual fields and an ophthalmologic examination should be done before surgery.[75,79] This assessment not only establishes a baseline, but also may help guide the surgical approach if one optic nerve is substantially impaired and the other has retained function. Consultation with endocrinologists is important, including obtaining a panel of laboratory studies to evaluate the pituitary function (see **Table 9.2 in Chapter 9**). Craniopharyngioma patients can be cortisol-deficient and profound deterioration can occur from apparently minor physiological stressors. The replacement of corticosteroids frequently averts disaster in these cases, and options include dexamethasone (1–4 mg intravenously) or hydrocortisone (30 mg/m^2). Lastly, although it is often not practical in the setting of an ill patient, those who come to medical attention in a more elective fashion may be candidates for a detailed neuropsychological evaluation, allowing caregivers and families to more effectively follow changes over the course of treatment and develop more tailored coping strategies.[79,80]

Radiographic Evaluation

An MRI scan is particularly useful for identifying tumors and delineating the relationship of the tumor to surrounding neurovascular structures, including the carotids and their branches, the optic apparatus, the pituitary gland and stalk, and the hypothalamus and ventricular system (see case figure). As in this patient, craniopharyngiomas may appear to be heterogeneous, with bright cystic components on T1- and T2-weighted images and solid portions of the tumor exhibiting variable enhancement after the administration of contrast. Obtaining MRI scans in axial, sagittal, and coronal planes with and without contrast is critical to preoperative planning and postoperative follow-up. For these same reasons, MR angiography (MRA) is helpful in delineating the vascular anatomy.

Specific to the decision to use a translaminar approach is the relationship of the optic chiasm to the tumor. When the bulk of the tumor is located posterior to the optic chiasm (as is the case in third ventricular tumors), the optic apparatus is often displaced anteriorly and thinned—a "prefixed" chiasm. Although many craniopharyngiomas are relatively midline, some may show asymmetry with associated rotation of the chiasm—an additional finding relevant for surgical planning that can be predicted with detailed preoperative MRI scans. Lastly, the length of the rostrocaudal window between the chiasm (caudally) and the anterior cerebral communicating artery (rostrally), as appreciated on the sagittal MRI scans, may also be useful for surgical planning.

A CT scan is also helpful in the diagnosis and surgical planning for patients with craniopharyngiomas. A distinguishing feature of these tumors is the presence of calcium, which may be difficult to detect on MRI. Regions of calcification are present in most pediatric tumors (up to 90%) and over half of adult lesions.[41,72,81] Preoperative radiographic visualization of solid calcium deposits (when present) is invaluable to the surgeon in determining the feasibility of specific operative approaches. This is especially relevant to operative planning for intraventricular lesions, as dense calcification may warn the surgeon that there may be profound challenges to the goal of surgical resection. In addition, CT is helpful in ascertaining the degree of pneumatization of the sphenoid, ethmoid, and frontal sinuses, information that is relevant to choosing the transsphenoidal approaches for sellar tumors, the transfrontal approaches for suprasellar tumors, and, particular to the case presented here, drilling down the planum sphenoidale to augment the visualization of retrochiasmatic lesions.

Preoperative angiography is generally not helpful in evaluating craniopharyngiomas. The tumors are usually fed by small vessels that are difficult to visualize, even with a dedicated angiogram, and there is no role for preoperative embolization. Most of the relevant structural anatomy can be better delineated with MRA, in which the parenchyma and tumor can be seen side by side with associated vessels.

Management

Althuogh this patient's tumor was identified in the outpatient setting, some children may present with rapid clinical deterioration. This is most commonly caused by hydrocephalus, and may require urgent decompression of the ventricular system with external catheters. In the setting of the rapidly deteriorating child, it is important to remember the potential need to administer stress-dose steroids. This case also serves to illustrate the potential need to place bilateral ventricular drains (or a unilateral drain with concomitant endoscopic septostomy), as the tumor's obstruction of both foramina of Monro may lead to catheter decompression of only the ipsilateral ventricle.

If possible, complex tumor resection should be delayed until the operation can be well thought out and an experienced and fully staffed operative team is available. A fresh and rested neurosurgical team is often in the best interest of both the surgeon and the patient.

Operative Planning

Once the tumor is identified, the primary objectives of craniopharyngioma treatment are restoring and preserving neurologic function with minimal morbidity. The debates regarding the most effective method to achieve this goal are substantial. The preferential use of specific treatments—radical surgery, subtotal resection, radiation, and the intracystic administration of chemotherapy or radioisotopes—may be influenced by both published data and institutional bias. Before undertaking an operation, neurosurgeons should define the goals of surgery. An important distinction is whether the objective is a complete resection or a planned subtotal debulking. This topic is controversial, with data supporting either strategy, and is beyond the scope of this chapter.[10,69,75,82–87] Here, we present an overview of one surgical technique—the translaminar approach—as illustrated by a specific case.

The Translaminar Approach

Operative Indications and Use

The primary goal of surgery is to resect the lesion while preserving vital neural and vascular structures. Factors such as anatomic constraints imposed by these vital structures or characteristics of the tumor (such as areas of calcification) may preclude a gross total resection, and the secondary goals of surgery may include reducing mass effect, debulking the tumor so that it becomes more amenable to radiation therapy (either through reduced size or by creating margins from vital structures to minimize dose effect), restoring patterns of CSF flow, or establishing a tissue diagnosis with pathological specimens. These goals are especially important with tumors akin to the one presented here, as they can present formidable challenges to the surgeon, with substantial risks to the patient.

The translaminar approach involves making an opening in the lamina terminalis to gain entry to the third ventricle. This approach is limited by a narrow angle of entry and a necessarily small working aperture, bounded by the optic apparatus, the nuclei of the hypothalamus, and the anterior cerebral arteries. Other than for the smallest lesions, it is often a poor choice as a sole route for tumor resection. However, when used in conjunction with other approaches (such as through the opticocarotid triangle or after drilling down the planum sphenoidale), the unique access afforded by the translaminar approach can markedly augment their effectiveness.

Indications for the translaminar approach include the presence of a prefixed chiasm, or a tumor location within the third ventricle or on the undersurface of the chiasm, in which case the opening of the lamina terminalis may allow better exposure of the tumor by allowing downward pressure on the tumor through the hypothalamic floor to deliver the mass into the already established infrachiasmatic exposure. The case presented here is challenging, and it is unlikely that a substantive resection could be achieved solely with a translaminar approach. However, when coupled with the other routes mentioned above (and potentially alternative trajectories, such as the transcallosal approach), safe resection of the mass might be achieved, either with a single or combined surgical procedure.

In addition to the anatomic indications discussed, the consistency of the tumor as estimated from imaging studies is an important factor to consider when selecting an approach. The presence of a mostly cystic and not heavily calcified tumor suggests that the translaminar route may be effective. Conversely, a heavily calcified or solid tumor will probably be difficult to resect through the small aperture afforded by this approach. As noted above, the tumor's appearance on preoperative CT scans will influence this aspect of preoperative planning.

Risks

Access to the lamina terminalis is usually obtained through a bifrontal or frontolateral approach, with the approach often augmented through removal of the orbital bar and roof to provide additional exposure from below. The risks to these approaches are discussed in greater detail elsewhere, but include CSF leakage (given the potential violation of the sinuses), injury to the olfactory nerves, and retraction injury to the brain (which can be minimized by diverting CSF through a catheter). When opening the lamina terminalis, care must be taken not to injure the optic chiasm (with risk to the bitemporal fields from midline damage), compress or avulse the anterior cerebral branches (which supply the optic system and anterior perforated substance), or cause harm to the hypothalamic nuclei. Although some authors have advocated sectioning of the anterior cerebral communicating artery to increase access through the lamina terminalis, that is not the practice at our institution.[88] Of particular note is the danger of traction injury to the structures out of view within the third ventricle from overaggressive tumor resection. These at-risk structures include the internal cerebral veins, the walls of the ventricle (including the thalamus, hypothalamus, and superior midbrain), the infundibulum, and vessels comprising the circle of Willis (especially in the setting of an incompetent floor of the third ventricle).

In addition to the surgeon making his or her own assessment of operative risk, it is important to have a candid discussion with the patient and the family before surgery to communicate the potential risks and benefits.

Preoperative Planning

The anesthesia and nursing team should be called in before the operation to review the treatment strategy and prepare the appropriate equipment. The anesthesia team should prepare for fluid shifts, possible pre- or intraoperative diabetes insipidus, the need for hormone replacement (especially stress-dose steroids), and blood loss, and anticipate a potential air embolus, particularly if midline exposures are done. Nursing staff can prepare the desired equipment, such as ventriculostomy catheters, specialized drill bits, the ultrasonic aspirator, frameless stereotaxy, intraoperative imaging (such as ultrasound, endoscopy, or dental mirrors) and specialized instruments such as specific retraction kits and small, long microdissectors (we often use transsphenoidal forceps and curettes in translaminar approaches). In addition, if transgression of the frontal air sinus is likely, an abdominal fat graft site can be prepared before starting the procedure.

Operative Approach

In this patient, the tumor is quite large and resection is likely to be challenging. Although many different approaches could be considered, the retrochiasmatic location of this tumor, coupled with its large size, suggests that surgical intervention is warranted. The goals in this specific case would be to alleviate the compression of peritumoral neural structures (thalamic and hypothalamic nuclei), restore CSF pathways, and remove as much tumor as possible, to either attempt a cure or, more likely, reduce the size to a smaller target for radiation. The success of the approach depends on the consistency of the tumor, as firm, calcified lesions are difficult and possibly unsafe to resect, whereas soft, suctionable tumors may be amenable to removal. It would be reasonable in this case to consider a preoperative ventriculostomy (perhaps aided by an endoscopic septostomy) and in some cases plan for access to a transcallosal route in the same sitting. Others might first attempt the translaminar approach and proceed to a transcallosal approach in a staged fashion as a separate procedure only if needed.

Here, we describe the subfrontal translaminar approach. The subfrontal approach allows for excellent visualization of the optic nerves, carotids, and, importantly, the lamina terminalis. This approach is useful for most craniopharyngiomas, albeit less so for isolated sellar lesions. It affords a wide range of potential approaches to the suprasellar region and can be easily combined with other approaches, such as the pterional, transcallosal intraventricular, and even the sellar (with drilling of the planum sphenoidale). The approach can be unilateral or bilateral, depending on the anatomy of the tumor. For retrochiasmatic and intraventricular tumors, removing the superior orbital rim and roof improves visualization while minimizing retraction on the frontal lobes. In this case, a bilateral frontal approach is used.

For patients with hydrocephalus, the placement of a preoperative drain may relax the brain and facilitate visualization with minimal retraction. A bicoronal incision is then marked out, with preparation to include the possibility of a pterional extension if needed. In patients with a large frontal air sinus, a site for an abdominal fat graft is readied.

The patient is pinned in extension with the head midline to allow the frontal lobes to fall away from the floor of the anterior fossa. After the incision is made, the pericranium is preserved by elevating the scalp flap in anticipation of the need for a vascularized pedicle to cover the frontal sinus. In a unilateral case, the operating table can be rotated to vary lines of sight while the surgeon remains in a comfortable operating position, seated or standing. The dural opening should be low to the floor of the anterior fossa and, in the case of bilateral exposure, care should be taken to preserve at least one olfactory nerve.

If the orbital rim and roof are removed, the surgeon should attempt to avoid injury to the periorbita, as fat can be troublesome to retract and can result in significant postoperative bruising and ocular ecchymosis. Gentle downward retraction on the orbit can greatly enhance visualization of the tumor, although some patients may experience bradycardia with compression of the eye. This will often resolve with slight repositioning of the retractor.

Once the dura is opened, the operating microscope is used and the CSF cisterns are opened to further relax the brain. It is our practice to avoid using mannitol if possible, given the ability to achieve good relaxation with proper positioning and the removal of CSF, and also given the potential issues with diabetes insipidus perioperatively. Draining the cyst contents can help relax the tight brain, but we prefer to maintain the tumor anatomy through the initial dissection, if possible, as the taut cyst provides good countertraction and a convenient dissection plane. Ultimately, however, cysts need to be drained, which can be accomplished with direct entry or aspiration with a fine needle. Placement of cottonoids around the cyst may help prevent the spread of the irritating cyst contents in the subarachnoid space, theoretically reducing the likelihood of chemical meningitis and tumor seeding.

In this patient, opening of the lamina terminalis will be useful and essential. The thinned, often darkened area just above the chiasm can be incised, and in this patient the area will be full or bulging. We often employ an arachnoid blade to make a rostrocaudal opening. The inferior extent of the opening is limited by the chiasm, whereas the rostral opening is restricted by the anterior cerebral communicating artery and the anterior commissure of the frontal lobes. Care must be taken to avoid blind traction on or injury to the walls of the third ventricle, as hypothalamic injury can be devastating, and thus self-retaining retractors are not placed within the laminar opening. This is equally important to prevent injury to vessels (especially the internal cerebral veins) and especially relevant in the setting of adherent or heavily calcified tumors. Gentle downward pressure on the tumor from the lamina terminalis can sometimes deliver the lesion into the more accessible subchiasmatic space, allowing other approaches to become more useful.

Employing a dental mirror or angled endoscope can substantially aid in visualizing difficult regions of the operative field. Drilling of the planum sphenoidale can increase the working room, allowing greater access to the sella when the chiasm is prefixed. When drilling in this area, the surgeon must be aware that the ethmoid or sphenoid sinus can be entered and appropriate steps must be taken to prevent a CSF leak if a breach occurs—namely, packing the sinus with fat or muscle and covering the defect with tissue, preferably vascularized pericranium and fibrin glue.

In this case, gentle, piecemeal resection of the tumor, if soft, may result in substantial debulking. The decision as to when to stop debulking often requires the surgeon's experienced judgment. Intraoperative imaging with either ultrasound or MRI can often be of great help in these cases, and, when available, both are used routinely in these cases because of the difficulty in visualizing the most superior extent of these large tumors.

Immediate Postoperative Care

After surgical resection of a craniopharyngioma, patients are usually monitored in the intensive care unit. Primary concerns center on the management of hormonal replacement (especially with regard to diabetes insipidus and stress-dose corticosteroids), repeated assessment of visual function (monitoring for hemorrhage or blood pressure–dependent changes to eyesight), and documentation of the level of consciousness (watching for delayed hydrocephalus and the effects of hypothalamic injury). Postoperative imaging is useful as a baseline, and is performed on our service either in the operating room or within 48 hours of the end of surgery. An ongoing discussion among the intensive care staff, nurses, and the neurosurgical team is critical to maximize communication and maintain a unified approach to the often difficult management issues that problems like postoperative diabetes insipidus can raise regarding fluid management.

Conclusion

Craniopharyngiomas remain one of the most challenging brain tumors, particularly when found in association with a prefixed chiasm and located totally within the third ventricle. The use of the translaminar approach offers neurosurgeons a route by which to attack these lesions. Detailed preoperative assessment, including MRI, CT, and clinical evaluations (endocrine and visual), is critical to developing a sound surgical strategy. The translaminar approach is most effective when coupled with other routes of access to the tumor. The ability to combine the translaminar approach with other surgical approaches, along with a clear understanding of potential complications such as traction injuries, leads to the safest and most effective surgical care being provided to the patient.

Craniopharyngioma: Choosing the Optimal Neurosurgical Approach

James T. Rutka and Osaama H. Khan

The topic of craniopharyngioma is steeped in a rich history in the neurosurgical literature and archives. In the days of Dandy,[89] this tumor was known as a hypophyseal ductal tumor. Dandy described his experiences with this predominantly childhood tumor, including a description of its predominant localization in the intracranial compartment, the presence of dark-colored cystic fluid containing cholesterol crystals, and various neurosurgical approaches used to reach the tumor itself. Dandy did not hesitate to move aside or resect structures that were in his way, such as the optic or olfactory nerve, to gain access and remove as much of the tumor as possible. Since Dandy's time, there have been numerous advances in our understanding of this disease and its treatment. This section of the chapter establishes the principles for the neurosurgical resection of craniopharyngiomas and offers a balanced perspective on the selection of approaches according to important clinical and neuroimaging features.

Incidence and Etiology

Craniopharyngiomas account for 3% of intracranial tumors[90] and 6 to 8% of pediatric brain tumors.[91] No underlying causes for their development have been consistently identified. On rare occasions, craniopharyngiomas have occurred in siblings,[92–94] but limited genetic studies suggest that this type of tumor is sporadic, not one that has genetic inheritance patterns.

Natural History

The natural history of craniopharyngiomas has not been entirely elucidated, but good evidence shows that both cystic and solid elements of the tumor have a significant potential to grow **(Fig. 10.4)**. If a craniopharyngioma is detected incidentally on imaging studies, then there is an option for follow-up with close serial imaging to more fully delineate its growth rate. As most craniopharyngiomas show growth of both cystic and solid elements over time, however, neurosurgical planning should be done early to maximize the opportunities for successful eradication or control of the lesion.

Classification System

Craniopharyngiomas can be classified according to their site of origin: sellar, prechiasmatic, or retrochiasmatic.[95,96] Sellar craniopharyngiomas present predominantly with endocrinopathy, prechiasmatic lesions with visual failure, and retrochiasmatic lesions with endocrinopathy and raised intracranial pressure because they often invaginate the floor of the third ventricle and grow toward and eventually occlude the foramina of Monro bilaterally.

In recent times, craniopharyngiomas have been classified on the basis of their relationship to the infundibulum.[97,98] This classification system is reasonable, but at times the precise localization of the infundibulum cannot be determined even with thin-slice MRI, given the large size and regional invasiveness of these tumors. In either case, craniopharyngiomas arise in the basal forebrain region, and the physician must appreciate and preserve, when possible, the important regional neuroanatomy, including the pituitary gland and stalk, the hypothalamus, the intracranial carotid artery, the A1 and A2 segments of the anterior cerebral artery, the M1 branch of the middle cerebral artery, and the first, second, and third cranial nerves.

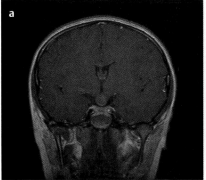 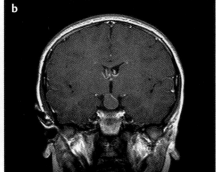 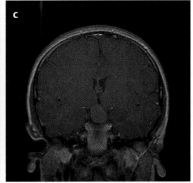

Fig. 10.4a–c Serial MRI scans of a craniopharyngioma found during the workup of a patient with headaches. Images were repeated at 6 months **(b)** and 10 months **(c)**, respectively. Although the patient had no neurologic or endocrinologic abnormalities, surgery was chosen because of progressive growth, with encroachment into the hypothalamus at 10 months.

Clinical Investigation

If a child is identified with a craniopharyngioma, then a series of examinations and investigations are recommended before surgery. These include neurologic, neuro-endocrinologic, neuro-ophthalmologic, neuroradiological, and neuropsychological assessments. A neuropsychological examination should be done before surgery because the basal forebrain structures and the mesial temporal lobes may be affected by treatment; thus, it is prudent to determine, if possible, the patient's preoperative neuropsychological status. Such an assessment is especially recommended for young children who may be candidates for radiation therapy at a later stage.

Treatment Options

The treatment options for craniopharyngiomas include conservative management, surgery (biopsy or open resection), chemotherapy (including intracystic therapy), radiation therapy, and hormonal therapy. In this context, hormonal therapy refers to the use of endocrine hormone replacement therapy to overcome deficiencies that can occur after treatment. Of the various hormone therapies, antidiuretic hormone replacement therapy may be most important in the early postoperative phase. Other hormones, such as growth hormone, thyroid hormone, and steroid hormones, are factored into the decision making in due course based on the results of serum hormone measurements in the postoperative period.

Neurosurgical Approaches

A myriad of neurosurgical approaches to craniopharyngiomas has been described. Some of the more commonly used approaches include the transsphenoidal, subfrontal, pterional, subtemporal, anterior intrahemispheric, intrahemispheric transcallosal, and endonasal endoscopic. In addition, for large tumors, a neurosurgeon may choose a combined approach, using, for example, an intrahemispheric transcallosal approach in conjunction with a pterional or subfrontal approach.[99] Recent reports from several centers describe the use of the endoscopic endonasal approach.[100–102]

The Case for Aggressive Neurosurgical Resection

Given the inexorable growth and neurologic deficits that can result from inadequately treated tumors, the case for aggressive neurosurgical resection of craniopharyngiomas has been made by several neurosurgeons in numerous centers.[11,86,103,104] Yaşargil and colleagues[11] reported on a series of 144 patients in whom craniopharyngiomas were aggressively resected. In this series, the recurrence rate was 7%, the morbidity was 16.7%, and the mortality was 2.1%. In the series by Hoffman and associates,[85] craniopha-

ryngiomas were aggressively resected toward gross total removal of the tumor. Despite what appeared to be a complete resection at surgery, however, the recurrence rate was 34%. Postoperative imaging studies could frequently predict which patients would have a recurrence of their craniopharyngioma.

In the series reported by Fahlbusch and coworkers,[9] the tumors were heavily weighted toward sellar craniopharyngiomas. As a result, a transsphenoidal approach could be used to reach these lesions, resection rates were high, and morbidity was low. In the follow-up report on this series, the gross total resection rate remained close to 89%.[105] The authors believed strongly that total resection was the treatment of choice, and radiotherapy should be reserved for tumor remnants or progression of disease after surgery.

Van Effenterre and Boch[2] reported on 122 patients who underwent aggressive resection. In their series, there was also a defined recurrence rate, but patients did well, suffering very few neurologic, endocrinologic, or ophthalmologic complications. In the study by Elliott and colleagues,[106] 86 patients underwent radical resection of craniopharyngiomas. These authors advocate radical surgery, and gross total resection was easiest at the first presentation, but there were three perioperative deaths. Subtotal resection, hydrocephalus, and the implantation of a ventricular peritoneal shunt were negative predictors of progression-free and overall survival. In the end, the authors recommended that, if aggressive surgery is necessary, it should be done by a neurosurgeon with considerable experience with this tumor.[86]

Our Preferred Neurosurgical Approach

At the Hospital for Sick Children in Toronto, Canada, we have typically used a unilateral subfrontal approach to remove craniopharyngiomas, primarily because of the midline position of the lesion, almost without exception. For this approach, the patient is placed in the supine position with the head tilted slightly backward. A bicoronal scalp incision is preferred, and a unilateral orbital osteotomy is done after a frontal craniotomy. When the dura is opened, there is an option to ligate the anterior superior sagittal sinus and divide the falx cerebri so as to facilitate brain relaxation. It is extremely important that the frontal lobe *not* be the object of a retraction injury at the end of the case. The CSF cisterns are opened widely so that brain relaxation can continue before tumor removal.

The operative corridor to the craniopharyngioma is then expanded under the operating microscope. Stepwise, the olfactory nerve, the intracranial carotid artery, and the optic nerve are first identified on the ipsilateral side (**Fig. 10.5**). In most cases, the tumor capsule is easily seen at this juncture. The carotid artery is typically followed distally to the A1 segment of the anterior cerebral artery, which crosses over the optic chiasm or tract, and the M1 segment of the middle cerebral artery. The same exposure is then done

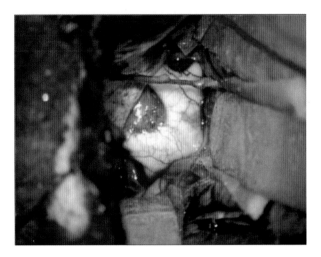

Fig. 10.5 Intraoperative image of a prechiasmatic craniopharyngioma through the subfrontal approach. The right olfactory nerve is seen superficially, with the tumor capsule surrounded by the optic nerves laterally and the optic chiasm posteriorly.

carefully on the contralateral side. For prechiasmatic lesions, dissection is performed predominantly anterior to the chiasm. Dissection within the opticocarotid triangle ensures the liberation of the tumor capsule from the optic apparatus beneath the optic nerve and chiasm. Early in the procedure, attempts are made to identify the pituitary stalk or infundibulum, which can be difficult, especially with large tumors.

For retrochiasmatic tumors, once the prechiasmatic space has been assessed to localize the tumor, then the lamina terminalis is exposed through gentle retraction on the frontal lobe. The lamina terminalis is typically exposed at the level of the anterior communicating artery and the junction of the A2 segments bilaterally (**Fig. 10.6**). The lamina terminalis is opened, and gentle dissection is performed to deliver the tumor capsule, the cyst wall, or both toward the midline. The operating microscope is used at high magnification as efforts are made to determine

whether the tumor adheres to the hypothalamus. Once sufficient microneurosurgical dissection has been done, gentle traction is applied to the tumor capsule with the micro-ring or equivalent forceps, and the tumor is delivered through the lamina terminalis. At the end of all procedures, it is wise to use mirrors or the curved endoscope to ensure that all tumor remnants and flecks of calcium have been removed (**Fig. 10.7**).

The Role of the Hypothalamus

A major determinant of the success of craniopharyngioma surgery is the integrity of the hypothalamus after the procedure. Recently, a classification system for craniopharyngiomas has been proposed based on the involvement of the hypothalamus. Puget and colleagues[96] described three categories of craniopharyngioma based on preoperative MRI findings. A class 0 tumor does not involve the hypothalamus and is a true prechiasmatic craniopharyngioma (**Fig. 10.8**). These tumors can be removed safely without fear of injury to the hypothalamus. Class 1 tumors have some involvement of the hypothalamus, usually on one side (**Fig. 10.9**). These cases can also be tackled surgically with expectations of a good outcome, but with some risk of injury to the hypothalamus and the development of obesity postoperatively. Class 2 tumors have potentially substantial involvement of the hypothalamus—the typical retrochiasmatic craniopharyngiomas—and surgery can be done, but the incidence of hypothalamic injury and obesity must be construed as a significant risk postoperatively (**Fig. 10.10**).

Endoscopic Endonasal Treatment of Craniopharyngiomas

Recently, Cavallo and colleagues[102] have described the use of the expanded endonasal approach for craniopharyngiomas. The approach they describe allows excellent visibility and access to the midline corridor up to the level of the third ventricle. But one of the problems described in this

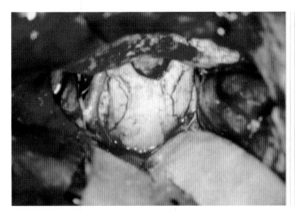

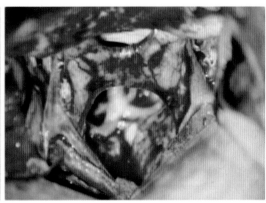

a

b

Fig. 10.6a,b Intraoperative images of the translamina terminalis approach to remove a retrochiasmatic craniopharyngioma. **(a)** The tumor capsule can be seen. **(b)** The tumor was debulked through resection of the lamina terminalis and the basilar complex can be seen in the distance.

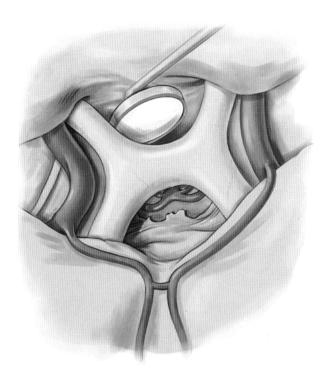

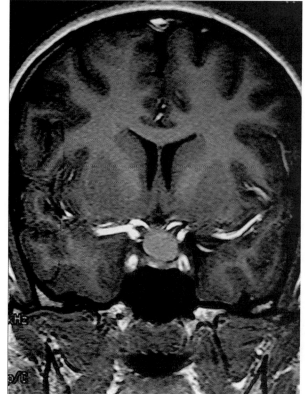

Fig. 10.7 Artistic illustration showing the use of a mirror to ensure adequate debulking of a craniopharyngioma. Note the bilateral carotids, the A1 and A2 segments, and the optic chiasm. Deep to the resected Liliequist membrane is the basilar complex. (From Cook DJ, Rutka JT. Craniopharyngioma: neurosurgical management. In: Hanna EY, DeMonte F, eds. Comprehensive Management of Skull Base Tumors. New York: Informa Healthcare, 2009:573-581. Reprinted by permission.)

Fig. 10.8 Coronal MRI of a class 0 craniopharyngioma located in the prechiasmatic space.

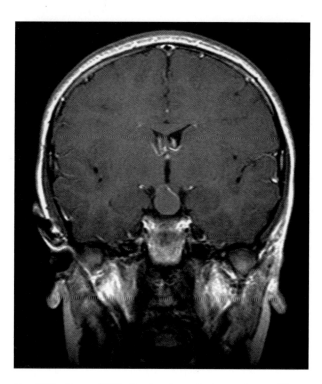

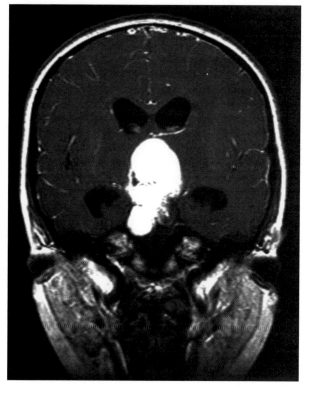

Fig. 10.9 Coronal MRI of a class 1 craniopharyngioma with encroachment into the hypothalamus (*right*).

Fig. 10.10 Coronal MRI of a class 2 craniopharyngioma that predominantly occupies the retrochiasmatic area with extensive involvement of the hypothalamus.

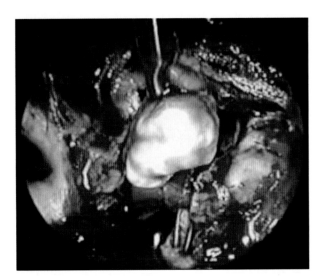

Fig. 10.11 Endoscopic endonasal image of forceps removing a cystic craniopharyngioma located in the sellar region. Care must be taken to avoid this method of resecting craniopharyngiomas known to have extensive calcification because of their adherence to nearby structures, most importantly the optic nerve and the hypothalamus.

series and with this approach in general is the early, relatively high rate of CSF leakage. In recent times, however, with the advent of the vascularized septonasal flap, the incidence of CSF leak has decreased significantly.[107] Leng and associates[101] have shown that minimal-access endoscopic and endonasal surgery for a craniopharyngioma can achieve high rates of gross total resection with low rates of CSF leakage. These authors claim that their results are very similar to those of transsphenoidal surgery reported in the past. We have found the endoscopic endonasal route to be particularly effective for recurrent craniopharyngiomas when there are remnants in the sella for which a transcranial approach would be rather difficult (**Fig. 10.11**).

Other Treatments for Craniopharyngiomas: Cystic Craniopharyngioma

It is not unreasonable to treat large cystic craniopharyngiomas with cyst-based therapy *ab initio*, which usually entails inserting a catheter into the tumor and attaching it to an Ommaya reservoir for repeated aspiration (**Fig. 10.12**). This strategy has worked well in several patients, but problems can occur with blockages or infection of the system itself. Several cystic sclerosing and ablative agents are available, including bleomycin, α-interferon, and radioisotopes such as phosphorus (^{32}P), iodine (^{125}I), and yttrium (^{90}Y). We have used bleomycin in cystic craniopharyngiomas, but because of its neurotoxicity, we now use α-interferon as the first agent of choice. Cavalheiro and colleagues[108] have reported excellent results related to this technique.

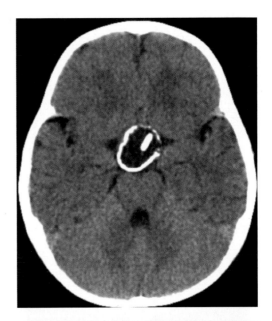

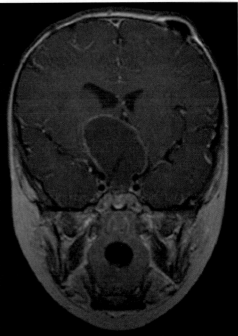

Fig. 10.12a,b An Ommaya reservoir is inserted into the cystic portion of a craniopharyngioma for repeated aspiration as clinically indicated. **(a)** Plain axial computed tomography shows a cystic lesion with calcifications. **(b)** The coronal T1-weighted MRI shows a left convexity extracranial reservoir. Both images show the catheter tip in place.

Radiation Therapy

Radiation treatment has been used for decades for patients with craniopharyngiomas. It can stabilize the tumor in 75% of patients. In the series by Merchant and colleagues,[84] limited surgery and radiation therapy were found to be preferable to radical surgery. Radiation therapy can potentially injure the mesial temporal lobes, and this risk must be factored into the patient's overall neuropsychological response after treatment as we continue to understand more about the results of craniopharyngioma treatments.

The experience with stereotactic radiosurgery is accumulating, and this modality appears to be best for small, solid residuals that are difficult to approach in other ways.[109] The problem with stereotactic radiosurgery is the relationship between the lesion and the optic nerves, hypothalamus, and cranial nerves. Niranjan and colleagues[110] have reported that stereotactic radiosurgery is safe and effective as a minimally invasive option for treating residual or recurrent craniopharyngiomas. Similarly, Veeravagu and associates[111] showed that the linear accelerator–based cyberknife can also be beneficial in stabilizing disease.

Neuropsychological Effects of Craniopharyngioma Treatment

There is no question that surgery in the basal forebrain and the area of the mesial temporal lobes can cause changes that affect the neuropsychology of a child. A retrospective review of 20 children from a single center failed to show any difference in neurobehavioral dysfunction at 36 months between patients undergoing partial resection and those undergoing gross total resection.[112] Carpentieri and associates[113] reported that craniopharyngioma patients had difficulty retrieving learned information. Memory recall was also disturbed in these children. A study from a series at our institution showed a decline in immediate verbal and visual memory in some children, and a slight diminution of the intelligence quotient in a prospective series.[85] It is important that families are made aware of the long-term side effects of treatment, not only in terms of cognitive changes but also of the potential to develop vascular malformations such as moyamoya disease, cavernomas, or secondary malignancies.

Conclusion

Can we predict which patients will do well and which will have difficulties after radical excision using data obtained preoperatively from our patients? The answer today is probably yes, and this answer hearkens back to the study by Puget and colleagues[96] and the role of the hypothalamus in this condition. Careful analysis of the preoperative imaging studies with fine cuts in the coronal plane can help the physician determine whether these lesions should be approached and, if so, what the anticipated morbidity might be with radical resection. Neurosurgeons are urged to carefully review all such data so that the best decisions can be made for their patients. Future research should focus on identifying markers for establishing prognostic factors, the long-term quality of life, supplementary outcome studies of patients undergoing subtotal resection complemented with cranial radiation, and novel pharmacological treatments.

References

1. Laws ER. Craniopharyngiomas in children and young adults. Prog Exp Tumor Res 1987;30:335–340
2. Van Effenterre R, Boch AL. Craniopharyngioma in adults and children: a study of 122 surgical cases. J Neurosurg 2002;97:3–11
3. Al-Mefty O. Less is less. J Neurosurg Pediatr 2010;6:401–402, discussion 402
4. Brunel H, Raybaud C, Peretti-Viton P, et al. Craniopharyngioma in children: MRI study of 43 cases. Neurochirurgie 2002;48:309–318
5. Duff J, Meyer FB, Ilstrup DM, Laws ER Jr, Schleck CD, Scheithauer BW. Long-term outcomes for surgically resected craniopharyngiomas. Neurosurgery 2000;46:291–302, discussion 302–305
6. Elliott RE, Wisoff JH. Surgical management of giant pediatric craniopharyngiomas. J Neurosurg Pediatr 2010;6:403–416
7. Chakrabarti I, Amar AP, Couldwell W, Weiss MH. Long-term neurological, visual, and endocrine outcomes following transnasal resection of craniopharyngioma. J Neurosurg 2005;102:650–657
8. Müller HL. Childhood craniopharyngioma—current concepts in diagnosis, therapy and follow-up. Nat Rev Endocrinol 2010;6:609–618
9. Fahlbusch R, Honegger J, Paulus W, Huk W, Buchfelder M. Surgical treatment of craniopharyngiomas: experience with 168 patients. J Neurosurg 1999;90:237–250
10. Wisoff JH. Surgical management of recurrent craniopharyngiomas. Pediatr Neurosurg 1994;21(Suppl 1):108–113
11. Yaşargil MG, Curcic M, Kis M, Siegenthaler G, Teddy PJ, Roth P. Total removal of craniopharyngiomas. Approaches and long-term results in 144 patients. J Neurosurg 1990;73:3–11
12. Hoffman HJ, De Silva M, Humphreys RP, Drake JM, Smith ML, Blaser SI. Aggressive surgical management of craniopharyngiomas in children. J Neurosurg 1992;76:47–52
13. Fukushima T, Hirakawa K, Kimura M, Tomonaga M. Intraventricular craniopharyngioma: its characteristics in magnetic resonance imaging and successful total removal. Surg Neurol 1990;33:22–27
14. Maira G, Anile C, Rossi GF, Colosimo C. Surgical treatment of craniopharyngiomas: an evaluation of the transsphenoidal and pterional approaches. Neurosurgery 1995;36:715–724
15. Golshani KJ, Lalwani K, Delashaw JB, Selden NR. Modified orbitozygomatic craniotomy for craniopharyngioma resection in children. J Neurosurg Pediatr 2009;4:345–352
16. Samii M, Bini W. Surgical treatment of craniopharyngiomas. Zentralbl Neurochir 1991;52:17–23
17. Konovalov AN, Gorelyshev SK. Surgical treatment of anterior third ventricle tumours. Acta Neurochir (Wien) 1992;118:33–39
18. Symon L, Sprich W. Radical excision of craniopharyngioma. Results in 20 patients. J Neurosurg 1985;62:174–181
19. Al-Mefty O, Ayoubi S, Kadri PA. The petrosal approach for the total removal of giant retrochiasmatic craniopharyngiomas in children. J Neurosurg 2007;106(2, Suppl):87–92

20. Hakuba A, Nishimura S, Inoue Y. Transpetrosal-transtentorial approach and its application in the therapy of retrochiasmatic craniopharyngiomas. Surg Neurol 1985;24:405–415

21. Laws ER Jr. Transsphenoidal microsurgery in the management of craniopharyngioma. J Neurosurg 1980;52:661–666

22. Baskin DS, Wilson CB. Surgical management of craniopharyngiomas. A review of 74 cases. J Neurosurg 1986;65:22–27

23. Cavallo LM, Prevedello D, Esposito F, et al. The role of the endoscope in the transsphenoidal management of cystic lesions of the sellar region. Neurosurg Rev 2008;31:55–64, discussion 64

24. Jane JA Jr, Kiehna E, Payne SC, Early SV, Laws ER Jr. Early outcomes of endoscopic transsphenoidal surgery for adult craniopharyngiomas. Neurosurg Focus 2010;28:E9

25. de Divitiis E, Cappabianca P, Cavallo LM, Esposito F, de Divitiis O, Messina A. Extended endoscopic transsphenoidal approach for extrasellar craniopharyngiomas. Neurosurgery 2007;61(5, Suppl 2)219–227, discussion 228

26. Dumont AS, Kanter AS, Jane JA Jr, Laws ER Jr. Extended transsphenoidal approach. Front Horm Res 2006;34:29–45

27. Gardner PA, Kassam AB, Snyderman CH, et al. Outcomes following endoscopic, expanded endonasal resection of suprasellar craniopharyngiomas: a case series. J Neurosurg 2008; 109:6–16

28. Kaptain GJ, Vincent DA, Sheehan JP, Laws ER Jr. Transsphenoidal approaches for the extracapsular resection of midline suprasellar and anterior cranial base lesions. Neurosurgery 2008;62(6, Suppl 3):1264–1271

29. Yamada S, Fukuhara N, Oyama K, et al. Surgical outcome in 90 patients with craniopharyngioma: an evaluation of transsphenoidal surgery. World Neurosurg 2010;74:320–330

30. Cappabianca P, Cavallo LM, Esposito F, de Divitiis E. Endoscopic endonasal transsphenoidal surgery: procedure, endoscopic equipment and instrumentation. Childs Nerv Syst 2004;20: 796–801

31. Hadad G, Bassagasteguy L, Carrau RL, et al. A novel reconstructive technique after endoscopic expanded endonasal approaches: vascular pedicle nasoseptal flap. Laryngoscope 2006; 116:1882–1886

32. Kassam AB, Thomas A, Carrau RL, et al. Endoscopic reconstruction of the cranial base using a pedicled nasoseptal flap. Neurosurgery 2008;63(1, Suppl 1):ONS44–ONS52, discussion ONS52–ONS53

33. Jane JA Jr, Prevedello DM, Alden TD, Laws ER Jr. The transsphenoidal resection of pediatric craniopharyngiomas: a case series. J Neurosurg Pediatr 2010;5:49–60

34. Jane JA Jr, Thapar K, Kaptain GJ, Maartens N, Laws ER Jr. Pituitary surgery: transsphenoidal approach. Neurosurgery 2002; 51:435–442, discussion 442–444

35. Komotar RJ, Starke RM, Raper DM, Anand VK, Schwartz TH. Endoscopic endonasal compared with microscopic transsphenoidal and open transcranial resection of craniopharyngiomas. World Neurosurg 2012;77:329–341

36. Al-Mefty O, Hassounah M, Weaver P, Sakati N, Jinkins JR, Fox JL. Microsurgery for giant craniopharyngiomas in children. Neurosurgery 1985;17:585–595

37. King JAJ, Mehta V, Black PM. Craniopharyngioma. In: Winn HR, ed. Youmans' Neurological Surgery, vol. 2, 6th ed. Philadelphia: Elsevier Saunders, 2011:1511–1522

38. Krisht AF, Ture U. Surgical approaches to craniopharyngiomas. In: Badie B, ed. Neurosurgical Operative Atlas, 2nd ed. New York: Thieme, 2007:9–16

39. Ohmori K, Collins J, Fukushima T. Craniopharyngiomas in children. Pediatr Neurosurg 2007;43:265–278

40. Samii M, Samii A. Surgical management of craniopharyngiomas. In: Schmidek HH, Sweet WH, eds. Operative Neurosurgical Techniques, 3rd ed. Philadelphia: WB Saunders, 1995:357–370

41. Samii M, Tatagiba M. Surgical management of craniopharyngiomas: a review. Neurol Med Chir (Tokyo) 1997;37:141–149

42. Steňo J. Microsurgical topography of craniopharyngiomas. Acta Neurochir Suppl (Wien) 1985;35:94–100

43. Steňo J, Malácek M, Bízik I. Tumor-third ventricular relationships in supradiaphragmatic craniopharyngiomas: correlation of morphological, magnetic resonance imaging, and operative findings. Neurosurgery 2004;54:1051–1058, discussion 1058–1060

44. Steňo J, Bízik I, Steňo A, Matejčík V. Craniopharyngiomas in children: how radical should the surgeon be? Childs Nerv Syst 2011;27:41–54

45. Türe U, Krisht AF. Craniopharyngiomas. In: Krisht AF, Tindall GT, eds. Pituitary Disorders: Comprehensive Management, 1st ed. Baltimore: Lippincott Williams & Wilkins, 1999:305–313

46. Yaşargil MG. Microneurosurgery, vol. IVB. Stuttgart: Georg Thieme Verlag, 1996

47. Yaşargil MG, Ture U, Roth P. Combined approaches. In: Apuzzo MLJ, ed. Surgery of the Third Ventricle, 2nd ed. Baltimore: Lippincott Williams & Wilkins, 1998:541–552

48. Zada G, Laws ER. Surgical management of craniopharyngiomas in the pediatric population. Horm Res Paediatr 2010;74: 62–66

49. Habrand JL, Ganry O, Couanet D, et al. The role of radiation therapy in the management of craniopharyngioma: a 25-year experience and review of the literature. Int J Radiat Oncol Biol Phys 1999;44:255–263

50. Kiehna EN, Merchant TE. Radiation therapy for pediatric craniopharyngioma. Neurosurg Focus 2010;28:E10

51. Stripp DC, Maity A, Janss AJ, et al. Surgery with or without radiation therapy in the management of craniopharyngiomas in children and young adults. Int J Radiat Oncol Biol Phys 2004; 58:714–720

52. Varlotto JM, Flickinger JC, Kondziolka D, Lunsford LD, Deutsch M. External beam irradiation of craniopharyngiomas: long-term analysis of tumor control and morbidity. Int J Radiat Oncol Biol Phys 2002;54:492–499

53. Yang I, Sughrue ME, Rutkowski MJ, et al. Craniopharyngioma: a comparison of tumor control with various treatment strategies. Neurosurg Focus 2010;28:E5

54. Albright AL, Hadjipanayis CG, Lunsford LD, Kondziolka D, Pollack IF, Adelson PD. Individualized treatment of pediatric craniopharyngiomas. Childs Nerv Syst 2005;21:649–654

55. Amendola BE, Wolf A, Coy SR, Amendola MA. Role of radiosurgery in craniopharyngiomas: a preliminary report. Med Pediatr Oncol 2003;41:123–127

56. Gopalan R, Dassoulas K, Rainey J, Sherman JH, Sheehan JP. Evaluation of the role of gamma knife surgery in the treatment of craniopharyngiomas. Neurosurg Focus 2008;24:E5

57. Kobayashi T, Kida Y, Mori Y, Hasegawa T. Long-term results of gamma knife surgery for the treatment of craniopharyngioma in 98 consecutive cases. J Neurosurg 2005;103(6, Suppl):482–488

58. Lee M, Kalani MY, Cheshier S, Gibbs IC, Adler JR, Chang SD. Radiation therapy and CyberKnife radiosurgery in the management of craniopharyngiomas. Neurosurg Focus 2008;24:E4

59. Ulfarsson E, Lindquist C, Roberts M, et al. Gamma knife radio-surgery for craniopharyngiomas: long-term results in the first Swedish patients. J Neurosurg 2002;97(5, Suppl):613–622

60. Zhang YQ, Ma ZY, Wu ZB, Luo SQ, Wang ZC. Radical resection of 202 pediatric craniopharyngiomas with special reference to the surgical approaches and hypothalamic protection. Pediatr Neurosurg 2008;44:435–443

61. Zuccaro G. Radical resection of craniopharyngioma. Childs Nerv Syst 2005;21:679–690

62. Elliott RE, Hsieh K, Hochm T, Belitskaya-Levy I, Wisoff J, Wisoff JH. Efficacy and safety of radical resection of primary and recurrent craniopharyngiomas in 86 children. J Neurosurg Pediatr 2010;5:30–48

63. Karavitaki N, Brufani C, Warner JT, et al. Craniopharyngiomas in children and adults: systematic analysis of 121 cases with long-term follow-up. Clin Endocrinol (Oxf) 2005;62:397–409

64. Dehdashti AR, de Tribolet N. Frontobasal interhemispheric trans-lamina terminalis approach for suprasellar lesions. Neurosurgery 2005;56(2, Suppl):418–424, discussion 418–424

65. Konovalov AN. Some problems of craniopharyngioma treatment. In: Broggi G, ed. Craniopharyngioma: Surgical Treatment. Berlin: Springer, 1995:88–96

66. Laws ER Jr, Jane JA Jr. Craniopharyngioma. J Neurosurg Pediatr 2010;5:27–28, discussion 28–29

67. Liu JK, Christiano LD, Gupta G, Carmel PW. Surgical nuances for removal of retrochiasmatic craniopharyngiomas via the trans-basal subfrontal translamina terminalis approach. Neurosurg Focus 2010;28:E6

68. Türe U, Yaşargil MG, Al-Mefty O. The transcallosal-transforaminal approach to the third ventricle with regard to the venous variations in this region. J Neurosurg 1997;87:706–715

69. Jane JA Jr, Laws ER. Craniopharyngioma. Pituitary 2006;9:323–326

70. Kanter AS, Sansur CA, Jane JA Jr, Laws ER Jr. Rathke's cleft cysts. Front Horm Res 2006;34:127–157

71. Louis DN, Ohgaki H, Wiestler OD, et al. The 2007 WHO classification of tumours of the central nervous system. Acta Neuropathol 2007;114:97–109

72. Zada G, Lin N, Ojerholm E, Ramkissoon S, Laws ER. Craniopharyngioma and other cystic epithelial lesions of the sellar region: a review of clinical, imaging, and histopathological relationships. Neurosurg Focus 2010;28:E4

73. Miller DC. Pathology of craniopharyngiomas: clinical import of pathological findings. Pediatr Neurosurg 1994;21(Suppl 1):11–17

74. Crotty TB, Scheithauer BW, Young WF Jr, et al. Papillary craniopharyngioma: a clinicopathological study of 48 cases. J Neurosurg 1995;83:206–214

75. Scott RM. Craniopharyngioma: a personal (Boston) experience. Childs Nerv Syst 2005;21:773–777

76. Karavitaki N, Brufani C, Warner JT, et al. Craniopharyngiomas in children and adults: systematic analysis of 121 cases with long-term follow-up. Clin Endocrinol (Oxf) 2005;62:397–409

77. Feletti A, Marton E, Mazzucco GM, Fang S, Longatti P. Amaurosis in infancy due to craniopharyngioma: a not exceptional but often misdiagnosed symptom. Neurosurg Focus 2010;28:E7

78. Sanford RA, Muhlbauer MS. Craniopharyngioma in children. Neurol Clin 1991;9:453–465

79. Waber DP, Pomeroy SL, Chiverton AM, et al. Everyday cognitive function after craniopharyngioma in childhood. Pediatr Neurol 2006;34:13–19

80. Müller HL, Bruhnken G, Emser A, et al. Longitudinal study on quality of life in 102 survivors of childhood craniopharyngioma. Childs Nerv Syst 2005;21:975–980

81. Samii M, Bini W. Surgical treatment of craniopharyngiomas. Zentralbl Neurochir 1991;52:17–23

82. Wisoff JH. Craniopharyngioma. J Neurosurg Pediatr 2008;1:124–125, discussion 125.

83. Sanford RA. Craniopharyngioma: results of survey of the American Society of Pediatric Neurosurgery. Pediatr Neurosurg 1994;21(Suppl 1):39–43

84. Merchant TE, Kiehna EN, Sanford RA, et al. Craniopharyngioma: the St. Jude Children's Research Hospital experience 1984-2001. Int J Radiat Oncol Biol Phys 2002;53:533–542

85. Hoffman HJ, De Silva M, Humphreys RP, Drake JM, Smith ML, Blaser SI. Aggressive surgical management of craniopharyngiomas in children. J Neurosurg 1992;76:47–52

86. Elliott RE, Hsieh K, Hochm T, Belitskaya-Levy I, Wisoff J, Wisoff JH. Efficacy and safety of radical resection of primary and recurrent craniopharyngiomas in 86 children. J Neurosurg Pediatr 2010;5:30–48

87. Craniopharyngioma in children. 41st annual congress of the French Society of Neurosurgery. Lisbon, Portugal, June 4-7, 1991. Neurochirurgie 1991;37(Suppl 1):1–174

88. Shibuya M, Takayasu M, Suzuki Y, Saito K, Sugita K. Bifrontal basal interhemispheric approach to craniopharyngioma resection with or without division of the anterior communicating artery. J Neurosurg 1996;84:951–956

89. Dandy W. Hypophyseal duct tumors. In Lewis D.: Practice of Surgery. Hagerstown, MD: WF Prior, 1938:598–560

90. Bunin GR, Surawicz TS, Witman PA, Preston-Martin S, Davis F, Bruner JM. The descriptive epidemiology of craniopharyngioma. Neurosurg Focus 1997;3:e1

91. Carmel PW, Antunes JL, Chang CH. Craniopharyngiomas in children. Neurosurgery 1982;11:382–389

92. Vargas JR, Pino JA, Murad TM. Craniopharyngioma in two siblings. JAMA 1981;246:1807–1808

93. Green DM. Childhood cancer in siblings. Pediatr Hematol Oncol 1986;3:229–239

94. Boch AL, van Effenterre R, Kujas M. Craniopharyngiomas in two consanguineous siblings: case report. Neurosurgery 1997;41:1185–1187

95. Pascual JM, González-Llanos F, Barrios L, Roda JM. Intraventricular craniopharyngiomas: topographical classification and surgical approach selection based on an extensive overview. Acta Neurochir (Wien) 2004;146:785–802

96. Puget S, Garnett M, Wray A, et al. Pediatric craniopharyngiomas: classification and treatment according to the degree of hypothalamic involvement. J Neurosurg 2007;106(1, Suppl):3–12

97. Qi S, Lu Y, Pan J, Zhang X, Long H, Fan J. Anatomic relations of the arachnoidea around the pituitary stalk: relevance for surgical removal of craniopharyngiomas. Acta Neurochir (Wien) 2011;153:785–796

98. Kassam AB, Gardner PA, Snyderman CH, Carrau RL, Mintz AH, Prevedello DM. Expanded endonasal approach, a fully endoscopic transnasal approach for the resection of midline suprasellar craniopharyngiomas: a new classification based on the infundibulum. J Neurosurg 2008;108:715–728

99. Filis AK, Moon K, Cohen AR. Synchronous ventriculoscopic and microsurgical resection of complex craniopharyngiomas. Pediatr Neurosurg 2009;45:434–436

100. Liu JK, Christiano LD, Patel SK, Eloy JA. Surgical nuances for removal of retrochiasmatic craniopharyngioma via the endoscopic endonasal extended transsphenoidal transplanum transtuberculum approach. Neurosurg Focus 2011;30:E14

101. Leng LZ, Greenfield JP, Souweidane MM, Anand VK, Schwartz TH. Endoscopic, endonasal resection of craniopharyngiomas: analysis of outcome including extent of resection, cerebrospinal fluid leak, return to preoperative productivity, and body mass index. Neurosurgery 2012;70:110–123, discussion 123–124

102. Cavallo LM, Prevedello DM, Solari D, et al. Extended endoscopic endonasal transsphenoidal approach for residual or recurrent craniopharyngiomas. J Neurosurg 2009;111:578–589

103. Weiner HL, Wisoff JH, Rosenberg ME, et al. Craniopharyngiomas: a clinicopathological analysis of factors predictive of recurrence and functional outcome. Neurosurgery 1994;35:1001–1010, discussion 1010–1011

104. Hoffman HJ. Craniopharyngiomas. The role for resection. Neurosurg Clin N Am 1990;1:173–180

105. Hofmann BM, Höllig A, Strauss C, Buslei R, Buchfelder M, Fahlbusch R. Results after treatment of craniopharyngiomas: further experiences with 73 patients since 1997. J Neurosurg 2012;116:373–384

106. Elliott RE, Sands SA, Strom RG, Wisoff JH. Craniopharyngioma Clinical Status Scale: a standardized metric of preoperative function and posttreatment outcome. Neurosurg Focus 2010;28:E2

107. Garcia-Navarro V, Anand VK, Schwartz TH. Gasket seal closure for extended endonasal endoscopic skull base surgery: efficacy in a large case series. World Neurosurg 2011

108. Cavalheiro S, Di Rocco C, Valenzuela S, et al. Craniopharyngiomas: intratumoral chemotherapy with interferon-alpha: a multicenter preliminary study with 60 cases. Neurosurg Focus 2010;28:E12

109. Selch MT, DeSalles AA, Wade M, et al. Initial clinical results of stereotactic radiotherapy for the treatment of craniopharyngiomas. Technol Cancer Res Treat 2002;1:51–59

110. Niranjan A, Kano H, Mathieu D, Kondziolka D, Flickinger JC, Lunsford LD. Radiosurgery for craniopharyngioma. Int J Radiat Oncol Biol Phys 2010;78:64–71

111. Veeravagu A, Lee M, Jiang B, Chang SD. The role of radiosurgery in the treatment of craniopharyngiomas. Neurosurg Focus 2010;28:E11

112. Anderson CA, Wilkening GN, Filley CM, Reardon MS, Kleinschmidt-DeMasters BK. Neurobehavioral outcome in pediatric craniopharyngioma. Pediatr Neurosurg 1997;26:255–260

113. Carpentieri SC, Waber DP, Scott RM, et al. Memory deficits among children with craniopharyngiomas. Neurosurgery 2001;49:1053–1057, discussion 1057–1058

Chapter 11

Resection of Gliomas in Eloquent Areas of the Brain

Case

A 35-year-old woman came to medical attention for a recent onset of seizures and headaches.

Participants

Glioma Resection in an Awake Patient with Cortical Stimulation: Mitchel S. Berger and Nader Sanai

Optimal Resection of Insular Glima with Image-Guided Technologies: Sanju Lama, Stefan Wolfsberger, and Garnette R. Sutherland

Glioma Resection in Eloquent Areas: Anatomical Basis and Resection with Tractography Studies: Uğur Türe and Pablo González-López

Moderator: Insular Tumors: Allan Friedman

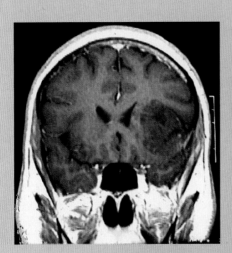 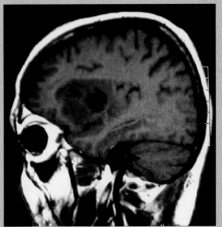

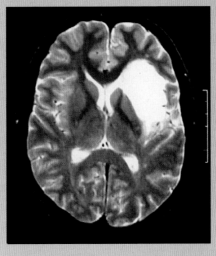

Glioma Resection in an Awake Patient with Cortical Stimulation

Mitchel S. Berger and Nader Sanai

The insular region remains one of the most challenging locations for aggressive resection of both low-grade and high-grade gliomas.[1-12] These tumors are entrenched in eloquent tissue and surrounded by microvasculature that serves critical language and motor systems.[13,14] Moreover, the insula itself is implicated in a variety of cognitive functions, including memory, drive, affect, gustation, and olfaction.[15-17] Given the potential involvement (and impairment) of these essential neural networks, controversy persists as to which treatment strategy is appropriate for patients with insular gliomas and how intervention can have an impact on patient outcomes. Although observation, stereotactic biopsy, radiosurgery, and microsurgical resection have all been proposed,[18-20] none has been studied in comprehensive detail in patients with insular gliomas. Insular gliomas are not rare, and, according to a recent epidemiological study by Duffau and Capelle,[21] account for up to 25% of all low-grade gliomas and 10% of all high-grade gliomas.

As we recognize the eloquence and complexity of the insular anatomy, we discern that insular gliomas can be distinguished from other gliomas in several respects. As suggested by epidemiological data, there is a clear propensity for low-grade histology that is unique to the insula. Although the etiologic cause of this predisposition is not yet understood, this phenomenon may indicate a particular microenvironment within the insula or address the very nature of the glioma cells of origin propagating these tumors. Additionally, many patients harboring these tumors experience a prolonged and slowly progressive clinical course that is generally less aggressive than patients with similar lesions in other locations. Among tumors with both low- and high-grade histologies, this unpredictable natural history is characteristic of insular gliomas. Recent analysis, however, suggests that an insular glioma's predilection for malignant transformation can be altered with aggressive cytoreduction.[22]

Case Discussion

Clinical Presentation

The patient's history provides important information regarding the likely diagnosis of the tumor, and the neurologic examination can reveal the lesion's location. Together with imaging, the history and physical examination are the foundation on which the perioperative assessment is established.

Patients with insular gliomas often come to medical attention because of an ictal event (seizure), a change in functional capacity (paresis, vision changes, etc.), or headache and cognitive impairment (increased intracranial pressure). The speed with which these problems evolve is often proportional to the aggressiveness of the tumor (e.g.,

a rapid evolution of signs portends a rapidly growing lesion). However, slow-growing or low-grade lesions can remain clinically silent until they reach a critical size, at which time small changes in tumor volume can generate dramatic neurologic symptoms. Because the chronicity of the history gives some indication of the anticipated growth rate of the tumor, it is very important to inquire about signs and symptoms that may be considered unremarkable or unrelated by the patient.

It is not uncommon, particularly in patients with low-grade insular gliomas, that symptoms precede identification of the tumor by many years. The most common undetected sign of a tumor is a partial seizure. Clues that suggest partial complex seizures include a history of problems in school or unexplained learning disabilities. A careful assessment of the patient's academic history or work performance can uncover early evidence of a tumor that remained undetected. A change in function or capacity to perform at a consistent level may be misinterpreted as the result of stress or inattention when, in fact, the impairments may be the result of partial seizures. In addition, the rapidity with which signs and symptoms evolve gives an indication of how quickly intervention is needed. Progressive changes in functional capacity or altered consciousness are indications for more rapid intervention.

Seizures are the most common sign of a tumor in patients with low-grade gliomas and are the first sign of a tumor in 80 to 90% of these patients. Because most of these tumors expand slowly, subtle changes in functional capacity are commonly overlooked or accommodated by the patient, and it is an ictal event that is the first indication of a structural problem. Progressive neurologic deficits occurring over a few days to weeks are more common in patients with high-grade gliomas. A more rapidly expanding mass lesion produces focal neurologic signs that bring the patient to medical attention.

Neurosurgical Management Paradigms

Once a diagnosis of insular glioma is suspected, surgical priorities should be directed toward establishing a diagnosis, relieving tumor mass effect, and maximizing cytoreduction. Surgical options for insular gliomas are limited to a biopsy versus resection. Stereotactic needle biopsy can obtain tissue for diagnostic purposes, but there is a risk of sampling error. In one recent study, overgrading of World Health Organization (WHO) grade II tumors occurred in 11% of cases and undergrading of WHO grade III gliomas in 28%.[23] Thus, histopathological diagnosis of gliomas with only stereotactic biopsy comes with a substantial risk of inaccuracy, particularly for tumors with low proliferative activity or for mixed gliomas. At present, the indications for a biopsy in a patient with a presumed insular glioma are a diffuse lesion, such as gliomatosis, and the patient's inability to undergo a definitive operation for medical reasons.

Microsurgical corridors to the insula include transcortical and transsylvian routes.[1,3,4,6,13,19] For select lesions, a transcortical "plus" operation allows the combined use of transcortical and transsylvian routes through a small split in the sylvian fissure. In a recent study comparing operative approaches to temporal mediobasal tumors, the transsylvian approach was associated with the highest combined rate of neurologic morbidity.[19] A transsylvian route may be effective, but the risk of vascular injury and pial transgression during the course of exposure is not insignificant. To illustrate this point, a recent retrospective study of patients with insular gliomas treated at a single center noted that the transition from transsylvian to transcortical approaches was associated with a concomitant decline in neurologic morbidity.[6] Nevertheless, the literature remains inconclusive for purely insular lesions, and therefore the use of a transcortical "windowing" technique or a transsylvian fissure split is a valid option.

The tumor's location and the patient's hemispheric dominance determine the selection of either general or awake anesthesia. Our protocol for awake neuroanesthesia has been previously described.[24] Patients are placed in a semilateral position with the head parallel to the floor. For tumors occupying the posterior aspect of the insula, turning the patient's head 15 degrees upward allows for tumor resection underneath the lip of functional cortex overlying the posterior insula. The vertex of the head is tipped 15 degrees toward the floor or toward the ceiling when the tumor is predominantly below or above the sylvian fissure, respectively (**Fig. 11.1**). After a tailored craniotomy, cortical and subcortical language are assessed and motor and sensory mapping are conducted as needed and according to previously reported protocols.[24] Once functional areas have been identified, transcortical windows above and below the sylvian fissure are created through nonfunctional cortex, taking care to maintain at least a 1-cm margin from any functional language site. For motor sites, however, the 1-cm rule need not apply. This "windowing" technique allows for tumor resection along the course of the uncinate fasciculus, generating suprasylvian and infrasylvian resection cavities that are eventually connected to one another underneath the skeletonized sylvian vessels (**Fig. 11.1**). Finally, identification of the lenticulostriate arteries[25] and motor mapping of the internal capsule[26] allow for delineation of the medial border of resection in most cases.

The Berger-Sanai Insular Glioma Classification System

For each patient, the insula can be divided into four zones and the tumor's location can be assigned to one or more of these zones (**Fig. 11.2**). Along the horizontal plane in a sagittal view, the insula is first bisected along the sylvian fissure. A perpendicular plane is then intersected with this at the level of the foramen of Monro. The resultant quadrants (anterior-superior, posterior-superior, posterior-inferior, and anterior-inferior) are designated zones I, II, III, and IV, respectively (**Fig. 11.3**). Tumors that occupy more than one zone are noted as such (e.g., zone I + II). When the tumor occupies all four zones, these insular gliomas are defined as "giant."

The anterior zones of the insula most frequently harbor insular gliomas. An analysis of the extent of resection, however, confirms that these zones are also most amenable to a greater extent of resection.[22] In contrast, more posterior lesions, such as those of zone II (posterior-superior), are associated with a lower mean extent of resection, likely because of their close proximity to the rolandic cortex, inferior parietal language sites, and the posterior limb of the internal capsule. Nevertheless, with the appropriate use of cortical and subcortical motor and language mapping techniques, a mean extent of resection of 67.4% can be achieved for zone III insular gliomas and a greater than 95% extent of resection for tumors in zone I.[22] Overall, it is feasible to aggressively resect gliomas of all grades in the insula, and the morbidity profiles reported in recent years

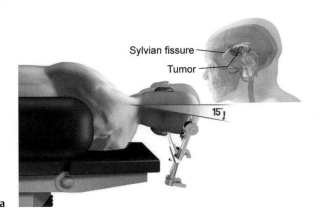
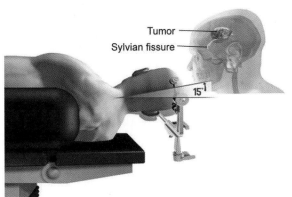

Fig. 11.1a–e The patient's position and microsurgical technique for transcortical resection of insular gliomas. For tumors primarily below the sylvian fissure, the head is tilted 15 degrees below horizontal **(a)**, while it is tilted 15 degrees above horizontal **(b)** for tumors primarily above the sylvian fissure. (*continued on next page*)

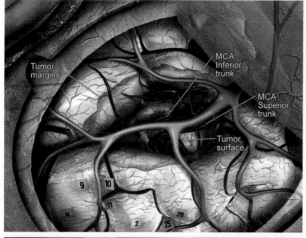

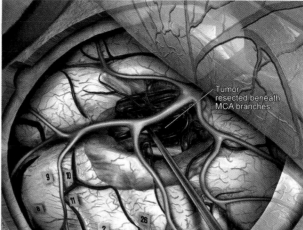

c

d

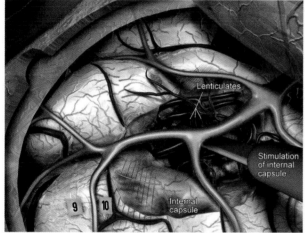

e

Fig. 11.1a–e (*continued*)   After cortical mapping identifies areas of nonfunctional cortex, a series of cortical windows **(c)** is made above and below the sylvian fissure. **(d)** Tumor resection traces the course of the uncinate fasciculus, eventually connecting the suprasylvian and infrasylvian windows. **(e)** Lenticulostriate arteries are identified at the medial margin of resection, along which the internal capsule can be subcortically stimulated. MCA, middle cerebral artery. (From Sanai N, Polley M-Y, Berger MS: Insular glioma resection: Assessment of patient morbidity, survival, and tumor progression. J Neurosurg 112(1): 1–9, 2010. Reprinted by permission.)

indicate that this can be done relatively safely and without the neurologic morbidity that detracts from the quality of life.[6,9,22,27]

Outcomes Analysis

The heterogeneous nature of gliomas is evidenced by the diversity in histology, genetics, and locations exhibited by these tumors. Our experience with insular gliomas suggests that this particular subtype behaves differently from tumors of a similar grade located elsewhere. Specifically, gliomas located in the insula are associated with a prolonged clinical course characterized by comparatively longer intervals of overall survival and progression-free survival. In recent studies of grade II and III gliomas in all locations, the median times to progression were 5.5 years[28] and 2.1 years,[29] respectively. Comparatively, patients with grade II and grade III insular gliomas described in recent work have had longer progression-free survivals.[22] The magnitude of difference, however, remains unclear, as most published studies have an insufficient duration of clinical follow-up. Nevertheless, such a unique natural history applies to grades II, III, and IV insular gliomas, raising the possibility that the insular microenvironment, a shared histopatho-

logical trait, or a combination of the two may be driving this clinical behavior.

Aggressive resection, however, cannot be advocated without evidence of an improved outcome. This remains one of the most challenging dilemmas in neurosurgical oncology, as much controversy surrounds the value of a greater extent of resection for gliomas.[30] In some studies, however, focusing the analysis on a homogeneous subset of gliomas reveals the unambiguous value of greater resection.[31] Whether this indicates the heterogeneity of gliomas or that certain subtypes are more amenable to resection remains unknown. Nevertheless, among purely insular gliomas, a statistical correlation between greater extent of resection and critical patient outcome parameters, including overall survival, progression-free survival, and malignant progression-free survival, has been shown.[22] This relationship exists among both low-grade and high-grade gliomas, consistent with the hypothesis that insular gliomas, irrespective of grade, follow an indolent clinical course that can be positively affected by aggressive resection. We recently reported that the interval to malignant progression among grade II insular gliomas is longer for patients who have had greater resection.[22] The biological basis for this alteration remains unclear, but may be related to the vol-

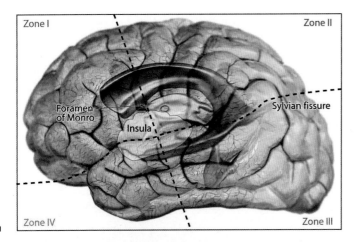

a

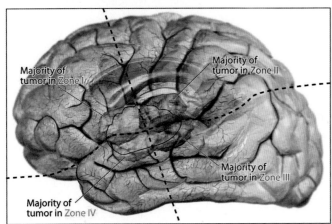

b

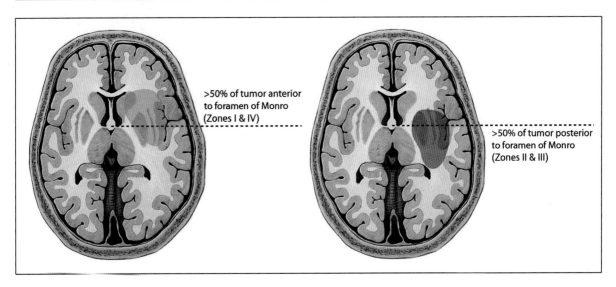

c

Fig. 11.2a–c   The Berger-Sanai insular glioma classification system. **(a)** Zones I to IV are divided along the line of the sylvian fissure and a perpendicular plane crossing the foramen of Monro. **(b)** The tumor's location is determined according to the location of the majority of the tumor mass. **(c)** Axial illustrations of zones I and IV, located anterior to the foramen of Monro, and zones II and III, located behind the foramen of Monro. (From Sanai N, Polley M-Y, Berger MS: Insular glioma resection: Assessment of patient morbidity, survival, and tumor progression. J Neurosurg 112(1): 1–9, 2010. Reprinted by permission.)

ume of residual tumor as a predictor of malignant transformation.[29] Given the dramatic differences in clinical behavior and outcome between grade II and III gliomas, this represents a potential shift in our concept of aggressive glioma resection. The ability to manipulate the natural history of these tumors makes a case for earlier intervention in the microsurgical treatment of insular gliomas and argues against the validity of a simple biopsy or a "wait-and-see" approach.

Conclusion

For the neurosurgeon, insular gliomas represent an opportunity to intervene and have an impact on outcome in several ways. Aggressive resection of insular gliomas of all grades can be accomplished with an acceptable morbidity profile and is predictive of an improved overall survival and progression-free survival. The extent of resection has been increasingly shown to correlate with an improved outcome,

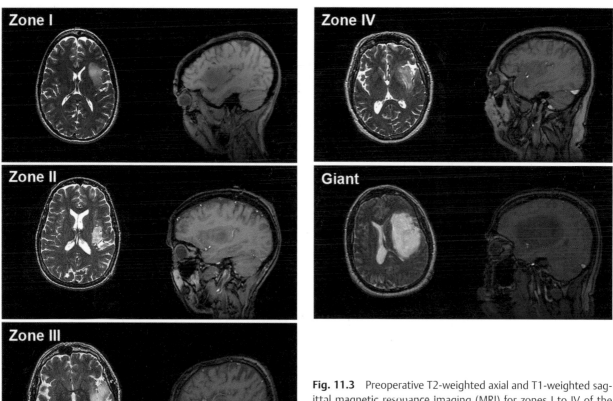

Fig. 11.3 Preoperative T2-weighted axial and T1-weighted sagittal magnetic resonance imaging (MRI) for zones I to IV of the Berger-Sanai insular glioma classification system. Giant tumors are those that occupy all four zones. (From Sanai N, Polley M-Y, Berger MS: Insular glioma resection: Assessment of patient morbidity, survival, and tumor progression. J Neurosurg 112(1): 1–9, 2010. Reprinted by permission.)

as well as with better seizure control and reduced malignant transformation rates. Neurologic morbidity can be minimized by combining traditional transcortical or trans-

sylvian neurosurgical approaches with intraoperative stimulation mapping to identify functional and nonfunctional sites in and around the insula.

Optimal Resection of Insular Glioma with Image-Guided Technologies

Sanju Lama, Stefan Wolfsberger, and Garnette R. Sutherland

The management of insular gliomas remains controversial primarily because of the relationship of the tumor to adjacent vessels and eloquent brain, resulting in various therapeutic options including observation, biopsy, subtotal resection, and resection with a volume reduction of greater than 90%. Observation has been recommended as insular gliomas have been found to generally follow a slow and protracted course. Because of the heterogeneous nature of gliomas, conventional magnetic resonance imaging (MRI) with contrast enhancement may underscore its true grade. Up to 10% of nonenhancing low-grade gliomas are subse-

quently classified as high grade.[32,33] Although subtotal resection is accompanied by a decreased operative risk, it may not have an impact on the patient's outcome or the tumor's progression to a higher grade.

There is a growing consensus that the extent of resection correlates with an improved outcome for patients with both low- and high-grade tumors and that gross total resection of a low-grade glioma decreases the probability of its malignant transformation.[22,28,30,34,35] Several groups have shown that low-grade insular and hemispheric gliomas can be safely approached, with a volumetric surgical resection of greater than 90% often achieved. Furthermore, investigators have suggested that the extent of resection of insular gliomas, irrespective of the grade, correlates with an improved outcome. However, because of the absence of randomized controlled clinical trials, establishing a definitive guideline for operative management remains controversial. Nevertheless, surgical excision is currently the preferred treatment option. Given the current evidence, maximal cytoreduction with the preservation of neurologic function can be considered the goal of modern glioma surgery.

Technological Advances in Glioma Surgery

Over the past decades, several surgical advances have made safe resection of these complex tumors feasible. These advances include pharmacological brain decompression, physiological monitoring of the speech cortex and motor tracts, awake craniotomy, improved instrumentation, surgical planning with advanced MRI sequences including functional magnetic resonance imaging (fMRI) and diffusion tensor imaging (DTI), surgical navigation based on optical or electromagnetic tracking, intraoperative magnetic resonance imaging (iMRI) to correct for brain shift, and, more recently, image-guided robotic technology for improved precision and accuracy.

Magnetic resonance imaging technology has been transported into the operating room to improve the intraoperative localization of lesions and control resection.[36–39] These systems were initially of an open configuration and contained relatively low field magnets. Signal-to-noise and contrast-to-noise ratios have improved with the evolution of iMRI systems to higher field magnets, which are not open. These closed systems interrupt surgery for imaging and are therefore generally used to evaluate the extent of surgery rather than to guide it. Despite this challenge, unsuspected residual tumor has been reported in up to 50% of cases in which MRI was used during dissection.[40] In a recent randomized clinical trial, the extent of resection and outcome were better in patients with gliomas treated with iMRI compared with conventional microsurgery.[41] Furthermore, iMRI together with multimodal neurophysiological monitoring have been shown to allow an extended and safe resection of gliomas near eloquent cortex.[42] In another study, among 89 patients with insular gliomas randomized to either microsurgery with iMRI or microsurgery alone, the extent of resection was greater in the iMRI-with-microsurgery group compared with the microsurgery-only group.[43] These studies indicate that the extent of resection is greater when using iMRI.

In an effort to increase the precision and accuracy of surgery, robotic technologies are being developed and merged with microsurgery,[44–48] and recent advances have initiated remote surgery with sensory immersive capabilities.[49,50] Posted at a workstation, the surgeon is able to take full advantage of imaging data while carrying out microsurgical dissection.

Patient Evaluation

The patient presented in this chapter is a 35-year-old woman with a recent onset of seizures and headache. It is assumed that her neurologic examination is unremarkable and that she is being treated with antiseizure medication. MRI studies show a large left nonenhancing cystic insular lesion consistent with a glioma (see images in the case description). The lesion spares the basal ganglia. The absence of significant contrast enhancement favors the diagnosis of a low-grade lesion.

It is recommended that the patient proceed to open surgery for definitive tissue diagnosis and gross total resection of the lesion. For surgical planning, further MRI studies are advised. The iMRI and image-guided robotic technology can be used to maximize safety and the extent of resection. For this patient, the goals of surgery are as follows:

- To obtain a definitive histopathological diagnosis for treatment planning
- To achieve maximal surgical resection of the tumor while preserving language and motor functions, which will improve the outcome, delay progression, and delay malignant transformation
- To potentially alleviate seizures and headache

Treatment Strategy

Surgical Approach

Surgical Anatomy of the Insula

Gliomas of the insular region pose a considerable surgical challenge relating to neural connectivity and vascular structures critical to language and motor function. Precise anatomic knowledge of the insula forms the foundation of surgical planning.

The insula is a well-defined anatomic structure buried deep within the sylvian fissure, covered by frontal, parietal, and temporal opercula.[51] It is triangular in shape, with the margin formed by the circular sulcus that is anatomically divided into anterior, superior, and inferior limiting sulci. There are two surfaces of the insula—anterior and lateral. The fronto-orbital operculum covers its anterior surface, whereas the lateral surface is covered by the frontoparietal operculum superiorly and the temporal operculum inferiorly.

Phylogenetically, the surface of the insula consists of mesocortex situated between the allocortex medially and the isocortex laterally. The allocortex consists of the amygdala and hippocampus, whereas the isocortex comprises the neocortex.[51] The vascular supply originates from 8 to 12 branches of the M2 segment of the middle cerebral artery.[52] The limen insulae, where the insular cortex is in continuity with the frontal operculum, is supplied by distal M1 branches and occasionally from the middle cerebral artery bifurcation. The insular arterioles supply the cortical and subcortical areas of the insular gyri and extreme capsule but not the external capsule, putamen, globus pallidus, or the internal capsule. This information is important, and with this knowledge the surgeon can perform coagulation with division of these arteries for tumor removal. The lenticulostriate vessels may be markedly displaced but they provide an important anatomic landmark during surgery, and they must be preserved.[26,53]

The normal insular cortex has been recognized for interoceptive awareness, that is, sensing the physiological condition of the body.[54] Functional MRI in humans has shown the insula and anterior cingulate cortex to be the critical and sole substrates for such awareness, and therefore to be important in representing the visceral state of the body.[55] Apart from language functions and sensorimotor integration, this region also accounts for cognitive and emotional processing; gustatory, auditory, and vestibular functions; and neuropsychiatric disturbances. Although data about the connectivity of the insula is sparse, DTI studies have shown important structural and functional connectivity.[56] The ventral-most anterior insula is functionally interconnected to the rostral anterior cingulate cortex, the middle and inferior frontal cortex, and the temporoparietal cortex. The dorsal posterior insula is connected to several cortical regions, such as the dorsal posterior cingulate, premotor, supplementary motor, temporal, and occipital cortical areas. Thalamic projections to and from the insula remain less clear in human studies, unlike in other species in whom complex, region-specific thalamic projections to both anterior and posterior insula have been described.[57]

Given the importance of the insula and its anatomic and functional relationship to the surrounding structures, it is necessary to obtain detailed preoperative clinical and imaging data on the patient before planning surgery. This information will help not only in planning the surgical resection of the lesion but also in anticipating potential complications for an optimal resection and outcome. With the appropriate use of technologies, surgical intervention can provide a definitive diagnosis of both the tumor type and grade and will decrease this patient's almost certainly elevated intracranial pressure, ultimately improving outcome.

Complementary Imaging

As part of the strategy for gross total tumor resection, diagnostic MRI studies are complemented with fMRI to delineate the speech and motor cortex.[58,59] From these regions of interest, a 3D DTI tractography is reconstructed to visualize the relationship of important fiber tracts that relate to the lesion[6]: the arcuate fasciculus, which is located in proximity to the superior limiting insular sulcus, and the corticospinal tract within the posterior limb of the internal capsule. By fusing the data available from these complementary imaging studies, the surgeon can outline the preoperative planning of the approach and the extent of resection.

It is probable that this chapter's patient has some bilateral representation for speech, given the location of the tumor and her sex.[60,61] Although not anticipated, fiber tracts within the neoplasm would limit tumor resection.[62]

Integration of the intraoperative imaging studies with the NeuroArm navigation system (IMRIS, Inc., Minneapolis, MN) further validates the accurate registration of the lesion's location and the associated anatomy of functional, vascular, and fiber tracts that are instrumental for safe resection.

Brain shift during surgery invalidates the navigation technology used for preoperative images.[63–65] Although three-dimensional reconstruction of fiber tracts provides an excellent pictorial representation of the otherwise not visible fiber pathways and direction within the white matter, there remains a variable degree of uncertainty as to a real-time verification of such pathways. In other words, are the fiber tracts in real time where they appear to be on images? If so, what is the margin of error for a fiber tract representation in DTI and real time?

Authors of cortical and subcortical stimulation studies, using a current intensity ranging from 2 to 8 mA, have reported the safe detection of fiber tracts at approximately a 5-mm distance from the site of stimulation.[66] In particular, investigators have shown the precise and alternate resection of thin tumoral layers with electrophysiological stimulation to detect pathways such as the pyramidal tract posteromedial to or the arcuate fasciculus superomedial to the lesion.[66,67] It has also been shown that the medial border of the resection is defined by the presence of the lenticulostriate arteries and functionally by the detection of the internal capsule and the pyramidal pathways.

Detecting Anaplastic Foci

Originating as histopathological low-grade tumors, gliomas have an inherent tendency to progress to malignant high-grade tumors over time. This progression originates in a localized tumor area because of focal genetic changes and causes the well-known tissue heterogeneity of gliomas.[68] Therefore, tissue sampling during open surgery may miss such an "anaplastic focus" in a large, otherwise low-grade tumor and delay the implementation of postoperative radiation and chemotherapy.

Identifying an anaplastic focus within a low-grade glioma is mandatory for tissue sampling. To accomplish this task, the following visualization modalities have been suggested:

- *Magnetic resonance tomography* shows areas of significant contrast-enhancement on T1-weighted MRI to indicate focal malignant progression and is routinely used to target tissue sampling. Most insular gliomas are nonenhancing; however, they may show the foci of a higher grade tumor.
- *Magnetic resonance spectroscopy* enables the intratumoral detection of the most malignant areas through the display of metabolite distribution. Proton magnetic resonance spectroscopy has been found especially useful for diffusely infiltrating gliomas with nonsignificant contrast enhancement.[69] The typical metabolite profile

of glioma tissue includes an increased choline peak (resulting from elevated turnover of the cell membrane), a decrease in *N*-acetylaspartate (because of impaired neuronal function), and a reduction in creatine (stemming from the hypermetabolic state).[70] Multivoxel spectroscopy, termed *chemical shift imaging*, has been successfully used for navigation-guided tissue sampling of the most malignant areas of gliomas.

- *Positron emission tomography* that uses amino-acid tracers such as [42]C-methionine or ^{18}F-fluoroethyl-L-tyrosine is an established modality for imaging malignant foci in diffusely infiltrating gliomas. These images can be used to define the target for neuronavigation systems that guide tissue sampling.[33]
- *Five-aminolevulinic acid* (5-ALA), a precursor of the porphyrin synthesis pathway, has been found to accumulate in malignant glioma cells as strongly fluorescing protoporphyrin IX.[33] Generally, if open neurosurgical resection of a low-grade glioma is attempted, the progressive brain shift usually renders navigation inaccurate and, consequently, precise tissue sampling becomes impossible. Incorporating 5-ALA into the procedure provides a more reliable intraoperative technique for visualizing anaplastic foci independent of brain shift. This compound can be excited with a violet-blue light source at 440 nm, and the resulting fluorescence at 635 nm then displays the anaplastic focus in an otherwise low-grade glioma. A recent study suggests that 5-ALA is a promising intraoperative marker for anaplastic foci in diffusely infiltrating gliomas with nonsignificant contrast enhancement on MRI independent from brain shift.

We recommend that the surgeon take full advantage of this variety of imaging modalities as well as other technolo- gies that will benefit neurosurgical planning and intervention. A high-field movable 3.0 T iMRI system, robot-assisted neuronavigation, and image-guided microsurgery with electrophysiological monitoring present a safe multimodal method for the surgical treatment of insular lesions. This approach provides both a mechanism for maximum control of resection and a more comprehensive framework for preserving the patient's neurologic function and quality of life.

Operative Management

After the patient is positioned and anesthesia is induced, images are acquired for surgical planning at the iMRI suite **(Fig. 11.4)**. These images—T1-weighted with contrast enhancement, T2-weighted, and DTI—are used for robot neuronavigation. Fusing the images facilitates the concurrent display of anatomic and functional information (with DTI tractography and fMRI) to set electronic tumor boundaries and no-go zones **(Fig. 11.5)** together with metabolic imaging data to assess and target an anaplastic focus.

A left frontotemporal craniotomy is performed in the usual fashion. The dura is opened in a cruciate manner to expose the sylvian fissure and the adjacent frontal and temporal opercula. The left sylvian cistern is opened to allow brain decompression.

At this stage of the procedure, the robot is brought to the surgical site and re-registration is done **(Fig. 11.6)**. Robotic dissection complemented with an assisting surgeon begins within the left sylvian cistern, and the M1 and M2 segments of the middle cerebral artery are defined together with the lenticulostriate and insular branches. Branches to the insula arising from the M2 segment are coagulated and divided. The tumor is entered at the predefined target

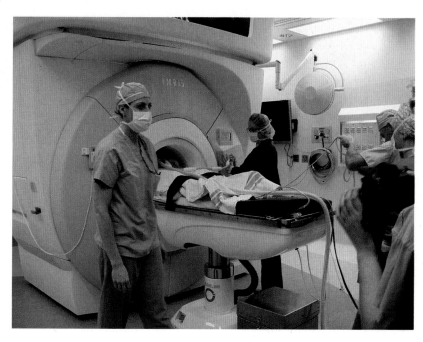

Fig. 11.4 Surgical planning for intraoperative MRI, showing the magnet moved into position over the patient.

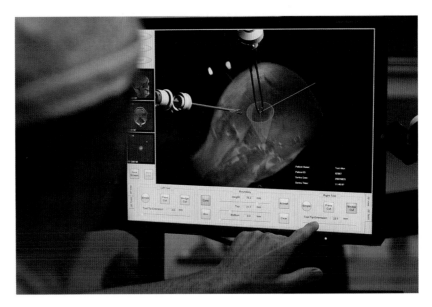

Fig. 11.5 MRID display for the NeuroArm showing the electronic surgical corridor. Robotic instruments are able to be manipulated only within the preset corridor.

point and initial biopsy specimens are obtained from the pre-registered areas of highest metabolic activity and sent to the lab for histopathology analysis, including frozen section. The tumor is debulked starting from the central aspect of the neoplasm with the aid of the robotic suction tool (**Fig. 11.7**). At progressive stages of the procedure, the robot and microscope are removed from the operative site and the magnet is returned for interdissection T1-weighted, T2-weighted fluid-attenuated inversion recovery (FLAIR), and DTI magnetic resonance imaging studies. Once these data are obtained, the magnet is removed from the operating room and re-registration to the updated images is done. Dissection continues out toward the tumor–brain interface defined on the MRI studies. As dissection approaches the

corticospinal tract visualized on DTI tractography, the margin of safety is assessed with subcortical electrical stimulation. Resection is limited upon attainment of motor stimulation with 5 to 7 mΛ.[71,72]

Discussion

The surgical treatment of gliomas in eloquent cortex has remained controversial, with recent meta-analysis data supporting extensive resection.[30] The anatomic location of the lesion, however, poses a significant challenge in preserving function, specifically in relation to speech and motor power. After a thorough preoperative workup, a representative tissue biopsy of the lesion and the intent to

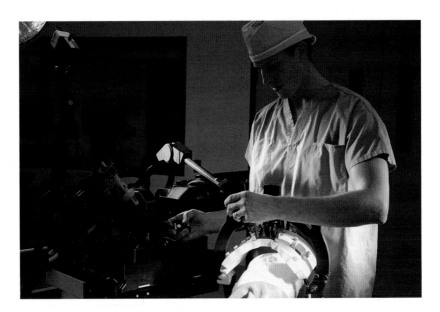

Fig. 11.6 Registration of the NeuroArm to intraoperatively acquired MRI studies.

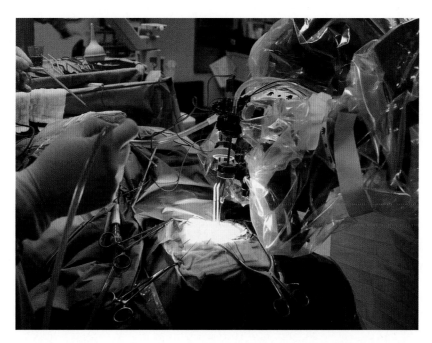

Fig. 11.7 The NeuroArm performing surgery. The right arm holds a bipolar forceps and the left a suction tool.

carry out maximum resection are currently considered the goals of modern glioma treatment. The use of important surgical adjuncts—intraoperative electrophysiological monitoring and precise and accurate microsurgical techniques such as MRI-compatible surgical robots—maximizes resection and functional outcome concurrently. Such technology incorporates a high level of finesse and dexterity into the surgical procedure, which is essential for the optimal management of insular gliomas.

Interdissection MRI enables a near real-time assessment of brain shift as resection progresses. In a patient with an insular glioma, this is especially important because the surgeon relies on MRI-based cues to resect residual tumor, as visual and haptic feedback is somewhat limited within the white matter. As the surgeon approaches the tumor margin, intraoperative electrophysiological monitoring adds to the safety of the resection by providing important information about the integrity of white matter tracts as well as the proximity of these tracts to the surgical dissection.

The workstation allows the surgeon to take full advantage of imaging data during surgery. The workstation is completed by a robotic system that allows the surgeon to remotely perform the operation and effectively communicate with the surgical team. A combination of the improved precision and accuracy of the machines together with the dexterity and speed provided by the assistant surgeon optimizes the performance of surgery.

In a retrospective review of 104 patients with a low-grade glioma of the insular region, the extent of resection correlated with a progression-free interval.[22] This interval was defined as the time between initial surgery and the demonstration of an unequivocal increase in tumor on follow-up imaging, malignant progression, and/or death. In patients who underwent extensive resection (> 90%), malignant transformation of the tumor (selected for patients with grade II gliomas) was delayed, as shown by radiological enhancement on follow-up imaging studies, histopathological diagnosis of a higher grade on subsequent surgery, or both. Furthermore, extensive tumor resection has been shown to prolong the median time to disease progression.[28,29] It is important, however, to reiterate the notion that a lack of enhancement on MRI studies does not establish a definitive diagnosis of a low-grade lesion. The existing literature shows no definitive consensus on whether the extent of resection improves the patient's survival and quality of life. Current evidence from insular glioma surgery, however, provides mounting evidence for maximum resection.[22,30,66]

Seizures are one of the most common presentations of low-grade gliomas, and intractable seizures are observed in 10 to 20% of patients.[73–75] In insular gliomas, which make up approximately 15% of low-grade gliomas, seizures are a predominant presenting feature and greatly impair the patient's quality of life. One of the main indications for surgical removal of this lesion is therefore to render the patient free of seizures. The mechanism behind seizure activity and treatment strategies remains largely unknown.[76,77] Despite the technical challenge pertinent to the insula and the variable tumor grade, surgical removal has been shown to benefit this cohort of patients. In this context, we believe that removing an insular glioma should alleviate a patient's seizures.

The technique of language mapping historically evolved from epilepsy surgery, in which a large exposure allowed extensive mapping of multiple cortical regions for language and motor functions before surgery as well as intraoperatively through awake craniotomy.[78,79] A similar technique is widely used in surgeries related to lesions of the dominant hemisphere. Brain tumors have considerable topographic variability because of mass effect and functional reorganization that takes place over time through inherent plasticity mechanisms.[66,80] Furthermore, individual variation among patients in their language representation, whether lateralized or bilateral, cannot be emphasized too greatly. Therefore, the surgeon must take into account the various fMRI evidence of language function areas near the tumor tissue while planning the surgical resection. Irrespective of tumor type, the use of intraoperative cortical and subcortical stimulation to accurately detect functional regions and pathways remains a key factor in the safe removal of insular gliomas of the dominant hemisphere. Although an awake craniotomy allows the surgeon to assess and preserve these functions, a combination of image guidance, iMRI, and electrophysiological monitoring is preferred in the anesthetized patient. Surgical planning based on multimodal imaging, together with a fusion of technologies for precise and accurate excision of the target, can help the surgeon achieve the therapeutic goal of gross total resection. Although the possibility of functional brain tissue within the lesion remains a matter of debate,[62] continuous electrophysiological stimulation can potentially alleviate the risks of unwanted injury.

Earlier in the disease progression, insular lesions can be typically infiltrative in nature. As the disease progresses, however, it tends to displace structures, thus allowing more room for central debulking.[81,82]

A considerable number of patients have new neurologic deficits after an attempt at maximum surgical resection of insular gliomas.[30,83] This has been observed despite the use of electrophysiological monitoring, and is in part because of maximizing the resection to the functional boundaries intraoperatively. If such boundaries are respected with the application of modern surgical technology, such deficits can be expected to be transient and reversible. It is therefore important to include these variables in a neurologic rehabilitation management plan.

From what is currently known about insular gliomas and their surgical management, the indication for surgery for tissue diagnosis is apparent. The extent of resection for maximum benefit in terms of clinical outcome, such as tumor progression, malignant transformation, the propensity for seizures, and overall survival, remains a matter of debate and discussion. The general incidence of insular gliomas is relatively low, but the technical and surgical challenges of carrying out such resections are profound. Although the evidence appears to support the surgical resection of such a lesion, the complex nature of the disease warrants referral to neurosurgical centers of excellence for the best outcome.

Glioma Resection in Eloquent Areas: Anatomical Basis and Resection with Tractography Studies

Uğur Türe and Pablo González-López

The available imaging studies for the patient presented in this chapter indicate a nonenhancing intrinsic mass located in the anterior aspect of the left insula, showing paramagnetic features of hypointensity on the T1-weighted MRI sequence and hyperintensity on the T2-weighted sequence. The lesion spares the adjacent temporal, fronto-orbital, and frontoparietal opercula, and has a clear border with the putamen, which is pushed medially and posteriorly. The internal capsule, primarily the anterior limb, is also moved posteromedially. The clinical and radiological findings strongly suggest the diagnosis of a left insular, possibly low-grade, glioma.

Low-Grade Gliomas in Eloquent Areas

Brain tumors in eloquent areas present a great challenge for neurosurgeons because of the difficulty in removing them without causing neurologic disturbances. The integral management of these lesions entails using a variety of elements in an optimal perioperative approach: diagnostic and preoperative functional techniques, a clear understanding of neuroanatomy, intraoperative monitoring, and appropriate microsurgical technique. These elements all contribute to increasing the surgeon's experience and anatomic knowledge, which are the only constant tools.

In our experience, and supporting Yaşargil's findings, gliomas do not originate from highly functional areas such as the motor or primary visual cortex (Brodmann areas 4 and 17). These tumors mainly affect eloquent regions by directly compressing the surrounding areas.

Complete surgical resection seems to be the best treatment for low-grade glial tumors.[29,30,84–86] Until new treatments are developed, the cytoreduction provided by surgery will be of value because it collects material for diagnosis and research, alleviates both neurologic and irritating impairments (as well as symptoms of intracranial hypertension), and increases the time to malignant progression.[22,30] Following this line of reasoning, evidence supports the idea of resecting the largest possible volume of tumor.[30,87–89] But the price to pay for such radical resection may be an increase in morbidity, a fact that is most important when eloquent areas are involved. To combat this problem, a great number of imaging, neurophysiological, neurochemical, and surgical techniques have been recently developed and incorporated into the general management of these tumors, with the ultimate objective of optimizing the resection and extending it to the maximum while minimizing the eventual associated morbidity.[90–92]

Nevertheless, the diagnostic and therapeutic armamentarium for gliomas should never obscure or replace the surgeon's strong knowledge of neuroanatomy. In the human body, especially in the brain, pathology follows the anatomy, and neurosurgeons should therefore accurately study the different cerebral functional compartments. After observing and treating thousands of gliomas, Yaşargil and his colleagues introduced the concept of functional units. He argued that gliomas tend to initially develop in a single functional unit, pushing away the surrounding compartments according to the location where they grow. This general behavior seems to apply to almost all low-grade lesions and to high-grade gliomas during their initial stages. However, recurrent, irradiated, and high-grade lesions in advanced stages may transgress the borders of those functional compartments, a fact that reinforces the importance of a total resection during the first procedure.

In general, the term *eloquent area* in the human brain refers to those regions with clearly demonstrated high functionality, where surgical or pathological disruption will unfailingly lead to neurologic impairment. This definition of eloquence is misleading, however. In this sense, many territories that are not considered eloquent may require surgical corridors related to highly functional compartments, as well as neighboring vascular structures feeding distant eloquent regions. In this perspective, eloquent regions should include motor, speech, and visual cortical areas with their white matter pathways, such as the pyramidal tract, superior longitudinal fasciculus (SLF), and optic radiation, and also the central nuclei such as the thalamus, hypothalamus, and basal ganglia, and certain regions in the limbic and paralimbic territories, brain stem, and deep cerebellar nuclei and peduncles. In short, with respect to function, neighboring anatomy, and surgical approach, most central nervous system lesions can be considered related to eloquent areas.[93] The insular region perfectly illustrates this concept.

As it would be too extensive to describe the general surgical management of tumors in the so-called eloquent areas, we consider the surgery of insular tumors as the perfect paradigm to illustrate this topic.

The Insula: Anatomic Considerations

In about the fifth month of embryological development, the cortical shield covering the basal ganglia and outlining the internal capsule forms the insula. Later on, this primitive insula begins enfolding in a central position because of the disproportionate growth of the adjacent neocortical areas, and is finally covered by the frontal, parietal, and temporal opercula. The insula of Reil belongs to the paralimbic system and represents a transitional element between the allocortex and the neocortex of the human brain. The paralimbic areas are commonly termed *mesocortical* because of their intermediate cortical architectonic features, and include the orbitofrontal cortex, insula, temporal pole, and parahippocampal and cingulate gyri. The gradual cortical differentiation between the old, and centrally positioned, limbic brain and the new neocortical areas takes the insula as its anatomic and cytoarchitectural link.[94]

The insula has connections to and from a large number of different regions within the human brain, and several higher functions have been attributed to this hidden structure, such as temperature, touch, fear, conscious desires, olfactory and gustatory inputs, subjective emotional experiences, the perception of effort during exercise, the regulation of higher cognitive functioning, and the processing of pain, as well as somatic functions, autonomic regulation, verbal working memory, and secondary motor and language control.[95–99] Since the first insulectomies were done, however, some controversy has surrounded this area as a clearly defined functional entity. Surgery in this region may induce postoperative hemiparesis as well as different degrees of speech impairment when dealing with the dominant hemisphere. Mutism and apraxia after damage to the nondominant insula have also been reported. In most of these cases, however, postoperative pathological examination revealed damage to the surrounding opercular cortex and corona radiata, probably resulting from opercular and subcortical involvement of the lesion or direct surgical manipulation of these neural structures and ischemic injury from manipulation of the branches of the middle cerebral artery (MCA).[98,100–102]

The Sylvian Fissure

The insula remains hidden in the depths of the sylvian fissure and forms the medial aspect of the sylvian fossa. To approach it, the surgeon should open the sylvian fissure and interopercular sulci. The sylvian fissure is divided into two compartments. The anterior or sylvian stem runs from the bifurcation of the internal carotid artery just inferior to the sylvian vallecula and, following the path of the sphenoid wing, reaches the level of the pars triangularis at the frontoparietal operculum. It courses between the orbital gyri and the polar planum in the anterior aspect of the medial surface of the temporal operculum. The place where the anterior stem becomes the posterior or insulo-opercular compartment at the level of the pars triangularis is named the sylvian point, and is an important landmark when splitting the sylvian fissure.

The insulo-opercular section is divided into three main rami with a common origin at the level of the sylvian point. The horizontal ramus runs forward between the pars orbitalis and pars triangularis, whereas the ascending ramus

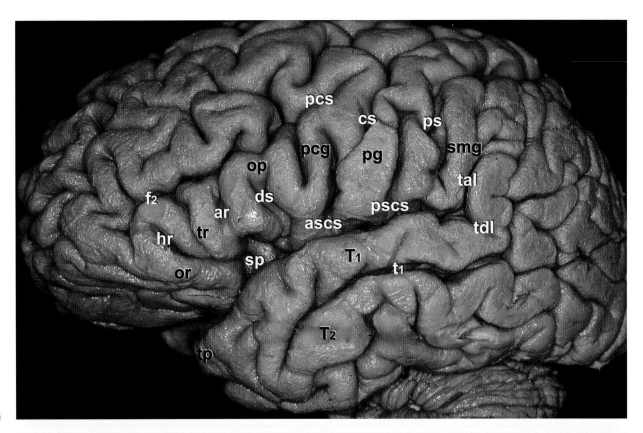

a

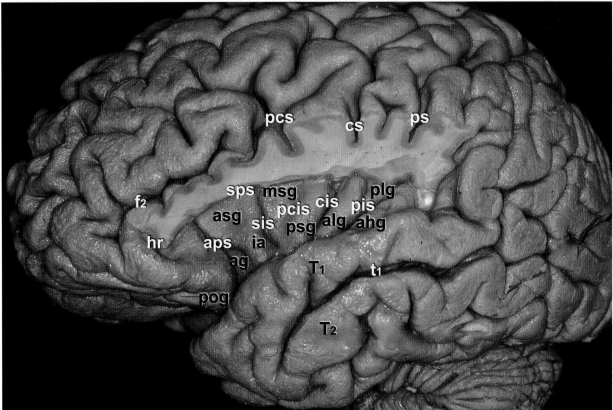

b

Fig. 11.8a–c Lateral view of the left hemisphere of a cadaveric specimen in which the main anatomic landmarks surrounding the sylvian fissure are marked. **(a)** The fronto-orbital, frontoparietal, and temporal opercula cover the insula. **(b)** The frontoparietal operculum has been removed, and the superior surface of the hidden insula is shown in the depth of the sylvian fissure.

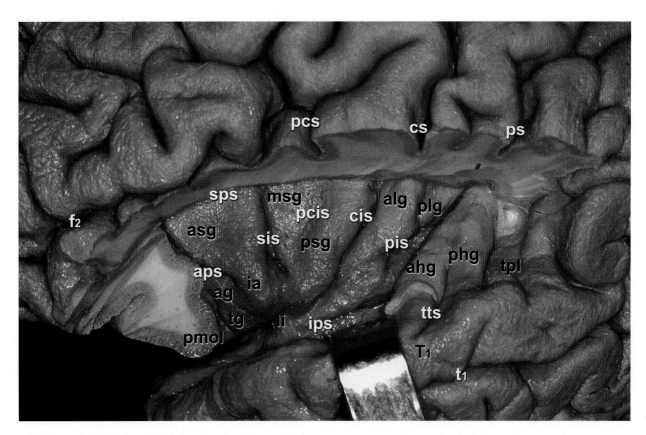

c

Fig. 11.8a–c (*continued*)   **(c)** A closer view in which the temporal operculum is being retracted downward to expose the entire surface of the insula. This maneuver provides a better view of the inferior surface of the insula to the level of the inferior peri-insular sulcus. Abbreviations in white letters denote sulci and fissures. ag, accessory gyrus; ahg, anterior Heschl's gyrus; alg, anterior long insular gyrus; aps, anterior peri-insular sulcus; ar, ascending ramus of the sylvian fissure; ascs, anterior subcentral sulcus; asg, anterior short insular gyrus; cis, central insular sulcus; cs, central sulcus of Rolando; ds, diagonal sulcus; f2, inferior frontal sulcus; hr, horizontal ramus of the sylvian fissure; ia, insular apex; ips, inferior peri-insular sulcus; li, limen insula; msg, middle short insular gyrus; op, pars opercularis; or, pars orbitalis; pcg, precentral gyrus; pcis, precentral insular sulcus; pcs, precentral sulcus; pg, postcentral gyrus; phg, posterior Heschl's gyrus; pis, postcentral insular sulcus; plg, posterior long insular gyrus; pmol, posteromedial orbital lobule; pog, posterior orbital gyrus; ps, postcentral sulcus; pscs, posterior subcentral sulcus; psg, posterior short insular gyrus; sis, short insular sulcus; smg, supramarginal gyrus; sp, sylvian point; sps, superior peri-insular sulcus; t1, superior temporal sulcus; T1, superior temporal gyrus; T2, middle temporal gyrus; tal, terminal ascending limb of the sylvian fissure; tdl, terminal descending limb of the sylvian fissure; tg, transverse insular gyrus; tp, temporal pole; tpl, temporal planum; tr, pars triangularis; tts, transverse temporal sulcus.

runs upward, separating the pars triangularis and pars opercularis. The posterior ramus runs backward in a moderate undulating path toward the supramarginal gyrus, where it opens into ascendant and descendant terminal limbs.[17] The posterior ramus is the longest of the fissure, and represents the cortical translation of the anteroposterior extension of the insula. It runs from the region of the pterion to its termination in the inferior parietal lobe, separating the frontoparietal and temporal opercula and forming the sylvian line. Its course seems partially broken by some subsulci that enter the frontoparietal and temporal opercula. The most constant subsulci are the diagonal sulcus in the pars opercularis, the anterior and posterior subcentral sulci delimiting the subcentral gyrus, and the side branch of the transverse temporal sulcus[17] (**Fig. 11.8**).

The Opercula

Three opercular lips join together at the level of the sylvian fissure, closing the direct line of visualization to the insula. The fronto-orbital operculum is formed by the posterolateral aspect of the orbital gyri, but mainly by the pars orbitalis of the inferior frontal gyrus. It is delineated by the posterolateral part of the transverse orbital sulcus and the horizontal ramus of the sylvian fissure. This breach represents the edge between the fronto-orbital (anterior) and the frontoparietal (posterior) opercula. The temporal operculum follows a more clearly delineated forward course from the inferior part of the supramarginal gyrus toward the temporal pole, all along the superior temporal gyrus. The only constant indentation of this path is created by the

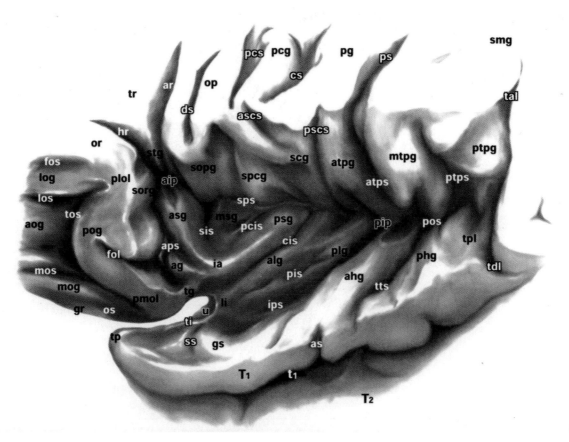

Fig. 11.9 Artistic rendering of the left insular region (artificial retraction of the opercula) with detailed nomenclature. Abbreviations in white letters denote sulci and fissures. ag, accessory insular gyrus; ahg, anterior Heschl's gyrus; aip, anterior insular point; alg, anterior long insular gyrus; aog, anterior orbital gyrus; aps, anterior peri-insular sulcus; ar, ascending ramus of the sylvian fissure; as, acoustic sulcus; ascs, anterior subcentral sulcus; asg, anterior short insular gyrus; atpg, anterior transverse parietal gyrus; atps, anterior transverse parietal sulcus; cis, central insular sulcus; cs, central sulcus of Rolando; ds, diagonal sulcus; fol, fronto-orbital limb; fos, fronto-orbital sulcus; gr, gyrus rectus; gs, gyri of Schwalbe; hr, horizontal ramus of the sylvian fissure; ia, insular apex; ips, inferior peri-insular sulcus; li, limen insula; log, lateral orbital gyrus; los, lateral orbital sulcus; mog, medial orbital gyrus; mos, medial orbital sulcus; msg, middle short insular gyrus; mtpg, middle transverse parietal gyrus; op, pars opercularis of F3; or, pars orbitalis of F3; os, olfactory sulcus; pcg, precentral gyrus; pcis, precentral insular sulcus; pcs, precentral sulcus; pg, postcentral gyrus; phg, posterior Heschl's gyrus; pip, posterior insular point; pis, postcentral insular sulcus; plg, posterior long insular gyrus; plol, posterolateral orbital lobule; pmol, posteromedial orbital lobule; pog, posterior orbital gyrus; pos, postinsular sulcus; ps, postcentral sulcus; pscs, posterior subcentral sulcus; psg, posterior short insular gyrus; ptpg, posterior transverse parietal gyrus; ptps, posterior transverse parietal sulcus; scg, subcentral gyrus; sis, short insular sulcus; smg, supramarginal gyrus; sopg, subopercular gyrus; sorg, suborbital gyrus; spcg, subprecentral gyrus; sps, superior peri-insular sulcus; ss, sulci of Schwalbe in the polar planum; stg, subtriangular gyrus; t1, superior temporal sulcus; T1, superior temporal gyrus; T2, middle temporal gyrus; tal, terminal ascending limb of the sylvian fissure; tdl, terminal descending limb of the sylvian fissure; tg, transverse insular gyrus; ti, temporal incisura; tos, transverse orbital sulcus; tp, temporal pole; tpl, temporal planum; tr, pars triangularis of F3; tts, transverse temporal sulcus. (From Türe U, Yaşargil DC, Al-Mefty O, Yaşargil MG. Topographic anatomy of the insular region. J Neurosurg 1999;90:723. Reprinted by permission.)

connection of the transverse gyri of Heschl with the superior temporal gyrus (**Figs. 11.8c, 11.9**).

Certain parts of these opercular segments are highly functional, representing some eloquent areas. The pars opercularis and the posterior segment of the pars triangularis of the frontoparietal operculum are frequently known as Broca's speech area in the dominant hemisphere. The subcentral gyrus represents the junction of the precentral and postcentral gyri of the central lobe, and so it belongs to the primary motor and somatosensory areas. The inferior aspect of the supramarginal gyrus and sometimes the posterior part of the superior temporal gyrus are commonly termed Wernicke's area in the dominant hemisphere, which is also related to speech functions. Finally, the transverse gyri of Heschl in the superior face of the superior temporal gyrus represent the primary auditory areas. Because of their high level of function, protecting these areas during insular tumor surgery is one of the challenges of these procedures.

The Insular Surface

The insula itself has a pyramidal triangular surface delimited by the anterior, superior, and inferior peri-insular sulci. The limen insula is located at the anterobasal part of the insula, which consists of a narrow strip of olfactory cortex acting as the junction between the sylvian vallecula, the insula, and the fronto-orbital and temporal poles. The central sulcus of the insula separates the insula into anterior and posterior portions. The anterior insula is composed of three short insular gyri (anterior, middle, and posterior) and in some cases also by the transverse and accessory insular gyri. The transverse gyrus runs in a fronto-medial direction toward the posteromedial orbital lobule, whereas the accessory gyrus joins the anterior portion of the anterior short gyrus with the suborbital gyri. The anterior and posterior short gyri are constant whereas the middle short gyrus is frequently found to be underdeveloped. These gyri join inferiorly to form the insular apex, which is the most superficial portion of the insula. The confluence of the anterior and superior peri-insular sulci coincides with the connection of the anterior short gyrus and the subtriangular gyrus at the so-called anterior insular point. The posterior insula generally contains two long gyri and is limited superiorly by the superior peri-insular sulcus and inferiorly by the inferior peri-insular sulcus, which join together at the posterior insular point **(Figs. 11.8c, 11.9)**.

The Insula as It Relates to the Opercula

A three-dimensional (3D) understanding of the architecture of the sulci and gyri of the medial aspects of the opercula is imperative. Their relationships to the insular surface remain constant and they may provide useful anatomic landmarks during surgical exploration. Two suborbital gyri (superior and inferior), located at the medial aspect of the fronto-orbital operculum, cover the anterior surface of the insula. The medial expression of the pars triangularis (subtriangular gyrus), pars opercularis (subopercular gyrus), precentral (subprecentral and subcentral gyri), and postcentral gyri (subcentral and anterior transverse parietal gyri), as well as the superior aspect of the supramarginal gyrus (anterior, middle, and posterior transverse parietal gyri) cover the superior surface of the insula. The polar planum (which consists of the sulci and gyri of Schwalbe), anterior and posterior transverse gyri of Heschl, and the temporal planum all together form the medial aspect of the temporal operculum and cover the anterior perforated substance and the inferior surface of the insula[17] **(Figs. 11.8b,c, 11.9)**.

Subinsular Anatomy

The subinsular region is composed of a sequence of layers of white matter and deep nuclei. Just underlying the insular cortex, the associated fiber system connecting the insula with the neighboring opercula is termed the extreme

capsule. The claustrum is a thin layer of gray matter mainly located deep in the anterior insula just beneath the extreme capsule, and separates it from the external capsule. The external capsule is the theoretical edge of the subcortical insular tissue, and this capsule differentiates it from the next deep layer, which is composed of the lateral aspect of the putamen. Growing insular tumors push medially but respect the putamen, which is a wonderful deep anatomic landmark, especially in the central aspect of the insula.[103]

Vascularization

The insula receives its blood supply from the leptomeningeal branches of the M2 segment of the MCA.[103] The M1 segment courses laterally within the sylvian vallecula all along the sylvian stem, and the lateral lenticulostriate arteries (LLAs) appear arising from this segment.[14] This origin of the LLAs may represent a valuable landmark during tumor resection in the anteroinferior aspect of the insula **(Fig. 11.10)**. The M1 segment turns approximately 90 degrees around the limen insula, forming the genu, where the main bifurcation occurs. This bifurcation has been highlighted as one of the main deep anatomic landmarks, and the surgeon must remember that, although in most cases it takes place at the level of the genu, it is also possible to find it distally or proximally.[14] Early small branches arise from the bifurcation, or even proximal from M1, to feed the limen insula. Along the cortical course in the anterior insula, the inferior and superior M2 trunks give off several main branches before becoming M3.

The lateral orbitofrontal artery supplies the anterior peri-insular sulcus and the accessory and transverse gyri. One of the most constant branches should be the prefrontal artery, which has been found in the anterior insular point, reaching the lateral hemispheric surface at the level of the sylvian point. The prefrontal, precentral, and central arteries usually extend small perforators to supply the anterior insula. The central artery runs along the central insular sulcus, which is the most vascularized region of the insula.[14] The anterior and posterior parietal arteries usually supply the anterior long gyrus and some direct branches to the posterior short gyrus, whereas small perforators coming from the temporo-occipital, angular, and posterior temporal arteries feed the posterior long gyrus. At the anteroinferior aspect of the insula, the main blood supply comes from the anterior and middle temporal arteries **(Fig. 11.10a)**.

Approximately 96 (range 77–112) insular arteries arise from the M2 segment and supply the insula.[14] These small and middle perforators must be identified during surgery, then coagulated and cut from their origin in the main branches to correctly devascularize the tumor. Careful attention must be paid to a special pattern of long perforators arising from the same M2 branches. These arteries have larger calibers, which are their specific features that extend as far as the corona radiata. These long perforators are mostly located in the posterior half of the central insular sulcus and on the long gyri, and special attention must be

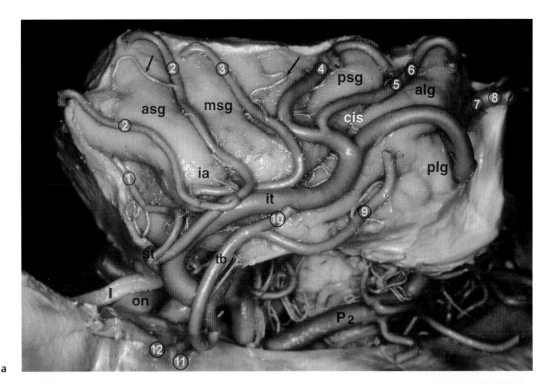

a

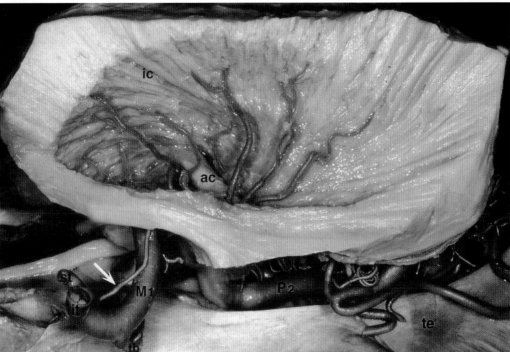

b

Fig. 11.10a,b Photographs of brain specimens. The insula is shown after removal of the frontal, parietal, occipital, and temporal lobes from the peri-insular sulci. The arteries of the insula originate from the M2 segment. **(a)** The insulo-opercular arteries (*arrows*) supply the insula and operculum. **(b)** Fiber dissection of this area reveals vascularization of the lentiform nuclei (which have been removed) and vascularization of the internal capsule by the lateral lenticulostriate arteries (LLAs; *arrow*), which arise from the M1 segment. 1, lateral orbitofrontal artery; 2, prefrontal artery; 3, precentral artery; 4, central artery; 5, anterior parietal artery; 6, posterior parietal artery; 7, angular artery; 8, temporo-occipital artery; 9, posterior temporal artery; 10, middle temporal artery; 11, anterior temporal artery; 12, temporal polar artery; ac, anterior commissure; alg, anterior long insular gyrus; asg, anterior short insular gyrus; cis, central insular sulcus; I, olfactory nerve; ia, insular apex; ic, internal capsule; it, inferior trunk of M2; M1, M1 segment of the MCA; msg, middle short insular gyrus; on, optic nerve; P2, ambient segment of the posterior cerebral artery; plg, posterior long insular gyrus; psg, posterior short insular gyrus; st, superior trunk of M2; tb, temporal branch of the MCA; te, tentorium. (From Türe U, Yaşargil MG, Al-Mefty O, Yaşargil DC. Arteries of the insula. J Neurosurg 2000;92:682. Reprinted by permission.)

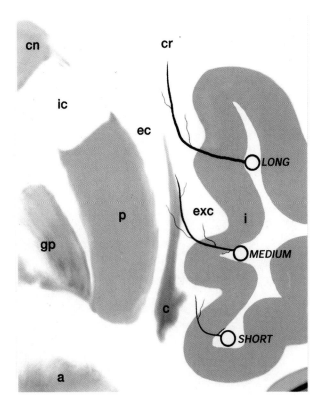

Fig. 11.11 Drawings showing that 85 to 90% of insular arteries are short and supply the insular cortex (i) and extreme capsule (exc); 10% are medium sized and supply, in addition, the claustrum (c) and external capsule (ec); and the remainder (3 to 5%) are long and extend as far as the corona radiata (cr). a, amygdala; ic, internal capsule; cn, caudate nucleus; gp, globus pallidus; p, putamen. (From Türe U, Yaşargil MG, Al-Mefty O, Yaşargil DC. Arteries of the insula. J Neurosurg 2000;92:686. Reprinted by permission.)

paid when tumor removal is performed at this level. Damage to these thin vessels may provoke severe corona radiata infarctions and consequent hemiparesis[14] **(Fig. 11.11)**.

The insular veins follow a parallel course to the insular sulci, draining into collecting veins along the superior and inferior peri-insular sulci. These collecting veins usually join together at the level of the anterior third of the inferior peri-insular sulcus, and travel deep through the stem of the sylvian fissure to join the deep sylvian vein just beneath the MCA. The sylvian vein frequently drains into the basal vein, but in some cases it drains into the sphenoparietal sinus. Sometimes there is a connection between the most rostral insular veins and the superficial system through the frontosylvian veins.

Insular Tumors

Total resection of an insular tumor is one of the most delicate neurosurgical procedures, and has long fascinated neurosurgeons because of the microsurgical skills required and the challenging approach. Reaching the insular surface involves splitting the sylvian fissure, which entails careful

dissection of the sylvian superficial and deeply located arteries and veins while the highly functional opercular lips are delicately protected. Medial resection of these tumors is a very important step, and special care must be taken because of the tumor's close relationship to important structures such as the LLA, basal ganglia, and internal capsule.[14,17,103]

In the 1950s, Penfield and Faulk[104] directly stimulated the insular cortex in awake patients and followed with various degrees of insular resection in certain patients with epilepsy, reporting no immediate neurologic deficits. Because of the lack of microsurgical techniques, these first procedures required a huge anterior temporal lobectomy to expose the insular surface. Following the same philosophy, Guillaume and colleagues[105] performed transopercular approaches (frontal or temporal depending on the electrocorticographic activity) to reach the insula.

Yaşargil and Reeves introduced the use of the microsurgical transsylvian approach and provided the first reported series of limbic and paralimbic tumors, including 57 insular and parainsular tumors[106] to which 93 more cases were recently added.[103] The vast majority of patients (93% with benign tumors, 91% with malignant ones) had good outcomes with acceptable seizure-free rates. These first encouraging results, reported after the advent of microsurgical techniques, prompted many neurosurgeons to take a renewed interest in insular tumor surgery.[1,12,27,81] Still, however, many controversies surround the optimal treatment of these lesions and different options, such as observation, stereotactic biopsy, radiosurgery, and direct surgery, have been proposed.[18–20]

Recent studies have analyzed the extent of resection and other important factors, such as overall survival and progression-free survival, showing better results in patients with insular low-grade gliomas when compared with gliomas with the same histological features in different locations.[22,29,30] Sanai and associates[22] analyzed the impact of the extent of resection in 104 patients undergoing surgery for insular gliomas, reporting better general outcomes when more extensive resections were achieved. Thus, it seems that a careful and gross total removal of insular tumors is safe and feasible, and may provide strong benefits in terms of survival and the alleviation of symptoms. Consequently, microsurgical removal appears to be the most appropriate first option for a patient with a symptomatic insular glioma. To achieve this goal, the surgeon's experience, neuroanatomic knowledge, and training, aided by some recently improved perioperative tools, are the key points.

In their initial stages, insular tumors seem to respect the cytoarchitectonic barriers of the brain, but after surgery, radiotherapy, or even spontaneously in cases of advanced high-grade gliomas, these edges may be blurred. After years of experience with hundreds of insular tumors, Yaşargil and Reeves[106] described these tumors' propensity to grow within the confines of the allocortical and mesocortical zones, sparing the neocortical and medial structures such as the basal ganglia and internal capsule. Their observations emphasize the idea that these tumors stay within their phylogenetic zones instead of spreading to neighboring zones even when they grow to huge sizes. Following this line of reasoning, Yaşargil described four general growth patterns: (1) a group of tumors mainly confined to the insula, (2) another group expanding to the basal orbitofrontal region, (3) tumors growing in the insula and invading the temporal pole area, and (4) a group of tumors growing through both the basal orbitofrontal and temporal pole areas. In our experience, however, in a few cases insular tumors may extend into the medial aspect of the frontoparietal opercula, which present one of the most difficult surgical explorations.

Clinical Presentation

Insular tumors are often discovered as medium or large lesions. It is quite uncommon to discover small ones, probably because of the indolent course they follow until they reach a significant volume. Thus, significant mass effect, compression, and shifting of the ipsilateral basal ganglia and ventricular system may occur in a patient with no clinical signs. Recently, however, improvements in diagnostic methods have allowed for earlier diagnosis.

The most common clinical spectrum for insular tumors includes the presence of seizures (33–98% of patients). These seizures are mostly complex partial (34–60%), generalized (27.5–30%), and simple partial (8–13%),[1,5,26,27,30,94,103,107–109] and appear as medically refractory epilepsy in a relatively high number of patients (12–60%),[1,5,108] a fact that by itself should be considered an indication for surgery.

Uncommon presenting symptoms include such neurologic impairments as hemiparesis and dysphasia, as well as symptoms of intracranial hypertension. Although underestimated, the presence of psychological alterations is quite common in patients with insular tumors, and special care should be paid to detect these abnormal behaviors (organic psychosis, anxiety, personality changes, and sexual dysfunction).[1,5,26,27,30,94,103,107–109] Neurologic impairment and symptoms stemming from intracranial hypertension are generally related to high-grade tumors, whereas low-grade gliomas generally course more indolently, with a history of atypical seizures and psycho-emotional disturbances usually described by the patient's family.[1,106] The large mass effect, as well as a possible extension beyond the insular functional unit, may easily explain the different behavior of the higher grades.

The Decision to Operate

The treatment of patients with insular tumors has changed drastically in the past two decades, mainly because of technological developments in neuroimaging and the surgical armamentarium. The benefits provided by these technical upgrades have generally improved the decision-making process (diagnosis, treatment, and prognosis) for intrinsic brain tumors. However, this evolution must be clearly understood because the leap in quality may also present more complex decisions.

The decision to operate must be made on an individual basis, attending to the patient's symptomatology, the tumor's topography and accessibility, and the surgeon's ability. Clinicians must be aware of their limitations before making any kind of decision. As mentioned earlier, insular tumors either produce intermittent but recurrent symptoms or are asymptomatic. Furthermore, they are located deep in the floor of the sylvian fissure and are completely covered by highly eloquent neurovascular structures. These general features seem to diminish their accessibility, and many surgeons recommend a biopsy of large, dominant-hemisphere insular tumors to prevent postoperative deficits. Nevertheless, this approach does not provide any benefit when compared with complete removal.[98,106]

A classic option sometimes offered to patients with insular gliomas is the wait-and-see strategy. Most low-grade insular gliomas grow slowly and are not as aggressive as tumors in other locations. This slow growth allows the surgeon, and especially the patient, to postpone the inevitable decision. This strategy surely will help the patients recover from their acute psychological trauma after being informed of their recently diagnosed tumor. Patients with these tumors can be followed closely for a while, and the decision to operate can be made calmly if images show progression or seizures do not respond to antiepileptic drugs. Nevertheless, the unpredictable natural history of these lesions must also be taken into consideration when choosing the optimal treatment, and surgery presents the safest therapeutic option. Some exceptions to this strategy are the presence of large or hemorrhagic tumors, as well as lesions causing an important mass effect. Generally, when either low-grade or high-grade tumors have these features, patients are more likely to undergo surgery.

In patients with seizures, low-grade insular gliomas have refractory epilepsy rates of up to 60%. In such patients, microsurgical excision has been promoted as the only solution, with good results. Thus, when pharmacologically refractory seizures are present, the decision to operate seems clear. With regard to other features, Simon and colleagues[5] showed that patient selection is an important factor determining functional outcomes. In this sense, most young patients with WHO grade I to III gliomas who are free of neurologic deficit are the ideal candidates for surgical resection, achieving a 3-month postoperative Karnofsky score of 80 to 100. Thus, the ideal candidates for surgery can be described as follows: young patients in good clinical condition with low-grade neuroimaging signs, patients with intractable epilepsy, and patients in good general condition with important mass effect and symptoms of intracranial hypertension. But patients with high-grade tumors are also candidates for surgery despite their worse prognosis when general conditions allow a surgical procedure. Accepting the intrinsic difficulty of this kind of procedure, for the patient described in this chapter, we would choose total tumor removal through a microsurgical pterional transsylvian approach designed to spare the healthy neighboring neurovascular structures as much as possible.

We will discuss and illustrate our preoperative and surgical approach for a patient who was operated on by the senior author (U.T.) and who is very similar to the patient presented in this chapter. She is 41 years old, and was diagnosed after presenting with an 18-month history of dizziness. In the previous weeks, her family also witnessed some partial seizures during these episodes of dizziness.

The patient presented to our center after having been followed in a different department. Because of the presence of seizures and an area of minimal contrast enhancement on the MRI, we recommended surgery **(Fig. 11.12)**.

Preoperative Studies

The preoperative workup after the decision to operate is an important therapeutic step. During this stage, the surgeon should carefully study all available information about the

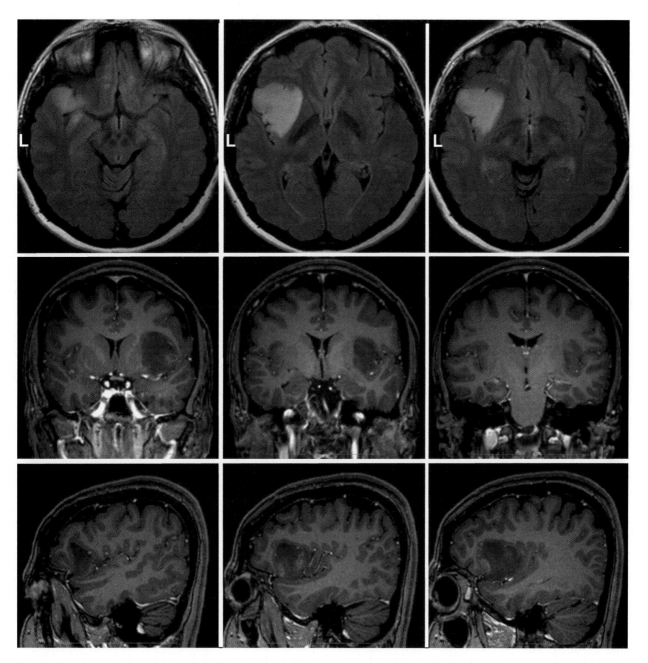

Fig. 11.12   *Top row:* Preoperative MRI findings through a fluid-attenuated inversion recovery (FLAIR) sequence in the axial plane where a hyperintense signal is seen, mainly located in the anterior aspect of the left (L) insula and showing clear delimitation with the lateral aspect of the putamen, which is pushed slightly posteromedially. *Middle and bottom rows:* Three-dimensional T1-weighted turbo field echo (TFE) sequence with contrast in the coronal and sagittal planes. A hypointense signal shows a clear delimitation within the borders of the anterior, inferior, and superior peri-insular sulci. These radiological features suggest the diagnosis of an anterior insular glioma. The posterior insular point is spared by the tumor.

patient, and combine this information with his or her previous experience and neuroanatomic knowledge to create a virtual 3D image of the tumor location and to note the potential pitfalls that could appear during surgery. To that end, the most helpful information might be inferred from the clinical records, but especially from the imaging studies.

Neuroimaging with MRI improves the accuracy of diagnosis and remains indispensable for surgical planning. Currently, modern imaging techniques are necessary for several reasons: to detect or confirm a structural abnormality; to localize, assess, and characterize that abnormality; to plan the surgical approach and extension; to predict possible postoperative neurologic deficits; to orient the surgeon to the patient's metabolism and the metabolic composition of the tumor and its surroundings; to understand the 3D anatomic relationship between the tumor and eloquent areas of the brain (cortical and subcortical) through functional and anatomic sequences; and to evaluate the extent of resection intra- and postoperatively.

A careful examination of the coronal, axial, and sagittal views of the brain on MRI, as well with 3D multiplanar reconstructions if available, is very helpful in understanding and visualizing the shape, dimensions, intrinsic features, and volume of the tumor. These views can also define the tumor's relationships to the different aspects of the sylvian fissure and the superficial sylvian vein (SSV) and its tributaries; the lateral and medial aspects of the fronto-orbital, fronto-parietal, and temporal opercula; and the peri-insular and central insular sulci. Furthermore, the relationships with highly functional deep structures, such as the basal ganglia, internal capsule, the anterior perforated substance, and the LLA, can be also studied. The latter structures belong to different functional units, and are often displaced by the main volume of the tumor.

The challenge of determining the precise location and relationships of a brain tumor reaches its highest point in patients with insular gliomas because of their central and hidden location. Once the tumor is diagnosed, the next step is to define its accurate anatomic location. T1- and T2-weighted MRI sequences, including FLAIR, and T1-weighted sequences after gadolinium enhancement are recommended to help define the tumor's location. To precisely delineate tumors in the different insular regions, we obtain at least the T1- and T2-weighted sequences in the axial, coronal, and sagittal planes. After having grossly analyzed the main morphological and topographical features in these sequences, we review 3D multiplanar reconstructions done in 1-mm slices to accurately study the detailed relationships and the tumor's edges (**Fig. 11.12**).

Identifying the central insular sulcus is not easy, especially when the tumor involves the whole insula. When the tumor mainly involves one of the insular aspects, however, it is possible to identify the central insular sulcus in sagittal slices, thereby locating in these patients a greatly useful intraoperative landmark. One of the most relevant details during this careful inspection is an understanding of the position of the tumor within the peri-insular sulci and the adjacent

opercula. For this determination, the coronal and sagittal are the most appropriate views, on which we can discern whether the opercula are involved or just pushed to the level of the anterior, superior, and inferior peri-insular sulci.

Magnetic resonance imaging angiography enables the identification of the M2 and M3 arteries, which may also be of great interest. This is also the most appropriate way to discern the relative location of the anterior perforated substance and the LLA crossing it. The extended use of carotid angiography is now reserved only for special cases.[26] Some authors have proposed using other sequences, such as 3D 3T time-of-flight, which provides a nice three-dimensional display of the LLA and their relationships with the mediobasal aspect of the tumor.[25] All these imaging modalities produce useful information about the distribution of the main branches of the MCA and their relation to the insular surface. These data may help to distinguish between tumors that mimic the normal cortical architecture and vascular pattern and those that completely involve and hide the M2 branches.

Diffusion Tensor Imaging–Based Tractography

Diffusion tensor imaging–based tractography has recently been incorporated into the neurosurgical diagnostic armamentarium. DTI is able to detect the characteristics of water diffusion in tissue and display particular dimensional brownian motion. The diffusion of water particles is facilitated by the ordered distribution of neural fibers through the membranes covering the axons. This imaging modality displays the white-matter fiber tracts by selecting a place where they can be easily visualized and then constructing a 3D image of them. DTI enables the visualization of bundles of axons by selecting regions with the same values of fractional anisotropy as "seed" to the production of tracts in the 3D space.[110]

Tractography provides information about the normal course and the displacement or disruption of white-matter tracts around the tumor, as well as damage to these tracts from vasogenic edema or tumor infiltration. In neurosurgery, tractography is being used mainly to understand the subcortical relation between the tumor and clinically relevant white-matter fiber tracts.[111] But tractography is limited in areas where tracts cross tumors or peritumoral vasogenic edema, a fact that should be noted when choosing a place for the seed. However, a great number of fascicles can be visualized through DTI-based tractography, and several main fiber bundles are studied. The corticospinal tract contains motor fibers that pass through the corona radiata to join the internal capsule, from which they lead to the brain stem. The SLF contains the arcuate fasciculus, which joins Broca's and Wernicke's areas, which is of great interest in patients with tumors located in the surroundings of the inferior frontal, angular, and superior temporal gyri. The optic radiations are also especially important when dealing with tumors not only in the occipital but also deep in the temporal and parietal lobes.[112]

Surrounding white-matter fiber tracts, such as the internal capsule and the SLF, belong to different anatomic and functional compartments, and so they are not invaded by the tumor. In some cases, however, the posterior deep limit of the tumor underlying the posterior insular point might be closely related especially to the posterior limb of the internal capsule. Furthermore, in rare cases in which the medial aspect of the frontoparietal operculum is involved, "U" (short association) fibers between the insula and medial aspect of the frontoparietal operculum, which is actually the extension of the extreme capsule, could be invaded by the tumor. Even in these cases, the SLF is mainly spared. Thus, preoperative tractographic analysis of these bundles may provide surgeons with very useful information to improve their three-dimensional understanding of the tumor and surrounding structures (**Fig. 11.13**).

Three-Dimensional Anatomic Reconstructions

Before approaching the insula, some surface landmarks must be comprehensively studied. These include the opercular lateral surface and the anatomic variations of the sylvian fissure and the related SSV and tributaries. This study is better done with a 3D display of the cortical surface, which enables the surgeon to visualize all these data in a direct and easily integrated fashion. We recommend the use of a 3D T1-weighted turbo field echo (TFE) sequence to create these cortical reconstructions. A 3D T2-weighted image may be helpful in some cases because it shows the anatomic disposition of sulci and gyri with great accuracy. These sequences contribute to a 3D reconstruction of the brain, which helps the surgeon plan the approach and the transsylvian microsurgical technique (**Fig. 11.14**).

The imaging modalities described above provide the chance to link all these data in the surgeon's mind with his or her anatomic knowledge and experience from previous procedures and follow-up. The result is a perfect display of preoperative information, which is crucial for creating a 3D visualization of the tumor and surrounding neurovascular structures.

The Surgical Approach

For the surgical approach, the patient is placed in the supine position with the chest raised 15 degrees, and the head is secured with the Mayfield headrest and rotated approximately 30 degrees to the contralateral side. A slightly posteriorly extended fronto-parietotemporal incision is made. The temporal muscle is fully detached and retracted posteroinferiorly. Generally, one bur hole is made 3 to 4 cm posterior to the pterion. For older patients, especially women, three bur holes can be made to protect the dura, which can be quite thin and attached to the inner aspect of the bone. Two semicircular craniotomy lines are made superiorly and inferiorly to the level of the lateral aspect of the sphenoid wing. At this point, the surgeon begins working under the microscope, drilling the external line of the sphenoid bone.

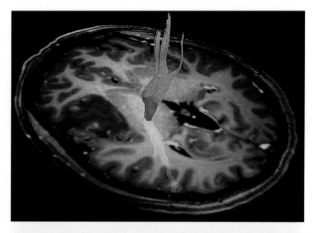

a

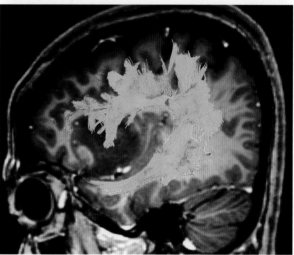

b

Fig. 11.13a,b Preoperative axial T1-weighted MRI of the presented patient. **(a)** Fibers of the left corticospinal tract (*pink*) are slightly displaced posteromedially by the tumor mass, which closely relates to the posterior insular point. **(b)** Preoperative sagittal T1-weighted MRI of the presented patient. Fibers of the left superior longitudinal fasciculus (*green*), which remain intact, are seen surrounding the left insular tumor.

Once the bone flap is removed, the remaining sphenoid wing is drilled away with the high-speed drill to allow appropriate retraction of the dural flap and a comfortable access to the sylvian point and adjacent posterior frontobasal region. The durotomy is made in a semicircular fashion with the base at the level of the sphenoid bone. A posterior rectilinear extension is made from the tip of the first incision and parallel to the sylvian fissure. This posterior extension allows a larger exposure of the posterior aspect of the sylvian fissure and a comfortable view of the frontoparietal and temporal opercula. The sylvian fissure remains a constant surface landmark that should be identified initially. Usually, this goal is easily achieved as the SSV delineates its lateral course. In a few patients, however, the SSV is absent or deeply located, or the outer arachnoid membrane is so thick that its course is obscured (**Fig. 11.15a**).

In addition to the information gotten from direct inspection of the sylvian fissure, we routinely use indocyanine

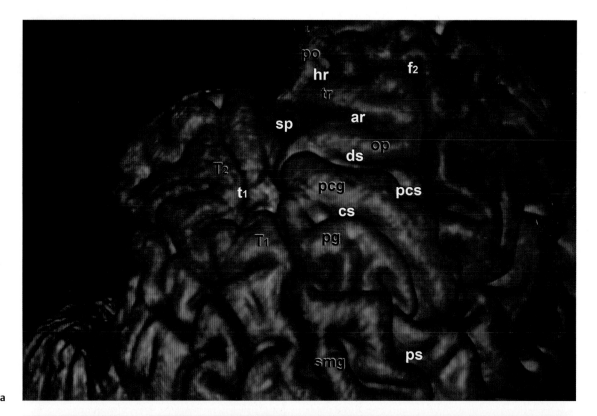

a

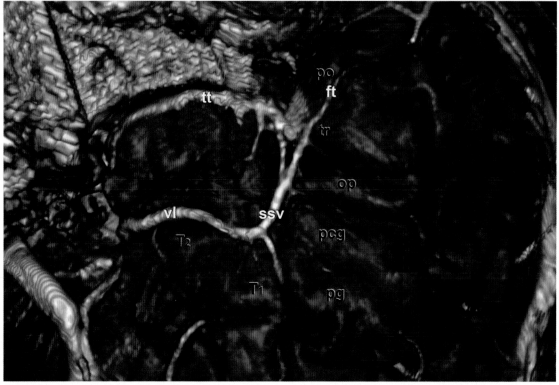

b

Fig. 11.14a,b Three-dimensional brain-surface reconstructions from the surgical perspective (left pterional) created from the three-dimensional T1-weighted TFE sequence of the presented case. These images highlight important anatomic landmarks without **(a)** and with **(b)** cortical vessel reconstruction. ar, ascending ramus of the sylvian fissure; cs, central sulcus; ds, diagonal sulcus; f2, inferior frontal sulcus; ft, frontal tributary branch of the superficial sylvian vein; hr, horizontal ramus of the sylvian fissure; op, pars opercularis; pcs, precentral sulcus; pcg, precentral gyrus; pg, postcentral gyrus; po, pars orbitalis; ps, postcentral sulcus; smg, supramarginal gyrus; sp, sylvian point; ssv, superficial sylvian vein; t_1, superior temporal sulcus; T_1, superior temporal gyrus; T_2, middle temporal gyrus; tr, pars triangularis; tt, temporal tributary branch of the superficial sylvian vein; vl, vein of Labbé.

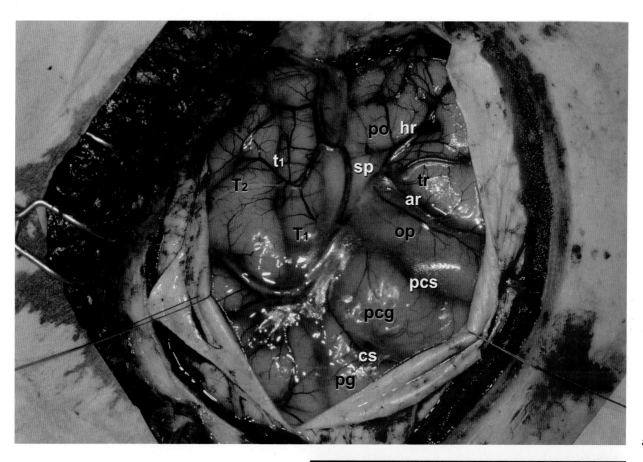

a

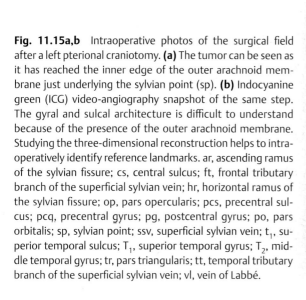

Fig. 11.15a,b Intraoperative photos of the surgical field after a left pterional craniotomy. **(a)** The tumor can be seen as it has reached the inner edge of the outer arachnoid membrane just underlying the sylvian point (sp). **(b)** Indocyanine green (ICG) video-angiography snapshot of the same step. The gyral and sulcal architecture is difficult to understand because of the presence of the outer arachnoid membrane. Studying the three-dimensional reconstruction helps to intraoperatively identify reference landmarks. ar, ascending ramus of the sylvian fissure; cs, central sulcus; ft, frontal tributary branch of the superficial sylvian vein; hr, horizontal ramus of the sylvian fissure; op, pars opercularis; pcs, precentral sulcus; pcq, precentral gyrus; pg, postcentral gyrus; po, pars orbitalis; sp, sylvian point; ssv, superficial sylvian vein; t_1, superior temporal sulcus; T_1, superior temporal gyrus; T_2, middle temporal gyrus; tr, pars triangularis; tt, temporal tributary branch of the superficial sylvian vein; vl, vein of Labbé.

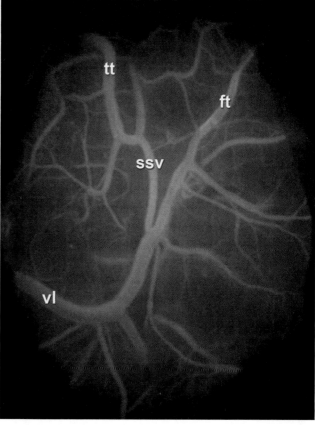

b

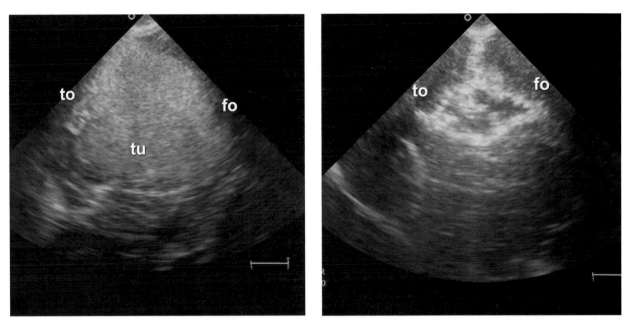

a   b

Fig. 11.16a,b   Photos from the ultrasonographic study of the left insular tumor and its relation to the sylvian fissure and the surrounding opercula before **(a)** and after **(b)** resection. fo, frontoparietal operculum; to, temporal operculum; tu, insular tumor.

green (ICG) video angiography. This tool provides information about the arterial and venous architecture, helping to verify the position of the sylvian fissure. M3 branches coming from the depth of the sylvian cistern reach the opercular surface and curve 90 degrees upward and downward to become M4.[14] However, the most useful information extracted from the ICG is a comprehensive understanding of the direction of venous flow and the presence of collaterals **(Fig. 11.15b)**. Once the venous anatomy is understood, we always use ultrasound to check the rostrocaudal extension of the tumor and its relation to the exposed sylvian fissure **(Fig. 11.16a)**. Careful analysis of the intraoperative ultrasound findings allows the surgeon to define the rostrocaudal tumor borders to determine the extension needed to open the sylvian fissure. In some cases, mainly when large tumors occupy the entire insular region, it may be necessary to open the whole length of the fissure.

The next recommended maneuver is to release cerebrospinal fluid from the basal cisterns to relax the brain. This goal can be achieved with the aid of fine bipolar coagulation forceps and a cotton pledget slightly introduced parallel to the posterior fronto-orbital gyrus until it reaches the lateral membrane between the optic and olfactory nerves. A small incision is then made to enter the carotid and chiasmatic cisterns, allowing the outflow of cerebrospinal fluid. This initial maneuver allows the release of cerebrospinal fluid when necessary during the procedure.

Splitting the Sylvian Fissure and Resecting the Tumor

With the aid of current microsurgical techniques and operative tools, the sylvian fissure can be precisely and suc-

cessfully split, avoiding injury to adjacent vital structures and thus preserving their function. The SSV is usually boxed in between the outer arachnoid membrane and the lateral sylvian membrane, which show some slight arachnoid bridges.[113] This venous system varies greatly in location, number, collaterals, length, and drainage routes. Although the clearest landmarks to define the components of the insulo-opercular segment of the sylvian fissure should be the pars triangularis, opercularis, and subcentral gyrus, this cortical architecture is not easily distinguished in the surgical field at exploration. Thus, a precise understanding of the regional venous anatomy remains imperative. Although the cerebral veins have a rich collateral system, we must precisely study the vascular patterns, combining our knowledge with the 3D reconstructions and the ICG video angiography to choose the exact point of entry to the arachnoid so that we can navigate through the fissure without disrupting the venous architecture. The incision is usually safely made in the frontal aspect of the fissure; however, variations in the venous flow patterns may require moving the SSV superiorly. In the rostrocaudal line, the fissure is usually incised at the level of the sylvian point, where the horizontal, ascending, and posterior rami of the sylvian fissure come together just below the tip of the pars triangularis.[103,114] Some landmarks can be helpful in locating this point. The sylvian venous confluence, where the temporal and frontal tributaries drain into the SSV, is several millimeters posterior to this area. Moreover, the prefrontal and middle temporal arteries usually emerge in the lateral hemispheric surface at this same level. The location of the sylvian point in reference to the pterion was shown to be just slightly posterior in the horizontal plane.[114] Its estimation is an acceptable point to start the splitting because

Broca's area is located in the dominant hemisphere just posterior to this point, and the subcentral gyrus still more posteriorly.[17] Large tumors, especially when located in the anterior insular region, could make the splitting easier and push the insular apex just under the outer arachnoid membrane at the level of the sylvian point (10% of cases) **(Figs. 11.14, 11.15)**.

Entering the sylvian fissure through the sylvian point and exploring in a deep direction soon exposes the insular apex, whereas the limen insulae and the main MCA division remain deeper, 10 to 20 mm perpendicular to the sylvian point itself. These neurovascular structures are the first reliable deep reference points. In most cases, however, it is not possible to visualize them without debulking the central tumor. After this initial debulking, dissection may continue over the surface of M1 to the bifurcation of the internal carotid artery. At this point, opening the fissure will move from inside to outside and the suprasellar cisterns can be reached. Every space gained in depth is maintained with round cottonoids, which facilitate the separation of the opercular lips and enable the surgeon to avoid the use of self-retaining retractors.

The posterior extension of the splitting depends on the vascular pattern and the posterior extension of the tumor. Generally, central debulking is performed posteriorly to gain access to the posterior aspect of the depth of the sylvian fossa. Posterior splitting of the fissure is done in the same manner, working from inside to outside. This extension exposes the lateral aspect of the insula. In general, the frontoparietal operculum covers more of the insular cortex surface compared with the temporal operculum,[17] and the distance from the lateral surface of the hemisphere at the level of the sylvian fissure slightly increases in a rostro-caudal direction. Thus, the depth of the interopercular sulci at the level of the suborbital gyri and polar planum is 10 to 20 mm, 25 to 40 mm at the level of the subopercular gyrus, and 35 to 50 mm at the level of the subcentral and transverse parietal gyri. This is the reason splitting the sylvian fissure is easier when starting at the level of the sylvian point, first directed anteromedially to open the stem and then posteriorly from the depth to the surface.

After enough of the sylvian fissure is split, debulking the central tumor is easier and the voluminous insular region relaxes. The transsylvian approach without the use of self-retaining retractors highlights the difficulty of not directly offering a wide view of the entire surface of the insula, forcing the surgeon to create small working spaces. These working spaces are maintained with two or three round cottonoids placed in strategic positions. When the tumor partially maintains the cortical insular anatomy, finding anatomic landmarks before resection becomes easier. The most appropriate strategy seems to be to locate the MCA bifurcation at the level of the limen insula, where devascularization of the most proximal short and medium insular perforators starts. Some tumors, however, break the pial edge, spreading along the sylvian fossa, or expand into the insular gyri so much that the M2 and its insular branches

remain encompassed by the tumor. In these situations tumor debulking starts without initial devascularization and it must be done with slight suction until the subpial level of the first arterial branch is encountered. Then, direct subpial devascularization can be achieved, and that branch can be subpially skeletonized toward its proximal segment, with pathological tissue removed until the MCA bifurcation is reached.

In any case, initial debulking is done at the level of the insular apex, where the superior and inferior trunks of the MCA give off their first main branches **(Fig. 11.10a)**. Some windows are created between these arteries, always achieving the same deep plane. During this first stage, all resection windows should be equally deep to preserve the orientation and keep a certain harmony. Before manipulating any important branch, we use the micro-Doppler to check its flow, and we check again after having worked on its surroundings, with the aim of learning how to deal with these vessels. Topical applications of papaverine are recommended to prevent vasospasm. During devascularization and tumor removal, or once it has been completed, the insular veins are coagulated.

With the initial central debulking at the level of the anteroinferior aspect of the insula (the inferior extension of the anterior and posterior short gyri), exploration of the peripheral regions around the peri-insular sulci is facilitated.

The inferior limb of the insular fossa is usually easier to explore because of its closer relationship with the central aspect of the insula (14.8 mm from the insular apex; 19.1 mm to the superior peri-insular sulcus).[17] With the aid of a flat cottonoid, the anteroinferior extension of the long gyri can be pushed downward, exposing the inferior trunk of the deep sylvian vein within the inferior peri-insular sulci. This anatomic landmark usually represents the inferior limit of the resection. In cases in which the polar planum is involved, however, the resection continues beyond this sulcus, following the tumoral tissue from the insula millimeter by millimeter. The most acceptable anatomic landmark deep in the anterior aspect of the inferior peri-insular sulcus is the dorsal surface of the amygdala, which is exposed only in patients in whom the tumor largely extends to the temporal pole.

Debulking and decompressing the central and inferior insular areas facilitates exploration of the anterosuperior and superior aspects, located beneath the fronto-orbital and frontoparietal opercula, respectively. It is extremely important to maintain a high level of concentration during all surgical steps, but we must sharpen our orientation especially in these last stages because tissue removal has distorted the anatomy and may confuse our vision. Thus, keeping in mind some anatomic landmarks is mandatory. The anterosuperior aspect of the tumor is the area around the anterior sylvian point. The prefrontal artery arising from the superior trunk usually takes this path to reach the cortical surface, whereas the lateral orbitofrontal branch, also arising from this trunk, follows the anterior peri-insular sulcus and can also be a valid landmark. The anterior peri-insular sulcus can seem quite deep, especially if the insular apex protrudes enough into the fissure. After this region is devascularized, the tumor is suctioned to the level of its extension. The posterior aspects of the superior and inferior peri-insular sulci are the most hidden areas in the insular region[17] and their surgical access remains quite difficult. Some authors propose opercular retraction, or even removal, to gain access to this region.[22,27] We believe these maneuvers may have important functional consequences and lead to speech impairment. Intraoperative speech disturbances have been reported during tumor removal in awake patients; these disturbances resolved after the retractors were removed.[1]

After having debulked the central, inferior, and antero-superior aspects of the tumor, a soft push of the posterior aspect downward with the aid of a flat cottonoid and the suction tube facilitates exposure of the region around the posterior insular point. Then devascularization is done as described. In this area, it is of extreme importance to recognize the presence of some long perforator insular arteries, which should be spared as they have been shown to reach the corona radiata[14] (**Fig. 11.11**). This is one of the most challenging steps of the surgery, but it is facilitated by the fact that the entire path of the M2 and M3 arteries has already been skeletonized. This posterior half of the superior peri-insular sulcus is located close to the pyramidal tract entering the posterior limb of the internal capsule. Damaging these fibers could also lead to serious postoperative neurologic impairment. Some intraoperative tools have been developed to prevent these problems, but no intraoperative device can yet distinguish this highly functional fiber system ideally. Motor evoked potentials seem an adequate tool to promptly detect any motor disturbance, but vascular damage cannot be repaired even when quickly recognized. On the other hand, the use of intraoperative motor evoked potentials can resolve motor impairment caused by manipulation and retraction maneuvers. Direct subcortical stimulation can theoretically predict the deep position of the motor fibers in the posterior limb of the internal capsule. Some surgeons use this intraoperative tool to carry out tumor removal as long as a positive response is noted. Although in the late postoperative period the neurologic impairment rates of these patients are equivalent to other reports, in the immediate postoperative period nearly 60% of these patients have worsening of their previous neurologic conditions.[27]

With the patient under general anesthesia, we routinely use direct subcortical stimulation in the posterosuperior limit of the lesion to assess our plan and the 3D picture we created in our minds, but the difference with the previously described practice is that our resection limit is given not only by the appearance of positive or negative responses but also by many other intraoperative tools and the tumor extension. We believe that none of these tools is solely reliable; therefore, surgeons must integrate all the data with their own experience.

The recent advent of DTI-based tractography represents a great advance in neurosurgical planning. This technique allows the surgeon to study the 3D relationships between the posterior limb of the internal capsule and the tumoral volume itself, as well as the SLF in the rare cases in which the frontoparietal operculum is involved. In our experience, this technique is still increasing its accuracy, and its main value is as a preoperative and postoperative tool. Its intraoperative use through its implementation in navigation systems cancels its accuracy during tumor removal due to the brain shift. Preoperative tractography is carefully analyzed to understand the deep relationships, but for the time being we pay special attention to the postoperative tractography, which allows us to integrate our preoperative thinking with the intraoperative findings and the postoperative result, thereby increasing our surgical experience and anatomic knowledge in real conditions.

Once the posterior tumor extension has been removed, we check the viability of the dissected MCA branches using the micro-Doppler, and apply topical papaverine if we suspect vasospasm. The LLA are the most appropriate anatomic landmarks in the anteroinferior region. Certain tumors may envelop these arteries, but no tumor goes further medially except the rare ones that originate from the putamen. A careful examination of this region under the microscope is mandatory with the goal of preserving all these arterial branches, as it has been widely reported that most of the definitive neurologic impairment after the resection of insular tumors is related to ischemic events. Obliteration of these branches may lead to different degrees of motor disturbances, including hemiplegia from deep strokes in the internal capsule. Again, combining anatomic knowledge with the available preoperative images and some intraoperative tools is the key to managing this stage. Using intraoperative micro-Doppler can help assess the position of the LLA, and although this finding cannot be realized in every case, the emergence of a group of radiating small veins indicates the close proximity of this deep arterial system. Some authors defend the use of awake procedures to check for possible worsening of certain functions, but those procedures can neither predict nor prevent ischemic events.

Every surgical step during insular tumor removal increases in difficulty, but the most challenging stage is dealing with the tumor borders and the healthy surrounding tissues. There is still no definite method to distinguish the border between the tumor and normal brain tissue, and surgeons must sharpen all their senses to detect changes in the color, consistency, and texture of the tumor tissue because this is often critical in determining when the resection should be stopped. Deep in the central region, the claustrum is very difficult to distinguish. This is the reason the lateral surface of the putamen is the basic anatomic landmark at which to stop the deep resection. Because of the different architecture between these compartments, the tumoral limit is always sharply defined in this region. Thus, the knowledge and experience gained enable the surgeon to appreciate the change in consistency, color, and vascular pattern when the putamen has been exposed. This is the only reliable method to define the medial limit of surgical resection.

Although ultrasonography is very helpful during the entire surgical procedure, its usefulness for checking the medial border is diminished because of artifacts from the tumor cavity when the ultrasound probe is applied over the sylvian fissure. For this reason, the probe should be applied over the opercula as far as possible from the sylvian fissure. Comparing the snapshot taken before resection with the postresection picture can be useful for experienced surgeons **(Fig. 11.16)**. But this intraoperative imaging device loses its usefulness in patients with previously irradiated tumors. Intraoperative MRI is another useful tool to determine the quality of surgical resection. Fluorescence-guided resection with 5-aminolevulinic acid allows the visualization of malignant tissue during surgery for glioblastomas. In our experience, this technique still has many pitfalls, such as a lack of visualization in deep locations and the danger of extreme resection relating to color changes in tumor borders.

Once the resection and hemostasis are complete, we routinely analyze the surgical field and cortical surface using ICG video angiography. This tool is mainly used to assess the arterial integrity as well as to check the optimal functioning of the venous anatomy. It also provides very important information about possible contusions in the healthy opercular tissues, representing a way to measure how delicate the surgical approach has been **(Fig. 11.17)**. Postoperative MRI is done the next day. A detailed MRI with fiber tractography is repeated routinely 2 or 3 months after surgery **(Figs. 11.18, 11.19)**. The histopathological examination in our presented case revealed a diffuse astrocytoma (WHO grade II); therefore, we did not recommend any adjuvant therapy.

Controversial Issues in Insular Tumor Surgery

The state of the art during any neurosurgical procedure is still the complete removal of the lesion while sparing the anatomy and functionality of the surrounding normal brain tissue. The following three steps aid in achieving this goal: first, making a corridor based on anatomic and cisternal principles to minimize disruption of the neighboring neurovascular structures; second, carrying out atraumatic manipulation along the narrow surgical corridor without rigid retraction; and third, preserving the normal surrounding structures and function as much as possible during tumor removal. The first surgical explorations of the insula were achieved after gross removal of the temporal or frontoparietal opercula (or both).[104,105] Some decades later, and with the advent of microsurgical techniques, Yaşargil[103,107] demonstrated the microsurgical transsylvian fissure approach as the optimal method of exploration for removing insular tumors. The fundamental principles of this atraumatic ap-

proach allow successful tumor removal without damaging the surrounding normal structures. Despite the good results provided by this concept, followed by anatomic resection of the tumor, in recent years some groups have shifted this anatomic concept to a functional resection. In this sense, these authors propose approaching the insular region through the removal of healthy tissue from the fronto-orbital, frontoparietal, or temporal opercula during awake procedures, justifying this method with a better and faster exposure of the insular surface.[1,12,22,27,108,110,115,116]

The most commonly reported neurologic impairments after insular tumor resection are hemiparesis and speech disturbances.[1,12,22,25-27,81,97,103,106] These complications are usually attributable to the disruption of healthy structures surrounding the insula or their blood supply, rather than the insula itself. Hemiparesis or speech disturbances may arise when the central or precentral arteries are inadvertently damaged or temporarily obstructed, or because of vasospasm.[81] The popularization of awake procedures makes possible intraoperative notification of some of the causes of speech disturbances. Some investigators have reported immediate postoperative speech impairment in their patients despite the fact that different stimulation tests were done in the removed opercular and insular cortex without any speech arrest. Some of these patients experienced speech dysfunction during tumor removal, which in certain cases resolved after the self-retaining retractors were removed from the opercula. Thus, it seems that the retraction of the opercula or the vasospasm caused by vascular manipulation, or both, might have contributed to these intraoperative disturbances,[1,81] but performing awake procedures did not predict their appearance.

Malak and colleagues[97] reviewed the temporary evolution of the most common neurologic impairments in different series, highlighting two important findings. First, the incidence of permanent deficit was lower (3% for hemiparesis and 1.4% in cases of speech problems) than immediately after the surgical procedure (17% for hemiparesis and 16% in cases of speech problems). Second, all cases of permanent disturbance were related to an infarct in the territory of the LLA. From these findings, it becomes clear that most transient motor and speech impairments are caused by direct or indirect injury to the opercular areas and temporary ischemia secondary to the M2 or M3 branches supplying these cortical regions, as well as ischemic deep areas from the surgical injury of the deep LLA. A possible risk that should also be considered comes from the fact that the medullary branches arising from the M4 segments travel through the opercula to feed certain areas of the corona radiata. The surgeon has no control over these small vessels during a transopercular approach. Thus, it seems clear that this transopercular corridor indefinitely requires awake surgery so that the surgeon can check the available functionality of the opercula. In our opinion, the discomfort for the patient and surgeon and the stressful atmosphere that these procedures entail do not justify removing healthy tissue to get a better initial view of the insular region. More-

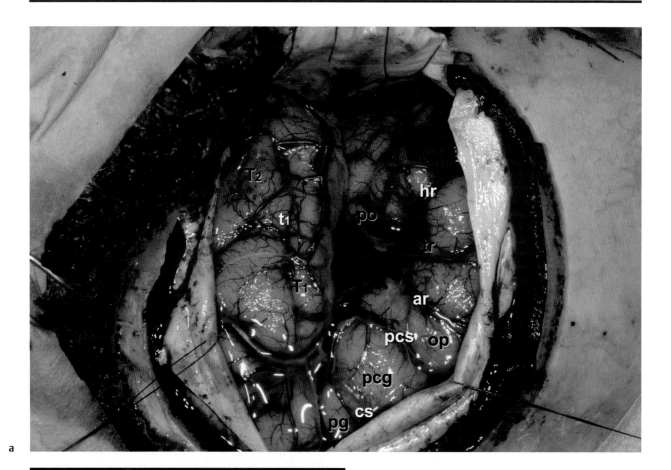

a

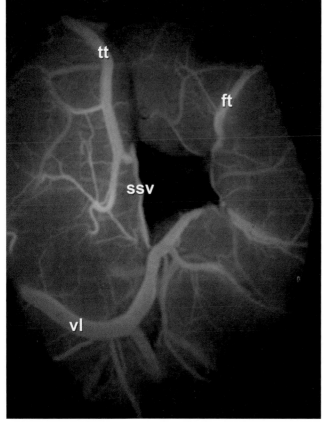

b

Fig. 11.17a,b Intraoperative photo of the surgical field just after tumor resection **(a)** and ICG video-angiography snapshot showing the vascular architecture of the same field **(b)**. The arachnoid incision and the creation of surgical windows to remove the tumor have been optimized, achieving an intact postoperative venous pattern without evident contusion at the surrounding opercula. ar, ascending ramus of the sylvian fissure; cs, central sulcus; ft, frontal tributary branch of the superficial sylvian vein; hr, horizontal ramus of the sylvian fissure; op, pars opercularis; pcs, precentral sulcus; pcg, precentral gyrus; pg, postcentral gyrus; po, pars orbitalis; ssv, superficial sylvian vein; t_1, superior temporal sulcus; T_1, superior temporal gyrus; T_2, middle temporal gyrus; tr, pars triangularis; tt, temporal tributary branch of the superficial sylvian vein; vl, vein of Labbé.

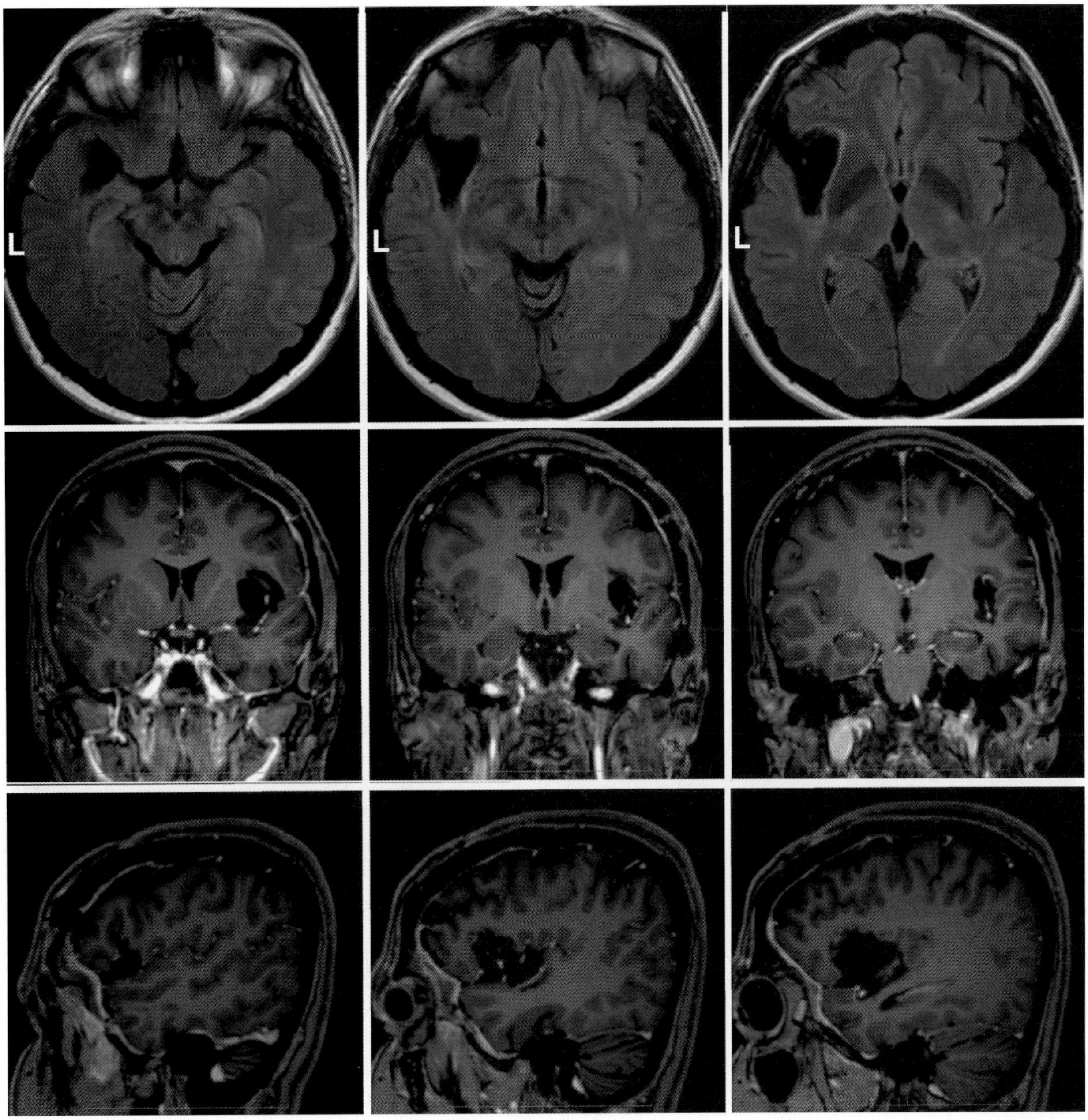

Fig. 11.18 *Top row:* The 2-month postoperative MRI findings through the FLAIR sequence in the axial plane show that the resection cavity is free of residual tumor and the medial structures have returned to their normal position. *Middle and bottom rows:* The 3D T1-weighted TFE sequences with contrast in coronal and sagittal planes. The resection cavity is seen at the level of the left (L) insula with no sign of residual tumor. The posterior edge is clean and free of tumor and the internal capsule is completely spared. Histopathological examination revealed a diffuse astrocytoma (WHO grade II); therefore, we did not recommend any adjuvant therapy.

over, as has been discussed, awake surgery does not prevent the most common definitive impairments mainly related to mechanical and vascular causes, which can be misinterpreted and limit the extent of resection.

Another important issue is the intraoperative control of the extent of resection and deep orientation during the procedure. Some groups support the use of intraoperative navigation and the implementation of the preoperative im-

ages tractography provides. In our opinion, these frameless stereotactic neuronavigation systems are of little use as the resection is less accurate after the durotomy and release of cerebrospinal fluid because of brain shift. The point remains to focus all our senses during the procedure, identifying as many anatomic landmarks as possible at every step to maintain orientation during resection. This approach allows us to go back and find these anatomic landmarks in

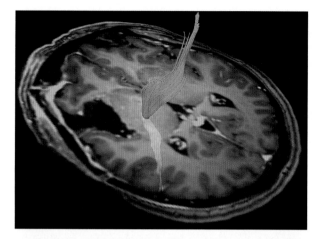

a

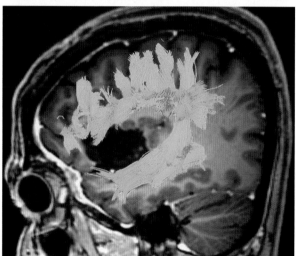

b

Fig. 11.19a,b **(a)** Postoperative axial T1-weighted MRI showing complete preservation of the posterior limb of the internal capsule (*pink*), which has recovered its natural location after tumor removal. **(b)** Postoperative sagittal T1-weighted MRI showing that fibers of the left superior longitudinal fasciculus (*green*) remain intact after tumor removal. The posterior insular point was spared because it was free of tumor.

case we lose orientation during any step. This is why it is so important to acquire extensive knowledge of neuroanatomy and follow the ordered steps we propose.

The valuable information provided by tractography combined with accumulated surgical experience and neuroanatomic knowledge is key to managing insular tumors. Some groups have suggested studying the location of deep structures, such as the posterior limb of the internal cap-

sule and the SLF, to carry out the resection until these fiber bundles are encountered during direct subcortical stimulation in awake patients. We believe there is no need for extreme subcortical resection of these healthy tissues, and that is the reason we argue for an anatomic approach (stay within the tumor volume). Moreover, insular tumor resection requires a calm environment and a high level of concentration to maintain the orientation during every step of the procedure, a goal difficult to achieve when dealing with awake patients. Some authors found that the number of intraoperative stimulations they performed was limited because patients in this situation could not easily tolerate a long surgical procedure.[116]

The point during any neurosurgical procedure is to offer our patients optimal treatment, and for that reason we must use the most delicate maneuvers. A quick surgery is the enemy of a carefully reasoned procedure, and every case requires an extremely high level of concentration during every step. Thus, a calm atmosphere and a relaxing environment are indispensable features in the operating theater.

Conclusion

A direct surgical approach is the most appropriate way to treat insular gliomas, and technical developments have provided many tools to assist the intraoperative management of these lesions. However, surgeons must assume that no decision should be based on the isolated findings provided by these devices, and the key point continues to be not only learning but also critiquing their results. The transsylvian avenue is the most appropriate surgical route to remove insular tumors and protect the healthy surrounding tissues. Despite the feasibility of removing these tumors without damaging the important microanatomic environment in which they are included, the surgeon's anatomic knowledge and microsurgical skills remain primary. Combining these features with preoperative, intraoperative, and postoperative modern devices will improve the surgeon's experience and provide a comprehensive understanding of this complex anatomic region.

We generally try to incorporate any novel device in our approach, but they must be considered as complementary, never indispensable, tools. None of these technologies by themselves determines a successful surgery; thus, we must learn from their results and confirm our previous thinking, but mainly we must critique and improve their functioning.

Moderator
Insular Tumors

Allan Friedman

Infiltrating gliomas have a predilection for the insula.[117] Twenty years ago, Yaşargil generated great excitement when he showed that surgery could safely be done on these "inoperable" tumors. Since that time, the relevant anatomy has been described in great detail and operative strategies have been honed.[118–122]

In this chapter, Türe and González-López summarized the previous publications on the essential anatomy a surgeon must master before contemplating surgery on insular gliomas. They went on to give the most thoughtful and detailed description of the transsylvian approach to insular tumors I have seen. Berger and Sanai reviewed the evidence supporting the benefits of aggressive resection of infiltrating gliomas. They reviewed their extensive experience with cortical and subcortical intraoperative mapping techniques and the risks associated with glioma surgery. They proposed an anatomic grading system to define the risks and relative chances of success in removing tumors from different regions of the insula, showing that tumors located in the posterior insula are less likely to be completely resected. Lama, Wolfsberger, and Sutherland showed us how advances in technology can improve operative results. Although their work employing intraoperative MRI is well known, their nascent work using robotics gives us a view of the future.

Anatomy

As stated in Türe and González-López's section, the key to insular glioma surgery is a good knowledge of anatomy. It would be hard to improve on their description; thus, I would like to emphasize some points. The gyral anatomy of the insula and sylvian fissure has been reviewed by Türe et al[123] and others.[124,125] The triangular-shaped insula is covered by the frontoparietal, temporal, and orbital opercula. The frontal operculum is parsed by the horizontal and ascending rami of the sylvian fissure into the pars orbicularis, triangularis, and orbitalis.[123] In most patients, the tip of the pars triangularis does not come in contact with the temporal operculum, and this arrangement provides a dependable route between the frontal and temporal opercula to the insula.[114,124] The distance from the cortical surface of the pars triangularis to the underlying superior limiting sulcus has been measured to be 2 cm in cadaver studies. The distance the surgeon must traverse from the cortical surface to the insula under the frontal operculum to the anterior end of the superior limiting sulcus is much greater in patients with large anterior insular tumors.[123,124,126] While opening the ascending ramus of the sylvian fissure would be a more direct route to the superior margin of the insula, such a maneuver risks injury to

crossing veins and damage to the pars opercularis and pars triangularis. The posterior orbital gyrus of the orbital opercularis is in continuity with the pars orbitalis or separated by the superficial orbital sulcus.[127] Extending the insular resection into the pars orbitalis and posterior orbital gyrus provides the surgeon access to the anterior aspect of insular tumors extending far into the inferior frontal lobe.

The surgeon must divide four layers of arachnoid when exposing the insula through the posterior ramus of the sylvian fissure.[113] The lateral-most projection of the insula is the insular apex, which usually involves the base of the middle short gyrus.[124] In large tumors, the insular apex may be just below the superficial sylvian veins. As the surgeon proceeds from anterior to posterior through the posterior ramus of the sylvian fissure, the distance between the frontoparietal and temporal opercula to the insula is deeper. Once the surgeon has reached the insula, the distance along the insula under the opercula to the superior and inferior limiting sulci is less posterior than anterior.

The anatomy and function of white matter tracts that surround the insula have been intensely studied over the past 5 years. The intact basal ganglia buffer the internal capsule from most low-grade insular tumors but the corona radiata containing the corticospinal fibers lies adjacent to the superior limiting sulcus at the level of the long insular gyri.[123,126,128,129] The third part of the superior longitudinal fasciculus lies deep to the frontoparietal operculum.[130] The inferior fronto-occipital fasciculus passes dorsal to the visual fibers in the temporal stem.[131,132]

Recently, a fiber tract that runs from the superior temporal lobe through the temporal stem and the extreme capsule to the frontal lobe has been described.[130] It is unclear whether these fibers differ from the interior fronto-occipital fasciculus. The inferior longitudinal fasciculus runs in the inferior lateral to the temporal horn, connecting the posterior temporal and occipital cortex with the temporal pole.[130,133] The middle longitudinal fasciculus runs lateral to the inferior frontal occipital fasciculus and predominantly connects fibers from the angular gyrus and posterior superior temporal lobe with the anterior superior temporal cortex.[134,135] Also running through the temporal stem are the optic radiations emanating from the lateral geniculate nucleus and passing over to the lateral surface of the lateral ventricle.

The lateral lenticulostriate arteries have been a concern to surgeons operating on insular gliomas. These vessels originate from M1, early frontal and temporal M1 branches, and proximal M2 branches. They pierce the anterior perforating substance and pass a short distance through the basal ganglia to reach the posterior limb of the internal capsule.[124,136] Thus, other than their short proximal passage from the middle cerebral artery through the basal white matter, the surgeon is unlikely to encounter these vessels lateral to the basal ganglia. What is of more concern is the vessels that originate from the distal M2 branches and provide blood supply to the corona radiata.[126,136]

The insula is supplied by about 100 small leptomeningeal vessels branching from the M2 arteries, which pass over the surface of the insula.[125,136] Most of these feeding vessels are small and should be coagulated and cut close to their origin to devascularize the tumor, thereby preventing inadvertent avulsion from their M2 origins when the tumor is manipulated. Larger perforating vessels are most prevalent penetrating the posterior long gyri and posterior superior limiting sulcus. They are described to be present in up to 25% of cadaver dissections.[124,125,128] In up to 5% of patients, these vessels have been shown to penetrate the corona radiata adjacent to the posterior limiting sulcus where corticospinal fibers are entering the posterior limb of the internal capsule.[95,125,136,137] These larger perforating arteries must be identified and preserved.[81]

The superficial sylvian veins can lie up to 4 mm below the posterior limb of the sylvian fissure and empty into the sphenoparietal sinus.[124] This position leads most surgeons who regularly open the sylvian fissure to expose aneurysms of the proximal middle cerebral artery or tumors originating from the sphenoid ridge to open the fissure superior to those veins. In fact, smaller purely insular tumors that reside posterior to the bifurcation of the middle cerebral artery are more easily approached by cutting the arachnoid on the temporal side of these veins.[129] This maneuver avoids the need to coagulate the veins passing over the frontal operculum. Temporal veins often drain into the vein of Labbé.[124] In practice, it is not uncommon to cut several windows in the arachnoid and work between the larger superficial veins. The superficial sylvian veins are sandwiched between an outer arachnoid membrane and a lateral arachnoid membrane.[113,138,139] Thus, the surgeon needs to cut both to enter the intraopercular space. As described by Inoue and colleagues,[113] the intermediate sylvian membrane spans the intraopercular space above the M2 branches and a medial sylvian membrane joins the frontoparietal operculum to the insula and must be divided to expose the superior insula. This last layer tends to hold the frontal parietal operculum against the insula.

Treatment Options

Observation alone is a decreasingly used option when a patient presents with a low-grade glioma. The extant literature indicates that, with longer follow-up, low-grade gliomas are likely to progress to a higher grade. There is no definitive study showing that early surgery improves outcome any better than surgery at the time of progression, but that question has not been well studied.[140,141]

A histological diagnosis is necessary before initiating therapy. Although a stereotactic biopsy is a low-risk procedure, these tumors are not necessarily homogeneous and a biopsy risks undergrading the tumor.[142]

Radiation Therapy

The efficacy of radiation therapy in prolonging progression-free survival has been shown in a randomized trial, but the efficacy of radiation in improving overall survival is derived from comparing case series. A study looking at administering radiation therapy at the time of diagnosis or withholding radiation until the time of disease progression showed no difference in overall survival.[143] Many centers do not initiate radiation therapy until the tumor has been shown to progress to avoid the delayed side effects of such therapy. Raising the dose from 50 to 60 Gy does not increase 5-year survival or progression-free survival but does increase the rate of radiation necrosis. Thus, the accepted dose is 50 Gy in 18-Gy fractions.[144,145]

Chemotherapy

Temozolomide has shown efficacy in 30 to 60% of patients harboring a low-grade tumor. Studies are in progress comparing the efficacy of this drug with the efficacy of radiation therapy.

Surgical Resection

The data supporting surgical resection of low-grade gliomas is compelling but based on uncontrolled case studies.[27,28,30,84,132,146–153] It is always possible that surgical resectability is a surrogate for a more compact, less invasive tumor with a natural better prognosis. It is clear that an oligodendroglioma histology and genetic marker such as IDH-1 and chromosome 1p/19q mutations portend an improved prognosis in patients with grade II gliomas.

Low-grade tumors vary from compact to diffuse. Most surgeons are more comfortable resecting visually abnormal tissue than normal-appearing tissue with a signal abnormality on T2-weighted MRI, but there is growing evidence that an extended resection improves prognosis. It is more difficult to get an MRI-complete resection with a diffuse tumor than with a well-circumscribed tumor.[154,155] Hentschel and Lang[81] used the sharpness of the border on a T2-weighted MRI to determine whether the tumor was circumscribed or diffuse. Skrap and associates[6] noted that tumors that were congruent on T1-weighted and on FLAIR MRI were most likely to be resectable. It is my experience that congruence on T1- and T2-weighted MRIs portends a tumor whose appearance is easier to differentiate from normal brain and that shows more complete resection on postoperative MRI scans.[155]

Surgical Therapy

Türe and González-López provided a very detailed description of the classic transsylvian approach to insular gliomas.

They operate with the patient under general anesthesia and guide the resection by anatomy and not physiology. Berger and Sanai advocate the use of functional mapping in awake patients. Functional mapping of the cortical and subcortical motor function has been well described. Although functional mapping of the cerebral cortex was made popular by the writings of Penfield, subcortical mapping of language function is a less standard procedure.

Duffau[27] has written extensively about mapping cortical and subcortical language at the time of surgery for a tumor in the dominant hemisphere. With other authors, he reports that subcortical stimulation of the suprasylvian white matter caused phonemic paraphasia, and stimulation of the inferior fronto-occipital tract caused semantic paraphasia. He describes a difficulty in articulation when stimulating the deep white-matter fibers of the parietal lobe adjacent to the sylvian fissure (superior longitudinal fasciculus) and phonemic paraphasia when more superior in the deep parietal white matter (arcuate fasciculus).[5] He has shown that stimulation along the inferior fronto-occipital fasciculus results in semantic paraphasia, but stimulation of the inferior and middle longitudinal fasciculi does not.[67,131–133] He indicates that stimulating above the temporal horn results in semantic paraphasia but stimulating lateral to the temporal horn does not.

In my hands, the results of subcortical stimulation are not quite as clean. Stimulation of the white matter deep to the parietal operculum sometimes results in phonemic paraphasia but more frequently results in hesitation or mechanical problems with speech. I have not seen the clear-cut ventral dorsal differences in responses reported by Duffau. Stimulation of the white matter lateral to the temporal horn but deep to the superior and inferior temporal sulci can result in semantic paraphasia in some patients. The removal of white matter in this area can result in a speech difficulty lasting up to 6 weeks. Thus, I have not been able to show that language function is confined to the classic inferior fronto-occipital fasciculus and does not extend into the longitudinal fasciculi in some patients.

Controversy remains as to the optimal approach to tumors in the sylvian fissure region that do not extend to a lateral cortical surface.[5,12,27,81,105,106,126,146,149] Türe and González-López advocate a purely transsylvian approach. Berger and Sanai prefer a transopercular transcortical approach.[22,27] Both approaches are valid. The approach a surgeon uses should be based on the expertise and experience of that surgeon. The references cited by Berger and Sanai favoring a transcortical approach are not convincing.

The transsylvian approach requires a wide separation of the three opercula from the insula extending to the limiting sulci. This requires meticulous and patient dissection. The transsylvian approach allows the surgeon to trace the M2 branches from the bifurcation of the MCA when the tumor has broken through the pia at the insula and surrounded these vessels. The approach also allows the surgeon to ligate the small leptomeningeal insular vessels as they come off the M2 arteries, and avoid the possibility of

these arteries being avulsed during tumor removal. The surgeon can trace the lenticulostriate vessels from their origin. Difficulties with this approach are that the surgeon is removing tumor through windows between the M2 branches and that exposure of the anterior superior corner of the insula requires significant manipulation of the frontal operculum. The transcortical approach opens a wide window into the tumor, but the surgeon is dependent on a subpial dissection to protect the branches of the MCA. Feeding vessels are encountered in the tumor.

I have adopted a hybrid approach. I operate on all large, dominant, diffuse insular tumors with the patient awake during resection of the tumor. While operating with the patient under general anesthesia is adequate for a well-circumscribed lesion, having the patient awake helps me when the borders of the tumor are less well defined. When resecting the margin of the tumor especially close to the temporal stem, the patient may develop difficulty with naming. With the patient awake, I can stop the resection at a time when the patient will most probably make a good recovery. If the patient suffers a deficit that I believe may be of vascular origin, I can use papaverine to mitigate any spasm and raise the patient's blood pressure. Although I have no controlled data, I believe that rapid intervention can limit the ischemic damage. I have two patients who have made a good functional recovery despite restricted diffusion in the corona radiata on the postoperative MRI. With an experienced surgical team, the patients can be kept comfortable and calm throughout the procedure.

I believe that the transcortical approach affords a better view of the anterior portion of a large tumor, and the transsylvian approach provides better control of the vasculature. I use a wide exposure at the insula to gain control of the vasculature, and a transcortical approach through the pars orbicularis and posterior orbital gyrus to remove large frontobasilar extensions without retracting the frontal operculum. I begin by opening the posterior ramus of the sylvian fissure, exposing the apex of the insula, the length of the inferior limiting sulcus, the inferior portion of the anterior limiting sulcus, and the posterior segment of the superior limiting sulcus as required to expose the posterior aspect of the tumor. If the tumor is small and does not have a large anterior, superior, or inferior frontal component, the transsylvian approach is sufficient to allow exposure of the anterior superior portion of the insula. If the tumor has a large superior component or if it has a large extension into the frontal lobe between the inferior frontal lobe and the lateral ventricle, I extend my corticotomy anterior to the anterior limiting sulcus into the posterior orbital gyrus and pars orbitalis of the frontal lobe, providing access to the mesial inferior frontal extension of the tumor. Lang and associates[126] reported that retracting the frontal operculum can lead to a language disturbance.

This approach provides an early definition of the sylvian arteries, the ability to ligate small insular leptomeningeal arteries as they branch from the M2 vessels, and the ability to identify and preserve any large artery perforating the superior insula behind the central sulcus. The extension into the pars orbitalis and posterior orbital gyrus allows me to remove the inferior medial tumor without significant manipulation of the frontal operculum. Intraoperative ultrasound helps avoid large surprises on postoperative studies.

Morbidity

It is clear that morbidity decreases with the experience of the surgeon.[5,6,95] Most surgeons have noted that operating on low-grade tumors has less morbidity than operating on high-grade tumors in this area.[5] I find that high-grade tumors are more difficult to separate from the lenticulostriate vessels. In patients with high-grade tumors infiltrating the basal ganglia, the surgeon must identify the lenticulostriate vessels proximal to the tumor in the basal ganglia and then follow them through an often vascular tumor. The lack of a preoperative deficit and younger age are associated with a lower surgical morbidity.[5]

The literature indicates a rate of 4 to 9% permanent morbidity from the surgical resection.[5,126] Most authors note significant numbers of transient postoperative language deficits when operating on the language-dominant insula.[67,126,133,156–159] It is my experience that, if the patient loses the ability to visually name but can read or repeat, the language function will return to baseline. Speech hesitation or dysarthria persists beyond classic expressive or receptive dysphasias.[22] Also of note is that the preoperative frequency of seizures improved in about 75% of patients.[5,12,22,27,129,159]

The extent of resection depends on patient selection as well as the surgeon's experience.[5,34,95] A survey of the extant literature indicates that 80% of patients can have a greater than 70% resection, with 90% resection in half of all patients.[5,126,130]

New Technology

Lama, Wolfsberger, and Sutherland address the technical advances that can aid in tumor resection, and Sutherland's pioneering work using intraoperative MRI is well known. A growing number of studies indicate its value in glioma surgery.[40,42,43] The question that confronts the surgeon is in the case of a diffuse glioma: Does further resection of an area of normal-appearing brain with an increased T2 signal have a significant risk of evoking a new neurologic deficit? The combination of awake surgery with intraoperative MRI remains challenging.

Robotic surgery is intriguing and can directly integrate the imaging studies to prevent the resection of functionally important brain tissue. I have had opportunities to experiment with a bimanual robot on a cadaver brain. The robotic arms were easy to use. Through a subtemporal approach, I was able to cut and re-anastomose a basilar artery. The problem was that the temporal lobe, which was outside the view of my camera, was pulped. There was insufficient constraint on the movement of the arms outside my field of vision. Considering the fact that much of insular tumor resection takes place underneath the three opercula, I do not believe that the robot is ready for use in this procedure. I look forward to the day that it is.

References

1. Lang FF, Olansen NE, DeMonte F, et al. Surgical resection of intrinsic insular tumors: complication avoidance. J Neurosurg 2001;95:638–650

2. Majchrzak K, Bobek-Billewicz B, Tymowski M, Adamczyk P, Majchrzak H, Ladziński P. Surgical treatment of insular tumours with tractography, functional magnetic resonance imaging, transcranial electrical stimulation and direct subcortical stimulation support. Neurol Neurochir Pol 2011; 45:351–362

3. Saito R, Kumabe T, Kanamori M, Sonoda Y, Tominaga T. Insulo-opercular gliomas: four different natural progression patterns and implications for surgical indications. Neurol Med Chir (Tokyo) 2010;50:286–290

4. Signorelli F, Guyotat J, Elisevich K, Barbagallo GM. Review of current microsurgical management of insular gliomas. Acta Neurochir (Wien) 2010;152:19–26

5. Simon M, Neuloh G, von Lehe M, Meyer B, Schramm J. Insular gliomas: the case for surgical management. J Neurosurg 2009;110:685–695

6. Skrap M, Mondani M, Tomasino B, et al. Surgery of insular nonenhancing gliomas: volumetric analysis of tumoral resection, clinical outcome, and survival in a consecutive series of 66 cases. Neurosurgery 2012;70:1081–1093, discussion 1093–1094

7. Talos IF, Zou KH, Ohno-Machado L, et al. Supratentorial low-grade glioma resectability: statistical predictive analysis based on anatomic MR features and tumor characteristics. Radiology 2006;239:506–513

8. Vanaclocha V, Sáiz-Sapena N, García-Casasola C. Surgical treatment of insular gliomas. Acta Neurochir (Wien) 1997; 139:1126–1134, discussion 1134–1135

9. Wu AS, Witgert ME, Lang FF, et al. Neurocognitive function before and after surgery for insular gliomas. J Neurosurg 2011;115:1115–1125

10. Yaşargil MG. Microneurosurgery, vol. 4. New York: Thieme, 1996

11. Yaşargil MG, von Ammon K, Cavazos E, Doczi T, Reeves JD, Roth P. Tumours of the limbic and paralimbic systems. Acta Neurochir (Wien) 1992;118:40–52

12. Zentner J, Meyer B, Stangl A, Schramm J. Intrinsic tumors of the insula: a prospective surgical study of 30 patients. J Neurosurg 1996;85:263–271

13. Tanriover N, Rhoton AL Jr, Kawashima M, Ulm AJ, Yasuda A. Microsurgical anatomy of the insula and the sylvian fissure. J Neurosurg 2004;100:891–922

14. Türe U, Yaşargil MG, Al-Mefty O, Yaşargil DC. Arteries of the insula. J Neurosurg 2000;92:676–687

15. Isolan GR, Bianchin MM, Bragatti JA, Torres C, Schwarts-

mann G. Musical hallucinations following insular glioma resection. Neurosurg Focus 2010;28:E9

16. Shelley BP, Trimble MR. The insular lobe of Reil—its anatomico-functional, behavioural and neuropsychiatric attributes in humans—a review. World J Biol Psychiatry 2004;5:176–200

17. Türe U, Yaşargil DC, Al-Mefty O, Yaşargil MG. Topographic anatomy of the insular region. J Neurosurg 1999;90:720–733

18. Mehrkens JH, Kreth FW, Muacevic A, Ostertag CB. Long term course of WHO grade II astrocytomas of the Insula of Reil after I-125 interstitial irradiation. J Neurol 2004;251:1455–1464

19. Schramm J, Aliashkevich AF. Surgery for temporal mediobasal tumors: experience based on a series of 235 patients. Neurosurgery 2007;60:285–294, discussion 294–295

20. Shankar A, Rajshekhar V. Radiological and clinical outcome following stereotactic biopsy and radiotherapy for low-grade insular astrocytomas. Neurol India 2003;51:503–506

21. Duffau H, Capelle L. Preferential brain locations of low-grade gliomas. Cancer 2004;100:2622–2626

22. Sanai N, Polley MY, Berger MS. Insular glioma resection: assessment of patient morbidity, survival, and tumor progression. J Neurosurg 2010;112:1–9

23. Muragaki Y, Chernov M, Maruyama T, et al. Low-grade glioma on stereotactic biopsy: how often is the diagnosis accurate? Minim Invasive Neurosurg 2008;51:275–279

24. Sanai N, Mirzadeh Z, Berger MS. Functional outcome after language mapping for glioma resection. N Engl J Med 2008;358:18–27

25. Saito R, Kumabe T, Inoue T, et al. Magnetic resonance imaging for preoperative identification of the lenticulostriate arteries in insular glioma surgery. Technical note. J Neurosurg 2009;111:278–281

26. Moshel YA, Marcus JD, Parker EC, Kelly PJ. Resection of insular gliomas: the importance of lenticulostriate artery position. J Neurosurg 2008;109:825–834

27. Duffau H. A personal consecutive series of surgically treated 51 cases of insular WHO grade II glioma: advances and limitations. J Neurosurg 2009;110:696–708

28. Smith JS, Chang EF, Lamborn KR, et al. Role of extent of resection in the long-term outcome of low-grade hemispheric gliomas. J Clin Oncol 2008;26:1338–1345

29. Keles GE, Chang EF, Lamborn KR, et al. Volumetric extent of resection and residual contrast enhancement on initial surgery as predictors of outcome in adult patients with hemispheric anaplastic astrocytoma. J Neurosurg 2006;105:34–40

30. Sanai N, Berger MS. Glioma extent of resection and its impact on patient outcome. Neurosurgery 2008;62:753–764, discussion 264–266

31. Lamborn KR, Chang SM, Prados MD. Prognostic factors for survival of patients with glioblastoma: recursive partitioning analysis. Neuro-oncol 2004;6:227–235

32. Scott JN, Brasher PM, Sevick RJ, Rewcastle NB, Forsyth PA. How often are nonenhancing supratentorial gliomas malignant? A population study. Neurology 2002;59:947–949

33. Widhalm G, Wolfsberger S, Minchev G, et al. 5-Aminolevulinic acid is a promising marker for detection of anaplastic foci in diffusely infiltrating gliomas with nonsignificant contrast enhancement. Cancer 2010;116:1545–1552

34. Claus EB, Horlacher A, Hsu L, et al. Survival rates in patients with low-grade glioma after intraoperative magnetic resonance image guidance. Cancer 2005;103:1227–1233

35. Yordanova YN, Moritz-Gasser S, Duffau H; Clinical Article. Awake surgery for WHO grade II gliomas within "non-eloquent" areas in the left dominant hemisphere: toward a "supratotal" resection. Clinical article. J Neurosurg 2011;115:232–239

36. Black PM, Moriarty T, Alexander E III, et al. Development and implementation of intraoperative magnetic resonance imaging and its neurosurgical applications. Neurosurgery 1997;41:831–842, discussion 842–845

37. Steinmeier R, Fahlbusch R, Ganslandt O, et al. Intraoperative magnetic resonance imaging with the Magnetom open scanner: concepts, neurosurgical indications, and procedures: a preliminary report. Neurosurgery 1998;43:739–747, discussion 747–748

38. Sutherland GR, Kaibara T, Louw D, Hoult DI, Tomanek B, Saunders J. A mobile high-field magnetic resonance system for neurosurgery. J Neurosurg 1999;91:804–813

39. Hall WA, Martin AJ, Liu H, Nussbaum ES, Maxwell RE, Truwit CL. Brain biopsy using high-field strength interventional magnetic resonance imaging. Neurosurgery 1999;44:807–813, discussion 813–814

40. Albert FK, Forsting M, Sartor K, Adams HP, Kunze S. Early postoperative magnetic resonance imaging after resection of malignant glioma: objective evaluation of residual tumor and its influence on regrowth and prognosis. Neurosurgery 1994;34:45–60, discussion 60–61

41. Senft C, Bink A, Franz K, Vatter H, Gasser T, Seifert V. Intraoperative MRI guidance and extent of resection in glioma surgery: a randomised, controlled trial. Lancet Oncol 2011;12:997–1003

42. Senft C, Forster MT, Bink A, et al. Optimizing the extent of resection in eloquently located gliomas by combining intraoperative MRI guidance with intraoperative neurophysiological monitoring. J Neurooncol 2012;109:81–90

43. Chen X, Meng X, Zhang J, et al. Low-grade insular glioma resection with 1.5T intraoperative MRI: preliminary results of a prospective randomized trial. AANS Annual Scientific Meeting, April 2012, Miami, Florida

44. Sutherland GR, Latour I, Greer AD, Fielding T, Feil G, Newhook P. An image-guided magnetic resonance-compatible surgical robot. Neurosurgery 2008;62:286–292, discussion 292–293

45. Hongo K, Kobayashi S, Kakizawa Y, et al. NeuRobot: tele-controlled micromanipulator system for minimally invasive microneurosurgery-preliminary results. Neurosurgery 2002;51:985–988, discussion 988

46. Nathoo N, Cavuşoğlu MC, Vogelbaum MA, Barnett GH. In touch with robotics: neurosurgery for the future. Neurosurgery 2005;56:421–433, discussion 421–433

47. Le Roux PD, Das H, Esquenazi S, Kelly PJ. Robot-assisted microsurgery: a feasibility study in the rat. Neurosurgery 2001;48:584–589

48. Pandya S, Motkoski JW, Serrano-Almeida C, Greer AD, Latour I, Sutherland GR. Advancing neurosurgery with image-guided robotics. J Neurosurg 2009;111:1141–1149

49. Sutherland GR, Latour I, Greer AD. Integrating an image-guided robot with intraoperative MRI: a review of the design and construction of neuroArm. IEEE Eng Med Biol Mag 2008;27:59–65

50. Sutherland GR. Surgeon at a Work Station: Information Age Surgery. Cureus Online J. 2012;1:1

51. Ribas GC. The cerebral sulci and gyri. Neurosurg Focus 2010;28:E2

52. Yaşargil MG, Krisht AF, Türe U, Al-Mefty O, Yaşargil DCH. Microsurgery of Insular Gliomas. Part II: Opening of the Sylvian Fissure. Contemp Neurosurg. 2002;24:1–6

53. Yaşargil MG. Insular Tumors. Microneurosurgery, vol. IVB. New York: Thieme, 1996:263–268

54. Craig AD. How do you feel? Interoception: the sense of the physiological condition of the body. Nat Rev Neurosci 2002; 3:655–666

55. Khalsa SS, Rudrauf D, Feinstein JS, Tranel D. The pathways of interoceptive awareness. Nat Neurosci 2009;12:1494–1496

56. Cauda F, D'Agata F, Sacco K, Duca S, Geminiani G, Vercelli A. Functional connectivity of the insula in the resting brain. Neuroimage 2011;55:8–23

57. Guldin WO, Markowitsch HJ. Cortical and thalamic afferent connections of the insular and adjacent cortex of the cat. J Comp Neurol 1984;229:393–418

58. Zacà D, Nickerson JP, Deib G, Pillai JJ. Effectiveness of four different clinical fMRI paradigms for preoperative regional determination of language lateralization in patients with brain tumors. Neuroradiology 2012;54:1015–1025

59. Pillai JJ. The evolution of clinical functional imaging during the past 2 decades and its current impact on neurosurgical planning. AJNR Am J Neuroradiol 2010;31:219–225

60. Shaywitz BA, Shaywitz SE, Pugh KR, et al. Sex differences in the functional organization of the brain for language. Nature 1995;373:607–609

61. Clements AM, Rimrodt SL, Abel JR, et al. Sex differences in cerebral laterality of language and visuospatial processing. Brain Lang 2006;98:150–158

62. Skirboll SS, Ojemann GA, Berger MS, Lettich E, Winn HR. Functional cortex and subcortical white matter located within gliomas. Neurosurgery 1996;38:678–684, discussion 684–685

63. Kuhnt D, Bauer MH, Nimsky C. Brain shift compensation and neurosurgical image fusion using intraoperative MRI: current status and future challenges. Crit Rev Biomed Eng 2012;40:175–185

64. Hill DL, Maurer CR Jr, Maciunas RJ, Barwise JA, Fitzpatrick JM, Wang MY. Measurement of intraoperative brain surface deformation under a craniotomy. Neurosurgery 1998;43: 514–526, discussion 527–528

65. Dorward NL, Alberti O, Velani B, et al. Postimaging brain distortion: magnitude, correlates, and impact on neuronavigation. J Neurosurg 1998;88:656–662

66. Duffau H, Peggy Gatignol ST, Mandonnet E, Capelle L, Taillandier L. Intraoperative subcortical stimulation mapping of language pathways in a consecutive series of 115 patients with grade II glioma in the left dominant hemisphere. J Neurosurg 2008;109:461–471

67. Bello L, Gallucci M, Fava M, et al. Intraoperative subcortical language tract mapping guides surgical removal of gliomas involving speech areas. Neurosurgery 2007;60:67–80, discussion 80–82

68. Paulus W, Peiffer J. Intratumoral histologic heterogeneity of gliomas. A quantitative study. Cancer 1989;64:442–447

69. Widhalm G, Krssak M, Minchev G, et al. Value of 1H-magnetic resonance spectroscopy chemical shift imaging for detection of anaplastic foci in diffusely infiltrating gliomas with non-significant contrast-enhancement. J Neurol Neurosurg Psychiatry 2011;82:512–520

70. Peeling J, Sutherland G. High-resolution 1H NMR spectroscopy studies of extracts of human cerebral neoplasms. Magn Reson Med 1992;24:123–136

71. Nossek E, Korn A, Shahar T, et al; Clinical Article. Intraoperative mapping and monitoring of the corticospinal tracts with neurophysiological assessment and 3-dimensional ultrasonography-based navigation. Clinical article. J Neurosurg 2011;114:738–746

72. Mikuni N, Okada T, Enatsu R, et al. Clinical significance of preoperative fibre-tracking to preserve the affected pyramidal tracts during resection of brain tumours in patients with preoperative motor weakness. J Neurol Neurosurg Psychiatry 2007;78:716–721

73. Berger MS, Ghatan S, Haglund MM, Dobbins J, Ojemann GA. Low-grade gliomas associated with intractable epilepsy: seizure outcome utilizing electrocorticography during tumor resection. J Neurosurg 1993;79:62–69

74. Zentner J, Hufnagel A, Wolf HK, et al. Surgical treatment of neoplasms associated with medically intractable epilepsy. Neurosurgery 1997;41:378–386, discussion 386–387

75. Isnard J, Guénot M, Ostrowsky K, Sindou M, Mauguière F. The role of the insular cortex in temporal lobe epilepsy. Ann Neurol 2000;48:614–623

76. Taillandier L, Duffau H. Epilepsy and insular grade II gliomas: an interdisciplinary point of view from a retrospective monocentric series of 46 cases. Neurosurg Focus 2009;27:E8

77. Haglund MM, Berger MS, Kunkel DD, Franck JE, Ghatan S, Ojemann GA. Changes in gamma-aminobutyric acid and somatostatin in epileptic cortex associated with low-grade gliomas. J Neurosurg 1992;77:209–216

78. Penfield W. Activation of the Record of Human Experience: Summary of the Lister Oration delivered at the Royal College of Surgeons of England on 27th April 1961. Ann R Coll Surg Engl 1961;29:77–84

79. Ojemann G, Ojemann J, Lettich E, Berger M. Cortical language localization in left, dominant hemisphere. An electrical stimulation mapping investigation in 117 patients. 1989. J Neurosurg 2008;108:411–421

80. Duffau H, Taillandier L, Gatignol P, Capelle L. The insular lobe and brain plasticity: Lessons from tumor surgery. Clin Neurol Neurosurg 2006;108:543–548

81. Hentschel SJ, Lang FF. Surgical resection of intrinsic insular tumors. Neurosurgery 2005;57(1, Suppl):176–183, discussion 176–183

82. Lang FF, Olansen NE, DeMonte F, et al. Surgical resection of intrinsic insular tumors: complication avoidance. J Neurosurg 2001;95:638–650

83. Gil-Robles S, Duffau H. Surgical management of World Health Organization grade II gliomas in eloquent areas: the necessity of preserving a margin around functional structures. Neurosurg Focus 2010;28:E8

84. Berger MS, Deliganis AV, Dobbins J, Keles GE. The effect of extent of resection on recurrence in patients with low grade cerebral hemisphere gliomas. Cancer 1994;74:1784–1791

85. Keles GE, Lamborn KR, Berger MS. Low-grade hemispheric gliomas in adults: a critical review of extent of resection as a factor influencing outcome. J Neurosurg 2001;95:735–745

86. Shaw EG, Berkey B, Coons SW, et al. Recurrence following neurosurgeon-determined gross-total resection of adult supratentorial low-grade glioma: results of a prospective clinical trial. J Neurosurg 2008;109:835–841

87. Giese A, Bjerkvig R, Berens ME, Westphal M. Cost of migration: invasion of malignant gliomas and implications for treatment. J Clin Oncol 2003;21:1624–1636

88. McGirt MJ, Chaichana KL, Attenello FJ, et al. Extent of surgical resection is independently associated with survival in patients with hemispheric infiltrating low-grade gliomas. Neurosurgery 2008;63:700–707, author reply 707–708

89. McGirt MJ, Chaichana KL, Gathinji M, et al. Independent association of extent of resection with survival in patients with malignant brain astrocytoma. J Neurosurg 2009;110:156–162

90. Price SJ, Jena R, Burnet NG, et al. Improved delineation of glioma margins and regions of infiltration with the use of diffusion tensor imaging: an image-guided biopsy study. AJNR Am J Neuroradiol 2006;27:1969–1974

91. Provenzale JM, McGraw P, Mhatre P, Guo AC, Delong D. Peritumoral brain regions in gliomas and meningiomas: investigation with isotropic diffusion-weighted MR imaging and diffusion-tensor MR imaging. Radiology 2004;232:451–460

92. Stummer W, Stocker S, Wagner S, et al. Intraoperative detection of malignant gliomas by 5-aminolevulinic acid-induced porphyrin fluorescence. Neurosurgery 1998;42:518–525, discussion 525–526

93. Türe U, Kaya AH. Principles for managing cavernous malformations in eloquent locations. In: Rigamonti D, ed. Cavernous Malformations of the Nervous Systems. Cambridge, England: Cambridge University Press, 2011:161–172

94. Kombos T, Süss O, Vajkoczy P. Subcortical mapping and monitoring during insular tumor surgery. Neurosurg Focus 2009;27:E5

95. Duffau H, Capelle L, Lopes M, Faillot T, Sichez JP, Fohanno D. The insular lobe: physiopathological and surgical considerations. Neurosurgery 2000;47:801–810, discussion 810–811

96. Kalani MY, Kalani MA, Gwinn R, Keogh B, Tse VC. Embryological development of the human insula and its implications for the spread and resection of insular gliomas. Neurosurg Focus 2009;27:E2

97. Malak R, Bouthillier A, Carmant L, et al. Microsurgery of epileptic foci in the insular region. J Neurosurg 2009;110:1153–1163

98. Roper SN, Lévesque MF, Sutherling WW, Engel J Jr. Surgical treatment of partial epilepsy arising from the insular cortex. Report of two cases. J Neurosurg 1993;79:266–269

99. Wu AS, Witgert ME, Lang FF, et al. Neurocognitive function before and after surgery for insular gliomas. J Neurosurg 2011;115:1115–1125

100. Berthier M, Starkstein S, Leiguarda R. Behavioral effects of damage to the right insula and surrounding regions. Cortex 1987;23:673–678

101. Starkstein SE, Berthier M, Leiguarda R. Bilateral opercular syndrome and crossed aphemia due to a right insular lesion: a clinicopathological study. Brain Lang 1988;34:253–261

102. Vignolo LA, Boccardi E, Caverni L. Unexpected CT-scan findings in global aphasia. Cortex 1986;22:55–69

103. Yaşargil MG. Microneurosurgery, vols. I–IV. Stuttgart: Georg Thieme, 1984–1996

104. Penfield W, Faulk ME Jr. The insula; further observations on its function. Brain 1955;78:445–470

105. Guillaume J, Mazars G, Mazars Y. Surgical indications in so-called temporal epilepsy. Rev Neurol (Paris) 1953;88:461–501, passim

106. Yaşargil MG, Reeves JD. Tumours of the limbic and paralimbic system. Acta Neurochir (Wien) 1992;116:147–149

107. Yaşargil MG, Krisht AF, Türe U, Al-Mefty O, Yaşargil DCH. Microsurgery of insular gliomas. Parts I–IV. Contemp Neurosurg. 2002;24:11–14

108. Duffau H, Moritz-Gasser S, Gatignol P. Functional outcome after language mapping for insular World Health Organization grade II gliomas in the dominant hemisphere: experience with 24 patients. Neurosurg Focus 2009;27:E7

109. Neuloh G, Pechstein U, Schramm J. Motor tract monitoring during insular glioma surgery. J Neurosurg 2007;106:582–592

110. Berger MS, Hadjipanayis CG. Surgery of intrinsic cerebral tumors. Neurosurgery 2007;61(1, Suppl):279–304, discussion 304–305

111. Kovanlikaya I, Firat Z, Kovanlikaya A, et al. Assessment of the corticospinal tract alterations before and after resection of brainstem lesions using diffusion tensor imaging (DTI) and tractography at 3T. Eur J Radiol 2011;77:383–391

112. González-Darder JM, González-López P, Talamantes F, et al. Multimodal navigation in the functional microsurgical resection of intrinsic brain tumors located in eloquent motor areas: role of tractography. Neurosurg Focus 2010;28:E5

113. Inoue K, Seker A, Osawa S, Alencastro LF, Matsushima T, Rhoton AL Jr. Microsurgical and endoscopic anatomy of the supratentorial arachnoidal membranes and cisterns. Neurosurgery 2009;65:644–664, discussion 665

114. Ribas GC, Ribas EC, Rodrigues CJ. The anterior sylvian point and the suprasylvian operculum. Neurosurg Focus 2005;18:E2

115. Kumabe T, Higano S, Takahashi S, Tominaga T. Ischemic complications associated with resection of opercular glioma. J Neurosurg 2007;106:263–269

116. Leclercq D, Duffau H, Delmaire C, et al. Comparison of diffusion tensor imaging tractography of language tracts and intraoperative subcortical stimulations. J Neurosurg 2010;112:503–511

117. Duffau H, Capelle L. Preferential brain locations of low-grade gliomas. Cancer 2004;100:2622–2626

118. Akert K. Das Limbische System. In: Zenker W, ed. Benninghoff Anatomie, vol. 3. Munich: Urban and Schwarzenberg, 1985:395–416

119. Yaşargil MG. Microneurosurgery, vol. IVB. New York: Thieme, 1996

120. Yaşargil MG, Wieser HG, Valavanis A, von Ammon K, Roth P. Surgery and results of selective amygdala-hippocampectomy in one hundred patients with nonlesional limbic epilepsy. Neurosurg Clin N Am 1993;4:243–261

121. Shafqat S, Hedley-Whyte ET, Henson JW. Age-dependent rate of anaplastic transformation in low-grade astrocytoma. Neurology 1999;52:867–869

122. Yaşargil MG. Insular tumors. In: Yaşargil MG, ed. Microneurosurgery, vol. IVB. New York: Thieme, 1996:263–268

123. Türe U, Yaşargil DC, Al-Mefty O, Yaşargil MG. Topographic anatomy of the insular region. J Neurosurg 1999;90:720–733

124. Tanriover N, Rhoton AL Jr, Kawashima M, Ulm AJ, Yasuda A. Microsurgical anatomy of the insula and the sylvian fissure. J Neurosurg 2004;100:891–922

125. Varnavas GG, Grand W. The insular cortex: morphological and vascular anatomic characteristics. Neurosurgery 1999; 44:127–136, discussion 136–138

126. Lang FF, Olansen NE, DeMonte F, et al. Surgical resection of intrinsic insular tumors: complication avoidance. J Neurosurg 2001;95:638–650

127. Ribas GC. The cerebral sulci and gyri. Neurosurg Focus 2010;28:E2

128. Yaşargil MG, von Ammon K, Cavazos E, Doczi T, Reeves JD, Roth P. Tumours of the limbic and paralimbic systems. Acta Neurochir (Wien) 1992;118:40–52

129. Vanaclocha V, Sáiz-Sapena N, García-Casasola C. Surgical treatment of insular gliomas. Acta Neurochir (Wien) 1997; 139:1126–1134, discussion 1134–1135

130. Schmahmann JD, Pandya DN, Wang R, et al. Association fibre pathways of the brain: parallel observations from diffusion spectrum imaging and autoradiography. Brain 2007;130(Pt 3):630–653

131. Duffau H, Peggy Gatignol ST, Mandonnet E, Capelle L, Taillandier L. Intraoperative subcortical stimulation mapping of language pathways in a consecutive series of 115 patients with grade II glioma in the left dominant hemisphere. J Neurosurg 2008;109:461–471

132. Martino J, Brogna C, Robles SG, Vergani F, Duffau H. Anatomic dissection of the inferior fronto-occipital fasciculus revisited in the lights of brain stimulation data. Cortex 2010;46:691–699

133. Mandonnet E, Nouet A, Gatignol P, Capelle L, Duffau H. Does the left inferior longitudinal fasciculus play a role in language? A brain stimulation study. Brain 2007;130 (Pt 3):623–629

134. Beauchamp MS, Yasar NE, Frye RE, Ro T. Touch, sound and vision in human superior temporal sulcus. Neuroimage 2008;41:1011–1020

135. Bernstein LE, Auer ET Jr, Wagner M, Ponton CW. Spatiotemporal dynamics of audiovisual speech processing. Neuroimage 2008;39:423–435

136. Türe U, Yaşargil MG, Al-Mefty O, Yaşargil DC. Arteries of the insula. J Neurosurg 2000;92:676–687

137. Kaneko N, Boling WW, Shonai T, et al. Delineation of the safe zone in surgery of sylvian insular triangle: morphometric analysis and magnetic resonance imaging study. Neurosurgery 2012;70(2, Suppl Operative):290–298, discussion 298–299

138. Yaşargil MG. Microneurosurgery, vol. I. New York: Thieme, 1984:5–53

139. Yaşargil MG, Kasdaglis K, Jain KK, Weber HP. Anatomical observations of the subarachnoid cisterns of the brain during surgery. J Neurosurg 1976;44:298–302

140. Recht LD, Lew R, Smith TW. Suspected low-grade glioma: is deferring treatment safe? Ann Neurol 1992;31:431–436

141. van Veelen ML, Avezaat CJ, Kros JM, van Putten W, Vecht C. Supratentorial low grade astrocytoma: prognostic factors, dedifferentiation, and the issue of early versus late surgery. J Neurol Neurosurg Psychiatry 1998;64:581–587

142. Woodworth GF, McGirt MJ, Samdani A, Garonzik I, Olivi A, Weingart JD. Frameless image-guided stereotactic brain biopsy procedure: diagnostic yield, surgical morbidity, and comparison with the frame-based technique. J Neurosurg 2006;104:233–237

143. van den Bent MJ, Afra D, de Witte O, et al; EORTC Radiotherapy and Brain Tumor Groups and the UK Medical Research Council. Long-term efficacy of early versus delayed radiotherapy for low-grade astrocytoma and oligodendroglioma in adults: the EORTC 22845 randomised trial. Lancet 2005;366:985–990

144. Shaw E, Arusell R, Scheithauer B, et al. Prospective randomized trial of low- versus high-dose radiation therapy in adults with supratentorial low-grade glioma: initial report of a North Central Cancer Treatment Group/Radiation Therapy Oncology Group/Eastern Cooperative Oncology Group study. J Clin Oncol 2002;20:2267–2276

145. Karim AB, Maat B, Hatlevoll R, et al. A randomized trial on dose-response in radiation therapy of low-grade cerebral glioma: European Organization for Research and Treatment of Cancer (EORTC) Study 22844. Int J Radiat Oncol Biol Phys 1996;36:549–556

146. Maldonado IL, Moritz-Gasser S, de Champfleur NM, Bertram L, Moulinié G, Duffau H. Surgery for gliomas involving the left inferior parietal lobule: new insights into the functional anatomy provided by stimulation mapping in awake patients. J Neurosurg 2011;115:770–779

147. Szelényi A, Bello L, Duffau H, et al; Workgroup for Intraoperative Management in Low-Grade Glioma Surgery within the European Low-Grade Glioma Network. Intraoperative electrical stimulation in awake craniotomy:

methodological aspects of current practice. Neurosurg Focus 2010;28:E7

148. De Witt Hamer PC, Moritz-Gasser S, Gatignol P, Duffau H. Is the human left middle longitudinal fascicle essential for language? A brain electrostimulation study. Hum Brain Mapp 2011;32:962–973

149. Desmurget M, Bonnetblanc F, Duffau H. Contrasting acute and slow-growing lesions: a new door to brain plasticity. Brain 2007;130(Pt 4):898–914

150. Duffau H. Awake surgery for nonlanguage mapping. Neurosurgery 2010;66:523–528, discussion 528–529

151. Metz-Lutz MN, Kremin H, Deloche G, Hannequin D, Ferrand I, Perrier-Palisson D. Standardisation d'un Test de Denomination Orale: Contrôle de l'áge, du Sexe et du Niveau de Scolarité Chez des Sujets Adultes Normaux. Rev Neuropsychologie 1989;1:316–326

152. Rossini PM, Tecchio F, Pizzella V, Lupoi D, Cassetta E, Pasqualetti P. Interhemispheric differences of sensory hand areas after monohemispheric stroke: MEG/MRI integrative study. Neuroimage 2001;14:474–485

153. Pouratian N, Bookheimer SY. The reliability of neuroanatomy as a predictor of eloquence: a review. Neurosurg Focus 2010;28:E3

154. Penfield W, Boldrey E. Somatic motor and sensory representation in the cerebral cortex of man as studied by electrical stimulation. Brain 1937;60:389–443

155. Deloche G, Hannequin D. DO 80: Test de Denomination Orale d'Images. Paris: Les Editions du Centre de Psychologie Appliquée, 1997

156. Cramer SC, Moore CI, Finklestein SP, Rosen BR. A pilot study of somatotopic mapping after cortical infarct. Stroke 2000;31:668–671

157. Ojemann G, Ojemann J, Lettich E, Berger M. Cortical language localization in left, dominant hemisphere. An electrical stimulation mapping investigation in 117 patients. J Neurosurg 1989;71:316–326

158. Oldfield RC. The assessment and analysis of handedness: the Edinburgh inventory. Neuropsychologia 1971;9:97–113

159. Duffau H. Brain plasticity and tumors. Adv Tech Stand Neurosurg 2008;33:3–33

Chapter 12

Approaches to a Colloid Cyst:
Transcranial vs. Endoscopic

Case

A 35-year-old man notes an ongoing headache and visual blurring.

Participants

The Cranial Approach for Resecting Colloid Cysts: Juraj Šteňo

Endoscopic Resection of Third Ventricular Colloid Cysts: Jalal Najjar, Emad T. Aboud, and Samer K. Elbabaa

Moderators: Approaches to Colloid Cysts: Endoscopic vs. Microsurgical Treatment: Engelbert Knosp and Aygül Mert

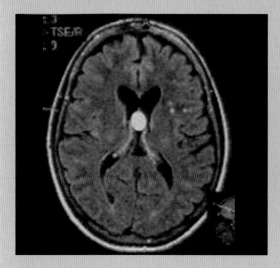

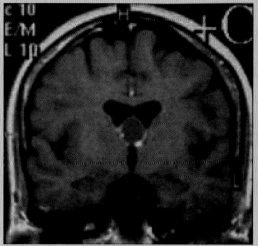

The Cranial Approach for Resecting Colloid Cysts

Juraj Šteňo

Making the Decision

The patient described in this case has symptoms of rather severely increased intracranial pressure. According to the T1-weighted and fluid-attenuated inversion recovery (FLAIR) magnetic resonance imaging (MRI), his lateral ventricles are enlarged because of obstruction of the foramina of Monro by a cystic lesion located in the anterior–superior part of the third ventricle. This lesion is apparently a colloid cyst, and the condition is life threatening. Observation only is very dangerous; without surgical treatment, the patient is endangered by the decompensation of intracranial hypertension with a sudden loss of consciousness and even death.[1] Two of 25 patients in our surgical series of colloid cysts were admitted to the hospital in a coma, necessitating emergency external ventricular drainage before the cyst was excised.

The Aim of Treatment

The chosen treatment should remove the obstruction of the cerebrospinal fluid pathways as well as relieve compression of the fornix by a tense cyst. The procedure should reach these goals as safely as possible and aim to prevent recurrence.

Topographical Features Relevant to Surgery

Colloid cysts are located inside the third ventricular cavity, most often in its anterior-superior compartment; the upper anterior part of the cyst is exposed at the foramina of Monro. A more posterior location of the cyst under the roof of the ventricle is rare. The orientation of the plane of the foramen of Monro, represented by its circumference, is oblique, tilting laterally and anteriorly. Its medial and posterior parts are located higher than the lateral and anterior borders. Consequently, the more lateral and anterior the point of entry at the surface of the brain, the more perpendicular and thus more suitable is the trajectory to the foramen of Monro. Therefore, the angle under which the foramen of Monro is exposed is more convenient with the transfrontal transventricular approach as compared with the transcallosal approach.

The fornix, the choroid plexus, and the veins of the venous angle are often displaced in a manner that leads to enlargement of the foramen. However, the foramen may also be narrowed or, rarely, practically occluded so the cyst wall cannot be seen from the frontal horn of the lateral ventricle. The distortion of the anatomic structures and the resultant shape of the foramina of Monro are usually asymmetrical, and preoperative MRI often cannot show the exact size of the foramina. The access to both foramina of Monro,

and thus the possibility of choosing the one that can better expose the cyst, is a great advantage of the transcallosal approach.

Obstruction of the cyst by the choroid plexus is easily solved through coagulation and dissection. More problematic is the covering of the upper part of the cyst by both halves of the fornix, which is distorted over the surface of the cyst. In one of our patients, the cyst was completely covered by the flattened halves of the fornix and the leaves of the septum. In such cases, the most convenient approach from the technical point of view is a midline dissection of the fornix.

In about a third of anatomic specimens, the venous angle is located posterior to the foramen of Monro; if necessary, the foramen may be enlarged through dissection of the choroid plexus on the forniceal side.[2]

Choosing the Type of Surgery

The surgeon can choose among four methods of treatment for patients with a colloid cyst: stereotactic aspiration[3]; endoscopy (through a working channel,[4,5] with the dual-port technique,[6] or through a neuro-endoport[7]); endoscope-assisted microsurgery through a craniotomy[8]; and microsurgery.[9–15] In the past, stereotactic aspiration was done without any visual control; later, a ventriculoscope was introduced to allow a view of the foramen of Monro and the capsule of the cyst.[16] Endoscopy offers non-stereoscopic monocular vision and one-handed manipulation; a wider tubular port (neuro-endoport) and the dual-port technique enable a bimanual surgical technique. Microsurgery and endoscope-assisted microsurgery through a craniotomy enable bimanual surgical manipulation under stereoscopic vision.

The disadvantage of monocular vision can be overcome through adequate experience with the endoscope. A more important drawback is the surgical manipulation with only one hand. The support and proprioceptive information provided by the second hand is invaluable during dissection of the structures, and is indispensable when structures must be pulled apart to stretch adhesions between them before cutting. Radical excision of the colloid cyst with microsurgical procedures can be achieved in all or almost all patients,[8,12,17–20] whereas remnants of the cyst after endoscopic procedures are found in a range of 4% of patients up to the majority of patients.[4,5,17,20,21] As might be expected, the recurrence rate after endoscopy is higher than after microsurgical resection.

Choosing the Surgical Approach

All surgical approaches to the third ventricle necessitate incision of the neural tissue, except for the supracerebellar subtentorial approach,[1,22] which is more convenient for reaching the posterior part of the third ventricular chamber. A consequence of surgical transgression of the cerebral cortex is the development of seizures; after transcortical approaches to the tumors of the third ventricle, they occur in 8.6 to 28% of patients.[23–25] After the transcallosal approach, they are rare.[12] An opposite proportion was found in a single series of patients with tumors in and around the lateral and third ventricles, in which the transcallosal approach carried a 4.4-fold increased risk of seizures.[26]

The experience described in series of patients with colloid cysts is the same as in the majority of reports of all patients with third ventricle tumors. Antunes and colleagues[27] reported seizures in two of 23 patients after the transcortical approach and in none of eight after callosotomy. Pamir and associates[12] noted seizures in one of 19 patients after the transcallosal excision of colloid cysts complicated by subsequent venous infarction of the superior frontal gyrus. We used the transcallosal approach in 45 of 141 patients with tumors of the third ventricle and transcortical approaches in 11 of these patients (10 transfrontal, one posterior after Van Wagenen). Epileptic seizures occurred in one patient treated with the transcallosal approach (2.2%) and in two patients treated with the transcortical approach (18%), and all three of these patients harbored gliomas.[28] Seizures did not occur in any of our patients with colloid cysts.

From the neuropsychological point of view, the anterior transcallosal route is a safe and feasible alternative to the transcortical approach.[29] The interhemispheric transfer of information is preserved as long as the splenium remains intact.[30] Partial sectioning of the corpus callosum does not cause significant neurologic deficits; however, if the surgery induces additional brain injury, the neurologic deficits can be more severe with a callosotomy.[31]

The Transcranial Approaches

We used the transfrontal-transventricular approach in three patients—in two after conversion from endoscopy to a craniotomy and in one to avoid the transection of a bridging vein. Likewise, the great majority of authors prefer the transcallosal approach, and we used it in 18 patients. Currently, we dissect the bridging veins from the dura even if the terminal part of the vessel runs between the dural layers (**Fig. 12.1**) or we open the dura atypically to reach the edge of the superior sagittal sinus. A sufficient callosotomy and complete removal of the cyst was possible when the anterior-posterior distance between the bridging veins at the sinus was as little as 20 mm.

The Transcallosal Approach

For the transcallosal approach, we adjust the placement of the craniotomy to the anatomy of the veins of the frontal lobe as shown by MRI. We use neuronavigation to find the most suitable trajectory from the convexity of the brain (as anterior as possible) via the corpus callosum (just behind the genu) to the foramina of Monro. The posterior border of the craniotomy rarely exceeds the coronal suture; it extends 1.5 cm across the midline medially.

After opening the dura with the base of the flap at the superior sagittal sinus, we proceed along the falx, separating the medial surface of the frontal lobe in the direction of the foramen of Monro. On the way down to the corpus callosum, fine adhesions are dissected between the medial surfaces of the frontal lobes and between the anterior cerebral arteries and the surrounding structures. Gradual evacuation of the cerebrospinal fluid while working with the suction in one hand and forceps in the other relaxes the brain sufficiently to prevent its compression by a retractor. Currently, we seldom use retractors during dissection. In a rare case, when the brain was too tight even after the patient's head was elevated, we punctured the frontal horn of the lateral ventricle and inserted a silicon tube, which we left in place until the end of tumor resection.

Once the corpus callosum is exposed, rolled cottonoids are introduced between the cingulate gyri in front of and behind the planned incision (**Fig. 12.2**). The callosotomy is made in the midline to prevent damage to the indusium griseum, as recommended by Winkler and colleagues.[32] We try to find an avascular zone but, rarely, a minute vessel has to be coagulated and transected. After sectioning the pia mater and some 1 to 2 mm of surface tissue approximately 8 to 10 mm long, we carry out blunt dissection by opening the arms of the forceps in the sagittal direction (**Fig. 12.3**). Additional cuts are made if necessitated by the location of the foramen of Monro. In patients with severe hydrocephalus and a thinned-out corpus callosum, a mere puncture with the tip of a fine forceps is sufficient to reach the frontal horn of one of the lateral ventricles or the space between the leaves of the septum pellucidum (**Fig. 12.4**). We fenestrate the septum in all patients to inspect both foramina of Monro and to choose the one that allows better

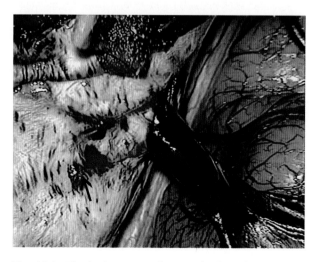

Fig. 12.1 The bridging vein draining the frontal lobe is dissected free from its attachment to the dura (*arrows*) up to its entry into the superior sagittal sinus.

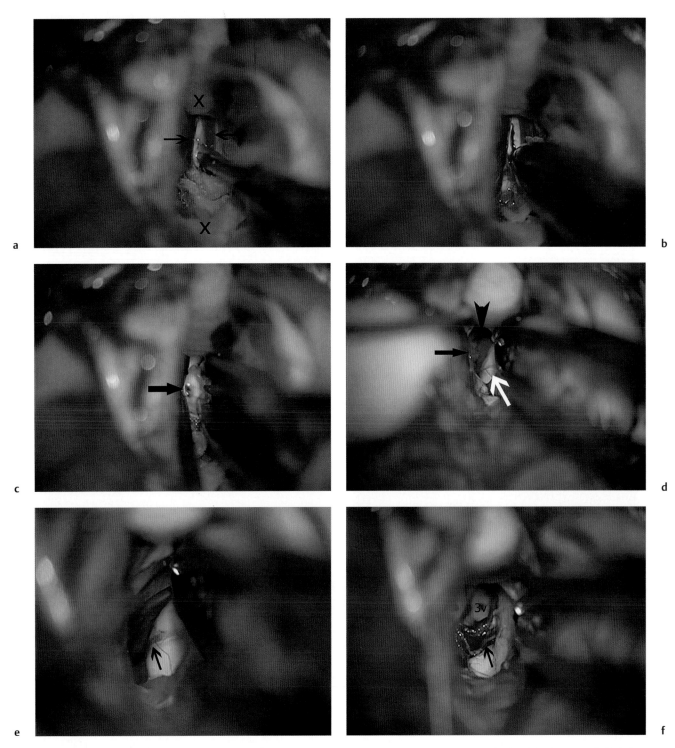

Fig. 12.2a–f Transcallosal transforaminal removal of the colloid cyst. **(a)** The incision into the superficial layer of the corpus callosum is between the pericallosal arteries (*arrows*). The cingulate gyri are held apart with cottonoid pads (*X*). **(b)** The forceps is introduced into the incision. **(c)** The ependyma (*arrow*) is exposed through blunt dissection. **(d)** The cyst (*arrowhead*) at the left foramen of Monro is covered by the body of the fornix medially (*white arrow*) and by the choroid plexus laterally (*black arrow*). **(e)** The small septal vein (*arrow*) pierces the fornix behind the anterior septal vein. **(f)** The cyst is completely removed, and the anterior and posterior (*arrow*) septal veins are preserved. 3v, the floor of the third ventricle.

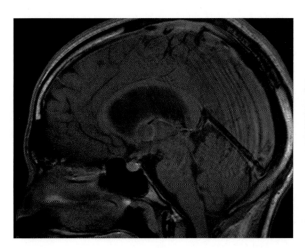
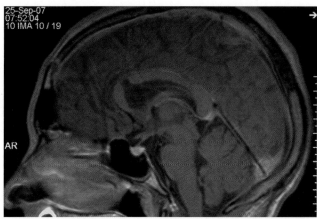

a   b

Fig. 12.3a,b   A colloid cyst of the third ventricle **(a)** removed through a short anterior callosotomy **(b).**

exposure, similar to the strategy used by Yaşargil and Abdulrauf.[14] We use the other foramen just to assess the completeness of cyst excision.

Dissection of the cyst usually starts with coagulation of the attached choroid plexus and with its dissection from the cyst wall. Opening the cyst and emptying its contents relieves tension and allows dissection of the capsule from the lower surface of the fornix and from the veins contributing to the venous angle. However small the foramen at the beginning, during dissection of the capsule from surrounding structures it always enlarges. Dissection of the choroid plexus in a posterior direction either from the forniceal or ventricular side (the subchoroidal approach[15]) further widens the exposure of the cyst. In cases with an atypical posterior variant of the venous angle, dissection of the plexus allows substantial enlargement of the approach.[2] In one of our patients, this maneuver allowed the safe removal of a cyst located posteriorly between the roof of the

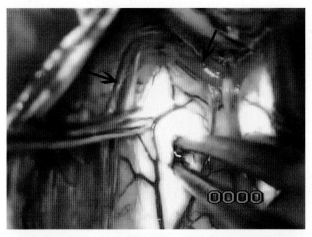
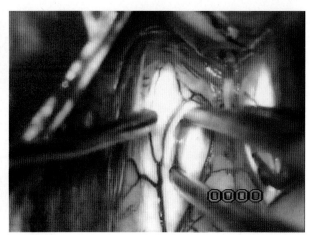

a   b

c

Fig. 12.4a–c   **(a,b)** The callosotomy is done through puncture of the thinned corpus callosum between the pericallosal arteries (*arrows*) with the forceps. **(c)** The leaves of the septum pellucidum (*arrowheads*) are spread apart.

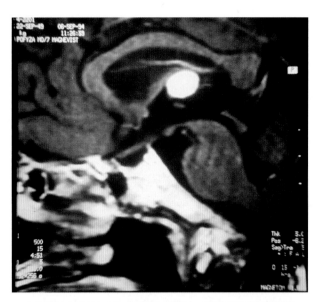

a

Fig. 12.5a–d **(a,b)** Atypical posterior location of a colloid cyst between the roof of the third ventricle and the interthalamic adhesion. **(c,d)** This lesion was removed after dissection of the posteriorly located venous angle via the transcallosal approach.

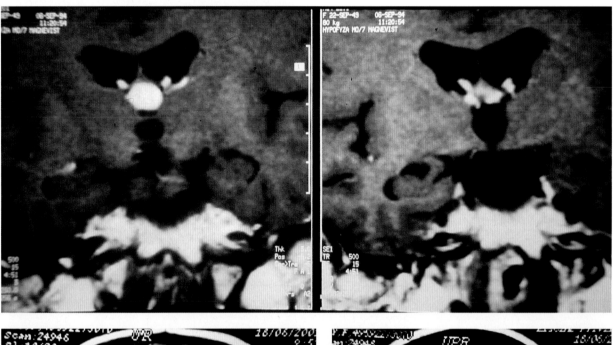

b

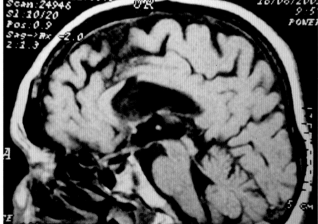

c

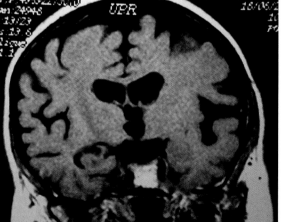

d

ventricle and the massa intermedia (adhesio interthalamica) **(Fig. 12.5)**. In one case, a minute vein of the septum pierced and apparently drained the fornix; on its way laterally to the venous angle, it firmly adhered to the surface of the cysts and its dissection and preservation required lengthy and meticulous technique **(Fig. 12.2e)**. After complete removal of the cyst, the lateral walls and the floor of the third ventricle come into view.

In three patients with both foramina of Monro no more than a slit, we used the interforniceal approach.[9] The body of the fornix was dissected at its midline raphe within the corridor bounded by the anterior commissure anteriorly and the choroid plexus at the foramen of Monro posteriorly. The anatomic situation, with the leaves of the septum being apart, helps the surgeon determine the precise orientation. After separation of the two halves of the fornix, the upper part of the cyst is exposed. Attachments to the lower surface of the fornix, the choroid plexus, and the veins are then dissected free and the cyst is removed. In a series of patients with cysts removed through the interforniceal approach, no permanent deficit was reported.[33] We observed temporary memory disturbances in two of our three patients. The disturbance was rather severe in one of them, and afterward we did not use this approach.

We achieved radical cyst resection in 21 patients treated microsurgically (including two patients after conversion of endoscopy to microsurgery because of venous bleeding) and in one of four with an accomplished endoscopic procedure **(Fig. 12.6)**. There was no permanent morbidity or mortality in the entire series. Temporary memory disturbances occurred in four patients—in two after resection of the cyst through the transcallosal transforaminal route and in two of three after the interforniceal approach. Meningitis occurred in one of two patients with external ventricular drainage, and repeated shunt revisions were necessary.

Avoiding Potential Complications

Preserving all bridging veins draining the frontal lobe prevents venous infarction. Dissection of the terminal parts of these veins from the dura or modified dural opening prevents their occlusion.

Surgical manipulation of the fornix should be as gentle as possible. Bilateral manipulation especially may lead to

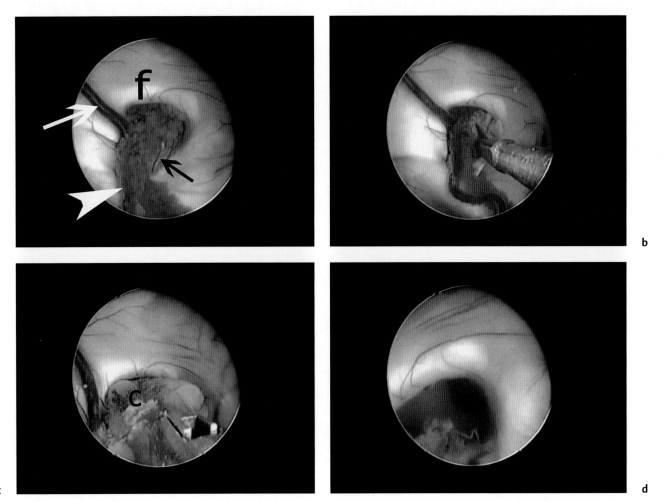

Fig. 12.6a–d Endoscopic removal of a colloid cyst through the right foramen of Monro. **(a)** At the foramen (f), the cyst (*black arrow*) is covered by the choroid plexus (*arrowhead*) and the ante-rior septal vein (*white arrow*) is beneath it. **(b)** Cutting the choroid plexus. **(c)** Removing the thick cyst contents. **(d)** The floor of the third ventricle seen through the emptied foramen of Monro.

the temporary impairment of short-term memory. Therefore, it is advisable to remove the tumor through one foramen of Monro and to use the other just to assess the completeness of resection, if necessary. The transforaminal exposure and resection of the cyst is preferable to the interforniceal approach. Traction on the veins contributing to the venous angle should be avoided as it may cause bleeding remote from the foramen of Monro. A two-handed operative technique increases the safety of tumor dissection.

A clean operative field during tumor removal prevents postoperative occlusion of the aqueduct, which necessitates diversion of the cerebrospinal fluid. Blocking the aqueduct during cyst removal with a cottonoid may be helpful. Avoiding the insertion of a cerebrospinal fluid shunt preoperatively should prevent all potential complications. Except for patients with decompensated intracranial hypertension, we prefer to start treatment by removing the tumor. An intraoperative ventriculostomy may be done if the brain is tight.

Closure of a callosotomy with fibrin glue is sometimes recommended. We always try to fill the intradural space with saline before the final dural stitch is taken to prevent collapse of the hemispheres and eventual bleeding from the stretched bridging veins.

Endoscopic Resection of Third Ventricular Colloid Cysts

Jalal Najjar, Emad T. Aboud, and Samer K. Elbabaa

Background

Colloid cysts derive their name from the Greek word *kollodes* (glue). They were first described as lesions within the third ventricle, but also appear in the fourth ventricle[34] and within the brain parenchyma.[35] There has even been one case of an olfactory groove colloid cyst that presented with cerebrospinal fluid rhinorrhea after eroding the dura of the anterior cranial fossa.[36]

Colloid cysts are benign, congenital epithelium-lined cysts that almost always arise in the anterior third ventricle. These rare tumors comprise 0.5 to 1% of all intracranial tumors and 15% of all intraventricular tumors. Colloid cysts are considered a potential cause of sudden death and acute neurologic deterioration,[37,38] which occurs in one third of symptomatic patients. Among all cases of sudden death, 10 to 15% had a colloid cyst at autopsy.[37] Both brain herniation and spinal infarction as a result of acute hydrocephalus have been described,[39] and neurogenic pulmonary edema has also been mentioned as the mechanism triggering sudden death.[40] On rare occasions, a colloid cyst may spontaneously resolve or rupture asymptomatically.[41]

Different surgical approaches have been described for resecting colloid cysts. The goal of any planned surgery is to achieve gross total resection with no residual capsule. Serial follow-up MRI studies are used to rule out any recurrence. The choice of any surgical approach should be geared toward avoiding complications and minimizing the manipulation of brain tissue and vasculature. Postoperative complications may include seizures, disconnection syndrome, memory difficulties, meningitis, and venous infarction.

A review of most published articles would indicate that the microsurgical resection of colloid cysts leads to better gross total removal than the endoscopic approach. On the other hand, endoscopic resections create fewer complications in general. The endoscopic approach is becoming more effective and well accepted as gross total resection is achieved with a low risk of complications.

In 1921, Dandy accomplished the first successful resection of a colloid cyst through a transcortical approach, and the transcallosal approach was first described by Greenwood in 1948. In the past 20 years, endoscopic approaches have become more popular. Other approaches include stereotactic aspiration and the infratentorial supracerebellar approach.[22]

Pathophysiology

Colloid cysts enlarge through an increased secretion of mucinous fluid from the lining of the epithelial cell wall. In addition, cyst cavities may be filled with blood and degradation products such as cholesterol crystals. Different theories exist concerning the origin of these lesions, which may include primitive neuroepithelium, ependyma, choroid plexus epithelium, and paraphysial tissue. But there is no structural or immunohistochemical evidence to support an ependymal or choroid plexus origin.[42] Some studies conclude that colloid cysts of the anterior third ventricle are clearly distinct from both the choroid plexus and ependyma, and therefore are not a developmental or degenerative product of these structures.[43] Tsuchida and colleagues[44] suggested a nonneuroepithelial origin of colloid cyst epithelium, underscoring its similarity to respiratory mucosa of the trachea and sphenoid sinus.

Historical Perspective

Surgical approaches to lesions located in the anterior and middle portions of the third ventricle are challenging, even for experienced neurosurgeons. Various approaches through

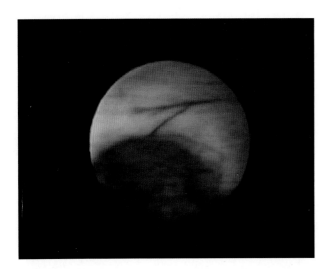

Fig. 12.7 Endoscopic view of a colloid cyst at the roof of the third ventricle with its choroid attachment at the right foramen of Monro.

the foramen of Monro, the choroidal fissure, the fornices, the lamina terminalis, and, rarely, the supracerebellar infratentorial route have been described in numerous publications.[2] Wallmann first reported the case of a colloid cyst in 1858 in a man with urinary incontinence and ataxia.[45] In 1921, Walter Dandy accomplished the first successful resection of a colloid cyst through a transcortical approach. He described a transcortical-transventricular approach to the third ventricle as partially resecting the frontal lobe to remove a colloid cyst. In 1949, James Greenwood[46] reviewed 60 colloid cyst cases, in which 15 were successfully removed. He concluded that surgical removal must be accomplished without damage to the walls of the third ventricle, as the attachments of the colloid cyst to the wall of the third ventricle are fragile. He described the cyst's movement as a ball valve at the level of the foramen of Monro, suggesting that the surgical approaches should be either transcortical or through the corpus callosum. His report described the importance of delivering the cyst only after removing the adjacent choroid plexus (**Fig. 12.7**).

Microsurgical Approaches

Early reports of the transcortical approach recommended its use in patients with hydrocephalus, and the common complications included the increased risk of seizures as well as infections. The transcallosal approach is commonly used to gain access to the third ventricle, but also has some disadvantages. Complications include direct or manipulation injury of the superior sagittal sinus and bridging veins, sometimes leading to sinus thrombosis and venous stroke. Some authors advocate the use of a large bone flap to avoid direct retraction of the sinus; others suggest the use of preoperative magnetic resonance venography for optimal evaluation of the venous anatomy and surgical planning.[47] Other complications include bleeding or spasm of the peri-

callosal arteries because of manipulation or chemical irritation from the contents of the cyst.[48] Forniceal injury can cause severe short-term memory loss and disconnection syndrome.[49]

Ulm and colleagues[50] have detailed the limitations of the transcallosal transchoroidal approach to the third ventricle. They concluded that the exposure of the anterior third ventricle was limited by the columns of the fornix and by the presence of parietal cortical draining veins.

Anatomic Considerations: Pendulous Pathology

Colloid cysts have been described as a pendulous pathology in the third ventricle. This theory correlates with the symptoms of patients, which are likely caused by intermittent obstruction of the foramen of Monro and include paroxysmal headaches that last from seconds to minutes and are initiated, exacerbated, or relieved by a change in the position of the head.[51] The pendulous theory also explains the spontaneous collapsing and floating of the cyst capsule by pulsations in cerebrospinal fluid after surgical aspiration of the cyst's contents. The cyst wall has no attachments except at its origin. Commonly, there is a firm attachment to the adjacent choroid plexus. Using a microsurgical technique, most neurosurgeons deliver the cyst from the third ventricle into the lateral ventricle and follow with careful coagulation and cutting of the attachment to the choroid plexus.

Endoscopic Resection: Signs for Safe Removal

En bloc resection of an intact colloid cyst was described in early surgical reports, starting in 1948 with Greenwood. Keeping the contents within the cyst without aspiration and delivering the whole cyst from the third ventricle to the lateral ventricle remains a popular technique and is practiced by many neurosurgeons during microsurgical resection.

In our early endoscopic experience with 10 colloid cyst resections, we observed that the cyst capsule slightly adheres to the ependyma of the roof of the third ventricle or foramen of Monro. After the cyst's contents are aspirated, the capsule is pendulous and floats between the lateral and third ventricles because of cerebrospinal fluid pulsation. Usually, there is a single attachment to the choroid plexus at the roof of the third ventricle. Delivering the residual cyst from the third ventricle to the lateral ventricle has been described by many neurosurgeons (**Figs. 12.8, 12.9**).

The Roof of the Third Ventricle: Anatomic Layers and Variations

The surgeon must recognize that the roof of the third ventricle consists of five layers. The first, superior layer is the fornix, and the second is the superior membrane of the tela

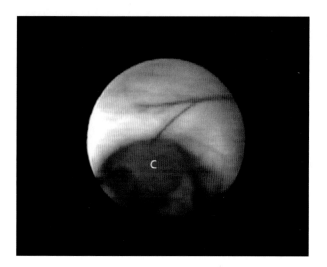

Fig. 12.8 Endoscopic view of a colloid cyst during its delivery from the third ventricle into the lateral ventricle through the foramen of Monro. C, colloid cyst.

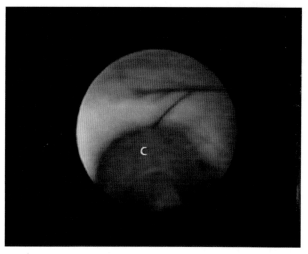

Fig. 12.9 Endoscopic view of a colloid cyst during its delivery from the third ventricle into the lateral ventricle through the foramen of Monro. C, colloid cyst.

choroidea. Third is the vascular layer, which consists of the internal cerebral veins and the medial posterior choroidal artery and its branches. The fourth layer is the inferior membrane of the tela choroidea, and the fifth layer is the choroid plexus, which is in continuity with the choroid plexus of the lateral ventricle.[52]

Türe and associates[2] investigated the variations in the subependymal veins of the lateral ventricle in the region of the foramen of Monro, as these structures are intimately involved in surgical exposure of the third ventricle. Based on their cadaveric study, the authors advocated opening the choroidal fissure as far as the junction of the anterior septal vein and internal cerebral vein to enlarge the foramen of Monro posteriorly. This technique allows adequate access to the anterior and middle portions of the third ventricle without injuring vital neural or vascular structures.

Attachment of the Cyst Wall to the Choroid Plexus: Surgical Considerations

Almost all colloid cyst resection techniques describe the final attachment of the colloid cysts as choroidal with small feeding vessels, and in most cases there is no significant difficulty or morbidity with this final stage of resection. Rhoton[53] described this final stage as coagulating the final remnant of the attachment of the cyst to the choroid plexus. Hernesniemi and colleagues[13] published a large series of 134 colloid cysts resected through the transcallosal approach. They describe the final stage as follows: "The attachments of the lesion to the roof of the third ventricle have to be coagulated and resected to avoid bleeding from the small vessels."

Konovalov and Pitskhelauri[22] also describe the final stage of colloid cyst resection through the infratentorial supracerebellar approach: "The capsule of the colloid cyst is dissected. After the colloid is aspirated and the dense contents

of the capsule are removed, the tumor is mobilized and separated from the choroidal plexus. The area of attachment of the colloid cyst to the plexus and small feeder vessels crossing from plexus to cyst are well visualized. These vessels are cauterized and divided, and the capsule of the cyst is removed."

Our Series

Over the past 15 years, about 150 neuroendoscopic procedures have been performed at our institution by the first author. Most cases involved the management of hydrocephalus. Cysts in 28 patients were removed endoscopically as primary treatment. The age range of patients was 12 to 65 years, and all patients were symptomatic with hydrocephalus. The cysts ranged in size from 6 to 36 mm, and all patients underwent preoperative imaging studies as part of the workup (**Figs. 12.10, 12.11, 12.12**). Presenting symptoms included progressive and intermittent headaches, vomiting, and blurred vision. One patient had undergone previous placement of a ventriculoperitoneal shunt at another institution. The shunt was complicated by an infection, which necessitated its removal and external drainage before our endoscopic procedure. Three patients required shunt placement after the endoscopic resection of the cyst, in one case because of incomplete resection.

In our early experience with 10 cases, we used the traditional technique of puncturing the cyst capsule followed by aspiration of the contents with a 2-mm needle prior to delivery of the cyst to the lateral ventricle. Maintaining the cyst intact without spilling the contents into the ventricular system can prevent chemical irritation or even chemical meningitis. The mucinous contents are occasionally solid and difficult to aspirate. On rare occasions, such contents can lead to the formation of an intraventricular granuloma.[54]

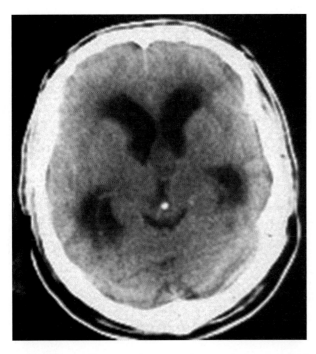

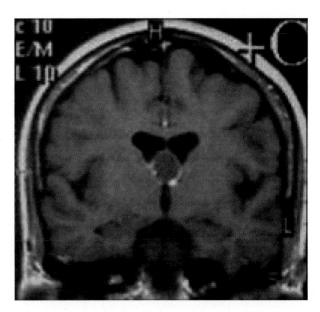

Fig. 12.11 Coronal magnetic resonance imaging (MRI) (T1 sequence) showing a colloid cyst at the roof of the third ventricle with moderate obstructive hydrocephalus.

Fig. 12.10 Axial computed tomography scan showing a colloid cyst in the third ventricle with severe obstructive hydrocephalus.

If the initial endoscopic exposure of the cyst reveals complete obstruction of the foramen of Monro, we coagulate the choroid plexus to increase exposure and maintain hemostasis. The cyst walls are then pushed away from the ependymal surface of the third ventricle while we apply coagulation. The cyst contents are then aspirated. Once the cyst is partially evacuated, it is sequentially mobilized into the foramen with flexible or rigid grasping forceps, where further aspiration, coagulation, and removal can be done.

Over the past 6 years, our technique has evolved and we now advocate removing the cyst without opening the capsule—the en bloc technique. The operative time is reduced by two thirds with the en bloc compared with the traditional technique. We treated 18 patients using this technique, with overall better results, a shorter operative time, and a decreased complication rate. As most cysts are larger than the lumen of the endoscope itself, we remove the endoscope with the forceps simultaneously, holding the cyst through the working channel. We follow this maneuver by rapidly exploring the surgical bed and foramen of Monro to control any bleeding with multiple rounds of irrigation with lactated Ringer's solution (**Fig. 12.13**).

After the cyst has been delivered extracranially, we explore the cyst and capsule to check for tears that might suggest a residual component. In most cases, we find a component of the choroid plexus firmly attached to the

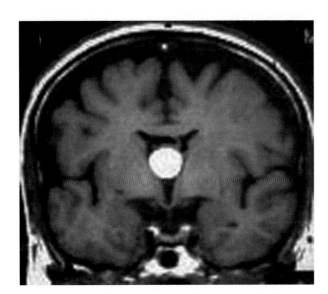

Fig. 12.12 Coronal MRI (T1 sequence) showing a colloid cyst at the roof of the third ventricle without obstructive hydrocephalus.

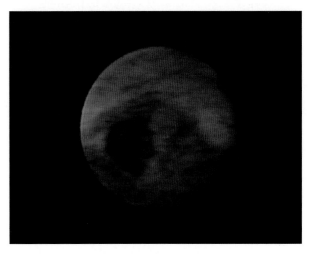

Fig. 12.13 Endoscopic view of the foramen of Monro after complete cyst excision and multiple rounds of irrigation.

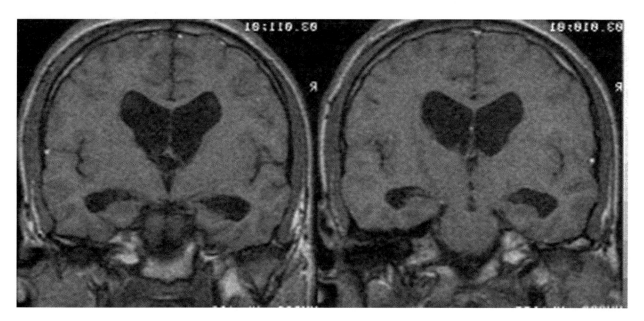

Fig. 12.14   Postoperative coronal MRI (T1 sequence) showing complete endoscopic resection of a cyst with no residual component.

capsule of the cyst. In three patients, we prolonged irrigation of the ventricular system when the mucinous contents of the cyst spilled into the ventricles during the final stage of removal, which was likely due to a tear in the capsule.

In all of our endoscopic cases, bleeding at the level of attachment to the roof of the third ventricle was successfully managed with repeated and prolonged rounds of irrigation to wash out the ventricle. In three patients, we kept an external ventricular drain in place for 2 or 3 days. These drains were removed after a computed tomography (CT) scan confirmed no residual intraventricular hemorrhage.

Major complications were encountered only during our early endoscopic experience and included one case of hemiparesis from injury by the aspiration needle. The hemiparesis completely resolved after 3 months. Other complications included two cases of short-term memory deficit, which resolved within 1 week, and one case of chemical meningitis, which was treated successfully.

Two patients had incomplete resection. One underwent microsurgical resection because of the firm cyst contents and attachment; the other had placement of a shunt. Follow-up MRI studies showed no further growth in the patient requiring a shunt. Overall, no recurrence was noted in the en bloc resection group, data that was confirmed with serial MRI studies during the 6 years of clinical and radiographic follow-up **(Fig. 12.14)**.

Endoscopic en bloc resection can be done safely, even for colloid cysts of large diameter (up to 36 mm in our series). We recommend aborting the en bloc technique if there is significant adhesion of the capsule to the ependyma of the foramen of Monro or neighboring structures.

Conclusion

Colloid cysts are known as nonvascular lesions with mucinous contents and a fragile attachment to the roof of the third ventricle. The adjacent choroid plexus has both an anatomic and a debatable histopathological relationship to these cysts. Microsurgical resection remains an excellent treatment modality with a low risk of residual or recurrent cysts, but with potential complications.[55,56] Endoscopic resection includes two main options. The first technique involves cyst aspiration and decompression followed by a delivery of the cyst through the foramen of Monro. The second technique uses en bloc resection. Intraoperative observations, such as the degree of attachment to the roof of the third ventricle or choroid plexus, may have an impact on the technique used for endoscopic resection. In our endoscopic series, en bloc removal was associated with a low but acceptable complication rate. The en bloc technique was also associated with very good complete resection outcomes and long radiographic evidence of no recurrence.

We believe that endoscopic resection of colloid cysts should be considered as the first option for all symptomatic patients with associated hydrocephalus and when appropriate endoscopic surgical expertise, setup, and equipment are available. Microsurgery remains an excellent option for patients with smaller ventricles, and at institutions without appropriate endoscopic experience or setup. Microsurgery also remains a good alternative when the endoscopic technique is aborted because of intraoperative findings that contradict safe endoscopic removal.

Approaches to Colloid Cysts: Endoscopic vs. Microsurgical Treatment

Engelbert Knosp and Aygül Mert

The Objective

Endoscopy has become an important tool in neurosurgery over the past two decades, but because of technical constraints and the lack of adequate instruments, the indications for endoscopic neurosurgery are still limited. Surgery in preformed spaces such as ventricles is an ideal indication for endoscopic procedures. Unlike intraventricular tumors, colloid cysts are a favorite target for endoscopic surgery, and they have been approached and removed successfully through this route for more than 20 years. Nonetheless, there is still controversy about the value of endoscopic removal of colloid cysts. In my opinion, there are two main reasons for this controversy: a general reluctance to use endoscopes in daily neurosurgical practice, and technical constraints such as inadequate instruments. Thus, the debate regarding the best technique to solve the problem of colloid cysts still awaits resolution.

Over the decades, the choice for treating colloid cysts has always been influenced by the highest technical standards, initially the transcortical approach by Dandy. In the microsurgical era, the transcallosal approach has become the gold standard for treatment.[56] The more favored, less traumatic approaches to this benign lesion in the third ventricle use frame-based stereotactic equipment.[57] Today, frameless neuronavigation provides sufficient accuracy to reach deep-seated lesions with minimal damage during the approach. Because of a high rate of recurrence, stereotactic puncture of such cysts has been abandoned.[16] In contrast, endoscopic surgery, also regarded as a minimally invasive technique, offers a direct view of important structures, including the cyst, the fornix, and the ventricular veins. And like stereotactic procedures, it offers a much greater chance to remove the cyst completely. A disadvantage of the endoscopic method, however, is that the cyst is not radically resected in all patients.[5,7,20,21,58]

Microsurgical resection still offers the best chance for complete resection of colloid cysts in the third ventricle[1,8,13,18,19,56,59] (**Table 12.1**). A transcortical approach, perpendicular to the largest entrance plane of the foramen Monro, offers the best view to the critical structures around the third ventricle. The shortcoming of this approach, however, is the higher rate of postoperative epilepsy. In my opinion, the interhemispheric transcallosal approach offers a lot of advantages compared with the transfrontal transcortical approach. With the transcallosal approach, both foramina of Monro can be seen or used for cyst re-

section. Furthermore, this approach can also be used in patients with normal and small ventricles and is not restricted by the size of the cyst or the consistency of the cyst's contents.

Our Experience

Over a period of 10 years (2002–2012), we treated 28 patients with colloid cysts at the Medical University Clinic in Vienna. Nine patients (32%) presented in an acute or periacute clinical stage with raised intracranial pressure, and six were unconscious at the time of admission. The majority of these patients were treated with acute extraventricular drainage and the cyst was resected directly. In one patient, the 5-mm cyst was an incidental finding, and the patient had headache without raised intracranial pressure. Cases like this one will be increasingly detected with the frequent use of CT and MRI.

The goal of treatment is to restore the cerebrospinal fluid pathway through both foramina of Monro by resecting the colloid cyst, and this can be done in all cases. The majority of our patients underwent microsurgery through either a transcallosal approach (24 patients) or transcortically (three patients). Most frequently, we used the transcallosal approach as described by Yaşargil but with some modifications. The most relevant modification was to use the endoscope to assist microsurgical resection (seven cases). An endoscope with an angulated shaft and 30- or 45-degree lenses works best during regular microsurgical dissection. Endoscopes can provide important anatomic information from the third ventricle during the resection, for example, a view of the contralateral foramen of Monro. But its most important function is to verify the completeness of resection and inspect the ventricles to detect blood clots at the end of the procedure. Without the help of endoscopes with angulated lenses, inspecting the roof of the third ventricle is more difficult and requires manipulation of the fornix. We later modified this approach by turning the patient's head 90 degrees to the side of the planned approach and elevating it 45 to 60 degrees, instead of keeping a straight and slightly elevated head position. This position facilitates interhemispheric dissection, as gravity allows the hemisphere rather to fall away from the falx, eliminating the need for active retraction.

The results and complications of our series are listed in **Table 12.2**. All but seven of our patients had hydrocephalus, which was transient because the cyst was totally resected. Shunt placement was never necessary.

Table 12.1 Reports of Treatments of Colloid Cysts

	Šteňo	Najjar, Elbabaa	Knosp	Horn et al[20]	Hellwig et al[5]	Lewis et al[59]	Hernesniemi et al[13]	Shapiro et al[15]	Engh et al[7]	Charalampaki et al[8]	Mathiesen et al[16]	Desai et al[18]	Sampath et al[19]	Boogaarts et al[21]	Teo[60]
No. of cases	21	28	28	55	20	15	134	57	32	28	16	105	10	90	18
Transcallosal approach	18	–	24	27	–	8	134	57	–	–	–	62	10	–	–
Transcortical approach	3	–	–	–	–	–	–	–	–	–	26	31	–	–	–
Endoscopic approach	1 (3ᵃ)	28ᵇ	4	28	20	7	–	–	32	28	–	–	–	90	18
Radicality of excision (%)	100	89 2 recur	89.3 2 recur	94 micro 53 endosc	0 1 recur	100	100 1 recur	89.5	96.9	100	0	96.8	100	51.3	100
Conversion	3	2	–	–	–	–	–	–	–	–	5	–	–	2	–
Minor complications	–	3	3	6	3	6	8	2	6	2	0	27	2	14	2
Mortality	–	–	–	–	–	–	–	–	–	–	1	7	–	1	–
Hemiparesis	–	1	–	1 endosc	–	–	1	–	–	–	–	–	1	1	1
Transient memory deficit	4	4	4	–	–	3	4	1	2	–	3	14	1	7	1
Permanent memory deficit	–	2	2	2 endosc	4	1	–	–	–	7	4	2	7	1	–
Epilepsy	–	–	–	2 micro	–	–	–	–	–	–	–	8 endosc	–	1	–
Shunt placement	1	1	–	6	1	1	17	3	–	3	3	23	1	3	–
Other major complications	–	–	–	–	–	–	–	–	–	1	5	–	–	–	–

Abbreviations: recur, recurrence; micro, microsurgical approach; endosc, endoscopic approach.

ᵃTwo of three colloid cysts were converted from an endoscopic to the microscopic technique; one case was finished endoscopically.

ᵇTen cases traditional and 18 en bloc endoscopic resections.

232

Table 12.2 Results and Complications

	Šteňo	Najjar and Colleagues	Knosp and Mert
Number of cases	21	28	28[a]
Transcallosal approach	18	–	24
Transcortical approach	3	–	–
Endoscopic approach	1 (3[b])	28[c]	4
Radicality of excision	100%	89%	82%[d]
Conversion	3	2	–
Minor complications	–	–	3
Mortality	–	–	–
Hemiparesis	–	1	–
Transient memory deficit	4	–	4
Permanent memory deficit	–	–	6
Epilepsy	–	–	–
Shunt placement	1	1	–

[a]Seven of 28 endoscopic-assisted microsurgical resections.

[b]Two of three colloid cysts were converted from an endoscopic to the microscopic technique; one case was finished endoscopically.

[c]Ten cases traditional and 18 en bloc endoscopic resections.

[d]92% radicality of resection for transcallosal approaches.

Choosing a Microsurgical or Endoscopic Approach

The participants in this debate are well-known experts in their field: Šteňo, who presents a very balanced argument with a clear preference for microsurgical resection, and Najjar and colleagues, who discuss the endoscopic treatment of colloid cysts.

The Transcallosal Approach

Šteňo, an expert in the treatment of tumors in the third ventricle, discusses the microsurgical approaches to remove colloid cysts. He presents a series of 21 patients with colloid cysts, 18 of whom underwent microsurgery through the interhemispheric transcallosal approach. In three patients, he used the transcortical approach, including two conversions from an initial endoscopic approach.

Based on his long experience and his thoroughly presented discussion of the advantages and disadvantages of either approach, he came to the conclusion that the transcallosal is the best choice for resecting colloid cysts. A transcortical approach was chosen only if severe obstacles like veins were encountered (one patient) or if an endoscopic approach had been converted to a microsurgical technique (two patients). He comments critically on his own experience with the endoscopic technique and its shortcomings, and this experience underscores his argument that the bimanual technique is mandatory for a safe and successful resection. Another key argument favoring

the microsurgical technique is that it provides a greater chance of complete resection. The higher rate of postoperative epilepsy was another point favoring the transcallosal approach.

I agree with Šteňo that a transcallosal approach is more flexible because both foramina are amenable for resecting the cyst. After inspecting both foramina, one can decide which foramen is more suitable for removal. Anatomic details, the thickness of the cyst wall, and the degree to which the cyst adheres to the fornix are important pieces of information that cannot be determined by imaging. After the cyst is resected, the third ventricle can be inspected from either side to confirm complete resection. This advantage of seeing both sides should not tempt the surgeon to use both sides for resection, which would damage both fornices. The advice not to use an interforniceal approach is well supported because two of three patients experienced a severe memory deficit from splitting of the fornix.

Šteňo also included his experience with three colloid cysts approached endoscopically, a choice that demonstrates a further dilemma for many neurosurgeons. Many want to offer a patient the least invasive technique, and many realize the advantages of using an endoscope, but the learning curve is significant. In two cases, Šteňo had to convert from the endoscopic to an open transcortical microsurgical technique because of insufficient control of bleeding. In these patients, the problem could be managed microscopically, resulting in no clinical deficit.

The Endoscopic Approach

Najjar and colleagues present their series of 28 patients with colloid cysts treated exclusively with the endoscope. The cysts ranged in size from 6 to 32 mm. The authors note that colloid cysts differ not only in size and in the consistency of the contents, but also in the intensity with which they adhere to the roof of the third ventricle.

In their initial experience, Najjar and colleagues first drained the cysts to facilitate the piecemeal resection of its wall. But the small size of the endoscope makes this procedure time-consuming, and complete resection was not possible in all patients. With increasing experience, these authors realized that the cyst's adhesion to the third ventricle is not always tight. This observation is important, but has dangerous implications. These surgeons have changed their technique so that they now pull the colloid cyst en bloc through the foramen of Monro into the lateral ventricle. By pulling the cyst further, they detach the cyst from the roof of the third ventricle and then deliver it together with the endoscope.

I have some concerns with this maneuver of pulling the cyst from the delicate layer of the roof of the third ventricle. Bleeding, which occurs easily after this procedure, is controlled with prolonged rinsing of the surgical bed. In my experience, controlling bleeding is a major problem during endoscopic procedures in preformed spaces like the ventricles. The view within the ventricles is immediately limited and the orientation during this so-called red-out situation is very difficult, sometimes even impossible, to determine. Successful coagulation is sometimes possible during endoscopic techniques, but there is no guarantee of this, especially if an artery within the third ventricle is the source of the bleeding. Patience, prolonged rinsing, and raising of the intraventricular pressure by forced rinsing are the methods of choice to stop venous bleeding. Only in cases of unusual bleeding at the site of attachment, which occurred in three of their 18 patients, did these authors place an intraventricular drain and leave it in for a few days.

Najjar and colleagues report better clinical results with fewer complications, and all resections were complete because they used en bloc resection. In addition, the duration of surgery was shorter. In general, these authors believe that the endoscopic resection of colloid cysts should be the first treatment choice for all symptomatic patients, provided that the surgeon has enough expertise.

Comparing the Series

If we compare both series, we note a comparable number of cases (21 for Šteňo and 28 for Najjar and colleagues) and no mortality in the treatment of this benign tumor. Major complications in the endoscopic series of Najjar and colleagues included one case of hemiparesis (3.6%) and two cases of transient memory deficit (7.1%). These complications occurred in the early endoscopic experience, during their learning curve for endoscopic surgery. Since these authors have started using en bloc resection (18 cases over the past 6 years), fewer complications were observed compared with the previous endoscopic technique. There were no minor complications. In Šteňo's series, four of the 21 patients (19%) had a transient memory deficit. No other complications were reported. In each series, a shunt was inserted after the cyst was removed, but none of the patients had seizures. Radical resection was achieved in all patients in Šteňo's series, regardless of the technique used, and in 89% of the patients treated with the endoscope by Najjar and colleagues. There were no differences in terms of recurrence.

The results shown by both experts are similar to the experience reported in most institutional series, and are too few to draw final conclusions. The most critical deficit after this surgery is in memory, which, according to the literature, is found in approximately 10% of patients in most series, regardless of the number of cases[5,7,16,20,21] (**Table 12.1**). The reason for the transient memory deficit in Šteňo's series was the use of a suboptimal approach in one patient and interforniceal dissection of the fornix in two patients. We fully agree with Šteňo that a maneuver to widen the approach to the third ventricle should not be done, at least not in patients with colloid cysts. Subchoroidal dissection is a better approach to enlarge the access to the third ventricle through the foramen of Monro, if the venous anatomy allows it.[2] In my opinion, it is better to stop surgery and leave parts of the cyst wall behind rather than risk damaging the fornix. Usually, gentle manipulation of the fornix, which can

be protected with cottonoids, and sharp dissection of the cyst wall from the choroid plexus, the roof of the third ventricle, or both, do not cause these deficits. I am surprised that en bloc resection of the cyst through the foramen of Monro, as shown by Najjar and colleagues, does not harm the fornix, especially when we read that colloid cysts up to 32 mm in diameter have been resected in this way.

A conversion from the intended approaches was necessary in two patients in each series. The reasons for changing from an endoscopic to a microscopic technique were severe adhesions and firm cyst contents in Najjar and colleagues' series and uncontrolled bleeding during surgery in three of Šteňo's cases when he started with the endoscope. The difficulty of maintaining exact hemostasis reflects a clear technical shortcoming of the endoscopic technique. Another shortcoming is the small size of the grasping forceps used to empty the cyst. If the cyst contents are hard, this procedure may be impossible. Severe adhesions are a problem regardless of the technique or approach, but bimanual dissection with forceps and scissors, instead of pulling and shearing, is definitely the safer method for dissection and resection.

Factors Influencing the Technique and Approach

The Necessity for Total Removal

If it is deemed necessary to remove 100% of the colloid cyst, the best option is to use a transcallosal approach with microsurgical techniques. This microsurgical technique allows the surgeon to enlarge the access to the third ventricle through subchoroidal dissection and also allows the inspection of both foramina to choose the one more favorable for resection with the possibility of verifying total resection from both sides. The transcallosal approach has a lower rate of postoperative epilepsy and is applicable in patients with slim ventricles.[18]

An alternative for achieving complete resection is the endoscopic en bloc resection described above, a procedure we do not recommend because of the risk of uncontrollable bleeding. It is reasonable to choose the endoscopic technique if you are convinced that subtotal removal, which occurs in 40% of cases, may be acceptable for the patient.[5,7,8,20,21,58] In this respect, "subtotal" means some remnants of the wall are left behind but not any residual contents after aspiration of the cyst. If unexpected problems occur, conversion to a transcortical approach is possible through minimal enlargement of the bur hole. Some of the patients who had subtotal endoscopic removal had to undergo a second operation during the follow-up period (1.5 months to 12 years).[5,21,58]

Hydrocephalus

Hydrocephalus is not a prerequisite for the endoscopic technique, but in my experience it facilitates the resection significantly, as in all patients in Najjar and colleagues' series, who presented with hydrocephalus. The presence of slim ventricles is a strong argument for a microsurgical approach, preferably the transcallosal.

The Side of the Approach

If an endoscopic or a transcortical approach is planned, the surgeon has to decide on which side to place the bur hole or minicraniotomy. The consensus is to prefer the nondominant side. Sometimes, however, the ventricles are asymmetrical. In these cases, I use the side of the enlarged ventricle regardless of the dominant side. Details seen best on T2-weighted MRI, such as unilateral enlargement of the foramen of Monro, an unusual site, or the size of the veins, may affect the decision about the side of the approach as well.

An Algorithm for the Decision

Theoretically, endoscopic resection of colloid cysts should be the first treatment option, as endoscopic surgery presents the least invasive procedure with a high, or at least acceptable, success rate. In my algorithm for decision making, the main concern in the treatment of patients with colloid cysts is a deterioration or loss of memory. Transient memory deficits are reported to occur in about 7% of patients and permanent memory deficits in about 5%, but in future reports memory deficits should be examined in more detail and include neuropsychological tests.[1,5,7,8,15,16,18,19,21,60]

The key issue in resecting colloid cysts is detachment of the lesion from the roof of the third ventricle with precise coagulation and without tearing and shearing the fornix

with sharp transection from the choroid plexus. These goals can still best be achieved through the bimanual microsurgical technique, which is why I prefer a microsurgical transcallosal approach.

Endoscopic assistance during microsurgical surgery is very helpful to delineate anatomic details, especially to view the roof of the third ventricle, and it proves the completeness of resection. With angled lenses, it is possible to gather this information without touching the fornix at all. I regard this as part of the concept of a minimally invasive technique, which should not be restricted to the size of the craniotomy only. Stereotactic puncture and emptying of the cyst, however, is an even less invasive procedure, but the recurrence rates are too high.[16] It is very reasonable to start with endoscopic cyst resection and convert to a microsurgical technique as soon as an unfavorable situation arises, such as very viscous or hard contents of the cyst, severe adhesions, or, as pointed out by Šteňo, profound bleeding.

Another disadvantage is the higher rate of residuals and recurrences after endoscopic resection of colloid cysts.[21,58] A larger series of endoscopically treated colloid cysts shows that cyst wall remnants are visible on postoperative MRI in up to 42% of patients. These remnants are often clinically silent. In half of patients, however, wall remnants led to recurrence of the cyst, and reoperation was necessary in 18% of patients.[21]

Because of these shortcomings, we still prefer microsurgery to remove colloid cysts, but this can be done with endoscopic assistance. With further development of the endoscopic technique, we expect it will become the first choice of treatment for patients with colloid cysts, as Najjar and colleagues have discussed in their section of the chapter.

References

1. Hernesniemi J, Leivo S. Management outcome in third ventricular colloid cysts in a defined population: a series of 40 patients treated mainly by transcallosal microsurgery. Surg Neurol 1996;45:2–14

2. Türe U, Yaşargil MG, Al-Mefty O. The transcallosal-transforaminal approach to the third ventricle with regard to the venous variations in this region. J Neurosurg 1997;87:706–715

3. Kondziolka D, Lunsford LD. Stereotactic management of colloid cysts: factors predicting success. J Neurosurg 1991;75:45–51

4. Schroeder HW, Gaab MR. Endoscopic resection of colloid cysts. Neurosurgery 2002;51:1441–1444, discussion 1444–1445

5. Hellwig D, Bauer BL, Schulte M, Gatscher S, Riegel T, Bertalanffy H. Neuroendoscopic treatment for colloid cysts of the third ventricle: the experience of a decade. Neurosurgery 2003;52:525–533, discussion 532–533

6. Bergsneider M. Complete microsurgical resection of colloid cysts with a dual-port endoscopic technique. Neurosurgery 2007;60(2, Suppl 1):ONS33–ONS42, discussion ONS42–ONS43

7. Engh JA, Lunsford LD, Amin DV, et al. Stereotactically guided endoscopic port surgery for intraventricular tumor and col-

loid cyst resection. Neurosurgery 2010;67(3, Suppl Operative):ons198–ons204, discussion ons204–ons205

8. Charalampaki P, Filippi R, Welschehold S, Perneczky A. Endoscope-assisted removal of colloid cysts of the third ventricle. Neurosurg Rev 2006;29:72–79

9. Apuzzo ML, Chikovani OK, Gott PS, et al. Transcallosal, interfornicial approaches for lesions affecting the third ventricle: surgical considerations and consequences. Neurosurgery 1982;10:547–554

10. Yaşargil MG. Microneurosurgery. Stuttgart: Georg Thieme Verlag, 1996

11. Mathiesen T, Grane P, Lindgren L, Lindquist C. Third ventricle colloid cysts: a consecutive 12-year series. J Neurosurg 1997;86:5–12

12. Pamir MN, Peker S, Ozgen S, Kiliç T, Türe U, Ozek MM. Anterior transcallosal approach to the colloid cysts of the third ventricle: case series and review of the literature. Zentralbl Neurochir 2004;65:108–115, discussion 116

13. Hernesniemi J, Romani R, Dashti R, et al. Microsurgical treatment of third ventricular colloid cysts by interhemispheric far lateral transcallosal approach–experience of 134 patients. Surg Neurol 2008;69:447–453, discussion 453–456

14. Yaşargil MG, Abdulrauf SI. Surgery of intraventricular tumors. Neurosurgery 2008;62(6, Suppl 3):1029–1040, discussion 1040–1041

15. Shapiro S, Rodgers R, Shah M, Fulkerson D, Campbell RL. Interhemispheric transcallosal subchoroidal fornix-sparing craniotomy for total resection of colloid cysts of the third ventricle. J Neurosurg 2009;110:112–115

16. Mathiesen T, Grane P, Lindquist C, von Holst H. High recurrence rate following aspiration of colloid cysts in the third ventricle. J Neurosurg 1993;78:748–752

17. Grondin RT, Hader W, MacRae ME, Hamilton MG. Endoscopic versus microsurgical resection of third ventricle colloid cysts. Can J Neurol Sci 2007;34:197–207

18. Desai KI, Nadkarni TD, Muzumdar DP, Goel AH. Surgical management of colloid cyst of the third ventricle—a study of 105 cases. Surg Neurol 2002;57:295–302, discussion 302–304

19. Sampath R, Vannemreddy P, Nanda A. Microsurgical excision of colloid cyst with favorable cognitive outcomes and short operative time and hospital stay: operative techniques and analyses of outcomes with review of previous studies. Neurosurgery 2010;66:368–374, discussion 374–375

20. Horn EM, Feiz-Erfan I, Bristol RE, et al. Treatment options for third ventricular colloid cysts: comparison of open microsurgical versus endoscopic resection. Neurosurgery 2007;60:613–618, discussion 618–620

21. Boogaarts HD, Decq P, Grotenhuis JA, et al. Long-term results of the neuroendoscopic management of colloid cysts of the third ventricle: a series of 90 cases. Neurosurgery 2011;68:179–187

22. Konovalov AN, Pitskhelauri DI. Infratentorial supracerebellar approach to the colloid cysts of the third ventricle. Neurosurgery 2001;49:1116–1122, discussion 1122–1123

23. Bruce DA. Complications of third ventricle surgery. Pediatr Neurosurg 1991-1992–1992;17:325–330

24. Apuzzo MLJ, Litofsky NS. Surgery in and around the anterior third ventricle. In: Apuzzo MLJ, ed. Brain Surgery: Complication Avoidance and Management, vol. 1. New York: Churchill Livingstone, 1993:541–579

25. Villani R, Papagno C, Tomei G, Grimoldi N, Spagnoli D, Bello L. Transcallosal approach to tumors of the third ventricle. Surgical results and neuropsychological evaluation. J Neurosurg Sci 1997;41:41–50

26. Milligan BD, Meyer FB. Morbidity of transcallosal and transcortical approaches to lesions in and around the lateral and third ventricles: a single-institution experience. Neurosurgery 2010; 67:1483–1496, discussion 1496

27. Antunes JL, Louis KM, Ganti SR. Colloid cysts of the third ventricle. Neurosurgery 1980;7:450–455

28. Šteňo J, Šteňová J, Bízik I. Tumors of the third ventricle. [Article in Slovak] Cesk Slov Neurol Neurochir. 2009;72:302–315

29. Woiciechowsky C, Vogel S, Meyer BU, Lehmann R. Neuropsychological and neurophysiological consequences of partial callosotomy. J Neurosurg Sci 1997;41:75–80

30. Bogen JE. Physiological consequences of complete or partial commissural section. In: Apuzzo MLJ, ed. Surgery of the Third Ventricle, 1st ed. Baltimore: Williams & Wilkins, 1987:175–195

31. Kasowski H, Piepmeier JM. Transcallosal approach for tumors of the lateral and third ventricles. Neurosurg Focus 2001;10:E3

32. Winkler PA, Ilmberger J, Krishnan KG, Reulen HJ. Transcallosal interforniceal-transforaminal approach for removing lesions occupying the third ventricular space: clinical and neuropsychological results. Neurosurgery 2000;46:879–888, discussion 888–890

33. Amar AP, Ghosh S, Apuzzo MLJ. Ventricular tumors. In: Winn HR, ed. Youmans' Neurological Surgery, 5th ed., vol. 1. Philadelphia: WB Saunders, 2003:1237–1263

34. Jan M, Ba Zeze V, Velut S. Colloid cyst of the fourth ventricle: diagnostic problems and pathogenic considerations. Neurosurgery 1989;24:939–942

35. Müller A, Büttner A, Weis S. Rare occurrence of intracerebellar colloid cyst. Case report. J Neurosurg 1999;91:128–131

36. Alexiou GA, Zigouris A, Pahaturidis D, et al. Olfactory colloid cyst. Clin Neurol Neurosurg 2007;109:902–904

37. de Witt Hamer PC, Verstegen MJ, De Haan RJ, et al. High risk of acute deterioration in patients harboring symptomatic colloid cysts of the third ventricle. J Neurosurg 2002;96:1041–1045

38. Ryder JW, Kleinschmidt-DeMasters BK, Keller TS. Sudden deterioration and death in patients with benign tumors of the third ventricle area. J Neurosurg 1986;64:216–223

39. Siu TL, Bannan P, Stokes BA. Spinal cord infarction complicating acute hydrocephalus secondary to a colloid cyst of the third ventricle. Case report. J Neurosurg Spine 2005;3:64–67

40. Findler G, Cotev S. Neurogenic pulmonary edema associated with a colloid cyst in the third ventricle. Case report. J Neurosurg 1980;52:395–398

41. Annamalai G, Lindsay KW, Bhattacharya JJ. Spontaneous resolution of a colloid cyst of the third ventricle. Br J Radiol 2008; 81:e20–e22

42. Grigoriu C, Dumitrescu D, Florea I, et al. The colloid cyst of the third ventricle—a potential life threatening benign tumour. Rom J Leg Med. 2009;17:7–12

43. Kondziolka D, Bilbao JM. An immunohistochemical study of neuroepithelial (colloid) cysts. J Neurosurg 1989;71:91–97

44. Tsuchida T, Hruban RH, Carson BS, Phillips PC. Colloid cysts of the third ventricle: immunohistochemical evidence for non-neuroepithelial differentiation. Hum Pathol 1992;23:811–816

45. Hall WA, Lunsford LD. Changing concepts in the treatment of colloid cysts. An 11-year experience in the CT era. J Neurosurg 1987;66:186–191

46. Greenwood J Jr. Paraphysial cysts of the third ventricle; with report of eight cases. J Neurosurg 1949;6:153–159

47. Garrido E, Fahs GR. Cerebral venous and sagittal sinus thrombosis after transcallosal removal of a colloid cyst of the third ventricle: case report. Neurosurgery 1990;26:540–542

48. Webb AJ, Gillies MJ, Cadoux-Hudson TA. Acute vasospasm following transcallosal resection of a xanthogranulomatous colloid cyst of the 3rd ventricle. Clin Neurol Neurosurg 2010; 112:512–515

49. Gaab MR, Schroeder HW. Neuroendoscopic approach to intraventricular lesions. J Neurosurg 1998;88:496–505

50. Ulm AJ, Russo A, Albanese E, et al. Limitations of the transcallosal transchoroidal approach to the third ventricle. J Neurosurg 2009;111:600–609

51. Armao D, Castillo M, Chen H, Kwock L. Colloid cyst of the third ventricle: imaging-pathologic correlation. AJNR Am J Neuroradiol 2000;21:1470–1477

52. Rhoton AL Jr. Microsurgical anatomy of the third ventricular region. In: Apuzzo MLJ, ed. Surgery of the Third Ventricle. Baltimore: Williams & Wilkins; 1987:570–590

53. Rhoton AL Jr. The lateral and third ventricles. Neurosurgery 2002;51(4, Suppl)S207–S271

54. Lavrnic S, Stosic-Opincal T, Gavrilovic S, et al. Intraventricular textiloma with granuloma formation following third ventricle colloid cyst resection—a case report. Cent Eur Neurosurg 2009; 70:86–88

55. Yaşargil MG. Microneurosurgery, vol. IVB. Stuttgart: Georg Thieme Verlag, 1996

56. Symon L, Pell M, Yasargil MG, et al. Surgical techniques in the management of colloid cysts of the third ventricle. Adv Tech Stand Neurosurg 1990;17:121–157

57. Ostertag CB, Kreth FW. The stereotactic approach to colloid cysts. In: Al-Mefty O, Origitano TC, Harkey HL, eds. Controversies in Neurosurgery. New York: Thieme, 1996:32–34

58. Longatti P, Godano U, Gangemi M, et al; Italian neuroendoscopy group. Cooperative study by the Italian neuroendoscopy group on the treatment of 61 colloid cysts. Childs Nerv Syst 2006; 22:1263–1267

59. Lewis AI, Crone KR, Taha J, van Loveren HR, Yeh HS, Tew JM Jr. Surgical resection of third ventricle colloid cysts. Preliminary results comparing transcallosal microsurgery with endoscopy. J Neurosurg 1994;81:174–178

60. Teo C. Complete endoscopic removal of colloid cysts: issues of safety and efficacy. Neurosurg Focus 1999;6:e9

Chapter 13

Management of Unruptured Anterior Communicating Aneurysms: Coiling vs. Clipping vs. the Natural History

Case

A 40-year-old woman with no family history of intracranial aneurysms presents with an incidental 7-mm anterior communicating artery (ACoA) aneurysm. She has never smoked cigarettes. The treatment of this and other patients with incidental unruptured aneurysms is largely dependent on the natural history. This chapter discusses the controversies and the most current views on the natural history of intracranial aneurysms.

Participants

Endovascular Treatment of Unruptured Aneurysms: Aditya Bharatha, Timo Krings, and Karel terBrugge

Surgical Clipping of Unruptured Anterior Communicating Artery Aneurysms: Ali F. Krisht

Management of Unruptured Anterior Communicating Aneurysms: Natural History: Ning Lin and Rose Du

Moderator: Management of Unruptured Anterior Communicating Aneurysms: Coiling vs. Clipping vs. the Natural History: Robert F. Spetzler

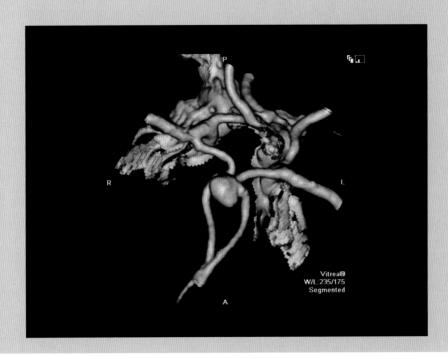

Endovascular Treatment of Unruptured Aneurysms

Aditya Bharatha, Timo Krings, and Karel terBrugge

The optimal treatment of patients with an asymptomatic saccular unruptured intracranial aneurysm (UIA) remains controversial. The most significant complication is rupture and subarachnoid hemorrhage (SAH) with its attendant morbidity and mortality. Hence, the goal of therapy is to identify those patients in whom the risks posed by the aneurysm itself outweigh the risks of possible treatment options and, where treatment is indicated, to identify the optimal strategy among the choices available.

Unruptured intracranial aneurysms are not rare. Based on autopsy and angiographic series, estimates of their prevalence have ranged greatly—from less than 1% to more than 10% depending on the patient population and study methodology. As expected, retrospective autopsy series have yielded the lowest apparent prevalence, whereas prospective angiographic series show the highest. A large systematic review of available series estimates their prevalence in the general population at around 2%.[1] Aneurysms are more common in women, patients with polycystic kidney disease, older patients, and those with a first-degree relative with an aneurysm or SAH. Other risk factors consistently associated with aneurysm formation are cigarette smoking, hypertension, and excessive alcohol use.[2]

When considering whether to treat a patient with a UIA, a crucial piece of information is the natural history of the lesion, specifically the likelihood of rupture. The International Study of Unruptured Intracranial Aneurysms (ISUIA) investigators have published the largest retrospective and prospective studies of the natural history of UIAs: ISUIA-I, with 1,449 patients and > 12,000 patient-years of follow-up,[3] and ISUIA-II, with 1,692 patients and > 6,500 patient-years of follow-up,[4] respectively. Based on a mean follow-up of 8.3 years, the annual rate of rupture in patients in ISUIA-I was 0.3%, 1%, and 0.05% for aneurysms greater than, equal to, or less than 1 cm, respectively. Aneurysms in the posterior circulation and posterior communicating artery were associated with higher risk. In the group of patients who received conservative treatment in the prospective ISUIA-II, the mean rate of SAH per patient-year was 0.8% over a mean follow-up of 4.1 years. The cumulative 5-year risk of bleeding for anterior circulation aneurysms was 0% for aneurysms smaller than 7 mm (1.5% in those with previous fully treated aneurysmal SAH), 2.6% for aneurysms 7 to 12 mm, and 14.5 to 40% for larger aneurysms. For posterior circulation and posterior communicating artery aneurysms, the 5-year rupture rates ranged from 2.5% for aneurysms smaller than 7 mm to 50% for giant aneurysms. These data have supported a more conservative approach to small anterior circulation aneurysms in recent years, with the caveat that a 0% rate of rupture of aneurysms smaller than 7 mm in ISUIA-II is implausibly low given that, in clinical

series of ruptured aneurysms, these make up 35 to 50%,[5] pointing to possible selection bias.

Wermer and colleagues[6] have published a meta-analysis of 19 studies (including the ISUIA data) published between 1966 and 2005, with a total of 6,556 UIAs in 4,705 patients and a mean follow-up of 5.6 years. The overall risk of rupture per patient-year at risk was 1.2% in studies with a mean follow-up of less than 5 years, 0.6% in studies with a mean follow-up between 5 and 10 years, and 1.3% in studies with a greater than 10-year follow-up. Factors associated with greater risk were a size greater than 5 mm, symptomatic presentation, posterior circulation location, female sex, age greater than 60 years, and Japanese or Finnish descent. Smoking was also associated with greater risk, although this risk was not statistically significant.

Undoubtedly, other factors also influence the rate of rupture. Likely candidates include patient-specific factors such as background vasculopathy, hypertension, alcohol use and family history, and aneurysm-specific factors such as morphology (lobulation, daughter sac, aspect ratio[7]), hemodynamics, aneurysm growth rate, and multiplicity. The presence of mural thrombus and calcification also likely affects the rupture risk. Although the data supporting these variables remain inconclusive, they must be kept in mind in the clinical decision-making process.[8]

Next, we must consider the treatment risks and benefits. A systematic review of the literature describing coil embolization of UIAs published between 1990 and 2002 (1,379 patients in 29 studies) indicated an overall procedure-related permanent morbidity and mortality rate of 7% and 0.6%, respectively, with a reduced morbidity rate of 4.5% in later studies.[9] A large, retrospective, single-institution case series of all 173 UIA patients treated with endovascular means over a 12-year period from 1992 to 2004 indicated a procedure-related mortality rate of 0.5% and permanent morbidity rate of 2.5% (1% severe deficit).[10] In a consecutive series of 146 unruptured aneurysms treated with Guglielmi detachable coils (GDCs), Holmin and colleagues[11] report a mortality of 0% and permanent morbidity in 3.4%. Although these figures compare favorably to surgical series, no randomized clinical trial has directly compared the morbidity and mortality of endovascular versus surgical treatment in patients with UIAs. The International Subarachnoid Aneurysm Trial (ISAT) concluded that, in 2,143 patients with ruptured aneurysms in which surgical and endovascular treatment were judged to be in clinical equipoise, the rate of death or dependence at 1 year was significantly less in the endovascular group (24% versus 31%) with a lower cumulative mortality over 7 years.[12]

In ISUIA-II, the morbidity rates for surgical and endovascular therapy were prospectively compared in a nonrandomized group of patients, 1,917 of whom underwent surgery and 451 of whom had endovascular repair.[4] The risk of death or disability at 1 year was significantly less in the endovascular cohort than in the surgical group (12.6% and 9.8%, respectively; 10.1% and 7.1% in the group with previously treated aneurysmal SAH). Overall, the patients in the endovascular group were older and had larger aneurysms and a greater proportion of basilar and cavernous aneurysms. These results suggest that, when both treatments are feasible, the up-front risk from endovascular procedures is lower than that from surgery.

But what about efficacy? Considerations of treatment efficacy are limited by relatively small numbers of patients, the length of follow-up, and the mixing of ruptured and unruptured aneurysm data. It has been accepted that satisfactorily clipped aneurysms are effectively cured, and surgical series have indeed shown a very low re-rupture rate in follow-ups of patients with clipped aneurysms that have been completely excluded as shown by angiography. In one series of clipped ruptured aneurysms followed for a mean of 10 years, annual rates of 0.14% for recurrent SAH and 0.09% for asymptomatic regrowth were seen.[13] There has been concern regarding the long-term durability of endovascular treatment. Published rates of residual or remnant aneurysm after endovascular treatment have been in the range of 5 to 20%, recanalization rates in the range of 15 to 35%, and retreatment rates of up to 13%. A lower degree of aneurysm occlusion and recanalization are thought to be risk factors for re-rupture, although the data have been conflicting.[14,15]

Despite these findings, the rates of rebleeding have been low. In a retrospective analysis of 173 patients with coiled unruptured aneurysms treated at a single institution between 1992 and 2004 for a mean of 3.7 years, three aneurysms ruptured (0.5% annual rupture rate), and all of these were giant posterior circulation aneurysms.[10] In the series by Holmin and colleagues,[11] the retreatment rate was 12% and rebleeding occurred in only one patient (0.68% of coiled UIAs) at a median follow-up of nearly 5 years. The Cerebral Aneurysm Rerupture After Treatment (CARAT) investigators identified all aneurysmal SAH patients treated at their institutions between 1996 and 1998 and reviewed the results in 1,010 patients treated with either surgery (711) or coils (299) who were followed for a mean of 4.4 years.[16] The annual rates of retreatment were 13.3% for coiling and 2.6% for clipping in the first year, 4.5% and 0%, respectively, in the second year, and 1.1% and 0% thereafter. Although late retreatment was more common in the coil group, no late retreatment led to death or disability. Rates of rebleeding were low for both groups but were slightly lower in the surgical cohort; annual rates of re-rupture for coiling and surgery were 4.9% and 2%, respectively, in the first year and 0.11% and 0% in subsequent years. Combining these data with the re-rupture rates in the ISAT study shows that the early benefit of coiling would only be reversed after 70 years of follow-up. If we project this data onto the disability and death data from the ISUIA study, it appears

that the impact of retreatment would not outweigh the early benefit of coiling even after 100 years of follow-up. Thus, the rate of aneurysm rupture after treatment and the need for repeated treatment is somewhat greater for endovascular therapy, but the difference appears to be small in comparison with the lower rates of procedure-related morbidity.

From a health care system perspective, another question is whether the treatment of unruptured aneurysms is cost-effective in terms of its ability to reduce the costs of hospitalization and long-term care. An analysis using Dutch data showed that, for 50-year-old patients, treatment using both surgical and endovascular techniques was cost-effective for a wide range of rupture rate scenarios above 0.3% per year, and slightly more so in women.[17]

Finally, in applying this disparate information to specific clinical scenarios, it is important to consider the data from the literature in the context of patient-specific, aneurysm-specific, and treatment-specific factors to provide individualized recommendations regarding treatment (**Fig. 13.1**).

Patient-specific factors relating to life expectancy are crucial parameters in determining the appropriateness of UIA treatment. In patients of advanced age or with significant comorbidities, the reduced life expectancy of the patient may result in the up-front risk of treatment exceeding the potential beneficial reduction in risk of SAH. Nonmodifiable risk factors for rupture, such as female sex and etiologic factors, and modifiable risk factors that may increase the risk of rupture, such as smoking, alcohol use, and hypertension, should also be taken into account. Idiosyncratic factors, such as excessive or debilitating anxiety pertaining to a small unruptured aneurysm, may result in the need to consider treatment for patients who might otherwise be followed. Patient factors can also influence the choice of therapy. Excessive tortuosity of the extracranial vessels can render endovascular treatment difficult or impossible, favoring surgery in some cases. Some patients may reject the idea of follow-up and the possibility of recurrence that goes with endovascular treatment. On the other hand, significant comorbidity may render a patient unable to tolerate the stresses of conventional surgery, making endovascular treatment more attractive.

Next, aneurysm-specific factors must be integrated. As discussed above, size plays an important but by no means exclusive role. In addition to influencing predictions about the risk of rupture, aneurysm size can influence the patient's choice of therapy. Coiling of very small aneurysms (< 2–3 mm) has been associated with an increased risk of rupture, whereas coiling of giant aneurysms has been associated with coil compaction and recanalization. Morphological factors can influence whether coiling is possible and whether assistive techniques such as balloon remodeling or stent-assisted techniques are required. Important parameters that can predict immediate post-coiling occlusion rates include the absolute size of the neck, the dome-to-neck ratio, the aneurysm's shape, and the incorporation of branch vessels.[18]

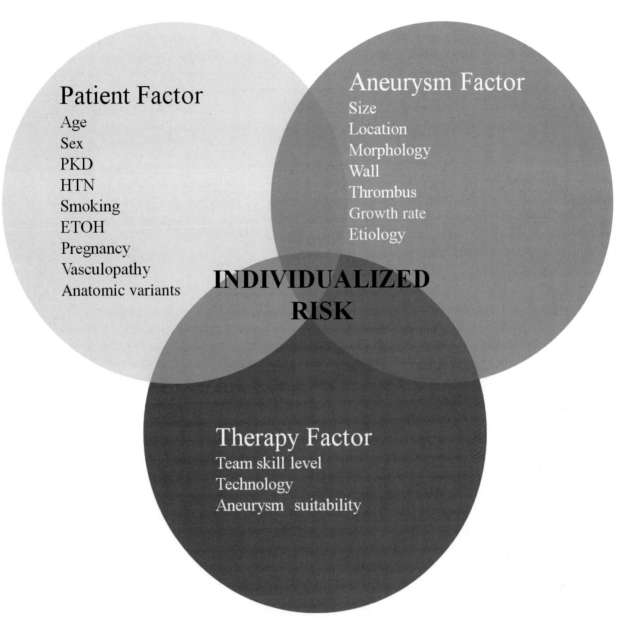

Fig. 13.1 Factors to be considered in providing patients with an individualized treatment recommendation. ETOH, ethyl alcohol consumption; HTN, hypertension; PKD, polycystic kidney disease.

The aneurysm's location is another important factor. The general rule of thumb is that basilar termination aneurysms, which are difficult to access through surgery, are often more suited for endovascular treatment. Aneurysms of the middle cerebral artery bifurcation often have an unfavorable geometry of branch vessels and are surgically accessible; hence, they are often (but not always) better suited to clipping. For aneurysms in other locations, both treatments are often possible. For example, for distal or peripheral aneurysms, both clipping and endovascular vessel sacrifice are possibilities. For anterior and posterior communicating artery aneurysms, both treatments can often be considered. In many cases, clinical, morphological, and local endovascular or surgical experience are the deciding factors. In other words, factors related to the patient and

the aneurysm need to be considered in the context of the technology available and institutional expertise (therapy factors). With the advent of new technologies, the repertoire of both surgical and endovascular therapies will continue to expand. Examples include the recent advances in flow-diverting stents and cerebrovascular bypass procedures.

With regard to the clinical case presented with this chapter, a presumably healthy 40-year-old woman with a greater than 30-year life expectancy and an anterior circulation aneurysm 7 mm in diameter, we would expect the cumulative risk of rupture to exceed 15 to 30%, which is much greater than the risk posed by endovascular or surgical treatment. In this location, both surgery and coiling are feasible, but we would want to offer the most effective treatment with the lowest risk. For patients in whom both options are equally feasible, we would advocate coiling given the lower up-front risks. However, in this case, based on the image provided, incorporating the A2s into the neck may increase the risks of coiling both in terms of thrombo-embolic complications and residual aneurysm, and this aneurysm is also quite suitable for surgery. Therefore, this case ultimately highlights how important it is that decisions regarding the choice of treatment be made in a systematic manner, based on careful analysis of the patient, the aneurysm, and all of the available therapeutic options.

Surgical Clipping of Unruptured Anterior Communicating Artery Aneurysms

Ali F. Krisht

In the past, a patient diagnosed with a UIA was considered to be a person walking around with a ticking time bomb in his or her head. Recent reports and studies, however, suggest that the natural history of unruptured aneurysms may be more benign than what was previously thought.[3,4,19–21] This is especially so when dealing with small aneurysms. Investigators from the ISUIA suggested that aneurysms arising from the posterior communicating artery or the basilar tip region are more prone to bleed than aneurysms arising from other locations in the anterior circulation.[3,4]

This assessment included aneurysms involving the ACoA complex. But as most neurosurgeons dealing with ruptured aneurysms on a routine basis know, lesions of the ACoA account for a large percentage of patients arriving in the emergency room with a ruptured aneurysm.[1,22–25] In addition, the ISUIA study included a relatively smaller number of ACoA aneurysms when compared with most surgical series. This may very well suggest that the majority of ACoA aneurysms present with rupture and a smaller number present in a nonruptured state (**Fig. 13.2**).

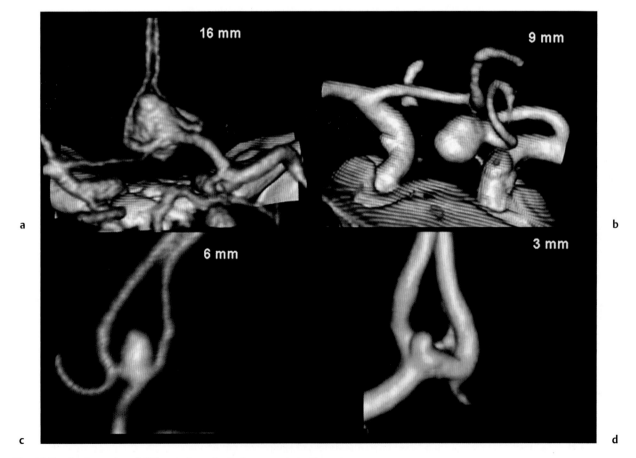

Fig. 13.2a–d Examples of different sizes of anterior communicating artery aneurysms.

The initial results of the ISUIA determined that the annual rupture rate of anterior circulation aneurysms smaller than 10 mm was a low 0.05%. This rate jumped significantly to 1% per year for aneurysms greater than or equal to 10 mm in size. Based on these statistical findings, the trend has been to leave small ACoA aneurysms untreated because of their extremely low risk of rupture. Further analysis of the ISUIA patients followed for 5 years suggested that aneurysms smaller than 10 mm in size should be subdivided into two groups, those less than 7 mm and those between 7 and 10 mm. This subdivision was proposed because the annual rupture rate of aneurysms between 7 and 10 mm jumped to 2.6%, whereas the annual rupture rate for aneurysms less than 7 mm remained at 0%. These findings led to a series of publications in *Stroke* in 2005 entitled "Patients with Small, Asymptomatic, Unruptured Intracranial Aneurysms and No History of Subarachnoid Hemorrhage Should Be Treated Conservatively."

Most neurosurgeons who regularly treat patients with aneurysms have a problem with such conclusions, in part because the ISUIA has predominantly focused on size in drawing its conclusions. Although the size of the unruptured aneurysm is a factor to be considered in the decision-making process, it should not always be considered the primary factor. The majority of lesions in several reported series of ruptured aneurysms were small. In addition, there is a long list of factors that may play a role in the etiology of aneurysmal rupture[7,26–55] **(Table 13.1).** For most of these factors, the extent of their influence on the rupture rate is not known. Defining how these various factors influence the activity within an aneurysm may one day help us differentiate between active and inactive aneurysms. With regard to ACoA aneurysms, several studies reached conclusions contrary to those of the ISUIA. In a meta-analysis of natural history studies, Mira and colleagues[56] found that the risk of rupture for unruptured anterior communicating artery aneurysms was twice that of other locations (95% confidence interval, 1.29–3.12). Furthermore, in a study from Japan involving 13 hospitals, Yonekura[57] reviewed the rupture rates of aneurysms less than 5 mm in size. This study included 329 patients with 380 aneurysms and a mean follow-up of 13.8 months. The author found that the annual rupture rate was 0.8%, but 18 of the aneurysms had enlarged (seven grew more than 20 mm) during the study period and were treated because of concern about their growth and the possibility of rupture. This approach obviously created a bias in the final annual rupture rate, which means the figure of 0.8% is probably an underestimate of the real rupture rate if those 18 aneurysms had been left untreated. The author also found that the risk of enlargement and rupture was influenced by the location at the ACoA complex in addition to other factors.

To recommend treatment for any patient with an unruptured aneurysm, it is clear that the proposed treatment must have a much higher chance for a better outcome than the natural history. For this reason, when we evaluate a patient with a small aneurysm of the ACoA, we

Table 13.1 Factors that May Influence Aneurysm Rupture

The hemodynamics, shape, and growth rate of the aneurysm

Multiple aneurysms

The regional perfusion pressure

The volume–pressure relationship

Wall thickness

The relationship of the aneurysm to the parent vessel

The genetic makeup of the vessel wall

The patient's ability to repair

The patient's use of tobacco, alcohol, or both

Elevated blood pressure

take into consideration the following factors for the following reasons:

Patients who are younger have a longer life expectancy and a higher cumulative risk of rupture during their lifetime. According to findings in studies by Juvela and colleagues[40–42,58,59] in Helsinki, the 30-year rupture rate of aneurysms in general was 30.3%. Therefore, patients who are in their 40s have a greater than 30% chance of rupture during their lifetime. In other words, they have up to a 15% chance of dying or being severely disabled. This risk should be an indication for initiating treatment. Whether the treatment should be through microsurgical clipping or endovascular means is the subject of the moderator's comments at the end of this chapter.

Other factors that have previously been noted to influence the rate of rupture include a history of heavy cigarette smoking, a family history of aneurysms, and untreated or uncontrolled hypertension. More recently, several studies suggested that the morphological features of the aneurysm, especially those related to size, may correlate with aneurysmal rupture.[60]

One of the most important factors yet to be evaluated for its influence on the rupture rate is the quality of the wall of the aneurysm. Until now, we have had no way to evaluate or assess this quality. In a pilot study at our institution, we reviewed the occurrence of a "blistering" type of change in 100 patients with UIAs treated through microsurgical clipping. In 90% of the cases examined, there was a significant weak spot in the aneurysmal wall that might later be the location for a potential rupture. This observation emphasizes our lack of knowledge about which aneurysms will bleed and which will not.

Because of the complexity of the facts described here, it continues to be very difficult for the treating neurosurgeon to decide whether a small UIA should be treated or left alone. Therefore, to help surgeons make a more educated decision, we evaluated our experience with surgical clipping of unruptured aneurysms as it compares with a 10-year survival for patients with unclipped aneurysms.[61]

This study was conducted in 116 consecutive patients with 148 aneurysms. These aneurysms were divided into the four groups defined by the ISUIA: small, medium, large, and giant aneurysms. We then statistically analyzed the severe morbidity and mortality expected to occur if our cohort of patients had been included in the ISUIA and were not operated on. These results were compared with the surgical outcomes in our patients. The analysis showed a statistically significant difference in the morbidity rate, but surgical intervention had a positive and significant impact on the mortality rate.

In conclusion, contrary to the ISUIA results, ACoA aneurysms are more common clinically and have a higher rate of rupture than what was reported in unruptured aneurysm studies. For this reason we should have a low threshold for treating them, especially in younger patients. We strongly advocate microsurgical clipping because nowadays, and in experienced hands, it has a very low rate of morbidity and mortality and it is superior to coiling in its durability and in providing patients with peace of mind, especially in terms of the future need for retreatment or the possibility of bleeding.

Management of Unruptured Anterior Communicating Aneurysms: Natural History

Ning Lin and Rose Du

The prevalence of cerebral aneurysms is estimated to be 1 to 2% in the general population[1,62,63] and could be higher in the elderly.[64] The management of an incidentally discovered intracranial aneurysm remains one of the most controversial topics in neurosurgery. Therapeutic options such as microsurgical clipping or endovascular coiling are offered to eradicate the potential risk of aneurysm rupture, which results in SAH and can lead to devastating morbidity and mortality. These interventions, however, also carry certain risks, and in some situations may do more harm than good. Therefore, it is essential to understand the natural history of UIAs and carefully balance the risks and benefits of all treatment options offered to a patient.

Observational Study and Meta-Analysis

The natural history of a UIA can ideally be assessed by a prospective, randomized trial. Nevertheless, given the severe consequence of SAH and the generally low incidence of aneurysmal rupture, clinicians and surgeons have been reluctant to perform such a study.[65] Instead, several observational cohort trials and meta-analyses have been conducted and published in the last decade; these represent our best knowledge in estimating the bleeding risk of UIAs **(Table 13.2)**.

The most widely cited reports are probably the two seminal papers by the ISUIA investigators.[3,4] The first study, ISUIA-I, consisted of a retrospective analysis of 1,449 patients harboring 1,937 unruptured aneurysms for a follow-up duration of 8.3 years.[3] These patients were purposefully divided into two groups: group 1 contained 727 patients with no history of aneurysmal SAH, and group 2 contained 722 patients who had previous aneurysmal SAH but recovered well (Rankin scale 1–2). In group 1, the annual rupture

rate was 0.05% for aneurysms smaller than 10 mm and 1% for aneurysms equal to or larger than 10 mm. In group 2, the annual rupture rate was 0.5% for smaller aneurysms and 1% for larger aneurysms. These results were drastically lower than the majority of those from previous, smaller-scale observational studies.[26,59,66–68] After the study, many questions were raised regarding selection bias, censoring during the follow-up period, and the composition of aneurysms in different locations.[19,64,69,70] Consequently, there was a strong demand for a larger, better designed study to further address the natural history of UIAs.

The second study (ISUIA-II) from the same group of investigators was published in 2003 and consisted of a prospective analysis of 1,692 patients with 2,686 aneurysms for a follow-up period of 4.1 years.[4] The patients were again divided into two groups based on SAH history, and the bleeding risk was stratified according to the location and size of the aneurysm. For patients with no SAH history (group 1, n = 1,077), the 5-year cumulative rupture rate for anterior circulation aneurysms (excluding cavernous aneurysms of the internal carotid artery) smaller than 7 mm was essentially 0%, and for posterior circulation aneurysms (including posterior communicating artery aneurysms) smaller than 7 mm, the cumulative rupture rate was 2.5%. For patients with a history of SAH (group 2, n = 615), the 5-year cumulative rupture rates for small anterior and posterior circulation aneurysms were 1.5% and 3.4%, respectively. In addition, the cumulative rupture rates were 2.6%, 14.5%, and 40%, respectively, for anterior circulation aneurysms measuring 7 to 12 mm, 13 to 24 mm, and ≥ 25 mm, and were 14.5%, 18.4%, and 50%, respectively, for posterior circulation aneurysms in the same size categories. These results provided better estimates of the natural history of UIAs compared with the retrospective portion of the study;

Table 13.2   Recent Studies of the Natural History of Unruptured Intracranial Aneurysms

Study	Year	Number of Patients	Type of Study	Rupture Rate and Other Findings
ISUIA-I[3]	1998	1,449	Retrospective	For aneurysms < 10 mm, the rupture rate was 0.05% per year if there was no prior SAH history, 0.5% if there was SAH history. For aneurysms ≥ 10 mm, the rupture rate was 1% for both groups.
ISUIA-II[4]	2003	1,692	Prospective	For anterior circulation aneurysms, the 5-year cumulative rupture rates were 0%, 2.6%, 14.5%, and 40% for aneurysms < 7 mm, 7–12 mm, 13–24 mm, and > 24 mm, respectively. For posterior circulation aneurysms, the 5-year cumulative rupture rates were 2.5%, 14.5%, 18.4%, and 50% for the same size categories.
Juvela et al[41]	2008	142	Prospective	The cumulative rupture rates for all aneurysms were 10.5% at 10 years, 23% at 20 years, and 30.3% at 30 years.
Sonobe et al[76]*	2010	374	Prospective	The overall rupture rate was 0.54% per year. The rupture rate was 0.34% per year for single aneurysms and 0.95% for multiple aneurysms.
Rinkel et al[1]	1998	3,907	Meta-analysis	The overall rupture rate was 1.9% per year. The rupture rate was 0.7% per year for aneurysms ≤ 10 mm, and 4.0% per year for aneurysms > 10 mm.
Mira et al[56]	2006	1,414	Meta-analysis	The rupture rate for ACoA aneurysms was 2.2% per year. ACoA aneurysms were twice as likely to rupture than aneurysms in other locations (RR = 2.0, 95% CI = 1.29–3.12).

Abbreviations: ACoA, anterior communicating artery; CI, confidence interval; RR, relative risk; SAH, subarachnoid hemorrhage.

*The study included only aneurysms < 5 mm in size.

nevertheless, ISUIA-II was still plagued by significant selection bias and design flaws. Of particular concern was the large number of patients who were initially managed conservatively but received treatment during the follow-up period (534 patients, or 31.6%). Moreover, there was a disproportionately low percentage of ACoA aneurysms in the study population (10.3%), well below what was estimated in the general population. Finally, the percentage of ruptured aneurysms smaller than 7 mm was much less than would be expected based on the ISAT, in which more than 90% of ruptured aneurysms were smaller than 10 mm.[12,71] This preponderance of small ruptured aneurysms is corroborated by other studies[1,72,73] and is not explained by the proportion of small aneurysms in the ISUIA study. Hence, it is highly likely that the study underestimated the bleeding risk in some groups of UIAs, and caution should be taken when applying these results to evaluate a specific unruptured aneurysm.[65,74,75]

Juvela and colleagues[41,72] in Helsinki, Finland, conducted a comprehensive observational trial, which was not constrained by the same selection bias and high crossover rate as the ISUIA because of a specific department policy prior to 1979 that all intracranial aneurysms be managed conservatively. The authors evaluated 142 patients with 181 aneurysms for a mean duration of 18.1 years. They reported cumulative rupture rates of 10.5% at 10 years after the diagnosis of a UIA, 23% at 20 years, and 30.3% at 30 years for the entire group, which translated into roughly 1% per year. The Helsinki series was of much smaller scale than the ISUIA and had its own flaws because of the homogeneity of the study population (all Finnish) and the fact that the vast

majority of patients had a history of SAH (131/142, 92%) from a separate aneurysm. Nevertheless, it remains the best designed and executed investigation to date because of its complete follow-up information and essentially zero crossover rate during the long observation period.

Given the focus on aneurysm size in the ISUIA, a recent trial performed by 12 national hospitals in Japan intended to address the rupture risk of small aneurysms (< 5 mm).[76] The authors prospectively followed 374 patients for 3.5 years. These patients harbored 448 small aneurysms, and seven patients suffered SAH, which translated into an annual rupture rate of 0.5% per year for all aneurysms. Ten of these patients underwent surgical or endovascular treatment during the follow-up period (for a crossover rate of 2.7%) because of aneurysmal growth or at the surgeon's discretion, constituting a much smaller proportion compared with the ISUIA.

Several meta-analyses of historic trials also provided insight into the risk of bleeding for UIAs. Rinkel and colleagues[1] published a comprehensive analysis of the prevalence and natural history of UIAs by exhaustively reviewing the literature published from 1955 to 1996. The authors identified nine studies totaling 3,907 patients and reported an overall rupture rate of 1.9% per year for all aneurysms. In particular, the rupture rate was 0.7% for aneurysms < 10 mm and 4% for aneurysms ≥ 10 mm. Moreover, the authors reported a roughly 1.1% per year rupture rate for all anterior circulation aneurysms and 4.4% per year for posterior circulation aneurysms. These results were in close agreement with those reported by Juvela and associates.[41,72] Another recent meta-analysis by Mira and colleagues[56] was intended to study the specific rupture risk of ACoA aneurysms because these were believed to be associated with a higher rupture rate than aneurysms in other locations but were underrepresented in large observational trials such as the ISUIA. The authors selected nine series published between 1987 and 2005; these series contained 1414 UIAs, 151 of which were ACoA aneurysms. The authors found that the relative risk of rupture of an ACoA aneurysm was nearly twice as high as that of aneurysms in other anterior or posterior circulations.

Other Risk Factors of Aneurysm Rupture

The rupture risk of an intracranial aneurysm depends on several demographic and biological factors in addition to the size and location of the aneurysm. The natural history of a UIA in a specific patient must be assessed with the clear understanding of his or her medical condition. For example, family history, female sex, multiple aneurysms, smoking, excessive alcohol consumption, the presence of daughter domes, and uncontrolled hypertension have all been shown to be predictors of an unfavorable natural history course[4,42,64,77–83] **(Table 13.3)**. The patient's age at the time of diagnosis is also of vital importance because a longer life expectancy usually places younger patients at a higher accumulated rupture risk than older patients. The Helsinki group, in fact, found that patient age was inversely associated with future aneurysm rupture.[42]

Active cigarette smoking is the most significant modifiable risk factor associated with aneurysm growth and rupture. Tobacco smoking is thought to accelerate the formation of atherosclerotic plaques, induce interstitial inflammation around intracranial vasculature, and weaken the vessel wall around the aneurysm. In the Helsinki series, active smokers were four times more likely to develop new aneurysms or exhibit aneurysmal growth during the follow-up period.[42,72] Similar results were found in respective studies done by investigators from the United States,[78] Sweden,[81] and Japan.[77] Smoking cessation is considered an important management step for patients harboring an UIA.

The relationship between the morphological parameters of an aneurysm and its rupture risk has only recently been systematically studied. Raghavan and colleagues[80] evaluated eight geometric factors in 27 aneurysms (nine ruptured, 18 unruptured) and found that ruptured aneurysms were associated with a significantly higher aspect ratio (aneurysm height divided by base diameter), undulation index (the roughness of the aneurysm's surface), and nonsphericity index (how nonspherical the aneurysm is). Dhar and associates[79] defined additional parameters while studying a larger group of 45 aneurysms (20 ruptured, 25 ruptured) and reported that the size ratio (maximum aneurysmal height divided by the average diameter of parent

Table 13.3 Demographic and Clinical Risk Factors Associated with Higher Rupture Rate

Risk Factors	
Demographic factors	Female sex[42,64]
	Age (inversely)[41,82]
Clinical factors	Hypertension[26,77,82]
	Active smoking[42,77,78,81]
	Family history[83,94]
	Multiple aneurysms[85,95]
	Posterior circulation aneurysms[1,4]
	Aneurysms > 7 mm[4,64]
	Unfavorable morphology[79,80]

and daughter vessels) was the most significant predictor of aneurysm rupture. In our series of 78 patients with middle cerebral artery aneurysms (43 ruptured, 35 unruptured),[84] a higher aspect ratio, a larger flow angle (the angle between the parent vessel and the axis of maximum aneurysmal height), and a smaller parent-to-daughter angle were strongly associated with aneurysm rupture. These simple morphological parameters could be used in conjunction with aneurysm size, location, and other demographic and clinical risk factors to evaluate the rupture risk of middle cerebral artery aneurysms.

Guidelines for the Management of Incidental Unruptured Intracranial Aneurysms

Although the optimal management of an incidental unruptured aneurysm remains controversial, a few groups have offered guidelines or recommendations for a general approach to these lesions **(Table 13.4)**. In 2000, the Stroke Council of the American Heart Association recommended intervention for all symptomatic aneurysms and asymptomatic aneurysms $\geq$ 10 mm while voicing caution for treating patients with asymptomatic aneurysms < 10 mm unless the patient has a history of SAH.[19] These suggestions were clearly influenced by the results of ISUIA-I and did not take into consideration the prospective portion of the ISUIA trial and other studies available after 2000. In 2008, a group of experts from Columbia University reviewed additional literature and published updated guidelines regarding the management of incidental UIAs.[64] Although these authors continued to advocate treatment for all symptomatic aneurysms and aneurysms $\geq$ 10 mm, they also recommended intervention for aneurysms $\geq$ 5 mm in patients younger than 60 years of age.

In practice, we concur with most of the recommendations from the Columbia group. We share their opinion that aneurysms should be treated aggressively in young patients and in those who experience excessive psychological

Table 13.4   Expert Recommendations for the Management of Unruptured Intracranial Aneurysms

	Stroke Council[19]	Columbia University[64]
Management of symptomatic UIAs	All symptomatic aneurysms should be treated.	All symptomatic aneurysms should be treated.
Management of small, asymptomatic UIAs	Aneurysms < 10 mm in patients without prior SAH history may be observed, but special consideration for treatment should be given to young patients, patients with aneurysms approaching 10 mm, and patients with unfavorable morphology or other risk factors.	Small incidental aneurysms < 5 mm should be managed conservatively. Incidental aneurysms ≥ 5 mm in patients younger than 60 years of age should be treated.
Management of large, asymptomatic UIAs	Large asymptomatic aneurysms > 10 mm should be treated with consideration of patient age and existing medical conditions.	Large incidental aneurysms > 10 mm should be treated in healthy patients younger than 70 years of age.
Treatment of patients with prior SAH history	Aneurysms in patients with prior SAH history carry a higher risk of rupture, particularly in the posterior circulation. They should be considered for treatment.	Not specified
Clipping versus coiling as the treatment of UIAs	Not specified	Microsurgical clipping should be the first choice in low-risk, young patients.

Abbreviations: UIA, unruptured intracranial aneurysm; SAH, subarachnoid hemorrhage.

stress from harboring a UIA.[64] Smaller aneurysms (< 5 mm) in patients with multiple risk factors, such as a positive family history, worrisome morphology, or active smoking, may also warrant early intervention **(Fig. 13.3)**. On the other hand, if the patient has no risk factors and the aneurysm does not have any unfavorable morphological features, an argument could be made to at least start with observation and then intervene if the aneurysm shows signs of growth. This approach requires vascular imaging at regular time intervals and close follow-up of the patient. Establishing mutual understanding and trust is essential for the successful treatment of patients with UIAs.

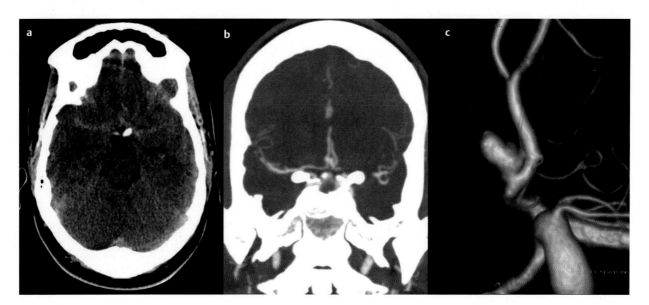

Fig. 13.3a–c   Radiological images of a 28-year-old woman who experienced a sudden onset of severe headache. The computed tomography (CT) scan **(a)** shows diffuse subarachnoid hemorrhage and hydrocephalus. The CT angiogram **(b)** and three-dimensional reconstruction of the cerebral angiogram **(c)** reveal an irregular 4-mm anterior communicating artery aneurysm.

Management of Unruptured Anterior Communicating Aneurysms: Coiling vs. Clipping vs. the Natural History

Robert F. Spetzler

The above three authored sections are remarkable in the similarity of their conclusions. Clearly, critical data are lacking to make a level I recommendation for the treatment of an asymptomatic 7-mm ACoA aneurysm in a 40-year-old woman without associated risk factors, making a consensus by these authors compelling.

The available data are confusing. The ISUIA provided conflicting rates of hemorrhage, depending on whether one considers the retrospective (ISUIA-I)[3] or prospective (ISUIA-II) trial.[4] In the retrospective study,[3] incidental aneurysms smaller than 10 mm were associated with a 0.05% rupture rate that jumped 10-fold in the prospective study.[4] These findings emphasize the dilemma associated with which numbers to use for making clinical decisions. One explanation is that the neurosurgeons were adept at selecting the most dangerous aneurysms for surgical treatment, thereby leaving patients with the aneurysms less likely to bleed available for the retrospective arm.[3] In the prospective study (ISUIA-II), there is significant bias in the small percentage of ACoA aneurysms entered,[4] that is, 10%. This percentage is much smaller than the percentage of small ruptured aneurysms found in clinical practice. Finally, there is the dilemma that more than 90% of aneurysms that become symptomatic with SAH are smaller than 10 mm in diameter.

Considering the Finnish and Japanese studies and the meta-analysis of rupture rates,[1,56,59,86] we can appreciate the difficulty of obtaining solid numbers on which to base clinical decisions. In contrast to the ISUIA, the Japanese study reported a much higher risk of rupture for ACoA aneurysms than those at other locations (2.2% per year, twice as likely as other sites).[56] That the best observational studies are consistent, with a predictable 0.5 to 1.0% or higher annual rate of hemorrhage for small aneurysms,[1,56,59,86] leads all three sets of authors to recommend treatment as a reasonable option.

The question then becomes which treatment option to choose. It is telling that the endovascular team recommends surgery as a primary consideration for this particular aneurysm because of the wide-based neck and the likely need for a more complex construct such as a stent. We all have our own biases, and mine are as deeply ingrained as anyone else's. However, our treatment recommendations should be based on the best available literature, and I believe the endovascular opinion is sound and on target in this case.

Let us briefly review the current landscape in terms of choosing whether to clip or coil an aneurysm. Two contemporary prospective studies have evaluated this issue: the ISAT and the Barrow Ruptured Aneurysm Trial (BRAT).[12,87–89] Both studies showed a benefit from coiling 1 year after treatment.[12,87] Neither study found a significant difference in clinical outcome between the two treatments at 5 and 3 years, respectively.[88,89] The ISAT study, however, did find a significant difference in the mortality rates between the two groups in favor of coiling. This difference, however, was based on pretreatment deaths related to the delay of more than 12 hours before clipping compared with those undergoing endovascular coiling. When this point is taken into account, there is no difference between the two treatment arms.[90] Furthermore, follow-up data from the ISAT study suggest that younger patients like the one presented for this discussion have better long-term outcomes with clipping compared with coiling.[91]

The entry criteria of the two studies differed markedly. The ISAT entered only 23% of eligible patients and excluded the vast majority of patients from the study.[12] The BRAT study randomized all eligible patients with SAH, irrespective of their anatomic presentation. This intent-to-treat design, however, led to a 38% crossover from the coiling group to the clipping group, mostly due to anatomic factors such as hematomas and the size of the aneurysm or the configuration of its neck.[87] The ISAT study had a profound effect on the management of aneurysms. In the United Kingdom, the rate of clipping declined from 51% to 31% and the rate of coiling increased from 35 to 68%.[92]

A recent, interesting study evaluated the actual results of change in practice patterns after the publication of the ISAT. O'Kelly and colleagues[93] retrospectively analyzed a cohort of adult patients with aneurysmal SAH who underwent treatment in Ontario between 1995 and 2004. Their goal was to determine whether endovascular occlusion of the ruptured aneurysm reduced the likelihood of readmission for SAH and the mortality rate compared with surgical occlusion. They counted 3,120 patients, 778 of whom had undergone coiling and 2,342 of whom had undergone clipping. In general, the rate of coiling tended to increase as the study years progressed. The marked difference in the mortality rate ($p < 0.0001$, 24.8% clipping versus 27.1% coiling) favored clipping. The rate of readmissions for SAH also significantly favored clipping (1.8%) compared with coiling (3.06%). Endovascular coiling was associated with a 25% increased risk of death or recurrent SAH.[93] In contrast to the ISAT,[12] in which coiling was done significantly earlier than clipping, the study by O'Kelly and colleagues showed that the time from admission to treatment was 2.68 days for coiling versus 1.99 days for the clipping group.[93] When a cohort of patients similar to the ISAT patient population

Table 13.5 Advantages and Disadvantages of Clipping and Coiling

Treatment	Advantages	Disadvantages	Advances
Clipping	Better initial occlusion Lower recurrence rate Lower re-bleed rate Few exclusions	Higher initial morbidity and mortality More invasive Seizure and cognitive risks?	ICG Adenosine Less retraction
Coiling	Lower initial morbidity and mortality Less invasive	Less occlusion Higher re-bleed rate Increased morbidity and mortality with stents Higher recurrence rate	Many stents, new coils, flow diverters, glues, catheters, etc. Industry driven

Abbreviations: ICG, indocyanine green videography.

was analyzed from each treatment group, the benefit of clipping was no longer statistically significant. The difficulty and risk of generalizing results from studies with highly selected patient populations to general practice are obvious. Furthermore, both treatments have their own advantages and disadvantages **(Table 13.5)**. It is obvious that both treatment modalities need to be available to offer each patient the best possible care.

In conclusion, I agree with the opinions expressed by the other experts and would also recommend clipping as the preferred treatment for this particular patient. I strongly believe that collaborative evaluation, which includes access to both treatment modalities to obtain the best recommendations for any individual patient, is the hallmark of excellent patient care.

References

1. Rinkel GJ, Djibuti M, Algra A, van Gijn J. Prevalence and risk of rupture of intracranial aneurysms: a systematic review. Stroke 1998;29:251–256
2. Feigin VL, Rinkel GJ, Lawes CM, et al. Risk factors for subarachnoid hemorrhage: an updated systematic review of epidemiological studies. Stroke 2005;36:2773–2780
3. International Study of Unruptured Intracranial Aneurysms Investigators. Unruptured intracranial aneurysms—risk of rupture and risks of surgical intervention. N Engl J Med 1998;339:1725–1733
4. Wiebers DO, Whisnant JP, Huston J III, et al; International Study of Unruptured Intracranial Aneurysms Investigators. Unruptured intracranial aneurysms: natural history, clinical outcome, and risks of surgical and endovascular treatment. Lancet 2003;362:103–110
5. Weir B. Patients with small, asymptomatic, unruptured intracranial aneurysms and no history of subarachnoid hemorrhage should be treated conservatively: against. Stroke 2005;36:410–411
6. Wermer MJ, van der Schaaf IC, Algra A, Rinkel GJ. Risk of rupture of unruptured intracranial aneurysms in relation to patient and aneurysm characteristics: an updated meta-analysis. Stroke 2007;38:1404–1410
7. Ujiie H, Tamano Y, Sasaki K, Hori T. Is the aspect ratio a reliable index for predicting the rupture of a saccular aneurysm? Neurosurgery 2001;48:495–502, discussion 502–503
8. Lall RR, Eddleman CS, Bendok BR, Batjer HH. Unruptured intracranial aneurysms and the assessment of rupture risk based on anatomical and morphological factors: sifting through the sands of data. Neurosurg Focus 2009;26:E2
9. Lanterna LA, Tredici G, Dimitrov BD, Biroli F. Treatment of unruptured cerebral aneurysms by embolization with Guglielmi detachable coils: case-fatality, morbidity, and effectiveness in preventing bleeding—a systematic review of the literature. Neurosurgery 2004;55:767–775, discussion 775–778
10. Standhardt H, Boecher-Schwarz H, Gruber A, Benesch T, Knosp E, Bavinzski G. Endovascular treatment of unruptured intracranial aneurysms with Guglielmi detachable coils: short- and long-term results of a single-centre series. Stroke 2008;39:899–904
11. Holmin S, Krings T, Ozanne A, et al. Intradural saccular aneurysms treated by Guglielmi detachable bare coils at a single institution between 1993 and 2005: clinical long-term follow-up for a total of 1810 patient-years in relation to morphological treatment results. Stroke 2008;39:2288–2297
12. Molyneux A, Kerr R, Stratton I, et al; International Subarachnoid Aneurysm Trial (ISAT) Collaborative Group. International Subarachnoid Aneurysm Trial (ISAT) of neurosurgical clipping versus endovascular coiling in 2143 patients with ruptured intracranial aneurysms: a randomised trial. Lancet 2002;360:1267–1274
13. Tsutsumi K, Ueki K, Usui M, Kwak S, Kirino T. Risk of recurrent subarachnoid hemorrhage after complete obliteration of cerebral aneurysms. Stroke 1998;29:2511–2513
14. Johnston SC, Dowd CF, Higashida RT, Lawton MT, Duckwiler GR, Gress DR; CARAT Investigators. Predictors of rehemorrhage after treatment of ruptured intracranial aneurysms: the Cerebral Aneurysm Rerupture After Treatment (CARAT) study. Stroke 2008;39:120–125
15. Willinsky RA, Peltz J, da Costa L, Agid R, Farb RI, terBrugge KG. Clinical and angiographic follow-up of ruptured intracranial aneurysms treated with endovascular embolization. AJNR Am J Neuroradiol 2009;30:1035–1040
16. CARAT Investigators. Rates of delayed rebleeding from intracranial aneurysms are low after surgical and endovascular treatment. Stroke 2006;37:1437–1442

17. Greving JP, Rinkel GJ, Buskens E, Algra A. Cost-effectiveness of preventive treatment of intracranial aneurysms: new data and uncertainties. Neurology 2009;73:258–265

18. Kiyosue H, Tanoue S, Okahara M, et al. Anatomic features predictive of complete aneurysm occlusion can be determined with three-dimensional digital subtraction angiography. AJNR Am J Neuroradiol 2002;23:1206–1213

19. Bederson JB, Awad IA, Wiebers DO, et al. Recommendations for the management of patients with unruptured intracranial aneurysms: a statement for healthcare professionals from the Stroke Council of the American Heart Association. Stroke 2000; 31:2742–2750

20. Brett A. Unruptured intracranial aneurysms. N Engl J Med 1999;340:1441–1442

21. Caplan LR. Should intracranial aneurysms be treated before they rupture? N Engl J Med 1998;339:1774–1775

22. Rogers LA. Intracranial aneurysm size and potential for rupture. J Neurosurg 1987;67:475–476 (Letter)

23. Rinne J, Hernesniemi J, Niskanen M, Vapalahti M. Analysis of 561 patients with 690 middle cerebral artery aneurysms: anatomic and clinical features as correlated to management outcome. Neurosurgery 1996;38:2–11

24. Solomon RA, Correll JW. Rupture of a previously documented asymptomatic aneurysm enhances the argument for prophylactic surgical intervention. Surg Neurol 1988;30:321–323

25. Weir B, Disney L, Karrison T. Sizes of ruptured and unruptured aneurysms in relation to their sites and the ages of patients. J Neurosurg 2002;96:64–70

26. Asari S, Ohmoto T. Natural history and risk factors of unruptured cerebral aneurysms. Clin Neurol Neurosurg 1993;95:205–214

27. Austin GM, Schievink W, Williams R. Controlled pressure-volume factors in the enlargement of intracranial aneurysms. Neurosurgery 1989;24:722–730

28. Bonita R. Cigarette smoking, hypertension and the risk of subarachnoid hemorrhage: a population-based case-control study. Stroke 1986;17:831–835

29. Connolly ES Jr, Choudhri TF, Mack WJ, et al. Influence of smoking, hypertension, and sex on the phenotypic expression of familial intracranial aneurysms in siblings. Neurosurgery 2001; 48:64–68, discussion 68–69

30. Crompton MR. Mechanism of growth and rupture in cerebral berry aneurysms. BMJ 1966;1:1138–1142

31. de la Monte SM, Moore GW, Monk MA, Hutchins GM. Risk factors for the development and rupture of intracranial berry aneurysms. Am J Med 1985;78(6 Pt 1):957–964

32. Dickey P, Nunes J, Bautista C, Goodrich I. Intracranial aneurysms: size, risk of rupture, and prophylactic surgical treatment. Conn Med 1994;58:583–586

33. Eskesen V, Rosenørn J, Schmidt K. The influence of unruptured intracranial aneurysms on life expectancy in relation to their size at the time of detection and to age. Br J Neurosurg 1988; 2:379–384

34. Findlay JM, Deagle GM. Causes of morbidity and mortality following intracranial aneurysm rupture. Can J Neurol Sci 1998; 25:209–215

35. Forget TR Jr, Benitez R, Veznedaroglu E, et al. A review of size and location of ruptured intracranial aneurysms. Neurosurgery 2001;49:1322–1325, discussion 1325–1326

36. Freger P, De Sousa MM, Sevrain L, et al. Is it necessary to operate on asymptomatic aneurysms? Apropos of 114 surgically treated asymptomatic aneurysms. Neurochirurgie 1987;33: 462–468

37. Graf CJ; Analysis of the Cooperative Study of Intracranial Aneurysms and Subarachnoid Hemorrhage. Prognosis for patients with nonsurgically-treated aneurysms. Analysis of the Cooperative Study of Intracranial Aneurysms and Subarachnoid hemorrhage. J Neurosurg 1971;35:438–443

38. Hashimoto N, Handa H. The size of cerebral aneurysms in relation to repeated rupture. Surg Neurol 1983;19:107–111

39. Heiskanen O. Risk of bleeding from unruptured aneurysm in cases with multiple intracranial aneurysms. J Neurosurg 1981; 55:524–526

40. Juvela S. Risk factors for multiple intracranial aneurysms. Stroke 2000;31:392–397

41. Juvela S, Porras M, Poussa K. Natural history of unruptured intracranial aneurysms: probability of and risk factors for aneurysm rupture. J Neurosurg 2008;108:1052–1060

42. Juvela S, Poussa K, Porras M. Factors affecting formation and growth of intracranial aneurysms: a long-term follow-up study. Stroke 2001;32:485–491

43. Kamitani H, Masuzawa H, Kanazawa I, Kubo T. Bleeding risk in unruptured and residual cerebral aneurysms—angiographic annual growth rate in nineteen patients. Acta Neurochir (Wien) 1999;141:153–159

44. Kataoka K, Taneda M, Asai T, Yamada Y. Difference in nature of ruptured and unruptured cerebral aneurysms. Lancet 2000; 355:203

45. Leblanc R, Melanson D, Tampieri D, Guttmann RD. Familial cerebral aneurysms: a study of 13 families. Neurosurgery 1995; 37:633–638, discussion 638–639

46. Leblanc R, Worsley KJ. Surgery of unruptured, asymptomatic aneurysms: a decision analysis. Can J Neurol Sci 1995;22:30–35

47. Longstreth WT Jr, Nelson LM, Koepsell TD, van Belle G. Cigarette smoking, alcohol use, and subarachnoid hemorrhage. Stroke 1992;23:1242–1249

48. Peters DG, Kassam AB, Feingold E, et al. Molecular anatomy of an intracranial aneurysm: coordinated expression of genes involved in wound healing and tissue remodeling. Stroke 2001; 32:1036–1042

49. Teunissen LL, Rinkel GJ, Algra A, van Gijn J. Risk factors for subarachnoid hemorrhage: a systematic review. Stroke 1996;27: 544–549

50. Ujiie H, Tachibana H, Hiramatsu O, et al. Effects of size and shape (aspect ratio) on the hemodynamics of saccular aneurysms: a possible index for surgical treatment of intracranial aneurysms. Neurosurgery 1999;45:119–129, discussion 129–130

51. van Crevel H, Habbema JD, Braakman R. Decision analysis of the management of incidental intracranial saccular aneurysms. Neurology 1986;36:1335–1339

52. Weir BK, Kongable GL, Kassell NF, Schultz JR, Truskowski LL, Sigrest A. Cigarette smoking as a cause of aneurysmal subarachnoid hemorrhage and risk for vasospasm: a report of the Cooperative Aneurysm Study. J Neurosurg 1998;89:405–411

53. Yasargil MG. Microneurosurgery, vol. 2. Stuttgart: Thieme, 1984

54. Yasargil MG, Fox JL, Ray MW. The operative approach to aneurysms of the anterior communicating artery. In: Krayenbuhl H, ed. Advances and Technical Standards in Neurosurgery, vol. 2. New York: Springer-Verlag, 1975:113–170

55. Yasargil MG, Kasdaglis K, Jain KK, Weber HP. Anatomical observations of the subarachnoid cisterns of the brain during surgery. J Neurosurg 1976;44:298–302

56. Mira JMS, Costa FAD, Horta BL, Fabião OM. Risk of rupture in unruptured anterior communicating artery aneurysms: meta-analysis of natural history studies. Surg Neurol 2006;66(Suppl 3):S12–S19, discussion S19

57. Yonekura M. Small unruptured aneurysm verification (SUAVe Study, Japan)—interim report. Neurol Med Chir (Tokyo) 2004; 44:213–214

58. Juvela S, Porras M, Heiskanen O. Natural history of unruptured aneurysms. J Neurosurg 1994;80:773–774 (Letter)

59. Juvela S, Porras M, Heiskanen O. Natural history of unruptured intracranial aneurysms: a long-term follow-up study. J Neurosurg 1993;79:174–182

60. Rahman M, Smietana J, Hauck E, et al. Size ratio correlates with intracranial aneurysm rupture status: a prospective study. Stroke 2010;41:916–920

61. Krisht AF, Gomez J, Partington S. Outcome of surgical clipping of unruptured aneurysms as it compares with a 10-year non-clipping survival period. Neurosurgery 2006;58:207–216, discussion 207–216

62. Rinkel GJ. Natural history, epidemiology and screening of unruptured intracranial aneurysms. Rev Neurol (Paris) 2008;164: 781–786

63. Weir B. Unruptured intracranial aneurysms: a review. J Neurosurg 2002;96:3–42

64. Komotar RJ, Mocco J, Solomon RA. Guidelines for the surgical treatment of unruptured intracranial aneurysms: the first annual J. Lawrence Pool Memorial Research Symposium—Controversies in the Management of Cerebral Aneurysms. Neurosurgery 2008;62:193–194

65. Mocco J, Komotar RJ, Lavine SD, Meyers PM, Connolly ES, Solomon RA. The natural history of unruptured intracranial aneurysms. Neurosurg Focus 2004;17:E3

66. Dippel DW, Habbema JD. Natural history of unruptured aneurysms. J Neurosurg 1994;80:772–774

67. Nakagawa T, Hashi K. The incidence and treatment of asymptomatic, unruptured cerebral aneurysms. J Neurosurg 1994;80: 217–223

68. Wiebers DO, Whisnant JP, O'Fallon WM. The natural history of unruptured intracranial aneurysms. N Engl J Med 1981;304: 696–698

69. Kobayashi S, Orz Y, George B, et al. Treatment of unruptured cerebral aneurysms. Surg Neurol 1999;51:355–362

70. Ausman JI. The *New England Journal of Medicine* report on unruptured intracranial aneurysms: a critique. Surg Neurol 1999; 51:227–229

71. Molyneux AJ, Kerr RS, Yu LM, et al; International Subarachnoid Aneurysm Trial (ISAT) Collaborative Group. International subarachnoid aneurysm trial (ISAT) of neurosurgical clipping versus endovascular coiling in 2143 patients with ruptured intracranial aneurysms: a randomised comparison of effects on survival, dependency, seizures, rebleeding, subgroups, and aneurysm occlusion. Lancet 2005;366:809–817

72. Juvela S, Porras M, Poussa K. Natural history of unruptured intracranial aneurysms: probability of and risk factors for aneurysm rupture. J Neurosurg 2000;93:379–387

73. Schievink WI. Intracranial aneurysms. N Engl J Med 1997; 336:28–40

74. Kailasnath P, Dickey P. ISUIA-II: the need to share more data. Surg Neurol 2004;62:95

75. Chen PR, Frerichs K, Spetzler R. Natural history and general management of unruptured intracranial aneurysms. Neurosurg Focus 2004;17:E1

76. Sonobe M, Yamazaki T, Yonekura M, Kikuchi H. Small unruptured intracranial aneurysm verification study: SUAVe study, Japan. Stroke 2010;41:1969–1977

77. Inagawa T. Risk factors for the formation and rupture of intracranial saccular aneurysms in Shimane, Japan. World Neurosurg 2010;73:155–164, discussion e23

78. Connolly ES Jr, Poisik A, Winfree CJ, et al. Cigarette smoking and the development and rupture of cerebral aneurysms in a mixed race population: implications for population screening and smoking cessation. J Stroke Cerebrovasc Dis 1999;8:248–253

79. Dhar S, Tremmel M, Mocco J, et al. Morphology parameters for intracranial aneurysm rupture risk assessment. Neurosurgery 2008;63:185–196, discussion 196–197

80. Raghavan ML, Ma B, Harbaugh RE. Quantified aneurysm shape and rupture risk. J Neurosurg 2005;102:355–362

81. Koskinen LO, Blomstedt PC. Smoking and non-smoking tobacco as risk factors in subarachnoid haemorrhage. Acta Neurol Scand 2006;114:33–37

82. Nahed BV, DiLuna ML, Morgan T, et al. Hypertension, age, and location predict rupture of small intracranial aneurysms. Neurosurgery 2005;57:676–683, discussion 676–683

83. Brown BM, Soldevilla F. MR angiography and surgery for unruptured familial intracranial aneurysms in persons with a family history of cerebral aneurysms. AJR Am J Roentgenol 1999;173:133–138

84. Lin N, Ho A, Gross BA, Day AL, Du R. Simple morphological variables for predicting the rupture risk of middle cerebral artery aneurysms. Congress of Neurological Surgeons Annual Meeting, 2010, Abstract

85. Casimiro MV, McEvoy AW, Watkins LD, Kitchen ND. A comparison of risk factors in the etiology of mirror and nonmirror multiple intracranial aneurysms. Surg Neurol 2004;61:541–545

86. Juvela S, Porras M, Poussa K. Natural history of unruptured intracranial aneurysms: probability and risk factors for aneurysm rupture. Neurosurg Focus 2000;8:1

87. McDougall CG, Spetzler RF, Zabramski JM, et al. The Barrow Ruptured Aneurysm Trial. J Neurosurg 2012;116:135–144

88. Spetzler RF, McDougall CG, Albuquerque FC, Zabramski JM, Hills NK, Partovi S, Nakaji P, Wallace RC: The Barrow Ruptured Aneurysm Trial: Three year results. J Neurosurg 2013 Apr 26.

89. Molyneux AJ, Kerr RS, Birks J, et al; ISAT Collaborators. Risk of recurrent subarachnoid haemorrhage, death, or dependence and standardised mortality ratios after clipping or coiling of an intracranial aneurysm in the International Subarachnoid Aneurysm Trial (ISAT): long-term follow-up. Lancet Neurol 2009;8:427–433

90. Bakker NA, Metzemaekers JD, Groen RJ, Mooij JJ, Van Dijk JM. International subarachnoid aneurysm trial 2009: endovascular coiling of ruptured intracranial aneurysms has no significant advantage over neurosurgical clipping. Neurosurgery 2010;66: 961–962

91. Mitchell P, Kerr R, Mendelow AD, Molyneux A. Could late rebleeding overturn the superiority of cranial aneurysm coil embolization over clip ligation seen in the International Subarachnoid Aneurysm Trial? J Neurosurg 2008;108:437–442

92. Gnanalingham KK, Apostolopoulos V, Barazi S, O'Neill K. The impact of the international subarachnoid aneurysm trial (ISAT) on the management of aneurysmal subarachnoid haemorrhage in a neurosurgical unit in the UK. Clin Neurol Neurosurg 2006; 108:117–123

93. O'Kelly CJ, Kulkarni AV, Austin PC, Wallace MC, Urbach D; Clinical Article. The impact of therapeutic modality on outcomes following repair of ruptured intracranial aneurysms: an administrative data analysis. Clinical article. J Neurosurg 2010; 113:795–801

94. Ruigrok YM, Rinkel GJ, Wijmenga C. Familial intracranial aneurysms. Stroke 2004;35:e59–e60, author reply e59–e60

95. Inagawa T. Incidence and risk factors for multiple intracranial saccular aneurysms in patients with subarachnoid hemorrhage in Izumo City, Japan. Acta Neurochir (Wien) 2009;151: 1623–1630

Chapter 14

Treatment of Giant Ophthalmic Aneurysms

Case

A 35-year-old patient who smokes presented with grade I subarachnoid hemorrhage. On examination, the patient had a nasal visual field defect. Digital subtraction angiography and three-dimensional reconstruction delineated a giant right ophthalmic aneurysm.

Participants

Endovascular Treatment of Giant Ophthalmic Artery Aneurysms: Bradley A. Gross, Stephen V. Nalbach, and Kai U. Frerichs

Treatment of Giant Ophthalmic Aneurysms: Microsurgical Clipping: Ana Rodríguez-Hernández, Osman Arikan Nacar, and Michael T. Lawton

Treatment of Giant and Large Carotid Ophthalmic Artery (Paraclinoid) Aneurysms: A Combined Microsurgical and Endovascular Approach: Rami Almefty and Kenan I. Arnautovic

Treatment of Giant Aneurysms of the Carotid Ophthalmic Artery: The Pipeline Embolization Device: Christopher S. Ogilvy and Christopher J. Stapleton

Moderators: The Treatment of Giant Ophthalmic Artery Aneurysms: Mark J. Dannenbaum and Arthur L. Day

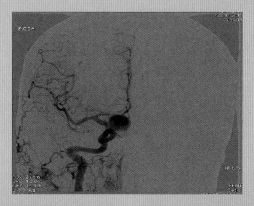

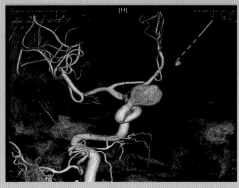
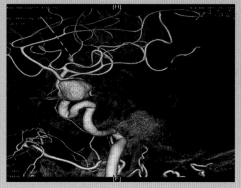

253

Endovascular Treatment of Giant Ophthalmic Artery Aneurysms

Bradley A. Gross, Stephen V. Nalbach, and Kai U. Frerichs

According to the International Study of Unruptured Intracranial Aneurysms, giant noncavernous aneurysms of the internal carotid artery (ICA) have an unfortunate natural history with an annual rupture rate of about 8%.[1] Unless treatment is contraindicated by the patient's age or numerous medical comorbidities, the incidental finding of these aneurysms strongly merits intervention.

The two standard treatment options for giant ophthalmic artery aneurysms include microsurgical direct clip ligation and endovascular coiling with or without adjunctive balloon remodeling or stenting.[2–9] Fortunately, most large and giant ophthalmic artery aneurysms are saccular, allowing for direct clip reconstruction without the need for revascularization techniques. Nevertheless, the ubiquitous need for an adjunctive anterior clinoidectomy in combination with the added challenge of clip reconstruction do add to the morbidity of the procedure as a result of cerebrospinal fluid leakage, thermal injury to the optic nerve, or perforator injury. In addition, proximal control essentially requires access to the cervical carotid artery. Not uncommonly, these giant aneurysms have some degree of calcification, a characteristic that can make microsurgical management treacherous if the calcification is present at the neck of the aneurysm. Modern, candid assessments of microsurgical morbidity after clipping of very large or giant anterior circulation aneurysms have reported major neurologic complication rates as high as 44% with concomitant systemic complication rates as high as 30%.[4] A recent report of very large or giant ophthalmic segment aneurysms treated surgically reported a 71% obliteration rate with a 14% visual complication rate and a 14% additional rate of hemispheric ischemia.[3]

Advantages of Endovascular Techniques

Ophthalmic artery aneurysms are advantageously located from an endovascular perspective. It is generally easy to gain access to these proximal lesions, and it is often feasible to successfully navigate a variety of adjunctive balloons or stents **(Fig. 14.1)**. Not surprisingly, the endovascular management of large and giant carotid-ophthalmic artery aneurysms has been associated with relatively low morbidity.[5,9] A recent report by Yadla and colleagues[9] compared microsurgical to endovascular results in the treatment of 170 patients with carotid ophthalmic aneurysms. The authors noted a greater rate of complications that was statistically significantly in the microsurgical cohort (26.1%) compared with the endovascular cohort (1.4%, *p* = 0.001). Specifically, of eight patients with giant ophthalmic aneurysms, two of three treated with clip ligation had major complications (visual loss), whereas none of the five treated with endovascular techniques had complications. Another

recent report described no complications or aneurysm ruptures after stent-coil treatment of seven very large or giant ophthalmic aneurysms (2 to 3.5 cm).[5]

Limitations of Endovascular Techniques

Endovascular coiling has not achieved similar rates of complete obliteration compared with surgical techniques,[5,8] but the clinical significance of this finding balanced against the impact of lower procedural morbidity remains to be elucidated. Preliminary studies have already shown some benefit to partial coiling.[10] In the Barrow Ruptured Aneurysm Trial, although the rates of aneurysm obliteration were not provided, none of the aneurysms treated with coil embolization re-bled over a 3-year follow-up period.[11]

The potential for recanalization and partial thrombosis of the aneurysm may also limit endovascular strategies. In addition, the clinical impact of endovascular coiling of symptomatic ophthalmic aneurysms remains controversial. One study of patients with large, symptomatic ophthalmic segment aneurysms treated with endovascular coiling reported visual improvement in 50%, stability in 25%, and worsening in 25%. Although these rates are generally lower than those seen in microsurgical cohorts, the contrast may not be as stark as expected. Visual worsening is seen in at least 10% of patients with symptomatic ophthalmic aneurysms in oft-cited surgical series.[2,3,7] Nevertheless, the ability to surgically decompress the optic apparatus has fueled an intuitive bias toward this approach for patients with symptomatic ophthalmic aneurysms.

Burgeoning Endovascular Techniques: Flow Diversion

Along with cavernous segment aneurysms, large and giant ophthalmic segment aneurysms are essentially the archetypal anterior circulation targets for emerging flow-diverting stent monotherapy.[12] This approach allows for the potential alleviation of mass effect from these aneurysms as a result of aneurysm involution after treatment. In the seminal Pipeline series of 53 patients harboring 63 intracranial aneurysms (30 large or giant), no major complications were reported and the angiographic obliteration rate was 95% at 1 year.[12] Although infrequent, cases of branch-vessel inclusion, including the ophthalmic artery, have been reported.[13] In one series of 19 paraclinoid aneurysms treated with the Pipeline embolization device (PED; Chestnut Medical Technologies, Menlo Park, CA), four patients showed angiographic occlusion of the ophthalmic artery at follow-up, though none were symptomatic.[13] Case reports of delayed hemorrhage have also surfaced[14]; however, the prevalence of this potentially devastating complication among larger

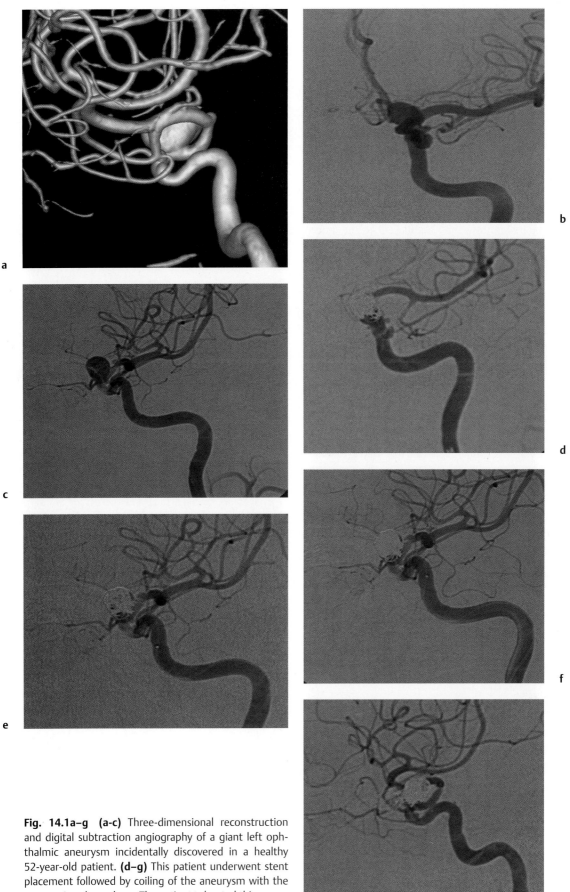

Fig. 14.1a–g (a-c) Three-dimensional reconstruction and digital subtraction angiography of a giant left ophthalmic aneurysm incidentally discovered in a healthy 52-year-old patient. **(d–g)** This patient underwent stent placement followed by coiling of the aneurysm with the progression shown here. The patient tolerated this procedure without incident and remains neurologically intact.

cohorts remains to be elucidated. Nevertheless, this technique is still in its infancy. Overall, it has shown considerable promise and is particularly germane in the consideration of treatment options for patients with large and giant ophthalmic segment aneurysms.

Treatment of Giant Ophthalmic Aneurysms: Microsurgical Clipping

Ana Rodríguez-Hernández, Osman Arikan Nacar, and Michael T. Lawton

Aneurysms arising from the ICA adjacent to the anterior clinoid process vary in their artery of origin, projection, and relationship to the dural rings and cavernous sinus.[15] These so-called paraclinoid aneurysms can be categorized as ophthalmic, superior hypophyseal, or variant aneurysms, with variant aneurysms including dorsal carotid aneurysms, carotid cave aneurysms, clinoidal segment aneurysms, and ventral carotid aneurysms (**Fig. 14.2**). These aneurysms originate on the ICA between the proximal dural ring and posterior communicating artery, either on the C6 segment of van Loveren's classification (between the distal dural ring and posterior communicating artery) or on the C5 segment (between the dural rings). Paraclinoid aneurysms account for 5% of all intracranial aneurysms, and giant, multiple, and bilateral aneurysms are frequent among them.[16–18] Their anatomic complexity, proximity to the optic nerve, and intimacy with the cavernous sinus makes these aneurysms surgically challenging despite the advances in microsurgical techniques.[19] This territory has been fertile ground for endovascular innovation and advancements, but the completeness of treatment, durability of endovascular repair, and visual outcomes with compressive lesions remain major concerns with this alternative modality.[3, 20] This section of the chapter highlights our surgical perspective on paraclinoid aneurysms.

Case Analysis

Diagnosis

The aneurysm in this chapter's presented case arises from the superior surface of the ICA, at the end of the siphon's curve, projecting superomedially in the direction of the blood flow around the bend. Aneurysms in this location with a clear relationship to the ophthalmic artery are considered ophthalmic artery aneurysms, whereas those arising on the superior surface but separate from the ophthalmic origin are categorized as dorsal ICA aneurysms. Dorsal carotid aneurysms are usually small, blister-shaped, and often caused by arterial dissection. The available images do not clearly reveal the origin of the aneurysm in this case, but the location, size, morphology, and projection are most consistent with an ophthalmic artery aneurysm.

The dome of an ophthalmic artery aneurysm usually has an impact on the lateral half of the optic nerve because

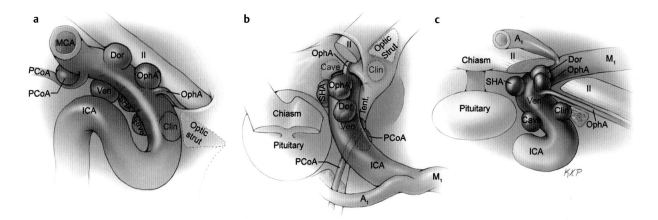

Fig. 14.2 The classification of paraclinoid aneurysms according to their location along the C5 and C6 segment of the internal carotid artery as viewed from lateral **(a)**, superior **(b)**, and anterior **(c)** perspectives. Clin, clinoid; Dor, dorsal; ICA, internal carotid artery; II, optic nerve; MCA, middle cerebral artery; OphA, ophthalmic artery; PCoA, posterior communicating artery; SHA, superior hypophyseal artery; Tent, tentorium; Ven, ventral.

the nerve angles medially along its course to the chiasm and ICA and curves laterally along its supraclinoid course. The optic nerve is typically displaced superiorly and medially, with its superolateral aspect pressed against the falciform ligament, provoking the nasal visual field defect in this patient.

Management Options

The goals of therapy are to protect the patient from aneurysm re-rupture and prevent further visual loss from the aneurysm's mass effect. Microsurgical clipping and endovascular coiling are both appropriate and available options, making the choice controversial.

Endovascular coiling is appealing because it is less invasive than an open craniotomy and has low rates of morbidity and mortality.[20] Despite this aneurysm's large size, the neck is small and well defined; there is a reasonable chance that dense packing can be done without a stent or balloon. However, rates of complete occlusion decrease with an increasing aneurysm size and range from 33 to 60% in giant aneurysms.[20–22] Endovascular therapy does not require any manipulation of the optic nerve as surgery does, but the mass effect on the optic apparatus remains after treatment and the likelihood of visual improvement is low. Heran and colleagues[6] and Sherif and associates[23] reported a 25 to 33% rate of visual deterioration after endovascular treatment of large or giant aneurysms of the ophthalmic artery. Only 50% of patients showed visual improvement after endovascular treatment and only when the carotid was occluded. Furthermore, the risk of aneurysm recurrence and retreatment is considerable, given this aneurysm's size, its location at a point of high hemodynamic stress, and its angulation between inflow and outflow arteries. The patient would require angiographic surveillance, with an estimated risk of recurrence of 20 to 40%. Additional retreatment is associated with some additional morbidity and may be more complicated when the aneurysm has grown.

New devices such as the PED are indicated for paraclinoid aneurysms like this one. Endoluminal flow diverters have performed favorably with these aneurysms, but the requirement of antiplatelet agents for at least 6 months limits their use in patients with subarachnoid hemorrhage. Treatment with a flow diverter would necessarily cover the ophthalmic origin, which could occlude the artery and cause new visual symptoms. In addition, long-term results are unclear. Delayed aneurysm ruptures have been reported after treatment with flow diverters, even among previously unruptured aneurysms.

Surgical results with ophthalmic aneurysms are excellent, with complete aneurysm occlusion rates in over 80 to 90% of patients, low rates of recurrence, and visual outcomes that are superior to those associated with endovascular therapy.[2,8,16,18,19,21,24,25] The anatomy of the paraclinoid region is complex, and safe dissection requires detailed knowledge of the dural rings, optic strut, cavernous sinus, and internal carotid artery.[26] These aneurysms cannot be thoroughly dissected without a complete anterior clinoidectomy; however, dissection must respect the delicacy and importance of the optic nerve.[15,27] Preserving the arachnoidal layers around the nerve and manipulating the ICA rather than the nerve translate into better visual results.[15]

Working with ophthalmic artery aneurysms is more favorable than working with other paraclinoid aneurysms because the dome is not intimately associated with the anterior clinoid process, complete circumferential dissection of the distal dural ring is not necessary, and a neck on the superior ICA wall is easier to clip than one on the medial ICA wall.[15] A distinct advantage of surgery is the ability to decompress the optic nerve by opening the optic canal and deflating the aneurysm after clipping. These maneuvers increase the likelihood of visual recovery. The potential benefits of optic nerve decompression after clipping must be carefully weighed against the risks of visual deterioration during the dissection. An optic nerve that is stretched and attenuated by a large ophthalmic artery aneurysm is particularly vulnerable to manipulation. An anterior clinoidectomy can affect the nerve because of heat or vibration from the drill, and dissection can cause perforator spasm or loss. Nonetheless, the risk of visual deterioration with ophthalmic artery aneurysms is around 2 to 4%.[23,27,28] However, more than 70% of patients with ophthalmic aneurysms experience visual improvement after surgery.[2] Technical advances have facilitated surgery. Hemostatic agents can be injected into the cavernous sinus to control bleeding, and indocyanine green dye provides quick, reliable information about carotid patency and aneurysm occlusion.

This chapter's case, a 35-year-old woman with no significant comorbidities and a large ophthalmic artery aneurysm, is an ideal candidate for microsurgical clipping. Surgery can produce a durable cure that will prevent rebleeding and might improve her vision. In contrast, endovascular treatment can be accomplished with a lower procedural risk, but may not improve her vision, would require angiographic follow-up, and would have a significant recurrence risk, and the patient might need retreatment during her lifetime. Therefore, the treatment of choice for this particular patient is microsurgical clipping.

Surgical Technique

Ophthalmic artery aneurysms are approached through a standard pterional approach. The patient is positioned with the anterior cranial fossa oriented vertically and the head rotated 30 degrees laterally. The cervical ICA is routinely prepared in all cases and advanced neck exposure should be considered in ruptured or giant aneurysms. Preparations for intraoperative angiography are made at the start of the procedure, although indocyanine green video-angiography has supplanted angiography in our practice.[15]

An anterior clinoidectomy and circumferential dissection of the distal dural ring are required for most cases of ophthalmic aneurysms to gain intracranial proximal control and allow the correct positioning of the clip blades.

The anterior clinoidectomy can be completed extradurally (the Dolenc approach),[27] but we prefer an intradural clinoidectomy because it allows the surgeon to visualize the aneurysm and enables immediate clipping if the aneurysm ruptures prematurely.[15]

The sylvian fissure is widely split to expose the arachnoid over the optic nerve and the supraclinoid segment of the ICA. The dura covering the anterior clinoid process is sharply incised in an arc that extends from the posterior tip of the clinoid to the lateral sphenoid ridge. A second dural incision is made from the middle of the first cut, arcing medially across the roof of the optic canal onto the planum sphenoidale to the medial aspect of the falciform ligament (**Fig. 14.3a**). The two dural flaps are elevated with round

knives and mobilized to expose the clinoid completely. A round, diamond-tipped drill bit (2 mm in diameter) is used to cavitate and then remove the clinoid process. Copious irrigation with cold saline and frequent pauses help dissipate the heat from the drill.

First, the optic canal is unroofed to provide early decompression of the optic nerve, which also improves its tolerance of further clinoidal dissection. Next, the cancellous core of the anterior clinoid process is cavitated with the drill, and its cortical margins are thinned to reduce the anterior clinoid attachments medially from the roof and lateral wall of the optic canal and inferiorly from the optic strut (**Fig. 14.3b,c**). Finally, circumferential dissection around the cortical margins of the anterior clinoid

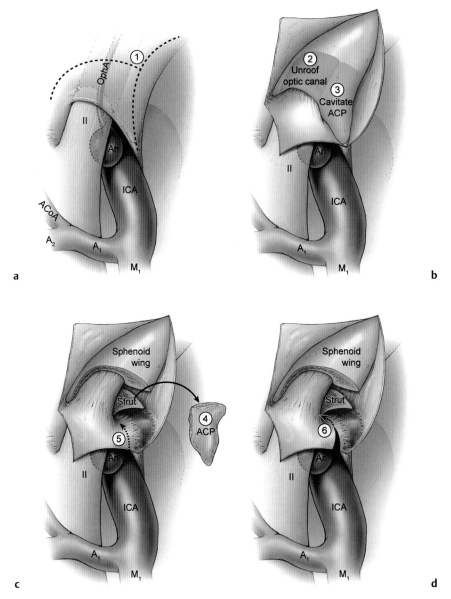

Fig. 14.3a–e   The microsurgical steps for the anterior clinoidectomy. **(a)** Incising the dura on the anterior clinoid process. **(b)** Unroofing the optic canal and cavitating the anterior clinoid process. **(c)** Removing the anterior clinoid process and opening the optic sheath. **(d)** Incising the distal ring superiorly. (*continued on next page*)

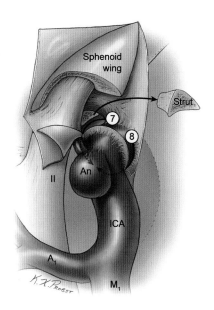

e

Fig. 14.3a–e (*continued*)   **(e)** Incising the distal dural ring medially first and then laterally and inferiorly. ACoA, anterior communicating artery; ACP, anterior clinoid process; An, aneurysm; ICA, internal carotid artery; II, optic nerve; OphA, Ophthalmic artery.

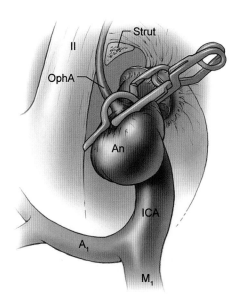

Fig. 14.4   The tandem clipping technique for a large ophthalmic artery aneurysm, with the fenestration encircling the origin of the artery and a stacked straight clip closing the fenestration. An, aneurysm; ICA, internal carotid artery; II, optic nerve; OphA, ophthalmic artery.

process loosens adhesions to the carotid-oculomotor membrane inferiorly, the sphenoidal dura laterally, the tentorial dura posteriorly, and the optic sheath medially, thus allowing the anterior clinoid process to be removed with minimal force. Final removal of the anterior clinoid process often provokes cavernous sinus bleeding, which is easily controlled with Nu-Knit packing or an injection of fibrin glue through the bleeding point in the carotid-oculomotor membrane.

The optic strut fills in the space in front of the clinoidal segment of the ICA, where the distal dural ring crosses the curve of the artery around the siphon. Bony reduction of the strut with a diamond-tip drill bit (1 mm diameter) allows the superior portion of the distal dural ring to be mobilized, opening an incision pathway for the microscissors. The operating table is rotated for a more lateral view under the optic nerve. Additional drilling of the strut is alternated with dural snips that follow the dorsal curve of the clinoidal ICA medially to the carotid sulcus **(Fig. 14.3d)**. The dissection should remain in the axilla of the ophthalmic artery to avoid the perforators arising from the shoulder to the undersurface of the optic nerve. Any needed manipulation should be done against the clinoidal ICA rather than against the optic nerve. The final medial cuts complete dissection of the upper half of the distal ring, untethering the ICA.

Dissection returns to the dural ring laterally to incise the lower half of the ring, again following the curve of the clinoidal ICA medially but now on its inferior surface **(Fig. 14.3e)**. It is difficult to join this inferomedial dissection with the previous superomedial cuts, but a completely cir-

cumferential incision of the ring is not needed with most ophthalmic artery aneurysms. In this particular case, the aneurysm has its neck on the superior wall of the carotid artery and the dome projects superiorly. Thus, an incision around the upper half of the distal ring may be enough for permanent clipping.

The aneurysm must be dissected proximally from the ophthalmic artery origin and distally from the superior hypophyseal artery and other medial perforators. The optic nerve poorly tolerates manipulation, particularly when it is already deflected, as in this patient. Instead, gentle pressure downward and slightly laterally moves the ICA after ring dissection to advance the proximal and distal neck dissection. If necessary, temporary clipping of the cervical ICA softens the aneurysm and permits more forceful manipulation.

Large or giant aneurysms like the one we are discussing are ideally clipped with a tandem clipping: first, a straight fenestrated clip to close the most medial part of the neck, followed by a second straight clip stacked over the fenestration to close it **(Fig. 14.4)**. This tandem clipping can leave residual aneurysm medially beneath the tips of the first clip. In this case, a third fenestrated clip with its fenestration encircling the blades of the initial clip would take care of that medial neck remnant. Indocyanine green video-angiography assesses the completeness of aneurysm occlusion and the patency of the parent vessels. Finally, as the aneurysm is causing a visual defect, it should be punctured, deflated, or debulked to relieve pressure on the optic nerve.

Conclusion

The large, ruptured ophthalmic artery aneurysm in this young patient is ideal for microsurgical clipping. Although the microsurgical treatment of aneurysms in this location is technically challenging and has some associated risks, meticulous dissection can yield a durable cure with a chance of visual recovery.

Treatment of Giant and Large Carotid Ophthalmic Artery (Paraclinoid) Aneurysms: A Combined Microsurgical and Endovascular Approach

Rami Almefty and Kenan I. Arnautovic

Case Analysis

This chapter's case presentation is a patient with a large, unruptured paraclinoid aneurysm with mass effect manifested by a visual field deficit and severe headaches associated with left retro-orbital pain (**Fig. 14.5**). The aneurysm size with its associated risk of rupture and the presence of mass effect necessitate treatment. The paraclinoid aneurysm is a challenging lesion because of its large size, wide neck, intimate relationship to the optic nerve, and difficulty for the surgeon to obtain proximal control. The combined use of endovascular and skull-base techniques, however, facilitates the process.

Operative Technique

The three major steps in the treatment strategy include acranio-orbital zygomatic approach, removal of the anterior clinoid process, and transfemoral endovascular balloon occlusion followed by distal control through direct temporary clipping and suction decompression of the aneurysm.

Cranio-Orbital Zygomatic Approach

The cranio-orbital zygomatic approach has been described in detail elsewhere.[29-33] The patient is placed in the supine position with a shoulder bump on the ipsilateral side. Intraoperative monitoring with electroencephalography, somatosensory evoked potentials, brainstem auditory evoked responses, and oculomotor nerve monitoring is done. The patient's head is turned 30 to 40 degrees, lowered to the floor, tilted 5 to 10 degrees, and fixed in a Mayfield head clamp (**Fig. 14.6**). The skin incision is begun at the level of the zygomatic arch 1 cm anterior to the tragus and continued behind the hairline to the opposite superior temporal line. The incision should avoid the frontal branch of the facial nerve and the superficial temporal artery. During dissection of the superficial and deep temporal fascia, care is taken to protect the frontal branch of the facial nerve and preserve the blood supply to the temporalis muscle. The zygomatic arch is then cut obliquely, allowing maximal downward reflection of the temporalis. A large pericranial graft is harvested for reconstruction of the anterior fossa floor and for closing the frontal and ethmoid sinuses, if nec-

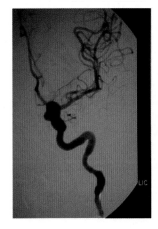
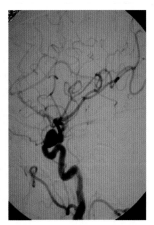

a

b

Fig. 14.5a–c **(a)** Large left paraclinoid aneurysm, oblique view of the four-vessel angiogram. **(b)** Lateral view of the same aneurysm.

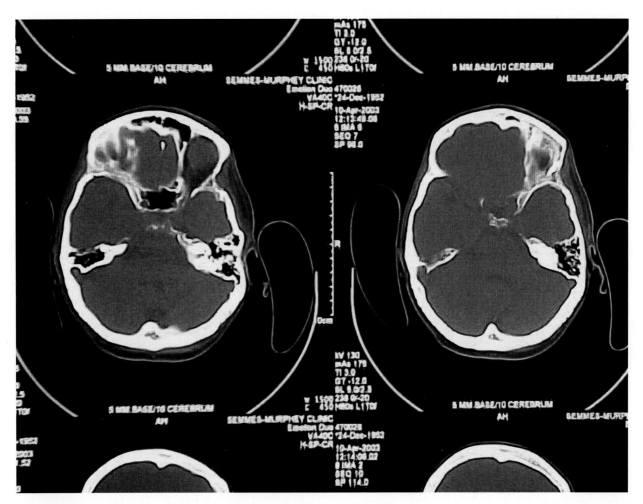

c

Fig. 14.5a–c (*continued*) **(c)** Axial computed tomography scan with bone windows. Note the left-sided anterior clinoid process. (From Arnautović KI, Al-Mefty O, Angtuaco E. A combined micro-surgical skull-base and endovascular approach to giant and large paraclinoid aneurysms. Surg Neurol 1998;50:504–520. Reprinted by permission.)

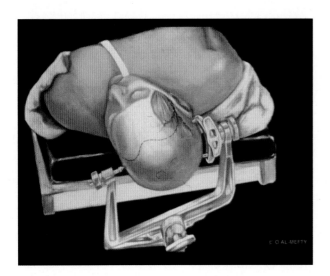

Fig. 14.6 Operative position of the patient for a right-sided cranio-orbital zygomatic approach. (From Arnautović KI, Al-Mefty O, Angtuaco E. A combined microsurgical skull-base and endovascular approach to giant and large paraclinoid aneurysms. Surg Neurol 1998;50:504–520. Reprinted by permission.)

essary. The supraorbital nerve is dissected away or freed from its foramen.

The craniotomy is done with three bur holes (**Fig. 14.7**). The first bur hole, the keyhole, is made just behind the zygomatic process of the frontal bone at the frontosphenoidal junction with the upper half opening into the anterior fossa and the lower half into the orbit (**Fig. 14.8**). Additional bur holes are made in the posterior temporal fossa and in the frontal bone above the supraorbital incisura and lateral to the nasion, with an attempt to avoid the frontal sinus. If the frontal sinus is encountered, the mucosa is stripped and packed with temporalis muscle. The bur holes are then connected with the craniotome. The final cut is made between the keyhole and the frontal hole and a spatula is used to protect the contents of the orbit. The remaining part of the orbital roof and lateral wall are then removed (**Fig. 14.9**).

Dissecting the Aneurysm

After the bone flap is removed, extradural dissection is done to expose the horizontal portion of the petrous ca-

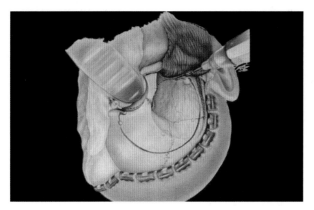

Fig. 14.7 Craniotomy for the cranio-orbital zygomatic approach. (From Arnautović KI, Al-Mefty O, Angtuaco E. A combined microsurgical skull-base and endovascular approach to giant and large paraclinoid aneurysms. Surg Neurol 1998;50:504–520. Reprinted by permission.)

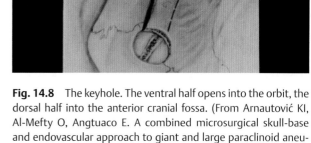

Fig. 14.8 The keyhole. The ventral half opens into the orbit, the dorsal half into the anterior cranial fossa. (From Arnautović KI, Al-Mefty O, Angtuaco E. A combined microsurgical skull-base and endovascular approach to giant and large paraclinoid aneurysms. Surg Neurol 1998;50:504–520. Reprinted by permission.)

rotid artery, providing an additional location for proximal control, if needed. The remaining roof and lateral orbit are removed in one piece. A diamond drill bit is used to remove the bony roof over the optic nerve and the anterior clinoid process. During drilling, the field is constantly irrigated to avoid thermal injury. If the anterior clinoid process is difficult to remove, dissection can be completed intradurally. In either case, the anterior clinoid process is removed entirely. If ethmoid air cells are encountered, they are obliterated to prevent a cerebrospinal fluid leak.

The dura is opened in a curvilinear fashion and reflected anteriorly. The sylvian fissure is widely split, at which point the aneurysm is encountered. The bridging veins of the temporal lobe are preserved and the arachnoid cisterns opened. The first few millimeters of the posterior communicating and anterior choroidal arteries are exposed, and space is

created for a temporary clip just proximal to the posterior communicating artery. The dura propria of the optic nerve is opened longitudinally along the entire length of the optic canal. This allows slight but significant mobilization of the optic nerve in the lateromedial direction, enabling dissection away from the aneurysm.

The ophthalmic artery origin is carefully dissected away from the aneurysm, and the distal dural ring is opened, exposing the proximal portion of the aneurysmal neck. The opening is extended toward the third cranial nerve. Venous bleeding may be encountered and is easily controlled with packing. The aneurysm is then dissected from its surrounding structures in a stepwise fashion. Papaverine is routinely applied to the ICA and its branches and repeated as necessary.

Endovascular Balloon Occlusion and Suction Decompression

At this point, femoral access is obtained and a 5-French, 100-cm arterial catheter is placed through a 6-French sheath. Once the catheter is correctly placed, it is exchanged for a 5-French double-lumen balloon catheter with a 300-cm exchange guidewire. The tip of the balloon catheter is positioned 2 cm above the carotid artery bifurcation and tested for proper intraluminal placement. Test inflation of the balloon is done under fluoroscopy to determine the necessary volume to occlude the ICA, typically 0.1 to 0.15 mL. A pressure drip infusion of normal saline is started to the distal arterial lumen to prevent clotting. Burst suppression with barbiturates is done for cerebral protection and the mean arterial pressure is elevated 10 to 20 mm Hg above baseline. The balloon is then inflated, achieving proximal control, and a temporary clip is placed just proximal to the posterior communicating artery to obtain distal control. Despite aneurysmal trapping, backflow through the superior hypophyseal and ophthalmic arteries prevents defla-

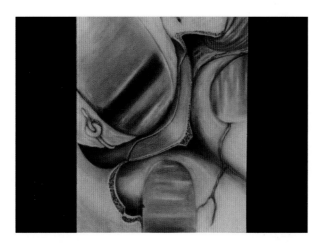

Fig. 14.9 Removing the remaining part of the orbital roof and lateral wall (right side). (From Arnautović KI, Al-Mefty O, Angtuaco E. A combined microsurgical skull-base and endovascular approach to giant and large paraclinoid aneurysms. Surg Neurol 1998;50:504–520. Reprinted by permission.)

tion of the dome. This problem is overcome with gentle and continuous hand retrograde suction decompression through the luminal end of the catheter (**Fig. 14.10**).

Aneurysm Clipping

The wall of the aneurysm is often thick and atherosclerotic, which distinguishes it from the thin parent artery and allows gentle compression of the aneurysmal sac. The aneurysm can be lifted to establish a plane between it and the ICA. At this point, the aneurysm is collapsed and carefully separated from the ICA, and the neck is dissected and permanently clipped. Often, multiple clips are needed to exclude the aneurysm and prevent the circulation pressure from opening or pulsating the blades of the clip. Placing the additional clip or clips parallel to or in the opposite direction and away from the parent artery should suffice. To eliminate any existing mass effect, the aneurysmal dome can be punctured or excised. In cases of severe thrombus or atherosclerosis, the dome of the aneurysm is opened and the contents evacuated. Once the clipping is complete, blood flow is reestablished and angiography is done to confirm that the aneurysm has been obliterated and the blood vessels are patent (**Figs. 14.10, 14.11**).

Rationale

The difficulty in treating these aneurysms is in gaining proximal control and relieving tension within the aneurysm to allow dissection and successful clipping. The combined approach detailed above offers several advantages. The cranio-orbital zygomatic approach provides superb access to the aneurysm, minimizes the need for brain retraction, and provides an excellent working angle. This approach also allows for additional sites for proximal control at the petrous and subclinoid ICA. Drilling the anterior clinoid process exposes the neck of the aneurysm. Transfemoral endovascular balloon occlusion and suction decompression makes obtaining proximal control safe and simple, and eliminates the need for a separate neck incision or direct carotid punc-

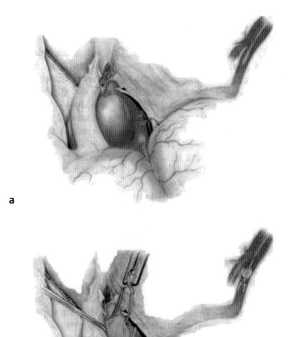

a

b

Fig. 14.10a,b The endovascular approach for proximal control of the right ICA. **(a)** The balloon is in position but still deflated. **(b)** The balloon is inflated for proximal control, the aneurysm is collapsed, and clipping is underway.

ture.[33,34] Suction decompression relieves the tension in the aneurysm and facilitates dissection and clipping.[35,36] Aneurysm puncture or excision relieves any mass effect, optimizing the patient's chances of visual recovery. Clipping definitively obliterates the aneurysm.[2,37–39] Endovascular access allows for immediate angiography to ensure obliteration of the aneurysm and good arterial filling.

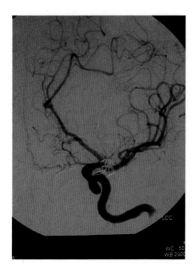
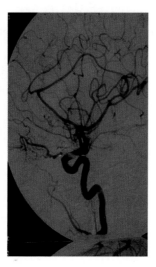

a

b

Fig. 14.11a–c **(a,b)** Postoperative oblique views of the four-vessel angiogram. (*continued on next page*)

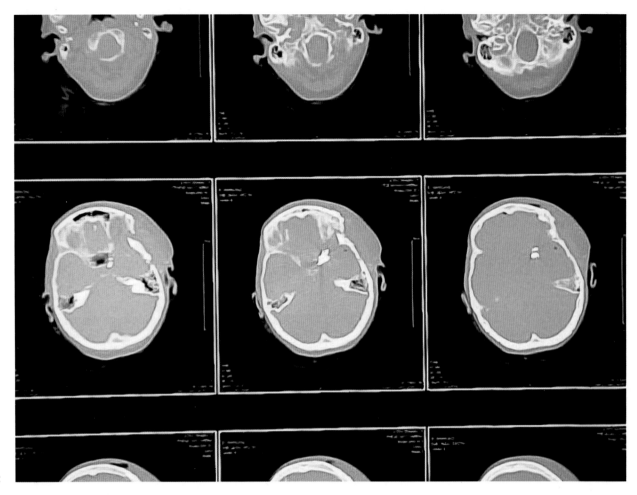

c

Fig. 14.11a–c (*continued*)   **(c)** Lateral postoperative axial computed tomography scan with bone windows showing the removed anterior clinoid process and the position of the clips.

Treatment of Giant Aneurysms of the Carotid Ophthalmic Artery: The Pipeline Embolization Device

Christopher S. Ogilvy and Christopher J. Stapleton

Illustrative Case

Here we present a different case from the one at the beginning of the chapter. A 50-year-old woman came to clinical attention after an episode of acute-onset loss of consciousness followed by persistent headaches. Computed tomography angiography of the head revealed a 22-mm partially thrombosed aneurysm of the left paraclinoid ICA without evidence of subarachnoid hemorrhage **(Fig. 14.12a,b)**. She was lost to follow-up until she appeared again with an acute myocardial infarction 6 years later. Computed to-

mography angiography of the head at that time showed a 47-mm aneurysm of the left paraclinoid ICA with associated hydrocephalus[40] **(Fig. 14.12c,d)**. A right occipital ventriculopleural shunt was placed given a decline in the patient's cognitive status and her complaints of gait instability and headaches. Her cognition and gait subsequently improved dramatically. Diagnostic cerebral angiography 9 months later showed the largely thrombosed aneurysm to have a residual filling volume of 7 × 8 × 10 mm **(Fig. 14.13a,b)**. An intraprocedural left ICA balloon test occlusion resulted in dysarthria, dysnomia, and a right facial

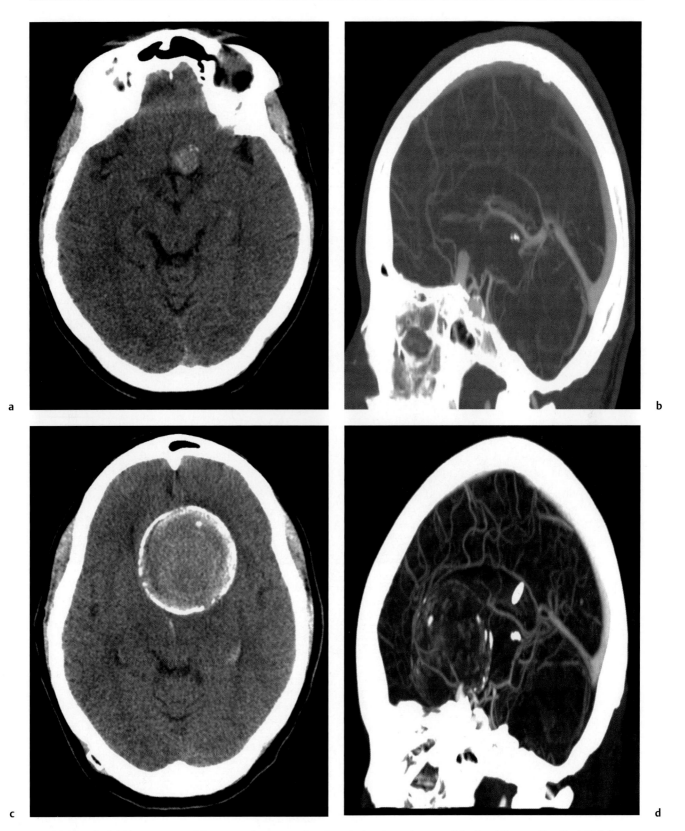

Fig. 14.12a–d **(a)** Noncontrast axial computed tomography of the head shows a 22-mm partially calcified lesion adjacent to the left suprasellar cistern. **(b)** Sagittal computed tomography angiography of the head shows a partially thrombosed 22-mm left ICA paraclinoid aneurysm. **(c,d)** A repeated computed tomography/angiography scan of the head 6 years after the initial diagnosis shows a 47-mm calcified and thrombosed left ICA paraclinoid aneurysm with associated hydrocephalus and displacement of adjacent vascular structures.

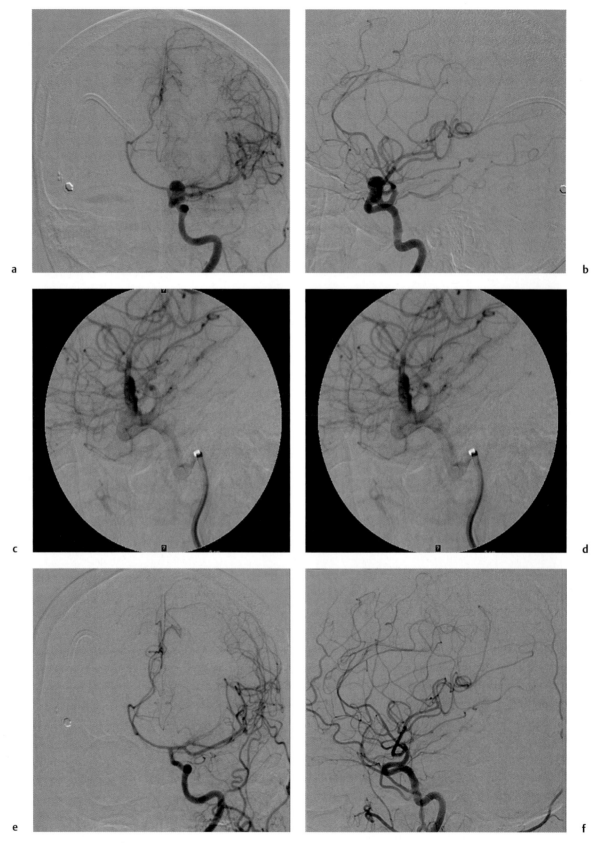

Fig. 14.13a–f **(a,b)** Anterior-posterior and lateral projections during diagnostic cerebral angiography showing the large left paraclinoid ICA aneurysm with a residual filling volume of 7 × 8 x 10 mm. **(c,d)** Lateral projections showing the placement of overlapping Pipeline embolization devices (PEDs) across the neck of the aneurysm (**c,** PED No. 1; **d,** PED No. 2). **(e,f)** Anterior-posterior and lateral projections at the 3-month follow-up diagnostic digital subtraction angiography showing complete occlusion of the left paraclinoid ICA aneurysm.

droop without peripheral limb weakness, circumstances that precluded the possible eventual sacrifice of the left ICA during treatment of the aneurysm.

Eight months later, the patient underwent the placement of two flow-diverting PEDs for definitive therapy (**Fig. 14.13c,d**). Follow-up cerebral angiography 3 months after PED placement showed complete occlusion of the giant left paraclinoid ICA aneurysm (**Fig. 14.13e,f**). She remained neurologically intact.

Pipeline Embolization Device Technology and Technique

The PED (ev3/Covidien Vascular Therapies, Mansfield, MA) is a braided mesh cylinder composed of 48 strands of 25% platinum and 75% cobalt-nickel alloy. The pore size is 0.02 to 0.05 mm.[41] The PED is packaged in an introducer sheath following attachment to a flexible delivery wire with radiopaque end markers. This packaged device can be loaded into standard microcatheters with an inner diameter of 0.027 inches or more. The device is properly positioned at the desired location in the vessel and, upon release from the delivery system, the implant expands to cover the neck of the target aneurysm, with metallic coverage approaching 30 to 35% of the total surface area. When it is deployed, the device is shortened by 50%, depending on the diameter of the device and the parent artery. Multiple PEDs can be placed and overlapped to aid in aneurysm thrombosis or to extend the construct length depending on the morphology of the aneurysm.[41,42] Ideally, the PED creates thrombosis within the aneurysm by introducing stagnant flow while maintaining the patency of critical arterial perforators.

Before undergoing endovascular treatment with PEDs, patients are treated with clopidogrel (75 mg daily) and aspirin (325 mg daily) for at least 72 hours. During the procedure, intravenous heparin is administered to a target activated clotting time of 250 to 300 seconds. Dual antiplatelet therapy is maintained for at least 6 months after the procedure.

The PED was approved by the Food and Drug Administration in April 2011 to treat unruptured large or giant wide-necked aneurysms of the petrous to superior hypophyseal ICA. Because antiplatelet therapy is necessary before and after application of the PED, the use of the device to treat ruptured aneurysms causing subarachnoid hemorrhage is off-label and carries the risk of worsening hemorrhage.

Results

Data Acquisition

To gather data about the use of PEDs, we searched the database of the National Library of Medicine to identify all articles pertaining to the use of PEDs to treat intracranial aneurysms. We analyzed all series describing neurologic outcomes and reviewed reference lists for additional arti-

cles not identified in the original search. Pertinent clinical characteristics extracted from each report included the patients' age and sex, the number of aneurysms treated, the aneurysm location and size, the number of PEDs used, PED-associated complications, and rates of aneurysm occlusion.

Data Summary

Table 14.1 summarizes the relevant clinical characteristics of patients described and aneurysms treated in previously published case series. In total, we identified 13 series between 2009 and 2012 in which more than 10 aneurysms were treated with the use of PEDs.[12,43–54] Eleven of these studies included aneurysms largely of the anterior intracranial circulation, with six of these 11 studies including a high proportion of specifically paraclinoid ICA aneurysms. Across all series, 11 to 89% of the aneurysms were small (< 10 mm), 11 to 56% were large (10 to 25 mm), and up to 47% were giant (> 25 mm). A single PED was used in 34 to 78% of cases, whereas two PEDs were used in 22 to 46% of cases, and three PEDs were used in up to 15.5% of cases. Periprocedural complications were noted in up to 22% of patients, and only one series included one delayed complication. Six of the 13 studies reported deaths associated with PED placement, although the overall mortality rate per series was 0 to 9%. Rates of aneurysm occlusion varied. At 6 months after the PED placement, eight of the 13 series showed a 54 to 94% rate of complete occlusion.

Aneurysm Size and Morphology

As a result of significant advances in endovascular neurosurgery over the past 20 years, endovascular therapies are now the treatment modality of choice for many patients with intracranial aneurysms, as borne out by the International Subarachnoid Aneurysm Trial (ISAT)[55] and the Barrow Ruptured Aneurysm Trial (BRAT).[11] Despite such advances and advantages, wide-necked, large, giant, and fusiform aneurysms can be difficult to treat with standard endosaccular endovascular techniques. The PED is an endoluminal strategy that allows for simultaneous aneurysm occlusion and vessel reconstruction. Although blood flow into the aneurysm is still possible immediately after the placement of a PED, the eventual stagnation of blood within the aneurysmal sac creates thrombosis.

In several publications documenting the Buenos Aires Pipeline experience,[12] the PED for the Intracranial Treatment of Aneurysms Trial,[44] and the Budapest experience with the PED,[48] and in the report by Lubicz and colleagues,[43] wide-necked (dome-to-neck ratio of < 2 mm or neck size > 4 mm) saccular aneurysms, nonsaccular aneurysms, and large and giant aneurysms represented specific sizes and morphologies of interest. Specifically, the authors of the Buenos Aires Pipeline experience reported that 89% of large aneurysms and 80% of giant aneurysms were completely occluded at the 6-month follow-up exam.[12] Similarly, McAuliffe and associates[51] found that 84% of large aneurysms

Table 14.1 Summary of the Relevant Clinical Characteristics of Patients Described and Aneurysms Treated in Previously Published Case Series

Author, Year	No. of Patients	No. of Aneurysms	Sex (%)		Aneurysm Location (%)			Aneurysm Size (%)		
			Male	Female	Paraclinoid	Anterior	Posterior	Small (< 10 mm)	Large (10–25 mm)	Giant (>25 mm)
Lylyk et al, 2009[12]	53	63	9	91	68	87	13	52	35	13
Lubicz et al, 2011[43]	20	27	30	70	44	96	4	89	11	0
Nelson et al, 2011[44]	31	31	29	81	77	93.5	6.5	64.5	29	6.5
Chan et al, 2011[45]	9	13	22	78	92	100	0	67	23	0
Colby et al, 2013[46]	34	41	21	79	90	90	10	51	44	5
Deutschmann et al, 2012[47]	12	12	25	75	75	92	8	75	25	0
Szikora et al, 2010[48]	18	19	–	–	–	95	5	26	53	21
Pistocchi et al, 2012[49]	26*	30*	57*	33*	0	100	0	67	33	0
Fischer et al, 2012[50]	88	101	49	51	–	78	22	–	–	–
McAuliffe et al, 2012[51]	54	57	18.5	81.5	–	81	19	32	56	12
Briganti et al, 2012[52]	273*	295*	21*	79*	–	87*	13*	11* (< 5 mm)	42* (5–15 mm)	47* (> 15 mm)
de Barros Faria et al, 2011[53]	23	23	48	52	4	9	91	30	30	40
Phillips et al, 2012[54]	32	32	34	66	0	0	100	–	–	–
Total	374	425	29#	72#	50#	77#	23#	55#	34#	10#

Abbreviation: PED, Pipeline embolization device.

*Results include data related to PEDs and Silk stents.

#Mean.

and 100% of giant aneurysms were entirely occluded 6 months after PED placement. As evidenced by these studies and our illustrative case, the use of PEDs for large and giant aneurysms in the paraclinoid ICA can be effective for complete aneurysm occlusion.

Aneurysm Location

Eleven of 13 case series in our study included aneurysms largely of the anterior intracranial circulation, according to the original Food and Drug Administration approval of April 2011. Data presented in **Table 14.1** show a high rate of aneurysm occlusion after PED placement in the anterior circulation, and specifically paraclinoid ICA, aneurysms. For instance, Lubicz and colleagues[43] examined 26 aneurysms of the anterior circulation (12 of the paraclinoid ICA) and noted a 78% complete occlusion rate at 6 months. On the other hand, Siddiqui and associates[56] recently reported their experience with PEDs in patients with large or giant fusiform aneurysms of the vertebrobasilar system. In their experience with six patients, four had died at the time of last follow-up with two of those deaths from post-PED aneurysm rupture.

Phillips and colleagues[54] reported on 32 posterior circulation aneurysms with a mean aneurysm size of 9.7 mm (range 2 to 30 mm), including 20 fusiform aneurysms. They

No. PEDs (%)			Complications (%)		Mortality (%)	Occlusion (%)			
1	2	3	Early (Periprocedural)	Late		Immediate	3 Months	6 Months	12 Months
70	27	3	0	0	0	8	56	93	95
78	22	0	10	0	5	0	–	78	–
58	36	3	6.5	0	0	–	–	93	–
54	46	0	0	0	0	–	–	54	69
73	21	3	12	0	3	3	–	–	–
–	–	–	8	0	0	17	–	67	92
37	37	15.5	22	0	5.5	21	–	94	–
67	33	0	7*	0	0	17	–	–	83
34	–	–	7	0	1	–	52	–	74
42	44	14	4	0	0	–	–	86	–
–	–	–	22*	0	6*	–	–	–	–
–	–	–	9	0	9	–	–	–	–
66	25	6	16	3	0	–	–	85	96
58#	32#	5#	9#	<1#	2#	11#	54#	81#	85#

report no deaths, but a 16% early morbidity rate. Overall, giant fusiform aneurysms of the posterior circulation often have a poor natural history. High rates of morbidity and mortality have been reported with both open surgical and endovascular techniques, and the optimal treatment strategy needs to be individualized to the specific patient and clinical situation.

A consideration specific to treating paraclinoid ICA aneurysms is the patency of the ophthalmic artery after the PED placement. Puffer and associates[13] evaluated this question in detail in 19 patients with 20 aneurysms. No change in ophthalmic artery flow was noted in 17 of 20 treated aneurysms. Two patients had delayed antegrade filling of the ophthalmic artery immediately after PED placement; one of them had retrograde flow from collateral vessels to the ophthalmic artery immediately after the device was applied. At follow-up (range 3 to 12 months), 13 of the 19 patients had normal antegrade flow, whereas four had ophthalmic artery occlusion. Despite changes in flow in the ophthalmic artery, none of the patients had visual symptoms associated with compromise of the ophthalmic artery.

Complications

In the case series available for examination, the overall periprocedural and delayed complication rate was low. Common periprocedural complications included in-stent thrombosis with or without resultant morbidity, transient or permanent neurologic deficits, and subarachnoid hemorrhage. Deaths were often the result of aneurysmal rupture. As evidenced in **Table 14.1**, the six case series with a majority of paraclinoid ICA aneurysms treated with PEDs had an overall early morbidity rate of less than 12% and a mortality rate of less than 5%.

Conclusion

The PED is an innovative endoluminal endovascular device used to treat intracranial aneurysms, specifically unruptured and of the anterior intracranial circulation. The advantage of the PED is in treating patients with large, giant, and wide-necked aneurysms in whom traditional coil em-

bolization or clip ligation would be difficult. Data reported in this review and indicated by our case illustration show that the PED is a safe and durable technology for unruptured paraclinoid aneurysms. More case reports and small case series are emerging regarding the use of this technology for ruptured lesions. Nonetheless, the exact risks and benefits of using the PED for ruptured lesions remain unknown. Future studies that more closely examine aneurysm size and morphology with respect to rates of occlusion and clinical outcome will help more clearly define the role of PEDs in treating intracranial aneurysmal disease.

Moderators
The Treatment of Giant Ophthalmic Artery Aneurysms
Mark J. Dannenbaum and Arthur L. Day

The above sections supporting microsurgical clip ligation alone, endovascular obliteration with coils with or without remodeling, combined microsurgery and endovascular therapy, and flow diversion are remarkable in that they demonstrate the tremendous disparity in treatment patterns for patients with giant ophthalmic segment aneurysms.

As new technologies have evolved, the debate between durability (open surgery) and minimal invasiveness (endovascular methodology) has grown. The current data for lesions of this type consist of a multitude of case series that report outcomes as treated through microsurgical,[17,25] endovascular,[5,6,20] or a combined[57] approach. All of the experts enlisted in this chapter are affiliated with established, high-volume cerebrovascular centers that offer a comprehensive array of treatment modalities for this disease process. Despite the ready access to all of these forms of treatment, however, a strong preference exists at each of their respective institutions.

Certainly, all of these modalities are useful for particular cases. The presence or absence of subarachnoid hemorrhage (including the resultant clinical grade), systemic comorbidities, visual loss, the specific type of aneurysm (saccular versus dissection), the specific segment (ophthalmic versus clinoidal), and the location within the ophthalmic segment (ophthalmic, superior hypophyseal, or dorsal variant) produce significant variations and difficulties that must be addressed according to the experience and expertise of the treating team.

In this chapter's case presentation, the following significant clinical and radiographic features were evident before treatment:

1. The patient has subarachnoid hemorrhage and a left-sided extraventricular drain is in place. She is apparently doing well clinically and has no spasm at present.

2. The patient is a woman in her mid-30s, with no major comorbidities and a long life expectancy.
3. The aneurysm is a saccular, dorsomedially projecting ophthalmic artery lesion of 22 mm with no major intraluminal thrombus or wall calcification.
4. The patient has clinical evidence of visual loss from visual apparatus compression (optic nerve or chiasm).

Under this specific set of circumstances, what is the best method of treatment?

Microsurgery

Microsurgery and clip ligation, including skull-base approaches for exposure, are a proven effective and durable means to permanently secure giant ophthalmic segment aneurysms.

The first series to define the microsurgical anatomy of the ophthalmic segment and meticulously analyze operative results reported outcomes in 54 patients treated surgically.[2] An overall excellent outcome, defined as no postoperative neurologic deficit, was achieved in 87% of patients. Ischemic injury and visual deficits occurred in six of the 54 patients in the series (11%), almost all in patients with very large or giant aneurysms of the superior hypophyseal artery. With further modification of clipping techniques, the risks of ischemic injury or visual loss, especially for ophthalmic artery variants, has been dramatically reduced, as a complex fenestrated clip reconstruction is not required, and the clip plane does not have a direct interface with the superior hypophyseal arteries.

This modality directly relieves mass effect and optic nerve compression by dividing the falciform ligament and collapsing of the aneurysm once clipped. The recovery of oculomotor nerve compression with posterior communicating aneurysms is very well documented, and the recovery of vision in surgical series appears superior to that of endovascular intervention for patients presenting with visual system compression.[58] Overall, 17 of 23 patients who presented with visual loss had improvement after clipping and decompression of the aneurysm. These results, too, have improved with further modification of the clipping techniques, particularly for superior hypophyseal lesions. In this series, three patients with no preoperative visual deficits developed increased visual deficits postoperatively and three experienced transient diplopia. In this group, endovascular intervention may be comparable or superior to open surgery.

More recently, Nanda and Javalkar[16] reported their experience in 80 patients with 86 ophthalmic segment aneurysms ranging from small to giant. They reported an 8.75% rate of visual deterioration after surgery, and a 2.5% permanent visual morbidity. No statistically significant difference in outcome was noted between giant and nongiant aneurysms, with 68 of the aneurysms treated in the series being large or giant. De Oliveira and colleagues[59] published a series focused on microsurgical treatment and outcomes in patients presenting with mass effect over the anterior optic pathways. Variables that influenced visual outcome included the size of the aneurysm, the duration of visual symptoms, aneurysmal wall calcification, and intraluminal thrombosis. Of the 15 patients in this series, seven had improved visual function after surgery, seven experienced complete recovery of preoperative visual deficits, and only one remained unchanged. Dehdashti and associates[3] evaluated the long-term visual outcome and aneurysm obliteration rates for very large and giant ophthalmic segment aneurysms in 38 patients, 21 of whom underwent surgical treatment (15 unruptured, six ruptured) and found an overall surgery-related visual complication rate of 14%.

One might propose that all ophthalmic segment aneurysms that produce symptomatic mass effect on the visual system should be dealt with microsurgically. It cannot be overemphasized, however, that such cases are complex and require experience and extensive knowledge of skull-base techniques. The surgeon must be skilled in the removal of the anterior clinoid process down to the base of the optic strut, without injury (thermal or traumatic) to the optic nerves and chiasm. Of equal importance is the delicate and precise micro-arachnoid technique used to define the aneurysmal neck, followed by very specific methods of clip placement without compromising the internal carotid, ophthalmic, and superior hypophyseal arteries and their branches supplying the visual system.

Endovascular Viewpoint

Less invasive technology is increasingly being used in all medical specialties. Specifically for ophthalmic segment aneurysms, multiple variables must be considered before the use of endovascular therapy. For large and giant aneurysms in this location, particularly those with partially thrombosed lumina, there is little debate that, with coil embolization alone, the likelihood of incomplete treatment and recurrence is very high.[60,61]

For those lesions presenting with mass effect on the visual system, the likelihood of improvement is not high with treatment through coil embolization alone. The dense packing needed to cure the aneurysm and the inflammatory response associated with expandable gel coils may promote chemical meningitis and actually worsen preexisting visual deficits.

One experienced and technically proficient endovascular group evaluated anatomic and visual outcomes after the coiling of large ophthalmic segment aneurysms.[6] The authors concluded that, in patients with anterior optic pathway compression, platinum coil therapy with ICA preservation did not greatly benefit vision; they advised that additional procedures may be needed. When endovascular trapping and ICA sacrifice were combined in those patients who could tolerate such treatments, good visual, clinical, and anatomic outcomes resulted.

More recently, the concept of flow diversion for aneurysms in this location has grown in popularity. The concept underlying this modality is the usage of a stent with a dense porosity that disrupts the laminar flow within an aneurysm and promotes spontaneous thrombosis and relief of mass effect while maintaining the patency of the parent vessel. Although this concept is intuitively appealing, it is not a practical treatment plan in the case of a *ruptured* large ophthalmic segment aneurysm with visual compromise because of the need for dual antiplatelet therapy (aspirin and clopidogrel) that must be maintained for a minimum of 3 to 6 months.

The treatment with flow diversion alone for our case example is appealing because it can potentially and gradually relieve the mass effect from the aneurysm over time. However, a multitude of reports are now surfacing that describe delayed aneurysm rupture, remote intraparenchymal hemorrhage, or both. Although the mechanism is not yet defined, the phenomenon is very real, and has caused a paradigm shift among many neuroendovascular physicians, whereby large and giant ophthalmic segment aneurysms are not treated with flow diversion alone, but rather through coiling in addition to flow diversion.

Conclusion

Both endovascular and microsurgical treatment of large and giant ophthalmic segment aneurysms have their roles in the management of these lesions; certainly, the surgical group must evaluate its results with rigorous scrutiny relative to acute outcomes as well as rebleeding risks, visual deficits, and long-term cure. We believe that the patient presented here should be treated surgically by a team experienced in skull-base techniques and clipping methods. There is insufficient evidence to support endovascular therapy as the first line of therapy for such a lesion presenting with the combination of optic pathway mass effect and subarachnoid hemorrhage. As more experience is gained with flow diversion, and more is understood regarding the underlying mechanism of delayed aneurysm rupture and remote intraparenchymal hemorrhage, this modality may become an appealing alternative to microsurgical clip ligation, particularly in patients who do not have subarachnoid hemorrhage.

References

1. Wiebers DO, Whisnant JP, Huston J III, et al; International Study of Unruptured Intracranial Aneurysms Investigators. Unruptured intracranial aneurysms: natural history, clinical outcome, and risks of surgical and endovascular treatment. Lancet 2003;362:103–110

2. Day AL. Aneurysms of the ophthalmic segment. A clinical and anatomical analysis. J Neurosurg 1990;72:677–691

3. Dehdashti AR, Le Roux A, Bacigaluppi S, Wallace MC. Long-term visual outcome and aneurysm obliteration rate for very large and giant ophthalmic segment aneurysms: assessment of surgical treatment. Acta Neurochir (Wien) 2012;154:43–52

4. Hauck EF, Wohlfeld B, Welch BG, White JA, Samson D. Clipping of very large or giant unruptured intracranial aneurysms in the anterior circulation: an outcome study. J Neurosurg 2008;109:1012–1018

5. Hauck EF, Welch BG, White JA, et al. Stent/coil treatment of very large and giant unruptured ophthalmic and cavernous aneurysms. Surg Neurol 2009;71:19–24, discussion 24

6. Heran NS, Song JK, Kupersmith MJ, et al. Large ophthalmic segment aneurysms with anterior optic pathway compression: assessment of anatomical and visual outcomes after endosaccular coil therapy. J Neurosurg 2007;106:968–975

7. Heros RC, Nelson PB, Ojemann RG, Crowell RM, DeBrun G. Large and giant paraclinoid aneurysms: surgical techniques, complications, and results. Neurosurgery 1983;12:153–163

8. Hoh BL, Carter BS, Budzik RF, Putman CM, Ogilvy CS. Results after surgical and endovascular treatment of paraclinoid aneurysms by a combined neurovascular team. Neurosurgery 2001;48:78–89, discussion 89–90

9. Yadla S, Campbell PG, Grobelny B, et al. Open and endovascular treatment of unruptured carotid-ophthalmic aneurysms: clinical and radiographic outcomes. Neurosurgery 2011;68:1434–1443, discussion 1443

10. Waldau B, Reavey-Cantwell JF, Lawson MF, et al. Intentional partial coiling dome protection of complex ruptured cerebral aneurysms prevents acute rebleeding and produces favorable clinical outcomes. Acta Neurochir (Wien) 2012;154:27–31

11. McDougall CG, Spetzler RF, Zabramski JM, et al. The Barrow Ruptured Aneurysm Trial. J Neurosurg 2012;116:135–144

12. Lylyk P, Miranda C, Ceratto R, et al. Curative endovascular reconstruction of cerebral aneurysms with the pipeline embolization device: the Buenos Aires experience. Neurosurgery 2009;64:632–642, discussion 642–643, quiz N6

13. Puffer RC, Kallmes DF, Cloft HJ, Lanzino G. Patency of the ophthalmic artery after flow diversion treatment of paraclinoid aneurysms. J Neurosurg 2012;116:892–896

14. Velat GJ, Fargen KM, Lawson MF, Hoh BL, Fiorella D, Mocco J. Delayed intraparenchymal hemorrhage following pipeline embolization device treatment for a giant recanalized ophthalmic aneurysm. J Neurointerv Surg 2012;4:e24

15. Lawton MT. Ophthalmic artery aneurysms. In: Lawton MT, ed. Seven Aneurysms: Tenets and Techniques for Clipping. New York: Thieme, 2010:121–146

16. Nanda A, Javalkar V. Microneurosurgical management of ophthalmic segment of the internal carotid artery aneurysms: single-surgeon operative experience from Louisiana State University, Shreveport. Neurosurgery 2011;68:355–370, discussion 370–371

17. Sharma BS, Kasliwal MK, Suri A, Sarat Chandra P, Gupta A, Mehta VS. Outcome following surgery for ophthalmic segment aneurysms. J Clin Neurosci 2010;17:38–42

18. Yasargil MG, Gasser JC, Hodosh RM, Rankin TV. Carotid-ophthalmic aneurysms: direct microsurgical approach. Surg Neurol 1977;8:155–165

19. De Jesús O, Sekhar LN, Riedel CJ. Clinoid and paraclinoid aneurysms: surgical anatomy, operative techniques, and outcome. Surg Neurol 1999;51:477–487, discussion 487–488

20. Loumiotis I, D'Urso PI, Tawk R, et al. Endovascular treatment of ruptured paraclinoid aneurysms: results, complications, and follow-up. AJNR Am J Neuroradiol 2012;33:632–637

21. Kolasa PP, Kaurzel Z, Lewinski A. Treatment of giant paraclinoid aneurysms. Own experience. Neuroendocrinol Lett 2004;25:287–291

22. Park HK, Horowitz M, Jungreis C, et al. Endovascular treatment of paraclinoid aneurysms: experience with 73 patients. Neurosurgery 2003;53:14–23, discussion 24

23. Sherif C, Gruber A, Dorfer C, Bavinzski G, Standhardt H, Knosp E. Ruptured carotid artery aneurysms of the ophthalmic (C6) segment: clinical and angiographic long term follow-up of a multidisciplinary management strategy. J Neurol Neurosurg Psychiatry 2009;80:1261–1267

24. Iihara K, Murao K, Sakai N, et al. Unruptured paraclinoid aneurysms: a management strategy. J Neurosurg 2003;99:241–247

25. Raco A, Frati A, Santoro A, et al. Long-term surgical results with aneurysms involving the ophthalmic segment of the carotid artery. J Neurosurg 2008;108:1200–1210

26. Giannotta SL. Ophthalmic segment aneurysm surgery. Neurosurgery 2002;50:558–562

27. Dolenc VV. A combined transorbital-transclinoid and transsylvian approach to carotid-ophthalmic aneurysms without retraction of the brain. Acta Neurochir Suppl (Wien) 1999;72:89–97

28. Khan N, Yoshimura S, Roth P, et al. Conventional microsurgical treatment of paraclinoid aneurysms: state of the art with the use of the selective extradural anterior clinoidectomy SEAC. Acta Neurochir Suppl (Wien) 2005;94:23–29

29. Al-Mefty O. The cranio-orbital zygomatic approach for intracranial lesions. Contemp Neurosurg. 1992;14:1–6

30. Al-Mefty O, Smith RR. Tailoring the cranio-orbital approach. Keio J Med 1990;39:217–224

31. Arnautović KI, Al-Mefty O, Angtuaco E. A combined microsurgical skull-base and endovascular approach to giant and large paraclinoid aneurysms. Surg Neurol 1998;50:504–518, discussion 518–520

32. Origitano TC, Anderson DE, Tarassoli Y, Reichman OH, al-Mefty O. Skull base approaches to complex cerebral aneurysms. Surg Neurol 1993;40:339–346

33. Smith RR, Al-Mefty O, Middleton TH. An orbitocranial approach to complex aneurysms of the anterior circulation. Neurosurgery 1989;24:385–391

34. Albert FK, Forsting M, von Kummer R, Aschoff A, Kunze S. Combined microneurosurgical and endovascular "trapping-evacuation" technique for clipping proximal paraclinoidal aneurysms. Skull Base Surg 1995;5:21–26

35. Batjer HH, Samson DS. Retrograde suction decompression of giant paraclinoidal aneurysms. Technical note. J Neurosurg 1990;73:305–306

36. Tamaki N, Kim S, Ehara K, et al. Giant carotid-ophthalmic artery aneurysms: direct clipping utilizing the "trapping-evacuation" technique. J Neurosurg 1991;74:567–572

37. Batjer HH, Kopitnik TA, Giller CA, Samson DS. Surgery for paraclinoidal carotid artery aneurysms. J Neurosurg 1994;80:650–658

38. Eliava SS, Filatov YM, Yakovlev SB, et al. Results of microsurgical treatment of large and giant ICA aneurysms using the retrograde suction decompression (RSD) technique: series of 92 patients. World Neurosurg 2010;73:683–687

39. Xu BN, Sun ZH, Romani R, et al. Microsurgical management of large and giant paraclinoid aneurysms. World Neurosurg 2010;73:137–146, discussion e17, e19

40. Kumar V, Ogilvy CS. Images in clinical medicine: giant intracranial aneurysm. N Engl J Med 2011;364:956

41. Kallmes DF, Ding YH, Dai D, Kadirvel R, Lewis DA, Cloft HJ. A new endoluminal, flow-disrupting device for treatment of saccular aneurysms. Stroke 2007;38:2346–2352

42. Kallmes DF, Ding YH, Dai D, Kadirvel R, Lewis DA, Cloft HJA. A second-generation, endoluminal, flow-disrupting device for treatment of saccular aneurysms. AJNR Am J Neuroradiol 2009;30:1153–1158

43. Lubicz B, Collignon L, Raphaeli G, De Witte O. Pipeline flow-diverter stent for endovascular treatment of intracranial aneurysms: preliminary experience in 20 patients with 27 aneurysms. World Neurosurg 2011;76:114–119

44. Nelson PK, Lylyk P, Szikora I, Wetzel SG, Wanke I, Fiorella D. The pipeline embolization device for the Intracranial Treatment of Aneurysms Trial. AJNR Am J Neuroradiol 2011;32:34–40

45. Chan TT, Chan KY, Pang PK, Kwok JC. Pipeline embolisation device for wide-necked internal carotid artery aneurysms in a hospital in Hong Kong: preliminary experience. Hong Kong Med J 2011;17:398–404

46. Colby GP, Lin LM, Gomez JF, et al. Immediate procedural outcomes in 35 consecutive pipeline embolization cases: a single-center, single-user experience. J Neurointerv Surg 2013;5:237–246

47. Deutschmann HA, Wehrschuetz M, Augustin M, Niederkorn K, Klein GE. Long-term follow-up after treatment of intracranial aneurysms with the Pipeline embolization device: results from a single center. AJNR Am J Neuroradiol 2012;33:481–486

48. Szikora I, Berentei Z, Kulcsar Z, et al. Treatment of intracranial aneurysms by functional reconstruction of the parent artery: the Budapest experience with the pipeline embolization device. AJNR Am J Neuroradiol 2010;31:1139–1147

49. Pistocchi S, Blanc R, Bartolini B, Piotin M. Flow diverters at and beyond the level of the circle of Willis for the treatment of intracranial aneurysms. Stroke 2012;43:1032–1038

50. Fischer S, Vajda Z, Aguilar Perez M, et al. Pipeline embolization device (PED) for neurovascular reconstruction: initial experience in the treatment of 101 intracranial aneurysms and dissections. Neuroradiology 2012;54:369–382

51. McAuliffe W, Wenderoth JD. Immediate and midterm results following treatment of recently ruptured intracranial aneurysms with the Pipeline embolization device. AJNR Am J Neuroradiol 2012;33:487–493

52. Briganti F, Napoli M, Tortora F, et al. Italian multicenter experience with flow-diverter devices for intracranial unruptured aneurysm treatment with periprocedural complications—a retrospective data analysis. Neuroradiology 2012;54:1145–1152

53. de Barros Faria M, Castro RN, Lundquist J, et al. The role of the pipeline embolization device for the treatment of dissecting intracranial aneurysms. AJNR Am J Neuroradiol 2011;32:2192–2195

54. Phillips TJ, Wenderoth JD, Phatouros CC, et al. Safety of the pipeline embolization device in treatment of posterior circulation aneurysms. AJNR Am J Neuroradiol 2012;33:1225–1231

55. Molyneux A, Kerr R, Stratton I, et al; International Subarachnoid Aneurysm Trial (ISAT) Collaborative Group. International Subarachnoid Aneurysm Trial (ISAT) of neurosurgical clipping versus endovascular coiling in 2143 patients with ruptured intracranial aneurysms: a randomised trial. Lancet 2002;360:1267–1274

56. Siddiqui AH, Abla AA, Kan P, et al. Panacea or problem: flow diverters in the treatment of symptomatic large or giant fusiform vertebrobasilar aneurysms. J Neurosurg 2012;116:1258–1266

57. Thorell W, Rasmussen P, Perl J, Masaryk T, Mayberg M. Balloon-assisted microvascular clipping of paraclinoid aneurysms. Technical note. J Neurosurg 2004;100:713–716

58. Chen PR, Amin-Hanjani S, Albuquerque FC, McDougall C, Zabramski JM, Spetzler RF. Outcome of oculomotor nerve palsy from posterior communicating artery aneurysms: comparison of clipping and coiling. Neurosurgery 2006;58:1040–1046, discussion 1040–1046

59. de Oliveira JG, Borba LA, Rassi-Neto A, et al. Intracranial aneurysms presenting with mass effect over the anterior optic pathways: neurosurgical management and outcomes. Neurosurg Focus 2009;26:E3

60. Li MH, Li YD, Fang C, et al. Endovascular treatment of giant or very large intracranial aneurysms with different modalities: an analysis of 20 cases. Neuroradiology 2007;49:819–828

61. Morishima H, Kurata A, Ohmomo T, et al. The efficacy of endovascular surgery for treatment of giant aneurysms with special reference to coil embolization for endosaccular occlusion. Interv Neuroradiol 1998;4(Suppl 1):135–143

Chapter 15

Treatment of Ruptured Wide-Neck Basilar Aneurysms

Case

A 40-year-old woman who smokes cigarettes and has hypertension presents with subarachnoid hemorrhage of Hunt and Hess grade I and Fisher grade I. The imaging studies include digital subtraction angiography and three-dimensional reconstruction.

Participants

Treatment of Ruptured Wide-Neck Basilar Aneurysms: Endovascular Treatment with Stent and Coil: Bernard R. Bendok, Salah G. Aoun, and Tarek Y. el Ahmadieh

Microsurgical Clipping of Ruptured Wide-Neck Basilar Aneurysms: Juha Hernesniemi and Miikka Korja

Moderators: Treatment of Ruptured Wide-Neck Basilar Apex Aneurysms: Shakeel A. Chowdhry and Peter Nakaji

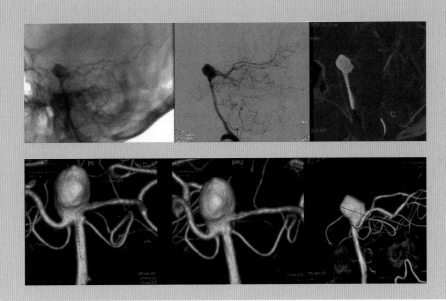

Treatment of Ruptured Wide-Neck Basilar Aneurysms: Endovascular Treatment with Stent and Coil

Bernard R. Bendok, Salah G. Aoun, and Tarek Y. el Ahmadieh

Basilar apex aneurysms pose unique challenges and technical issues from both the endovascular and surgical perspectives. Microsurgically these lesions can be difficult to treat, but not all basilar apex aneurysms pose the same degree of microsurgical difficulty. From an endovascular perspective, the dome-to-neck ratio, the absolute dome and neck sizes, and the relationship of the posterior cerebral artery (PCA) to the neck can all affect the acute and delayed risks and outcomes. The location of basilar tip aneurysms puts these lesions at a hemodynamic disadvantage vis-à-vis a recurrence risk because of the impact of blood flow on the behavior of the aneurysmal fundus and blood pulsations on the stability of the coil complex. Many factors can alter the therapeutic recommendations and risk–benefit analysis, including the aneurysm's neck and dome dimensions, the dome's projection, the PCA anatomy, the relationship of the neck to the posterior clinoid process, and the patient's age and comorbidities.

Case Discussion

In this interesting and challenging case, the dome of the aneurysm appears to be approximately 15 mm and the neck is likely greater than 6 mm depending on how it is measured. The PCAs are offset, with the left PCA being slightly higher in the craniocaudal dimension. The neck is approximately at the level of the posterior clinoid process, and the tilt of the dome is straight up. From a surgical perspective, the key determinant of risk is the anatomy of the perforators and the ability of the surgeon to preserve their patency without injury. From an endovascular perspective, the key determinant of risk in this case is the wide neck, which increases the likelihood of compromising the left PCA, coil herniation, incomplete aneurysm occlusion, and thromboembolic complications. The risk of recanalization is significant in this aneurysm given its size, and a stent may help attenuate this risk. Although early aneurysm repair has become the norm for most ruptured intracranial aneurysms, delayed treatment can be considered in select patients with highly complex lesions. An attempt should be made to treat this aneurysm, but difficulties encountered along the way may favor a delay in therapy.

From an endovascular perspective, there are six therapeutic options we would consider for this aneurysm and patient:

1. Coiling without an assist device
2. Balloon-assisted coiling with an attempt at complete occlusion
3. Stent-assisted coiling
4. Flow diversion
5. Coiling after partial clipping
6. Partial balloon-assisted coiling followed by delayed stent coiling

Microsurgical Clipping

Advances in microsurgical techniques, neuroanesthesia, and cranial-base approaches have improved microsurgical outcomes over the past two decades. An extended lateral transsylvian approach from the right would be our choice for this aneurysm. A zygomatic osteotomy with drilling of the posterior clinoid process may add additional welcome millimeters to the exposure. An extended subtemporal approach could be an alternative.

Clipping has the advantage of being associated with a minimal risk of recurrence if complete or near-complete occlusion is achieved. Additional benefits include less exposure to radiation when compared with endovascular approaches and less need for follow-up imaging. For a good outcome to be achieved, however, the precious perforators that emanate from the proximal P1s and occasionally the neck behind the aneurysm must be preserved. This simply cannot be compromised. If the aneurysm cannot be completely occluded during surgery, the neck can be narrowed with a clip followed immediately by aneurysm coiling. Hybrid surgical suites may allow for more efficient execution of this strategy.

Endovascular Treatment

The main advantage of the endovascular approach is the decreased risk of perforator injury. The endovascular options for this aneurysm are listed above, and their success depends on a thoughtful analysis of these options and execution of the chosen option with the least risk possible. Unlike for open surgery, a philosophy of staging should be considered if the total risk is acceptably low and, ideally, lower than a single-stage approach.

Coiling Without an Assist Device

Although coiling this aneurysm without an assist device may be potentially feasible with modern three-dimensional coils, we would be concerned about the significant risk of herniation of the coil loops into the parent vessels with the potential for thromboembolic complications. This approach would not be our first choice for this patient, although an attempt to see how the first coil behaves is not unreasonable. We would recommend having a balloon ready in the parent arteries.

Balloon-Assisted Coiling with an Attempt at Complete Occlusion

Balloon-assisted coiling allows for the potentially increased protection of the parent arteries during the coiling procedure and provides support for the coil complex until it is sufficiently stable to remain inside the aneurysm with a minimal risk of protrusion into the parent arteries. It also has the advantage of not requiring antiplatelet therapy after the coiling procedure, and has thus gained popularity for the treatment of ruptured wide-necked aneurysms. Additional potential benefits of using a balloon include a greater packing density and the prompt ability to address intraprocedural rupture. These would be welcome advantages in this challenging case. However, the rate of thrombus formation and thromboembolic complications may be high during balloon-assisted coiling procedures, especially with wide-necked compared with narrow-necked aneurysms. Certainly, if the coiling is going well, complete occlusion can be aimed for, but this could have the disadvantage of increasing thromboembolic risks from prolonged procedure time and the lack of preprocedural antiplatelet agents, which are generally avoided in the acute period of subarachnoid hemorrhage.

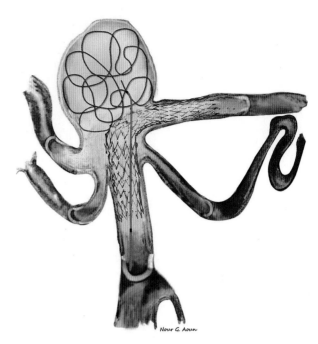

Fig. 15.1   Stent coiling with the first coil inside the aneurysm.

Stent-Assisted Coiling

Stent-assisted coiling would certainly simplify the coiling of this aneurysm from a technical standpoint, and we would guess that it could be done with one stent from the left PCA to the basilar artery **(Fig. 15.1)**. Y-stenting and waffle cone techniques would not be our first choice because of the added but likely unnecessary complexity. Our concern regarding this strategy stems from the now well-established body of literature that has shown increased morbidity and mortality with this approach because of the need for dual antiplatelet agents in the acute period of subarachnoid hemorrhage. External ventricular drain-related hemorrhages appear more likely and more morbid when dual antiplatelet agents are on board. The use of dual antiplatelet agents also complicates other potential procedures, such as tracheostomies and the placement of gastrostomy tubes. Certainly, there are scenarios in which there are no other good options and this increased risk becomes acceptable. On the surface, that does not appear to be the case here.

Flow Diversion

The use of flow diverters in the setting of subarachnoid hemorrhage has not yet been well evaluated. Risks include those related to the acute administration of antiplatelet therapy in an acute subarachnoid hemorrhage setting and those linked to the fact that the aneurysmal fundus is left unobliterated and may not thrombose with the concurrent platelet deactivation. The inability to easily reaccess

the dome adds a layer of concern that is problematic. Additional concerns include the potential for thromboembolic complications and parent-artery occlusion up to 2 years after placement of a stent. This has been noted days to weeks after the discontinuation of antiplatelet treatment. Considering the specific circumstances of this case, this may not be an optimal approach to treat the patient's aneurysm. Moreover, at the time of this writing, this patient's aneurysm would not meet the strict guidelines of the United States Food and Drug Administration (FDA) regarding the use of the currently available flow diverter. In our practice and hands, this strategy would be low on the list of options for this patient.

Coiling after Partial Clipping

On rare occasions, the findings at surgery can limit the surgeon's ability to close the neck of an aneurysm completely. The perforator anatomy and neck calcifications are the main determinants of this potential scenario. The good news is that even a partial reduction in the neck size in this case could potentially simplify the endovascular approach. Ideally, partial clipping should protect the higher P1. Coiling should be done immediately to prevent rehemorrhage. A hybrid operating room with immediate access to biplane angiography before the craniotomy is even closed would be ideal for this rare but potentially safe and effective scenario. Clearly, this approach is not without its own set of risks. The use of intravascular catheters without full anticoagulation may predispose to thromboembolic complications.

Partial Balloon-Assisted Coiling Followed by Delayed Stent Coiling

Partial balloon-assisted coiling followed by delayed stent coiling may be an excellent strategy here and the one we would favor. The key issue is determining what degree of partial coiling is enough to prevent rerupture in the ensuing several weeks until more definitive therapy is instituted. In our opinion, if the upper two thirds of the dome are well packed, with loose coiling in the lower third, the patient should be protected in the short term (**Fig. 15.2**) unless the rupture site is near the neck (which is very rare and is usually seen in the form of a suspicious daughter sac at the neck). This approach has the advantage of minimizing thromboembolic complications and limiting the procedure time. Placing only a few coils in the dome with significant residual interstitial filling, on the other hand, is not likely to be sufficient to prevent rehemorrhage. The use of antiplatelet agents becomes much safer after the acute period of subarachnoid hemorrhage (arbitrarily defined as 2 to 3 weeks after the initial hemorrhage). The end of the acute period implies that hydrocephalus, gastrostomy tube, and tracheostomy issues are dealt with to minimize the risk from dural antiplatelet therapy, which is needed for stenting. Stenting has the potential advantages of narrowing the neck, protecting the parent arteries, and increasing the packing density (**Fig. 15.3**). Our group has demonstrated an increased packing density, increased coil loop density at the neck, and better angiographic outcomes in an in-vitro model. Some studies suggest lower recanalization rates when stents are used. Whether the risk is increased by adding a stent remains controversial, and we would argue that the risk may actually be reduced by using a stent in this case.

Conclusion

Given the clinical presentation of the patient with subarachnoid hemorrhage and her young age, surgical clipping of the aneurysm as a means of providing a definitive cure might be considered as a first-line treatment, with potential perforator injury being the most significant potential risk. Endovascular treatment can be a safe and effective alternative, with thromboembolic complications and recurrence being the two most significant risks. The large size of this aneurysm and the wide neck with potential risk to the left P1 would not make this aneurysm an "equipoise case" in randomized trials of clip versus coil. In fact, viewing this case through the prism of "clip versus coil" may hinder the appreciation of creative solutions, which may be hybrid, staged, or both. The treating team must appreciate that managing this aneurysm carries significant risks, and that this risk should be put in compassionate perspective for the patient and her family. The question is which strategy offers the lowest possible risk profile with the greatest chance for both short-term and long-term success. In our opinion, complex aneurysms such as this should ideally be managed at centers with high levels of expertise in cerebrovascular cranial-base microsurgery as well as neurointerventional surgery. From an interventional perspective, the option we favor for this aneurysm is initial coiling with balloon assistance if feasible. Coiling at least two thirds of the dome should be the initial goal, with further coiling and stent assistance after the acute subarachnoid hemorrhage

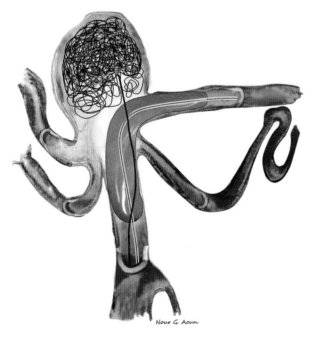

Fig. 15.2 Balloon remodeling with dense packing of the upper two thirds of the aneurysm and lower density packing of the lower third.

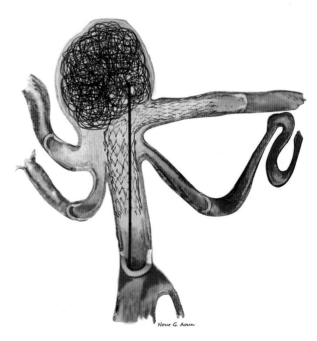

Fig. 15.3 The result of stent-assisted coiling.

period has passed. If the initial endovascular approach proves difficult and the risk seems to outweigh the benefit, then a microsurgical approach should be embraced.

Acknowledgment

The authors express gratitude to Miss Nour Aoun for her excellent illustrations.

Microsurgical Clipping of Ruptured Wide-Neck Basilar Aneurysms

Juha Hernesniemi and Miikka Korja

If only we could have back again many of those who were lost or badly hurt, for a second chance in the operative room with what we have learned.
—C.G. Drake, S.J. Peerless, and J.A. Hernesniemi, 1996

Our Approach

This aneurysm is a medium- to large-sized (around 15 mm in diameter) basilar bifurcation aneurysm projecting upward. The patient is young with a long life expectancy, and we would try to persuade her to stop smoking. To have the most permanent long-term result, we would suggest open microsurgery as the best option for perfect occlusion of this deadly sac. For more than 10 years, computed tomography (CT) angiography has served us as the most satisfactory diagnostic workup for cerebral aneurysms, because it

shows clearly the anatomic relationship between the aneurysm and the skull base. As far as we can assess the digital subtraction angiography images of the case, the base of the aneurysm appears to be at the level of the posterior clinoid process (see the figures presented with the case), but a good three-dimensional CT angiography image would give more information. The best projection for open microsurgery would be the forward projection of the sac, but this is the rarest type.

Because the base of the aneurysm is at the level of the posterior clinoid process and there are no other anterior circulation aneurysms, our approach is subtemporal (**Fig. 15.4**). The transsylvian route is mostly used in patients with basilar tip aneurysms with a high location, especially when the aneurysm is approximately 1 cm or more above the posterior clinoid process. The patient is placed in the

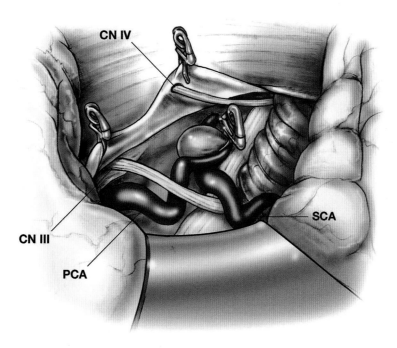

Fig. 15.4 The subtemporal approach requires slight retraction of the temporal lobe. The oculomotor nerve, which always lies between the P1 segment and the superior cerebellar artery (SCA), serves as a highway to the basilar bifurcation. The tentorial flap can be fixed with, for example, small Aesculap clips. CN, cranial nerve; PCA, posterior cerebral artery.

park-bench position, and the brain is slackened by an experienced neuroanesthesiologist, with simultaneous lumbar drainage of 50 to 100 mL of cerebrospinal fluid. The lumbar drain is always introduced by the operating neurosurgeon, as it gives a feeling of safety, comfort, and success for the surgery.

Merits of the Subtemporal Approach

Since the first successful subtemporal approach to a basilar bifurcation aneurysm by Olivecrona in Sweden in 1954, two basic surgical approaches have been widely used to attack basilar tip aneurysms: the subtemporal (since 1959 and mastered by Drake) and the transsylvian (frontotemporal or pterional described by Yasargil in 1976). Subsequently, numerous innovative microsurgical approaches have been tested for their value in the treatment. Both of these approaches are complex, and they destroy, more or less, some parts of the cranial base.

Some surgeons prefer the transsylvian approach because of its familiarity (it is used for anterior aneurysms) and because it possibly entails less retraction of the temporal lobe and causes fewer third nerve palsies. In our series and the series from London, Ontario, however, the subtemporal approach has been used in more than four fifths of patients with small and large basilar tip aneurysms. Patients with additional anterior circulation aneurysms in the middle cerebral or anterior communicating arteries should undergo the pterional approach, but internal carotid aneurysms can often be ligated through the subtemporal route rather easily. There is no doubt that many aneurysms arising from the basilar tip can be approached through most of the described, and often complex, operative techniques. The surgeon's preference or experience determines the choice of the safest technique. For a notable number of patients, however, only one approach can lead to accurate and safe clipping of the aneurysm.

A scrutiny of the 895 basilar bifurcation aneurysms operated on mainly at the teaching hospitals of the University of Western Ontario in London, Canada, between 1959 and 1992 showed that 137 were giant (25 mm or more) and were omitted from the analysis for obvious reasons. Incomplete radiological data or endovascular surgery excluded 63 more cases. Of those remaining, 440 patients with small (< 12 mm ie. ½ inch) and 255 patients with large (12–25 mm ie. ½ inch) basilar bifurcation aneurysms were analyzed. Of these, 95 patients underwent the transsylvian approach and 600 the subtemporal approach. The position of the basilar bifurcation and aneurysmal neck was assessed as follows:

1. Above the posterior clinoid process (more than 3 mm above the level of the posterior clinoid process)
2. At the posterior clinoid process (more than 3 mm above or below the level of the posterior clinoid process)
3. Below the posterior clinoid process (more than 3 mm below the level of the posterior clinoid process).

Most often, the right-sided subtemporal approach is used. If the projection or complexity of the aneurysm favors the left-sided approach, or a patient has a left oculomotor palsy, left-sided blindness or right hemiparesis, the approach under the dominant temporal lobe is preferred. Additional aneurysms in the anterior circulation have an important impact on the choice of operative side, and more than one fourth of patients eventually have a left-sided craniotomy. However, left-sided carotid aneurysms are often left for a second operation or conservative management. In our experience, the left-sided transsylvian route is slightly more uncomfortable than the right transsylvian approach for the right-handed surgeon.

Nowhere are the perforators more numerous or critical than at the basilar artery bifurcation. Most perforators can be dissected free with a tiny dissector after temporary occlusion or trapping of the basilar artery. The perforators in backward-projecting aneurysms can often be separated more easily than expected from the neck when the subtemporal approach is used. In these cases, a forward sac-tilting maneuver opens a clear space between the neck and the perforating branches. In spite of the complex perforator anatomy, most of these patients fare well. The transsylvian approach does not allow the same visualization behind the aneurysm, and the results of this approach were the poorest of all in the London, Ontario, series.

The outcome of surgery is best in patients with an aneurysm located above the posterior clinoid process, whatever the projection of the aneurysm and for both approaches. In the London, Ontario, series, the best results were seen in patients with forward-projecting aneurysms above the posterior clinoid process, and the worst for the same projection but below the posterior clinoid process. The worst combination of anatomic features was a very low location and forward projection. These aneurysms warrant the greatest respect among all basilar bifurcation aneurysms; the number of intraoperative aneurysm ruptures and inadvertent major vessel occlusions was highest in this subgroup. The transsylvian approach is inappropriate for most of these low-lying lesions, for it is difficult, if not impossible, to see the lesion without removing the dorsum sellae. The higher rate of low-lying lesions (32%) in the series of Drake and Peerless may be the result of a referral bias. In these series, the posterior clinoid process was never removed but instead avoided by selecting the proper approach. The complex anatomy of bilobular aneurysms is often best exposed from the lateral side, and the good results achieved in these rare aneurysms stem from the use of the subtemporal approach and two aneurysm clips, one for each lobe (necessary in four of 14 aneurysms in the series).

The higher the aneurysm lies above the dorsum sellae, the greater the retraction of the mesial temporal parahippocampal region must be during the subtemporal approach. If the neck of the sac reaches the apex of the interpeduncular space, the neck and perforators are more likely hidden by the mammillary bodies and peduncle. These rare cases with a very high bifurcation (< 1%) are preferentially approached after the sylvian fissure is split, and the surgeon eventually works above the carotid bifurcation or uses the lamina terminalis or interforniceal approach. The neck of an aneurysm is completely obliterated when the clip blades fall across the neck parallel to the posterior cerebral arteries, and then there is less risk of kinking the bifurcation; this is true particularly for aneurysms with large necks. This ideal placement is more readily achieved through the subtemporal approach. Clips placed perpendicular to this crotch often leave tags of the neck in front and behind ("dog ears"), as the sides of the neck are approximated and the bifurcation crimped. "Dog ears" of the residual neck may grow into new aneurysms.

Many recent series report that the transsylvian approach results in fewer third nerve palsies. In general, resolution of the third cranial nerve palsy is excellent even when complete paralysis exists postoperatively. After a few weeks or months, recovery is complete in practically all patients in whom no paresis exists preoperatively. When the basilar bifurcation aneurysm has been clipped through the pterional approach between the optic nerve and carotid artery, the likelihood of a postoperative oculomotor palsy is almost nonexistent. The use of very high magnification in operating on these aneurysms has markedly reduced the incidence of immediate oculomotor palsies.

In patients with unilateral carotid stenosis or occlusion, the subtemporal approach should be preferred. As in the transsylvian approach, carotid compression can cause complications and a carotid injury is a well-known complication. Admittedly, it is easier in acute and early aneurysm surgery to obtain space through a small subfrontal gap to open the lamina terminalis than to obtain room in the subtemporal approach. This can be facilitated by a ventricular tap and spinal drainage. Proximal control is easier in the subtemporal route than in the pterional one.

A "half-and-half" combination of the two approaches is useful when the transsylvian exposure does not allow visualization of the back of the neck of larger aneurysms, or when the neck has a more horizontal takeoff posteriorly. A mobile temporal pole may be readily displaced backward, but it is not wise to divide large temporal-sphenoidal veins, for severe temporal edema or hemorrhage may occur. Without these veins, the half-and-half approach is the ideal one, for it combines the good features while minimizing the drawbacks of both. If tethered by the veins, the pole may be elevated to allow dissection on either side of the third nerve behind the neck to clear the perforators. Then the clip may be applied from various angles with all vessels in view.

By deeply respecting the work and achievements of two great neurosurgeons, C.G. Drake and S.J. Peerless (personal communication), we finish this comment by citing their lifetime, never-to-be-repeated experience:

Nearly all (99%) of nongiant basilar bifurcation aneurysms can be visualized subtemporally regardless of

their size, height, direction or multilocularity. The inner third of the tent can be divided smoothly for very low necks and placement of a temporary basilar artery clip. There is no necessity to remove the posterior clinoid process or inner petrous apex. In fact, we do not understand the benefits of an extensive removal of an obstacle when you can evade it. Exactly, one of the great advantages of [the] subtemporal approach is its simplicity without extensive removal of [the] base of [the] skull. Replacement of the small bone flap gives excellent cosmetic results. Finally, control of forceful hemorrhage from inadvertent rupture of the aneurysm is far easier through the subtemporal rather than a transsylvian exposure. These advantages have outweighed the minor risks associated with temporal lobe retraction and the reported, more frequent, temporary third nerve paresis. The transsylvian exposure is suitable in 56% of basilar bifurcation aneurysms in our case series. It is most appropriate for single aneurysms with small necks lying in an ideal position near the level of the dorsum sellae and pointing upward. It is necessary for those rare, very highly located, single aneurysms, and more frequently for treating additional aneurysms of the anterior circulation in one sitting. Much of the merit of an approach is a matter of surgical experience. It is well known that there are different levels of manual skills. We always attempted to make these operations simpler, faster, and to preserve normal anatomy by avoiding resection of brain or sacrifice of veins. In most instances, the subtemporal route has served our patients well.

Discussion

It is our experience and belief that the difference in endovascular and exovascular routes is that nature has created a simple route for endovascular surgery, whereas an artificial route has to be created to the base of the aneurysm in microneurosurgery. It is also our belief that a perfect clip at the base of the aneurysm more likely creates a permanent occlusion of the aneurysm than is possible with endovascular means. Quite frankly, if open cerebrovascular microsurgery is to survive, we have to be both good and efficient. Because of the rarity of these hidden and complex aneurysms, many cerebrovascular neurosurgeons, instead of improving their operative skills, stopped placing the perfect clip at the base of these posterior circulation aneurysms and handed these patients over to their endovascular colleagues. Further, in many centers, endovascular treatment has completely replaced open microsurgery for posterior circulation aneurysms, and even for anterior circulation aneurysms. Many neurosurgeons send patients to endovascular treatment, not to more experienced cerebrovascular surgeons, for many reasons, not the least of which is pressure from their surroundings.

Much of the merit of any approach is a matter of surgical experience. We always attempt to make these operations simpler and faster, and to preserve normal anatomy by avoiding the destruction of the cranial base, brain, or veins. One of our secret weapons is good neuroanesthesia and avoiding brain compression. In this way, we still occlude the main part (> 80%) of posterior circulation aneurysms through open microsurgical means. The basilar bifurcation and its perforators are unforgiving for operative complications, but it did not prevent Drake and Peerless, and their students, from achieving excellent results in patients with these aneurysms.

Moderators

Treatment of Ruptured Wide-Neck Basilar Aneurysms

Shakeel A. Chowdhry and Peter Nakaji

The authors were presented with the challenging case of aneurysmal subarachnoid hemorrhage in a young patient secondary to a ruptured basilar apex aneurysm. The lesion has a favorable Hunt and Hess grade at the time of the patient's admission, and imaging reveals a superiorly projecting aneurysm of moderate size (15 mm) with a wide neck. Bendok and associates and Hernesniemi and Korja present eloquent arguments for endovascular and open surgical treatment, respectively.

Before the 1990s, open surgery was the only treatment option for this lesion. With the significant risk of rebleeding and the associated morbidity and mortality of aneurysmal subarachnoid hemorrhage from ruptured basilar apex aneurysms, neurosurgeons were driven to improve surgical techniques. Led by pioneers such as Charles Drake, approaches and techniques were devised to treat even very daunting lesions in this region. Even so, posterior circulation aneurysms, particularly those emanating from the basilar artery, are still associated with the highest surgical morbidity.

The advent of endovascular therapy offered an alternative and exciting treatment option. Since the initial FDA approval in 1995, endovascular outcomes have steadily improved commensurate with rapid advances in the development and refinement of interventional tools and embolic material. Recent studies, including the International Subarachnoid Aneurysm Trial and the Barrow Ruptured Aneurysm Trial, have found decreased morbidity with the endovascular treatment of ruptured posterior circulation aneurysms compared with open microneurosurgery. As Bendok and colleagues note, the assessment of procedural risk (endovascular versus microsurgical) requires an evaluation of different aspects of the aneurysm's morphology and anatomy. For any given aneurysm, the anticipated benefits and associated risks in the hands of the treating physician must be carefully weighed in selecting the appropriate treatment. Here, we discuss the microneurosurgical and endovascular treatment options, and conclude with our recommendation for this patient.

Surgical Occlusion

Microneurosurgical treatment involves direct visualization to occlude the neck of the aneurysm. As Bendok and colleagues note, microneurosurgery has also undergone advances in the past several decades. Refined microneurosurgical technique, improvements in neuroanesthesia, and multimodality neurophysiological monitoring have contributed to improved surgical outcomes. Furthermore, despite ongoing improvements in endovascular therapy, long-term durability remains superior with surgical clipping.

The key parameters to consider, arguably in decreasing order of importance, are the direction of the aneurysm's dome, the anatomic relationship to the posterior clinoid process, and the width of the aneurysmal neck. The orientation of the dome of the aneurysm is a critical aspect in the decision to operate on a basilar apex aneurysm. Aneurysms that point anteriorly or superiorly may allow for better visualization of the posteriorly projecting perforating arteries arising from the proximal posterior cerebral arteries and the basilar artery, thereby facilitating dissection and subsequent clip placement. Posteriorly projecting aneurysms may obstruct the visualization of some of these critical perforating arteries, thereby increasing the risk of inadvertent perforator occlusion. The base of the aneurysm is situated at the level of the posterior clinoid process, and satisfactory exposure of the basilar artery for temporary occlusion will likely necessitate removal of the posterior clinoid when approaching the aneurysm through an orbitozygomatic approach. Although cranial-base cerebrovascular surgeons routinely remove the posterior clinoid process, it does increase the risk of surgical morbidity, and this risk should be factored into the decision. On the other hand, particularly high basilar bifurcations situated well above the posterior clinoid process can be difficult to reach and may sway the pendulum toward endovascular therapy if the anatomy is otherwise amenable. Finally, the width of the neck, although often discussed in the decision-making process for endovascular therapy, does have an impact on

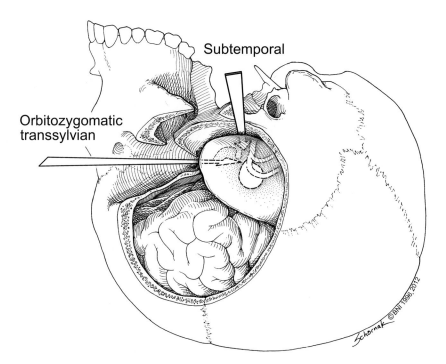

Fig. 15.5 The orbitozygomatic transsylvian approach provides a greater range of access to basilar apex aneurysms than afforded by the subtemporal approach, although the latter provides better access to the posterior aspect of the aneurysm's dome where the perforators are the hardest to visualize. (Courtesy of Barrow Neurological Institute.)

open surgical treatment as well. Indeed, narrow-necked aneurysms lend themselves toward both endovascular and open surgery. A wider neck means a longer distance to clear of perforators and to occlude with the surgical clip, which is made even more difficult by the small surgical corridors afforded by the approaches to this region.

Hernesniemi and Korja present a compelling argument for use of the middle fossa/subtemporal approach to treat this aneurysm. The subtemporal approach does allow for a direct lateral view at the level of the basilar apex and good visualization behind the aneurysm. This approach involves retracting the temporal lobe and is performed from the right side, when possible, to prevent placing the vein of Labbé of the dominant hemisphere at risk. Improvements in brain relaxation and neuroanesthesia have reduced retraction-related injury in this approach, but the working corridor remains relatively small, and subarachnoid hemorrhage and swelling can reduce this corridor further, particularly in a young patient. Although the subtemporal approach does allow for visualization of aneurysms below the posterior clinoid process, it is limited for viewing those originating well above the posterior clinoid.

We prefer to use the orbitozygomatic approach, an extension of the transsylvian approach, for basilar apex aneurysms **(Fig. 15.5)**. The approach provides a more inferior-to-superior trajectory toward the basilar apex, which permits access to aneurysms located above the posterior clinoid; nonetheless, those arising from a very high basilar apex can be difficult to reach with this approach as well. In the past, very high basilar apex aneurysms were reached through the adjunctive use of hypothermic circulatory arrest. In the present era, brief periods of relaxation for final clipping can be obtained with adenosine to stop the heart, but in general, surgical approaches that do not require these strategies are preferred. The orbitozygomatic approach is not associated with as significant a risk for oculomotor nerve palsy as is the subtemporal approach, but as Hernesniemi and Korja note, the oculomotor palsy, when present, is often temporary. In our experience, the orbitozygomatic approach allows for a larger working corridor and more surgical freedom **(Fig. 15.6)**. Direct visualization of the posterior aspects of the aneurysm is limited, but temporary clipping can soften the dome to allow it to be deflected to aid visualization. The orbitozygomatic approach does allow visualization of both sides of the neck, which are not easily seen with the subtemporal approach. The orbitozygomatic approach is restricted by the optic nerve and internal carotid artery, but these offer multiple windows and a variety of trajectories to the aneurysm's neck **(Fig. 15.7)**. Indeed, although there are advantages to placing the clip with the tines parallel to the posterior cerebral arteries, we have found that, with softening of the aneurysm, excellent closure without "dog-ear" remnants can be achieved with clip placement from front to back.

Regardless of the approach selected, the critical point of microneurosurgery is meticulous inspection of the per-

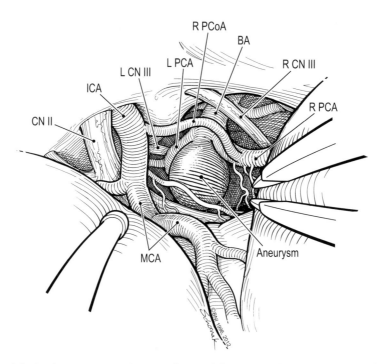

R PCoA
BA
L PCA
L CN III
R CN III
ICA
R PCA
CN II
MCA
Aneurysm

Fig. 15.6 The anatomy of the basilar apex as seen from a right orbitozygomatic approach through the oculomotor triangle. BA, basilar artery; CN, cranial nerve; ICA, internal carotid artery; L, left; MCA, middle cerebral artery; PCA, posterior cerebral artery; PCoA, posterior communicating artery; R, right. (Courtesy of Barrow Neurological Institute.)

forating arteries before and after clipping of the aneurysm. Digital subtraction angiography cannot be used to reliably evaluate the small perforating arteries. Indocyanine green angiography, however, can confirm the patency of perforating arteries but does require direct visualization of these vessels **(Fig. 15.8)**. In certain cases, the orbitozygomatic approach may be easily combined with a subtem-poral approach (otherwise known as the "half-and-half" approach) to view behind the aneurysm, which is particularly useful with posteriorly projecting aneurysms. The orbitozygomatic approach does not allow satisfactory visualization of aneurysms well below the posterior clinoid process. Midbasilar and vertebrobasilar junction aneurysms generally are accessed through the petrosal, retrosi-

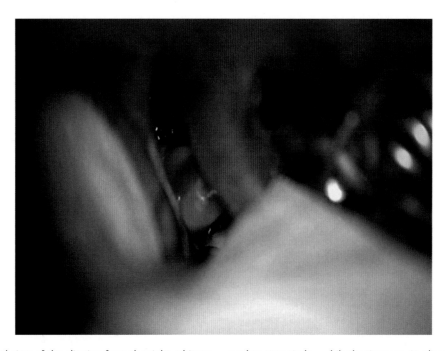

Fig. 15.7 Surgical view of the clipping from the right orbitozygomatic perspective. The clip in this case is advanced through the oculomotor window while the tines are visualized through the opticocarotid window. (Courtesy of Barrow Neurological Institute.)

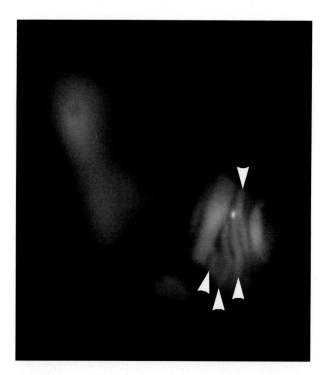

Fig. 15.8 Indocyanine green angiography shows that the perforators have been preserved (*arrowheads*) at the basilar apex after the clipping of a basilar apex aneurysm. (Courtesy of Barrow Neurological Institute.)

However, the morbidity of endovascular retreatment, when necessary, is usually low. Access is through the vertebral arteries, and significant stenosis of the vertebral artery origin or marked tortuosity may increase the difficulty of accessing the aneurysm. These access concerns are less likely in a patient as young as the one described. There may be an increased risk of dissection in patients with fibromuscular dysplasia.

The options for endovascular treatment have been well described, and we will expound briefly on these as well as other options. Coiling without an assist device would be done with the expectation of subtotal occlusion; the risk of coil herniation inferiorly with obstruction of flow into the PCAs would be a concern and would limit our ability to pack this aneurysm well. We would not recommend this as a first option.

The use of vessel-remodeling devices is associated with a higher morbidity than coiling without an assist device. Technological advances in design and development, however, have significantly reduced the morbidity associated with balloon remodeling. We would consider balloon-assisted coiling of the aneurysm with placement of the balloon extending from the basilar artery into the left PCA, with a second catheter or balloon in the right PCA to confirm patency and allow for more aggressive coil placement if the framing coils have formed an excellent basket (**Fig. 15.9**).

gmoid, or far lateral approaches if open surgical treatment is required.

Additional surgical options that should be presented in a thorough discussion of microneurosurgical therapy for this aneurysm include deconstructive therapy with occlusion of the basilar artery below the superior cerebellar arteries in patients with amenable anatomy. Based on results of an Allcock test, this surgical treatment may be augmented with a bypass as necessary, generally a superficial temporal artery-to-superior cerebellar artery bypass. We would not recommend this treatment as a first-line intervention for this patient.

Endovascular Occlusion

Bendok and colleagues present a thorough discussion of the endovascular treatment options for this patient. Indeed, the risk profile for endovascular treatment is different from that for microneurosurgery and includes inadvertent occlusion of a major branch or recanalization of the aneurysm. This aneurysm is fairly large, has a wide neck, and projects superiorly. During coil embolization of this aneurysm, the first priority must be to ensure the patency of both PCA branches. In general, endovascular therapy is associated with increased radiation exposure and a higher risk of initial incomplete occlusion, as well as a higher risk of recanalization, necessitating more frequent follow-up imaging compared with microneurosurgical treatment.

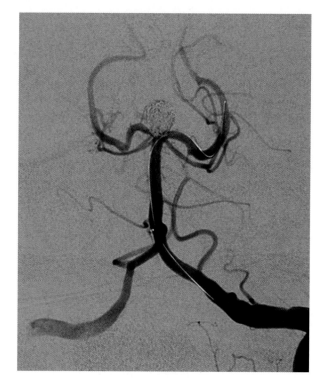

Fig. 15.9 A subtracted anteroposterior angiogram shows a basilar apex aneurysm at the conclusion of balloon-assisted coiling, with the supporting catheter in the basilar artery and the left posterior cerebral artery. (Courtesy of Barrow Neurological Institute.)

We routinely carry out coil embolization with the use of neurophysiological monitoring, which may be useful in detecting ischemia with balloon inflation. Complete occlusion would not be the expected outcome for this patient, however. Preventing the aneurysm from rerupture is the goal. Ultimately, recanalization and coil compaction is likely in this location, and retreatment at a later time (after the immediate sequelae of vasospasm have passed) would be planned. We agree with Bendok's plan and would anticipate the use of a stent with an extension into the left PCA during the delayed treatment. We prefer to place the patient on 1 week of dual antiplatelet therapy when possible rather than provide a bolus on the day of treatment. A balloon catheter would be placed in the other PCA for protection. But there are additional options. A dual-lumen balloon catheter could be used with the balloon situated at the neck of the aneurysm, although the particularly wide neck and risks associated with transient flow arrest in bilateral PCAs would be concerns with this option. This patient could be treated with a Y-stent construct (**Fig. 15.10**). If the posterior communicating arteries are large, they can be used to deliver a single stent from one PCA across to the other (T stent) (**Fig. 15.11**). We prefer not to use the "waffle cone" technique as we believe it drives blood flow to the base of the coil mass and would create a hemodynamic environment with a high risk of coil compaction and aneurysm recanalization (**Fig. 15.12**).

We would not pursue stent-assisted coiling in the acute period. Some authors have advocated its use in this setting, but we believe that the risks of hemorrhage, particularly if cerebrospinal fluid drainage is needed, are concerning for patients on dual antiplatelet therapy. Furthermore, the natural hypercoagulable state of a patient with subarachnoid hemorrhage dissuades us from placing fresh Nitinol. We also do not believe this aneurysm is amenable to flow

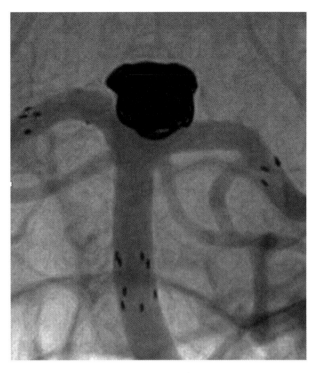

Fig. 15.10 An unsubtracted anteroposterior angiogram of a coiled basilar tip aneurysm with two stents in a Y-stent configuration. The stent markers can be seen in the basilar artery and both posterior cerebral arteries. (Courtesy of Barrow Neurological Institute.)

diversion and would not pursue this option. Another option not mentioned, Onyx HD 500, is also not suitable for this aneurysm and its use here would also be off-label and not recommended.

The final option proposed by Bendok and colleagues is an interesting one that warrants some discussion. Recon-

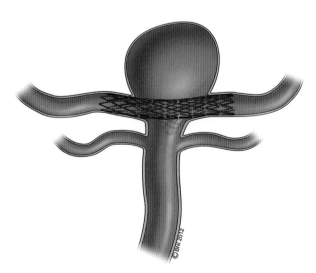

Fig. 15.11 Artist rendition of a T spanning from one posterior cerebral artery to the other. Placement requires a large posterior communicating artery through which the stent is delivered. (Courtesy of Barrow Neurological Institute.)

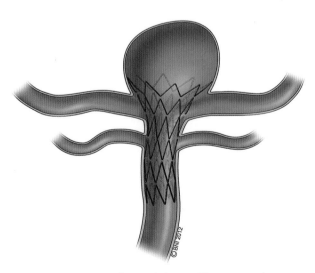

Fig. 15.12 Artist rendition of the "waffle cone" technique in which a stent is deployed within the basilar artery with the distal tines set in the proximal aspect of the aneurysm. (Courtesy of Barrow Neurological Institute.)

struction of the neck of the aneurysm can significantly reduce the risks of endovascular treatment and allow for a more dense packing of coils in the aneurysm, particularly across the neck. Indeed, with endovascular therapy in one's armamentarium, microneurosurgical treatment may be undertaken, and if proximal P1 perforators along the distal side of the aneurysm cannot be safely visualized and cleared, then subtotal occlusion of the aneurysmal neck may be a reasonable option. The remodeled neck may then be more amenable to aggressive embolization without the risk of coil herniation and could be embolized immediately with a good outcome.

One important point to consider in patients with large superiorly projecting basilar apex aneurysms is the delayed risk of settling of a large coil mass on the posterior cerebral arteries with external compression and flow limitation. This risk is likely reduced with stent-assisted coiling, but it has been described and would be of concern in patients with a larger aneurysm. We would not anticipate this to be a significant risk for the patient described.

A last critical point, regardless of the modality selected, is made by Hernesniemi and Korja about the modification of risk factors. A strong encouragement of smoking cessation is critical for these patients, particularly for achieving the best possible long-term outcome.

Conclusion

Both authors present excellent discussions of treatment options for this patient. A pure microneurosurgical approach is a good option in the hands of an experienced vascular neurosurgeon. The aneurysm may be approached through either a subtemporal or orbitozygomatic craniotomy, and the experience and comfort of the surgeon may be the deciding factor. The aneurysm has certain features amenable to open surgical treatment with respect to the direction of the dome and the location of the basilar bifurcation relative to the posterior clinoid process. A purely endovascular treatment is also a reasonable option for this patient. If treated in this way, we would recommend securing the aneurysm in the early period with balloon-assisted coiling followed by delayed, definitive stent-assisted coiling.

Our final recommendation is to pursue open surgical treatment for this patient through an orbitozygomatic approach because of her age and the Hunt and Hess grade of the lesion at the time of the patient's admission. We would anticipate complete closure of the aneurysm; however, if we were unable to visualize or protect distal perforators, then subtotal clipping with coil embolization would be our alternate strategy. Endovascular therapy as a first choice is eminently reasonable. Where locally available expertise strongly favors one approach or the other, the technique with the lower chance of morbidity is preferred. In any case, we concur with the other authors that aneurysms such as this should be treated in high-volume centers with expertise in both cerebrovascular microneurosurgery and neurointerventional surgery.

Recommended Readings

Amenta PS, Dalyai RT, Kung D, et al. Stent-assisted coiling of wide-necked aneurysms in the setting of acute subarachnoid hemorrhage: experience in 65 patients. Neurosurgery 2012;70: 1415–1429, discussion 1429

Bendok BR, Aoun SG. Flow diversion for intracranial aneurysms: optimally defining and evolving a new tool and approach. World Neurosurg 2011;76:401–404

Bendok BR, Getch CC, Parkinson R, O'Shaughnessy BA, Batjer HH. Extended lateral transsylvian approach for basilar bifurcation aneurysms. Neurosurgery 2004;55:174–178, discussion 178

Bendok BR, Hanel RA, Hopkins LN. Coil embolization of intracranial aneurysms. Neurosurgery 2003;52:1125–1130, discussion 1130

Chalouhi N, Jabbour P, Gonzalez LF, et al. Safety and efficacy of endovascular treatment of basilar tip aneurysms by coiling with and without stent assistance: a review of 235 cases. Neurosurgery 2012;71:785–794

Connolly ES Jr, Poisik A, Winfree CJ, et al. Cigarette smoking and the development and rupture of cerebral aneurysms in a mixed race population: implications for population screening and smoking cessation. J Stroke Cerebrovasc Dis 1999;8:248–253

de Oliveira JG, Beck J, Seifert V, Teixeira MJ, Raabe A. Assessment of flow in perforating arteries during intracranial aneurysm surgery using intraoperative near-infrared indocyanine green videoangiography. Neurosurgery 2008;62(6, Suppl 3):1300–1310

Drake CG, Hernesniemi JA, Peerless SJ. Selection of the surgical approach in basilar bifurcation aneurysms, 1993 (unpublished)

Drake CG, Peerless SJ, Hernesniemi JA, Yasargil MG. Surgery of Vertebrobasilar Aneurysms: London, Ontario Experience on 1767 patients. Vienna: Springer, 1996

Eddleman CS, Surdell D, Miller J, Shaibani A, Bendok BR. Endovascular management of a ruptured cavernous carotid artery aneurysm associated with a carotid cavernous fistula with an intracranial self-expanding Microstent and Hydrogel-coated coil embolization: case report and review of the literature. Surg Neurol 2007;68:562–567, discussion 567

Gruber DP, Zimmerman GA, Tomsick TA, van Loveren HR, Link MJ, Tew JM Jr. A comparison between endovascular and surgical management of basilar artery apex aneurysms. J Neurosurg 1999;90:868–874

Henkes H, Fischer S, Mariushi W, et al. Angiographic and clinical results in 316 coil-treated basilar artery bifurcation aneurysms. J Neurosurg 2005;103:990–999

Hernesniemi J, Vapalahti M, Niskanen M, Kari A. Management outcome for vertebrobasilar artery aneurysms by early surgery. Neurosurgery 1992;31:857–861, discussion 861–862

Hsu FP, Clatterbuck RE, Spetzler RF. Orbitozygomatic approach to basilar apex aneurysms. Neurosurgery 2005;56(1, Suppl):172–177, discussion 172–177

Jin SC, Ahn JS, Kwun BD, Kwon DH. Analysis of clinical and radiological outcomes in microsurgical and endovascular treatment of basilar apex aneurysms. J Korean Neurosurg Soc 2009;45: 224–230

Kellner CP, Haque RM, Meyers PM, Lavine SD, Connolly ES Jr, Solomon RA; Clinical Article. Complex basilar artery aneurysms treated using surgical basilar occlusion: a modern case series. Clinical article. J Neurosurg 2011;115:319–327

Krisht AF, Krayenbühl N, Sercl D, Bikmaz K, Kadri PA. Results of microsurgical clipping of 50 high complexity basilar apex aneurysms. Neurosurgery 2007;60:242–250, discussion 250–252

Lawton MT. Basilar apex aneurysms: surgical results and perspectives from an initial experience. Neurosurgery 2002;50:1–8, discussion 8–10

Lozier AP, Kim GH, Sciacca RR, Connolly ES Jr, Solomon RA. Microsurgical treatment of basilar apex aneurysms: perioperative and long-term clinical outcome. Neurosurgery 2004;54:286–296, discussion 296–299

Lusseveld E, Brilstra EH, Nijssen PC, et al. Endovascular coiling versus neurosurgical clipping in patients with a ruptured basilar tip aneurysm. J Neurol Neurosurg Psychiatry 2002;73:591–593

Mehra M, Hurley MC, Gounis MJ, et al. The impact of coil shape design on angiographic occlusion, packing density and coil mass uniformity in aneurysm embolization: an in vitro study. J Neurointerv Surg 2011;3:131–136

Ortiz R, Stefanski M, Rosenwasser R, Veznedaroglu E. Cigarette smoking as a risk factor for recurrence of aneurysms treated by endosaccular occlusion. J Neurosurg 2008;108:672–675

Pandey AS, Koebbe C, Rosenwasser RH, Veznedaroglu E. Endovascular coil embolization of ruptured and unruptured posterior circulation aneurysms: review of a 10-year experience. Neurosurgery 2007;60:626–636, discussion 636–637

Peerless SJ, Hernesniemi JA, Gutman FB, Drake CG. Early surgery for ruptured vertebrobasilar aneurysms. J Neurosurg 1994;80: 643–649

Pierot L, Cognard C, Spelle L, Moret J. Safety and efficacy of balloon remodeling technique during endovascular treatment of intracranial aneurysms: critical review of the literature. AJNR Am J Neuroradiol 2012;33:12–15

Piotin M, Blanc R, Spelle L, et al. Stent-assisted coiling of intracranial aneurysms: clinical and angiographic results in 216 consecutive aneurysms. Stroke 2010;41:110–115

Raabe A, Nakaji P, Beck J, et al. Prospective evaluation of surgical microscope-integrated intraoperative near-infrared indocyanine green videoangiography during aneurysm surgery. J Neurosurg 2005;103:982–989

Redekop GJ, Durity FA, Woodhurst WB. Management-related morbidity in unselected aneurysms of the upper basilar artery. J Neurosurg 1997;87:836–842

Rice BJ, Peerless SJ, Drake CG. Surgical treatment of unruptured aneurysms of the posterior circulation. J Neurosurg 1990;73: 165–173

Samson D, Batjer HH, Kopitnik TA Jr. Current results of the surgical management of aneurysms of the basilar apex. Neurosurgery 1999;44:697–702, discussion 702–704

Sanai N, Tarapore P, Lee AC, Lawton MT. The current role of microsurgery for posterior circulation aneurysms: a selective approach in the endovascular era. Neurosurgery 2008;62:1236–1249, discussion 1249–1253

Smith GA, Dagostino P, Maltenfort MG, Dumont AS, Ratliff JK. Geographic variation and regional trends in adoption of endovascular techniques for cerebral aneurysms. J Neurosurg 2011; 114:1768–1777

Vallee JN, Aymard A, Vicaut E, Reis M, Merland JJ. Endovascular treatment of basilar tip aneurysms with Guglielmi detachable coils: predictors of immediate and long-term results with multivariate analysis 6-year experience. Radiology 2003;226: 867–879

Yasargil MG, Antic J, Laciga R, Jain KK, Hodosh RM, Smith RD. Microsurgical pterional approach to aneurysms of the basilar bifurcation. Surg Neurol 1976;6:83–91

Chapter 16

Surgical Approaches to Basilar Tip Aneurysms

Case

A 45-year-old man who smokes cigarettes presents with subarachnoid hemorrhage of Hunt and Hess grade I and Fisher grade II. A left vertebral artery angiogram and a three-dimensional computed tomography angiography reconstruction show a broad-based basilar tip aneurysm.

Participants

The Pterional Approach to an Aneurysm at the Basilar Bifurcation: John L. Fox

The Cranio-orbital Zygomatic (COZ) Approach to Basilar Apex Aneurysms: Kaith K. Almefty and T. C. Origitano

The Transcavernous Approach to Basilar Aneurysms: Ali F. Krisht

The Pretemporal Approach to Basilar Aneurysms: Feres Chaddad, José Maria de Campos Filho, and Evandro de Oliveira

Moderators: Surgical Approaches to Basilar Apex Aneurysms: Duke Samson and Christopher S. Eddleman

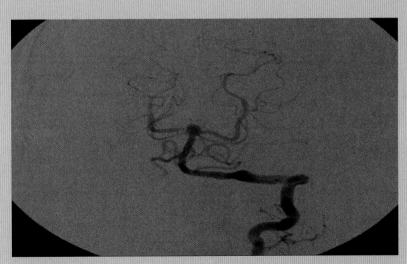

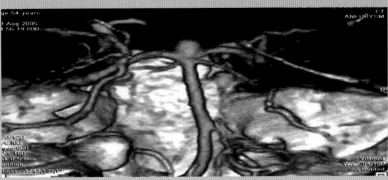

The Pterional Approach to an Aneursym at the Basilar Bifurcation

John L. Fox

Over the past few years, the pterional, or frontolateral, approach to the interpeduncular cistern has gained increasing acceptance.[1-6]

Surgical Approach

To visualize any targeted lesion in this cistern between the upper clivus and the midbrain, the surgeon must open a pathway between the sphenoid wing and the base of the sylvian fissure. Failure to drill the sphenoid wing and insufficient opening of the sylvian fissure under good magnification have been common causes of a surgeon's disappointment in using the pterional approach. **Figure 16.1a** illustrates the relationship of the aneurysm to cerebral structures as seen through a right pterional approach. **Figure 16.1b,c** shows the opening of the sylvian fissure.

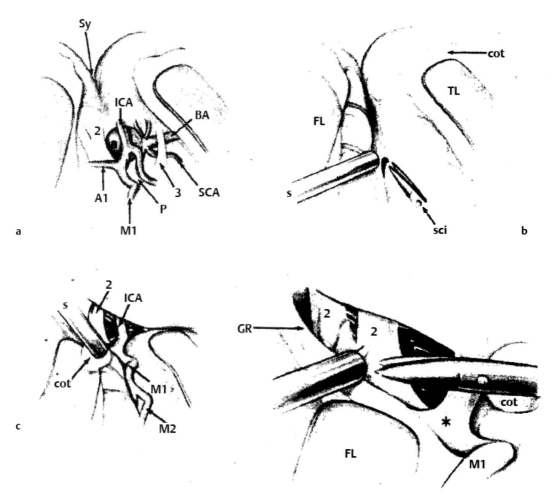

Fig. 16.1a–d **(a)** The projected relationship of an aneurysm at the basilar bifurcation to arteries and nerves as seen in the right frontotemporal or pterional approach after the sylvian fissure (Sy) is opened. Note the right A1 artery crossing the chiasm behind the optic nerve (2); the internal carotid artery (ICA) continuing toward the surgeon as the M1 artery; the right oculomotor nerve (3) arising from the midbrain and flanked by the posterior cerebral artery rostrally and the superior cerebellar artery (SCA) caudally (seen on the left side also); the termination of the basilar artery (BA); and the junction (p) of the right posterior communicating P1 and P2 arteries. **(b)** The arachnoid in the sylvian fissure is incised with microscissors (sci). The surgeon holds the suction tube (s) in the left hand. Self-retaining retractors support and separate the frontal lobe (FL) and temporal lobe (TL). cot, cotton ball. **(c)** The sylvian fissure has been opened widely, exposing M1 and M2 and the internal carotid artery (ICA), as well as the optic nerve (2). The tip of the suction tube (s) rests on a small dental cotton ball (cot). **(d)** The retractor is used to elevate the right frontal lobe (FL) and its gyrus rectus (GR) off the optic nerves (2) and chiasm. Arachnoid adhesions between the chiasm and frontal lobe are severed. The middle cerebral artery (M1) and bifurcation of the internal carotid artery (*) are in view. (From Fox JL. Microsurgical exposure of vertebrobasilar aneurysms. In: Rand RW, ed. Microneurosurgery, 3rd ed. St. Louis: CV Mosby, 1985:589–599. Reprinted by permission.)

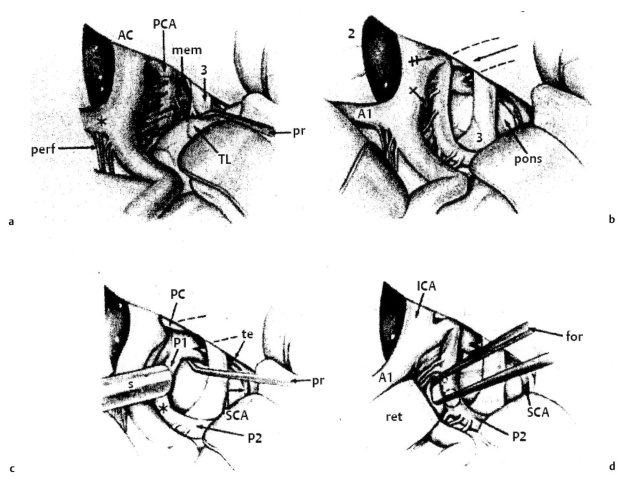

Fig. 16.2a–d **(a)** The posterior communicating artery (PCA) is followed back, and the uncus of the temporal lobe (TL) is dissected off the oculomotor nerve (*3*) with a microprobe (pr). In the background is the arachnoid membrane (mem) of Liliequist separating the chiasmatic and interpeduncular cisterns. Note the anterior clinoid process (AC) and the bifurcation of the internal carotid artery (*) and its perforators (perf). **(b)** The same view after the membrane of Liliequist and arachnoid adhesions have been cleared away. The origin of the right oculomotor nerve (*3*) is seen. The optic nerve (*2*), A1 artery, origin of the posterior communicating artery (*double-crossed arrow*), origin of the anterior choroidal artery (*single-crossed arrow*), rostral border of the pons, and tip of the basilar artery (*uncrossed arrow* shows its direction) are seen. The pituitary stalk and dome of this rostrally projecting aneurysm are hidden behind the arachnoid (*) between the optic nerve and the carotid artery. **(c)** The suction tube (s) is used to retract the internal carotid and posterior communicating arteries, exposing the right P1 artery, the right P2 artery, and their junction (*) with the posterior communicating artery. The posterior clinoid process (PC) hides part of the tip of the basilar artery in this view. A probe (pr) is used to lift the origin of the superior cerebellar artery (SCA). Note the edge of the SCA and the edge of the tentorium (te). **(d)** The bipolar forceps (for) is used to dissect arachnoid off the posterior communicating artery and its anterior thalamoperforators. Care must be taken not to perforate the adjacent dome of the aneurysm with the tips of the forceps. A narrow, self-retaining retractor (ret) is used to draw back the M1 artery and the internal carotid bifurcation. Also seen are the internal carotid artery (ICA) and the A1 artery. The P2 artery and the SCA flank the oculomotor nerve. (From Fox JL. Microsurgical exposure of vertebrobasilar aneurysms. In: Rand RW, ed. Microneurosurgery, 3rd ed. St. Louis: CV Mosby, 1985:589–599. Reprinted by permission.)

Figure 16.1d emphasizes the lysis of the arachnoid and adhesions between the optic nerve and the base of the frontal lobe.

In **Fig. 16.2**, we see the pathway taken caudally. The wide separation of the right frontal and temporal lobes with visualization of the middle cerebral artery is evident. The exposure is developed between the internal carotid artery and the oculomotor nerve; the posterior communicating artery is followed (**Fig. 16.2a,b**). Occasionally, the exposure is between the optic nerve and the internal carotid artery (rare in my experience). The rostral pons, the superior cerebellar artery, the origin of the oculomotor nerve, and the junction of the posterior communicating artery with the P1 and P2 portions of the posterior cerebral artery (PCA) are evident (**Fig. 16.2c,d**).

At times, the posterior clinoid process is in the visual field. In such uncommon cases, I use a small high-speed diamond drill to remove this projection. **Figure 16.3a** shows the aneurysm at the tip of the basilar artery coming into view between the retracted right internal carotid artery

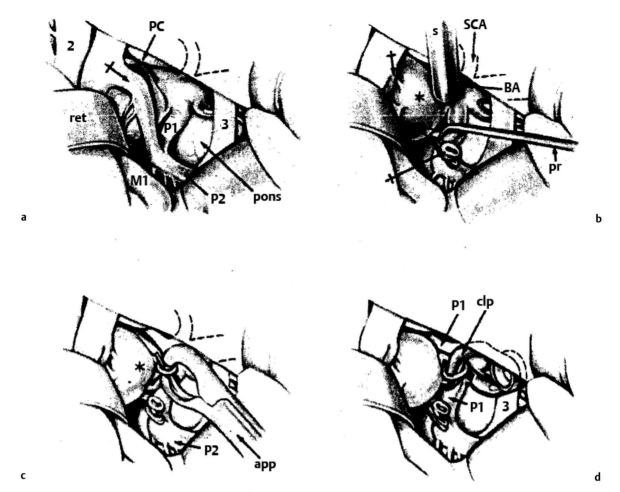

Fig. 16.3a–d **(a)** A narrow retractor (ret) is used to displace the internal carotid bifurcation and M1. The crossed arrow points to the posterior communicating artery lying lateral to the dome of the aneurysm. The optic *(2)* and oculomotor *(3)* nerves are seen. The posterior clinoid process (PC) hides part of the left P1 artery. The right P1 and P2 arteries and the rostral pons are seen. **(b)** The posterior communicating artery *(single-crossed arrows)* has been clipped with small, malleable, tantalum clips and severed to better expose the aneurysm (*). The suction tube (s) hides the junction of the left P1 and the aneurysm. The tip of the basilar artery (BA) is seen. The left superior cerebellar artery (SCA) is hidden. A probe (pr) is used to retract the right P1 artery to expose the posterior thalamoperforators. **(c)** A Yasargil clip straddles the neck of the aneurysm (*) before closure. The clip is in its applicator (app). The right P2 artery is seen. **(d)** The clip (clp) has been closed. Both P1 arteries and their perforators are preserved. The shank of the clip touches the oculomotor nerve *(3)*. (From Fox JL. Microsurgical exposure of vertebrobasilar aneurysms. In: Rand RW, ed. Microneurosurgery, 3rd ed. St. Louis: CV Mosby, 1985: 589–599. Reprinted by permission.)

and the oculomotor nerve. Often, the posterior communicating artery must be severed between small malleable clips (avoiding perforators) to gain an adequate view of the aneurysm **(Fig. 16.3b)**. After the aneurysm is separated from the posterior thalamic perforators, the neck is clipped **(Fig. 16.3c,d)**. A large aneurysm, such as that seen in the patient under discussion, often requires a long clip to be placed across the equator of the dome to collapse the aneurysm before clipping the neck. Otherwise, the clip on the neck will slip and occlude the P1 arteries.

Discussion

Samson and colleagues[7] and Wright and Wilson[8] have emphasized the importance of appreciating the relationship of the posterior clinoid process to the neck of the aneurysm on the lateral arteriogram. They concluded that the frontolateral approach is too difficult if the neck of the aneurysm lies below the level of the posterior clinoid process. With wide opening of the sylvian fissure, however, and excellent brain relaxation, I believe it is still usually possible to deal with these low-lying basilar tip aneurysms.

Yasargil and colleagues[6] preferred the frontolateral to the subtemporal route for the following reasons:

- There is less retraction pressure on the temporal lobe.
- The anatomy of the interpeduncular cistern is better seen (both P1 arteries and perforators) with a more frontal view of the aneurysm.
- The oculomotor and trochlear nerves are less disturbed.

- The surgeon can better treat additional aneurysms on the anterior circle of Willis at the same time.

The disadvantages of the frontolateral route may include the following:

- The internal carotid or M1 arteries must often be retracted (this is dangerous if the patient has atherosclerosis or if blood pressure drops very low).
- The posterior communicating or P1 artery must often be ligated and sectioned.
- The posterior clinoid process may be in the way of low-lying aneurysms at the basilar bifurcation.
- Aneurysms high up in the interpeduncular cistern that project backward are more difficult to visualize.
- Perforators between the posterior aspect of the aneurysm and the brain stem may be less easily seen in some cases.
- The working space between the internal carotid artery and the oculomotor nerve is confining, requiring expert microtechnique.

Some surgeons have used a modified approach that combines the pterional exposure with the subtemporal, usually resulting in posterior retraction of the temporal lobe rather than a true transsylvian exposure.[9,10] The supraorbital-pterional approach of Al-Mefty[11] provides further low-basal exposure of these lesions.

Early in my neurosurgical career, I operated on aneurysms at the basilar bifurcation through the standard subtemporal approach described by Drake.[12] After observing the techniques of Yasargil and colleagues[6] (who first used the pterional approach for those aneurysms), I changed to using the pterional approach because many patients had multiple aneurysms that could not all be clipped through the subtemporal approach during the same surgery. As I gained experience, I found myself more comfortable with the pterional approach and now rarely use the subtemporal approach to aneurysms in the interpeduncular fossa. In the patient described in this case, I would use the right pterional approach, operating when the patient is in good condition after the phase of vasospasm has passed.

The Cranio-orbital Zygomatic (COZ) Approach to Basilar Apex Aneurysms

Kaith K. Almefty and T. C. Origitano

Basilar apex aneurysms are among the most challenging cerebrovascular lesions because of their deep location, proximity to important and delicate neurovascular structures, and the surgeon's limited visibility and maneuverability. The surgical challenges have been exacerbated in the endovascular era as surgical treatment has often been reserved for the most complex geometrical lesions. The ideal surgical approach to these complex lesions should embody the following fundamental principles:

- Provide visualization and control of proximal and distal vasculature.
- Allow for the safe dissection of small perforating arteries.
- Maximize maneuverability and ergonomics for optimal dissection and clip placement with minimal brain retraction.[13]

The cranio-orbital zygomatic (COZ) approach achieves these tenets by providing a shorter and wider operative distance, early proximal and distal control, direct entry to the interpeduncular cistern, and multiple angles for viewing and dissecting, as well as minimizing brain retraction. An approach angle that is flat with the middle cranial fossa combined with the short, wide corridor enables the surgeon to place a hand in the middle cranial fossa for im-

proved control (**Fig. 16.4**). This approach provides clear visualization of the thalamoperforators, the neck and dome of the aneurysm, the anterior circulation, and both PCAs. In addition, the clip can be placed without compromising visualization or control.

Case Presentation and Description of the Cranio-orbital Zygomatic Approach

In this chapter's presented case, cerebral angiography with three-dimensional reconstruction delineates a broad-based aneurysm at the basilar apex (see the figures with the case presentation), and so this patient is considered high risk for endovascular treatment. We recommend that the patient undergo definitive clipping of the aneurysm through a right-sided COZ approach with removal of the posterior clinoid process and a transcavernous technique.

For this approach, the patient's head is placed in the Mayfield headrest (with all pins placed behind the ears if possible), slightly extended, and turned 30 degrees away from the operative side. A scalp incision is made 1 cm anterior to the tragus and continued behind the hairline to the midline. This incision can be extended toward the contralateral temporal line for additional exposure, and should be superficial to the pericranium and temporalis fascia.

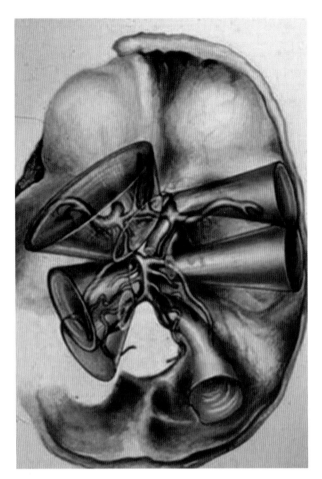

Fig. 16.4 Illustration showing the surgical approaches to the cerebral vasculature. The top left cone shows the cranio-orbital zygomatic (COZ) approach. The right top and middle cones show the pterional and subtemporal approaches, respectively. Note the short wide corridor to the basilar apex obtained with the COZ approach compared with the longer, more narrow corridors of the traditional approaches. (From Origitano TC, Anderson DE, Tarassoli Y, Reichman OH, Al-Mefty O. Skull base approaches to complex cerebral aneurysms. Surg Neurol 1993;40:339–346. Reprinted by permission.)

The subcutaneous flap is dissected sharply from the pericranium, and dissection is carried anteriorly to the prominence of the superior orbital rim. Further dissection in this plane is done posterior to the skin incision. A bicoronal incision is then made in the underlying pericranium, from temporal line to temporal line, based on the supraorbital blood supply. The large vascularized flap is then elevated, and the supraorbital arterial supply is preserved along the bilateral superior temporal lines. The supraorbital nerve should be identified along the medial third of the superior orbital notch. It may exit either through a notch or a true foramen. If through a notch, the nerve can be safely dissected free. If through a foramen, an osteotomy must be done around the foramen and the nerve dissected free with its bony attachment. The periorbita is detached from the

superior and lateral walls of the orbit and the scalp flap is reflected anteriorly.

To protect the frontotemporal branches of the facial nerve, the fat pad containing these branches is elevated with the superficial and deep layers of temporalis fascia. At a point 1.5 cm posterior to the lateral orbital rim, a 2-cm incision in the superficial and deep temporal fascia is made parallel with the zygomatic arch. In subperiosteal fashion, these layers are reflected with the fat pad and skin flap. The zygomatic arch is also dissected along its length in subperiosteal fashion. It is then sectioned obliquely at the malar eminence and the root of the zygoma. The temporalis muscle is incised posterior to the superficial temporal artery, elevated with subperiosteal dissection, and reflected downward.[14]

Bur holes are placed at the base of the zygoma and at the keyhole, which should expose both the dura and periorbita. An osteotomy is made on the lateral orbital rim and extended to the keyhole. The next cut extends from the zygomatic bur hole along the base of the temporal fossa to the sphenoid ridge. The sphenoid ridge is then removed with the high-speed drill, and this cut is connected to the keyhole. An osteotomy is then made from the temporal bur hole to the frontal bur hole and extended into the orbital roof. Next, an osteotomy is done from the keyhole through the orbital roof, extending medially. The skull flap can then be elevated, and the remaining portion of the roof and lateral orbit are removed in one piece with additional osteotomies. The first cut is in the roof of the orbit and extends posteriorly along but not into the ethmoid sinuses. The second cut is made at the base of the lateral wall of the orbit along the inferior orbital fissure. These cuts are then connected across the lesser sphenoid wing and the flap is elevated[15] (**Fig. 16.5**). The osteotomies can be tailored to individual aspects of the patient's anatomy and based on the surgeon's experience. They can be done as described above, or the orbitozygomatic osteotomy can be taken as a single piece or as two pieces (orbit and zygoma).

The medial aspects of the sphenoid wing are removed with the drill, which unroofs the superior orbital fissure. The optic canal is located medial to the superior orbital fissure at the apex of the orbit. It is opened extradurally and the optic strut is drilled, allowing for an extradural removal of the anterior clinoid process (**Fig. 16.6**). The dura is then opened with a curvilinear incision and reflected anteriorly. The surgeon can gain additional working space by depressing the orbit with anterior dural traction and fixation to further flatten the orbital trajectory.[16,17]

The sylvian fissure is widely dissected, allowing the temporal lobe to fall laterally and posteriorly. The tethering veins running from the sylvian fissure to the sphenoparietal sinus are dissected and preserved. The lateral and medial carotid cisterns, the lateral wall of the cavernous sinus, and the edge of the tentorial incisura are then exposed. The entrance of the third nerve into the cavernous sinus must be identified and will guide further dissection. Untether-

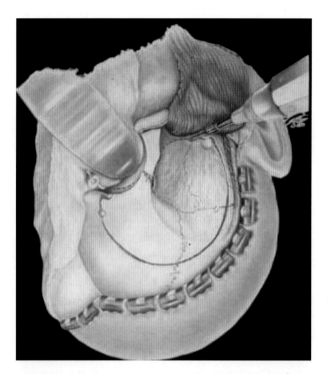

Fig. 16.5 Illustration of the COZ cuts. Bur holes are drilled in the temporal bone (the keyhole) and the frontal bone. Cuts are made as follows: from the lateral orbital rim to the keyhole, the zygomatic bur hole to the sphenoid ridge, the temporal bur hole to the frontal bur hole, the keyhole through the orbital roof extending medially, and the sphenoid ridge to the keyhole. (From Arnautovic KI, Al-Mefty O, Angtuaco E. A combined microsurgical skull-base and endovascular approach to giant and large paraclinoid aneurysms. Surg Neurol 1998;50:504–520. Reprinted by permission.)

ing the third nerve and opening the oculomotor foramen provides additional exposure and facilitates safe retraction of the nerve **(Fig. 16.7)**. Dissection is done along the third nerve toward the brainstem, and the origins of the PCAs and superior cerebellar arteries are identified. At this point, proximal control of the distal basilar artery should be established by identifying a "landing zone" for the application of a temporary clip. The posterior communicating artery is dissected from its origin on the carotid to the junction of the PCA. Beneath the posterior communicating artery, the interpeduncular cistern is approached obliquely from an anterior-to-inferior direction, and the posterior communicating artery is followed back to the PCA and the aneurysm. The superior aspect of the aneurysm is further dissected anterior to the third nerve in the interpeduncular cistern **(Fig. 16.8)**. The back wall of the aneurysm and the thalamoperforators may be dissected by working laterally and beneath the third nerve.

This exposure is typically sufficient for high-lying and normal basilar apex aneurysms; for low-lying aneurysms, additional exposure may be necessary. Skeletonizing and removing the posterior clinoid process may create further

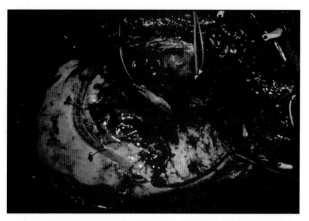

Fig. 16.6 Intraoperative photograph of the COZ craniotomy. The temporalis muscle is reflected inferiorly and out of the field of view. The orbital osteotomies have widened the transsylvian corridor.

anterior and lateral exposure **(Fig. 16.9)**. Exposing the proximal basilar artery for temporary clipping is possible at the level of the fifth nerve; cutting the tentorium behind the fourth nerve facilitates this by allowing for further inferior visualization[13,16] **(Fig. 16.10)**.

These maneuvers provide a wide exposure of the interpeduncular cistern with multiple viewing angles, allowing the surgeon to view the top of the basilar artery, the posterior communicating artery, and both PCAs. Clips may be applied in a lateral-to-anterolateral arc **(Fig. 16.11)**. If projecting dorsally, the aneurysm may be difficult to clip from this arc and a more lateral trajectory can be obtained by working through the ambient cistern. The COZ approach allows for this with minimal retraction of the temporal lobe.[16]

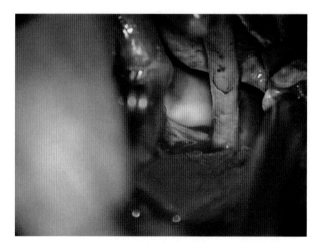

Fig. 16.7 The oculomotor foramen is opened, a maneuver that widens the depth of field and allows for safe manipulation of the nerve. Arrows: oculomotor nerve; arrows oculomotor foramen.

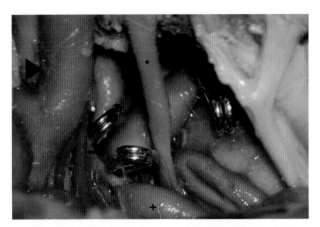

a

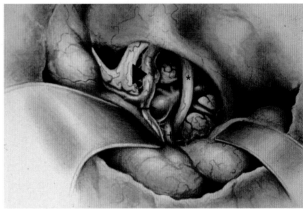

b

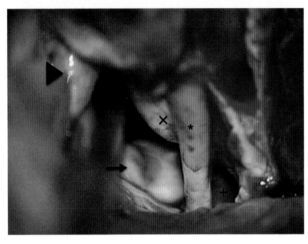

c

Fig. 16.8a–c (**a**) Anatomic dissection of the exposed basilar apex. The third nerve is in the foreground and guides the dissection. A clip, placed on the basilar artery inferior to the superior cerebellar arteries, provides proximal control. The bilateral posterior cerebral arteries are exposed and able to be controlled with temporary clips. The perforating arteries are well visualized. Illustration (**b**) and intraoperative photograph (**c**) are of similar views. Arrow, basilar tip aneurysm; arrowhead, internal carotid artery; *, oculomotor nerve; +, posterior cerebral artery; x, posterior clinoid. (Part **b** from Origitano TC, Anderson DE, Tarassoli Y, Reichman OH, Al-Mefty O. Skull base approaches to complex cerebral aneurysms. Surg Neurol 1993;40:339–346. Reprinted by permission.)

Discussion

The COZ approach, as described here and with variations by others,[13,14,16,18–20] provides distinct advantages in the clipping of basilar tip aneurysms as compared with the pterional and subtemporal approaches. The lateral subtemporal approach to basilar apex aneurysms provides the advantage of exposure to the posterior aspect of the aneurysm and to the thalamoperforators, but exposure of the apex and the contralateral P1 is limited. In addition, temporal lobe retraction is necessary and this approach may not be feasible in the setting of subarachnoid hemorrhage and cerebral swelling. The pterional approach provides access to the apex and contralateral P1, but limits the exposure to the back wall of the aneurysm. The trajectory is long, and aneurysms placed both high and low are not well visualized because of the one-directional, envelope-shaped field. The COZ approach provides both superior and posterior access and increases the number of viewing angles, fundamentally providing both the transsylvian and subtemporal avenues.[13,16] The wide exposure of the interpeduncular cistern allows access to the apex of the aneurysm, the carotid artery, and the posterior communicating and PCAs.[13,17] Temporary clipping distal or proximal to the superior cerebellar arteries is also possible (**Fig. 16.8**). The flat working area along the middle cranial fossa exposes the neck and the thalamoperforators. Untethering the

third nerve and drilling the posterior clinoid process opens up additional working angles and access to a low-lying bifurcation.[16,18]

The essential advantage of the skull-base approach is a shorter, wider corridor. This corridor provides the surgeon with greater visualization, maneuverability, control, and ergonomic advantages at the deepest and most delicate

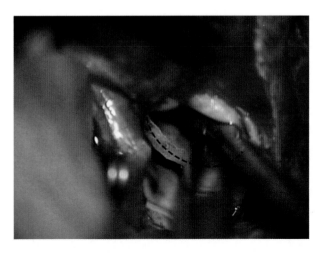

Fig. 16.9 The posterior clinoid is skeletonized and removed to allow additional anterior and lateral exposure.

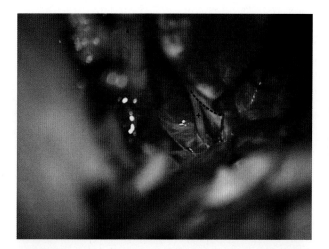

Fig. 16.10 The tentorium is cut posterior to the fourth nerve. This provides a wider exposure of the interpeduncular cistern and access to the proximal basilar artery to the level of the fifth nerve for temporary clip placement.

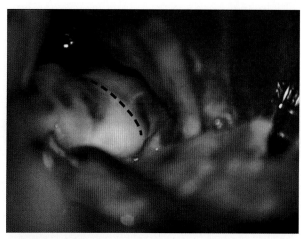

Fig. 16.11 The aneurysm is dissected with particular attention to the thalamoperforators, and the neck is prepared for clipping. A clip may be placed in an anterolateral trajectory. The dotted line indicates the location of clip placement.

points of dissection. The additional working angles ensure safer clipping with better visualization of the thalamoperforators and the contralateral P1.[13,15–17] Advancements in endovascular surgery have resulted in fewer basilar tip aneurysms treated through clipping. As a result, the aneurysms approached surgically are often complicated and present unique challenges, such as a large size, wide neck, and difficult projection. The advantages of the COZ approach are most profound in the surgical management of these complicated aneurysms, when both anterior and lateral dissection is necessary for safe and successful clipping.

The Transcavernous Approach to Basilar Aneurysms

Ali F. Krisht

Basilar apex aneurysms continue to be a treatment challenge.[21–26] The present trend is to refer most patients with basilar aneurysms, if not all, in some centers, for endovascular therapy. The problem with endovascular coiling of basilar aneurysms continues to be the question regarding curability and durability achieved with this treatment modality.[22–28] Reports indicate that recanalization and the need for future treatment occurs in as many as 20 to 30% of treated patients with basilar apex aneurysms.[29] This problem is further compounded by the finding that these aneurysms continue to have an annual risk of bleeding as high as 1.3% per year, which increases to 2.1% per year in partially coiled aneurysms. When this information is compared with the reported natural history of unruptured aneurysms,[30–32] it even raises the question of whether any protection is provided to an unruptured aneurysm with a coil.

Most basilar aneurysms have at least one criterion that predisposes them to a higher rate of failure with endovas-

cular therapy, such as a large or giant size, a wide dysmorphic neck, or both[27,29] (**Table 16.1**). Based on these findings, and making use of the advances in microsurgical techniques,[6,13,18,20,33–41] we have used the transcavernous approach to achieve a more durable outcome for patients with such difficult aneurysms.[42–44]

Table 16.1 Criteria for High Complexity

Criterion	Number	Percentage
Size (large/giant)	18/11	33/22
Posterior projecting dome	13	22
Low bifurcation	23	41
Wide dysmorphic base	20	35
Dolichoectasia	3	6

Surgical Technique

Craniotomy

The craniotomy used for the transcavernous approach is a frontotemporal craniotomy, which is like a modified pterional approach with a more temporal extension. To gain access to the pretemporal region, the zygomatic notch is drilled to allow more inferior reflection of the temporalis muscle. After the bone flap is raised, epidural hemostasis is established with tack-up stitches, and then, under the microscope, the sphenoid wing is drilled flat with the roof of the orbit. The posterior third of the roof and lateral wall of the orbital cone are removed either with a high-speed diamond drill or bone rongeurs. This removal of bone is extended medially to the level of the anterior clinoid process.

Removing the Anterior Clinoid Process

To ease the removal of the anterior clinoid process and to better expose it, pretemporal dural dissection is done at this stage. This dissection is started at the level of the orbitomeningeal artery, which is coagulated and cut (**Fig. 16.12**). From there on and along the temporal side, the dura propria of the temporal lobe is separated from the lateral wall of the cavernous sinus. The dissection is started at the level of the superior orbital fissure and extended laterally and posteriorly over the different branches of the trigeminal nerve. The dissection is then continued posteriorly to the level of the gasserian ganglion and Meckel's cave. To make this dissection easier, the middle meningeal artery is coagulated and cut from its course at the level of the foramen spinosum. Hemostasis within the cavernous sinus is established at this stage by injecting 1 cc of fibrin glue into the cavernous sinus proper between the V_1 and V_2 branches of the trigeminal nerve. After this stage of epidural dissection, the anterior clinoid process is removed.

From the surgical point of view, the anterior clinoid process has three main attachments. The first, its continuation with the orbital roof and the sphenoid wing, should have already been removed. The remaining two attachments are to the roof of the optic canal and the floor of the optic canal along its extension as the optic strut. Both attachments are drilled with a high-speed diamond drill with frequent stops and copious irrigation to prevent the generation of excessive heat, which may injure the optic nerve. Once these attachments are drilled, the tip of the anterior clinoid process becomes mobile and is easy to shell out from its dural attachments. Care is taken to dissect gently around the clinoidal segment of the carotid artery. The surgeon must also be cognizant of the extension of the clinoid attachment to the optic strut with the sphenoid sinus at the level of the opticocarotid angle. Occasionally, the clinoid process itself is pneumatized and the sphenoid sinus is immediately entered by just removing the clinoid tip. The importance of recognizing this anatomic variation is to pay attention to the obliteration of this window into the sphenoid sinus during closure. We usually apply a small piece

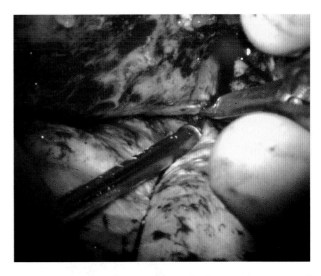

Fig. 16.12 Intraoperative photograph showing the cutting of the orbitomeningeal artery and the dural fold attaching the dura of the sphenoid wing to the periorbita.

of the temporalis muscle into the opening of the sphenoid sinus before the rest of the dura is closed (**Fig. 16.13**).

The Dural Opening

The dura is opened in a curved T fashion (**Fig. 16.14**). The vertical arm of the T extends along the indentation of the sphenoid ridge between the frontal and temporal lobes. This incision is extended all the way to the level of the oculomotor trigone. Opening the basal cisterns and releasing spinal fluid allows the brain to relax, facilitating visualization of the intradural course of the oculomotor nerve. The previous dissection of the lateral wall of the cavernous

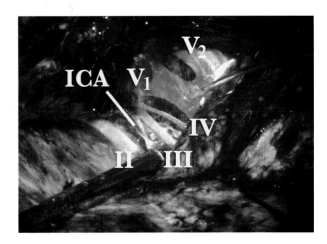

Fig. 16.13 The extent of the extradural pretemporal exposure after removing the anterior clinoid process. The photograph enhances the course of the optic nerve (II), the oculomotor nerve (III), the trochlear nerve (IV), the V_1 segment of the trigeminal nerve, and the V_2 segment of the trigeminal nerve. ICA, the location and course of the clinoidal segment of the internal carotid artery after removal of the anterior clinoid process.

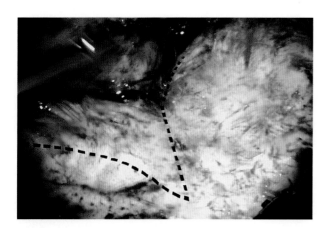

Fig. 16.14 Delineation of the dural opening.

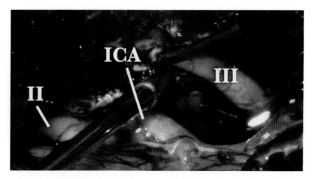

Fig. 16.15 Intraoperative photograph showing the sharp dissection of the intracavernous portion of the third nerve starting from the region of the oculomotor trigone. The intradural component of the third nerve is seen (III). ICA, internal carotid artery; II, optic nerve.

sinus already exposed the extradural component of the oculomotor nerve. At this stage, and under the microscope, both the intradural and extradural portions of the oculomotor nerve are visualized (**Fig. 16.15**). With a sharp microknife, the dura is then cut to further open the oculomotor canal from its intradural extension all the way to the level of the superior orbital fissure. A triangular piece of dura extending from the optic canal to the level of the oculomotor nerve is then removed and shaved from its attachment to the carotid dural ring.

Intradural Dissection and Exposure of the Aneurysm

Once epidural hemostasis is established and the dura is opened, the sylvian fissure is then opened from inside-to-outside, as described by Yasargil. Next, a self-retaining brain spatula is applied over the temporal lobe. We usually preserve the attachment of the temporopolar veins to the temporal dura and thus further cut the temporal dura under the temporal lobe and along its lateral extension. This maneuver leaves the temporal dura with the attached temporopolar veins on the surface of the temporal lobe and under the applied spatula. The temporal lobe posteriorly and laterally is gently retracted to allow a straight access from the pretemporal region to the interpeduncular fossa. The arachnoid along the skull base, including Liliequist's membrane, is dissected and cut, exposing the root of the oculomotor nerve to the level of its attachment with the brainstem (**Fig. 16.16a**).

At this stage, the surgeon assesses the level of the bifurcation in relationship to the posterior clinoid process. If the bifurcation is low, the posterior clinoid process is removed to allow better exposure of the bifurcation and the basilar trunk for application of the temporary clips. To remove the posterior clinoid process, the petroclival dura must be cut and removed, which leads to the posteromedial compartment of the cavernous sinus. In most cases, the previous injection of fibrin glue fills this compartment and provides adequate hemostasis. Occasionally, another injection of glue

is necessary before the dura is removed and the posterior clinoid bone is exposed.

Before the clinoid process is removed, the oculomotor nerve must be dissected from all its attachments along the oculomotor canal. Such dissection allows for easy mobilization of the third nerve, which can be moved from a medial to a lateral position to move the oculomotor nerve back and forth also from a medial to a lateral position. This maneuver prevents any permanent injury to the nerve and provides adequate exposure of the different corners of the posterior clinoid process. We used to drill the anterior clinoid process with a 1- or 2-mm high-speed diamond drill with frequent stops and copious irrigation. More recently, however, we have been using an ultrasonic aspirator, which alleviates the need for drilling. Once the posterior clinoid process is removed, the surgeon assesses the level and position of the basilar trunk. Careful dissection is done on the posterior aspect of the trunk to establish an adequate zone free of perforators where the temporary clips can be applied.

The clips are usually placed proximal to the takeoff of the superior cerebellar artery branches. The rationale behind this plan is to achieve proximal control but to continue to allow a small amount of collateral flow through the superior cerebellar artery system. This maneuver decreases the amount of flow within the aneurysm, softening it and making it more compressible during the initial application of a permanent clip to the neck. At the same time, it maintains a small amount of blood flow in the perforators, thereby improving the safety of the temporary occlusion should it be more prolonged than expected.

Cutting the Posterior Communicating Artery

The adequate exposure of the posterior aspect of the aneurysm to visualize the perforators arising from the P1 segment of the PCA may be enhanced by resecting the posterior communicating artery. This artery can be safely resected if coagulated and cut at the perforator-free zone,

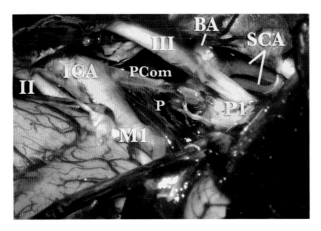

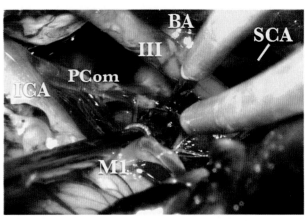

a

b

Fig. 16.16a,b **(a)** The exposure of the third nerve from the region of the brain stem to the level of the superior orbital fissure. The established view shows the full advantage of the approach, with the basilar trunk below the third nerve along the course of the basilar artery. The branches of the superior cerebellar artery are seen inferior to the third nerve. The aneurysm is hidden behind the posterior communicating artery. **(b)** Coagulating the posterior communicating artery at a perforator-free zone close to its junction with the posterior cerebral artery. BA, basilar artery; ICA, internal carotid artery; II, optic nerve; III, oculomotor nerve; M1, M1 segment of the middle cerebral artery; P, thalamoperforators of the posterior communicating artery (PCom); P1, posterior cerebral artery; SCA, superior cerebellar artery.

which is usually located at the junction of the posterior communicating artery and the PCA (**Fig. 16.16b**). This step is valuable for aneurysms that project posteriorly. This step is also valuable in enlarging the surgical field at its depth for patients in whom the posterior communicating artery is short and acts as a tension band by bringing together the PCA and the internal carotid artery.

Coagulating and resecting the posterior communicating artery in such cases enlarges the field by detaching and mobilizing the internal carotid artery anteriorly (**Fig. 16.17**). We have used this step in more than 35 patients with no significant sequelae. But this step is taken only when necessary and only if the P1 segment is larger in diameter than the posterior communicating artery.

Clipping

Once adequate exposure is achieved, a temporary clip is applied to the basilar trunk in a perforator-free zone. The microscope is then used to visualize the aneurysm's neck (**Fig. 16.18**). The aneurysm is now softer and more compressible, and the surgeon assesses the contralateral P1 segment of the left PCA and visualizes any perforators arising from this segment. The aneurysm is then dissected at its posterior aspect to better visualize the perforators that may be located in the neck region or sometimes attached to the dome of the aneurysm. This exploration should take 1 or 2 minutes, after which the temporary clips are removed. It can be repeated several times to gain as much information as possible about the location of the perfora-

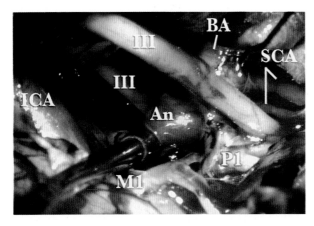

Fig. 16.17 An unobstructed view of the whole basilar apex after the posterior communicating artery is cut. The aneurysm is fully visualized with a 360-degree view. An, aneurysm; BA, trunk of the basilar artery; ICA, internal carotid artery; III, third nerve; M1, middle cerebral artery; P1, posterior cerebral artery; SCA, superior cerebellar artery.

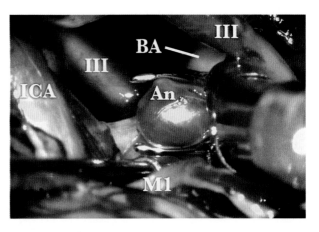

Fig. 16.18 The clip application with full visualization of the clip blades and the adjacent parent vessels. An unobstructed view can be achieved for most basilar aneurysms with this approach. An, aneurysm; BA, basilar artery; ICA, internal carotid artery; III, oculomotor nerves; M1, middle cerebral artery.

tors and to build a three-dimensional image in the neurosurgeon's mind of the exact dimensions of the aneurysm. It will also heighten the level of concentration of the different members of the team involved in this process, which includes the scrub nurse and the anesthesiologist.

Once the picture becomes clear, the temporary clips are applied to the basilar trunk, after which the first pilot clip is applied to the neck of the aneurysm. This clip is immediately explored to verify its location before the temporary clip is removed. This exploration may entail an attempt to puncture and shrink the aneurysm or sometimes apply a clip to the contralateral P1 segment of the PCA, once it is better visualized, to further deflate the aneurysm and reposition the clip. During this time, intraoperative monitoring of somatosensory evoked potentials, electroencephalography, and brainstem evoked responses is done continuously. Any changes in the electrophysiological monitoring may dictate a change in the plan, especially in relation to the time of application of the temporary clips.

Next, the temporary clips are removed and further assessment is done to ensure adequate clipping of the neck and to confirm that there are no perforators included in the clips. Adjustments are made accordingly. In most patients, we favor coagulating the aneurysm, which helps shrink the sac significantly and at the same time seals any rupture site. This step helps convert an acute rupture into a more elective situation, and provides a more relaxed atmosphere for the surgeon to better visualize the surrounding anatomy. With this step, the lesion is converted from a ruptured large aneurysm to an unruptured small aneurysm. This step allows better clipping of the aneurysm with no chance of any residual and with the ability to fully visualize the anatomy all around the neck.

If the aneurysm ruptures after the temporary clips have been applied, suction can be used to remove blood and prevent flooding of the field. Occasionally, the surgeon may need to immediately apply another clip to the contralateral P1 segment. This is the reason we ensure adequate removal of the posterior clinoid process to gain access to the contralateral P1 segment before attacking the aneurysm. If oozing continues before bleeding is controlled, the surgeon should not panic but should continue to visualize all the anatomy before taking any steps. If the aneurysm is bleeding, the brain is being perfused with adequate blood, which also means that prolonging temporary occlusion does not have a high risk of causing ischemia. The most common cause of injury is hasty clip application in reaction to the bleeding without proper visualization of where the clips are going.

Although many advocate the use of cerebral protection agents, we depend on neurophysiological monitoring for guidance. We do not use cerebral protection agents because they create a false sense of security with the assumption that the brain is protected. We depend instead on the efficient and safer steps in the clip application process. The surgeon should build the plan assuming ignorance about the extent of the collateral situation rather than on the false assumption of knowledge, and thus exercise more caution.

In the overall majority of patients, one temporary clip applied to the basilar trunk is enough to gain adequate hemodynamic control of the blood flowing to the aneurysm. Occasionally, and for a very short period of time, two additional clips are applied to both P1 segments to further coagulate and shrink the aneurysm before the final clip is applied. This procedure is done for no more than 2 minutes. Despite the presence of three clips, some flow still emanates from the superior cerebellar artery collateral system.

The main advantage of the transcavernous approach is that all the maneuvers described above can be done with full visualization of the anatomy in the interpeduncular fossa. The usually larger temporary clip applied to the basilar trunk is never in the way when working in the neck region. If two small clips are applied to the PCAs, they remain out of the way too.

Conclusion

The transcavernous approach demands the full dedication of the cerebrovascular neurosurgeon to understand the anatomic aspects of the skull-base region and to become familiar with the different steps involved in the approach. The mastery of such an approach demands frequent observation of other neurosurgeons who perform these procedures on a routine basis. The advantage gained is not only in treating basilar aneurysms but in treating different pathological entities that involve the anterior upper third of the posterior fossa region as well as the retrochiasmatic and interpeduncular fossa space. To assume that endovascular therapy should be used is the wrong approach because there are not enough microsurgeons who can achieve superior outcomes in patients with such difficult aneurysms. The correct approach should be to continue to aim at *curing* this problem and to achieve a more durable outcome by encouraging more young neurosurgeons who are interested in the cerebrovascular field to dedicate their time to developing the skills needed for such a result. There is no doubt that our patients need it and deserve it.

The Pretemporal Approach to Basilar Aneurysms

Feres Chaddad, José Maria de Campos Filho, and Evandro de Oliveira

Lesions that arise in the interpeduncular region, the superior aspect of the petroclival region, and the anterior segment of the tentorial incisura are very difficult to manage.[45] The most common lesions found in this region are aneurysms at the distal third of the basilar artery and tumors of the mesial aspect of the temporal lobe.

A great advance in the surgical treatment of basilar tip aneurysms occurred during the 1970s, when Yasargil[6,46] introduced the pterional approach and Drake[12,47] introduced the subtemporal approach. Sano[20] added his temporopolar approach in 1980. The pterional approach offers a straight downward view of the anterolateral aspect of the basilar bifurcation.[48] The subtemporal approach offers a lateral view of the interpeduncular fossa through retraction of the temporal lobe superiorly. The temporopolar approach consists of pulling back the temporal pole, thereby creating an anterolateral view of the interpeduncular fossa. The pretemporal approach, however, combines the advantages of these other approaches into one craniotomy.[49–51]

Operative Technique

For the pretemporal approach, the patient is positioned supine with the head elevated above the heart to improve venous return. The head is rotated approximately 20 degrees contralaterally and extended approximately 30 degrees, which brings the malar eminence to the highest point of the operative field.

The skin incision starts at the anterior segment of the tragus, extends above the ear, and curves toward the midline behind the hairline. Interfascial dissection is done to preserve the frontal branch of the facial nerve. The temporalis muscle is detached from the entire zygomatic bone and reflected over the horizontal portion of the zygomatic arch.

A frontotemporosphenoidal craniotomy is then done with one to four bur holes, depending on the degree of adherence between the dura and the bone. The first bur hole is made immediately below the most anterior limit of the superior temporal line and close to the zygomatic process of the frontal bone; this is the keyhole. The second bur hole is made on the frontal bone, 2 cm medial to the first one and above the superior orbital rim. The third hole is made below the superior temporal line at least 4.5 cm posterior to the first one. The fourth hole is made over the squamous part of the temporal bone at the level of the root of the zygomatic arch. The greater wing of the sphenoid and the squamosal part of the temporal bone are drilled out to expose the entire pole of the temporal lobe anteriorly and inferiorly. The orbital roof and the lesser sphenoid wing are also drilled. A large amount of bone resection provides better visualization of the anterior and inferior portions of

the temporal lobe and reduces the need for brain retraction **(Fig. 16.19)**.

The dura is opened with a curved incision from the frontal region to the level of the dural impression made by the sphenoid ridge. After that, the incision becomes straight and proceeds anteriorly toward the orbitomeningeal artery. To complete the exposure of the temporal lobe, another incision is made laterally and posteriorly, following the contours of the craniotomy.

Microsurgical techniques are used to access the interpeduncular cistern. The bridging veins draining the temporal pole to the sphenoparietal sinus and the veins from the orbital surface of the frontal lobe to the sphenoparietal and cavernous sinuses are sacrificed. The arachnoid that binds the uncus to the oculomotor nerve and to the tentorial edge is opened. To achieve good mobility of the temporal lobe, the ambient cistern and the arachnoid are dissected. After the cisternal opening, the temporal pole can be elevated superiorly and posteriorly to expose the interpeduncular region.

Clinical Case

A 45-year-old man arrived at the emergency room complaining of a sudden, mild headache. He had minimal nuchal rigidity. The computed tomography scan showed a subarachnoid hemorrhage at the basal cisterns less than 1 mm thick. Angiography of the cerebral vessels showed an aneurysm of the basilar tip. The patient was clinically well—grade I on the Hunt and Hess scale and grade II on the Fisher scale.

For such a patient, we have performed a pretemporal approach with microsurgical resolution of the aneurysm. It is also feasible to use the pterional approach for this patient.

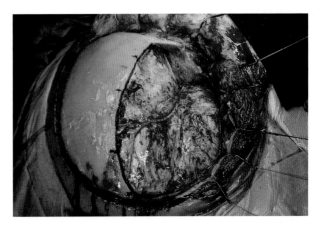

Fig. 16.19 In the pretemporal craniotomy, the greater and lesser wings of the sphenoid, the squamosal part of the temporal bone, and the orbital roof are drilled out.

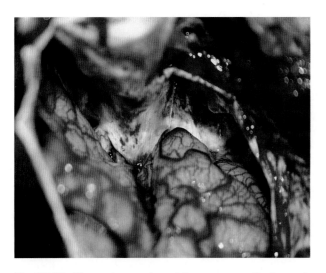

Fig. 16.20 The pretemporal craniotomy exposes the transsylvian, temporopolar, and subtemporal approaches.

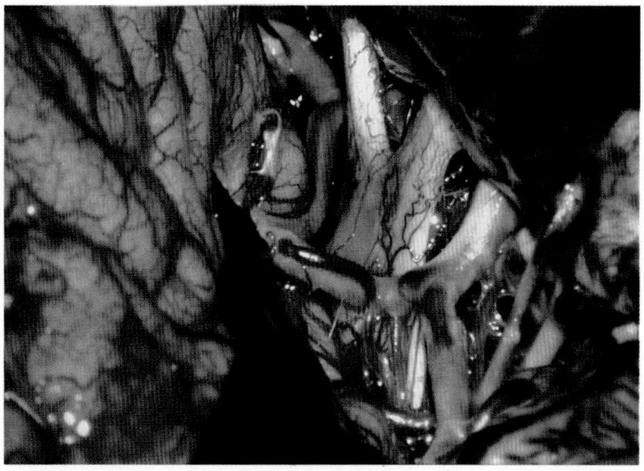

Fig. 16.21 The interpeduncular cistern can be accessed between the internal carotid artery and the optic nerve, between the internal carotid artery and the third nerve, and by retracting or opening the tentorium cerebelli lateral to the third nerve.

Discussion

The interpeduncular cistern can be reached through three different routes: between the internal carotid artery and the optic nerve, between the internal carotid artery and the third nerve, and by retracting or opening the tentorium cerebelli lateral to the third nerve.[52] The pterional approach exposes the aneurysm through the space between the internal carotid artery and the optic nerve or between the internal carotid artery and the third nerve. Both P1 segments of the PCAs can be seen, but unfortunately the perforators coming off the basilar tip behind the aneurysm cannot be well defined.[6,46] The temporopolar approach is a pterional craniotomy with a more extensive exposure of the temporal lobe. The temporal lobe is retracted posteriorly to expose the space between the third nerve and the free edge of the tentorium.[20]

The subtemporal approach offers a good lateral view of the basilar tip and the perforators, but the opposite P1 and the opposite thalamoperforating arteries are poorly visualized, and retracting the temporal lobe can injure the vein of Labbé.[12,47] The pretemporal approach is based on the extended resection of the sphenoid and temporal bones, the wide opening of the basal cisterns, and detachment from the frontal lobe to the temporal lobe. It combines the multiple angles of view offered by the pterional and subtemporal approaches (**Fig. 16.20**). The interpeduncular cistern can be reached through an anterolateral route and obliquely from below (**Figs. 16.21, 16.22, 16.23**). Depending on the intraoperative need, the subtemporal route can also be used.

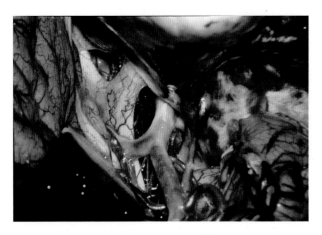

Fig. 16.22 The pretemporal approach allows a large exposure of the basal cisterns and visualization of the carotid artery and its bifurcation, the optic nerve, and the third nerve.

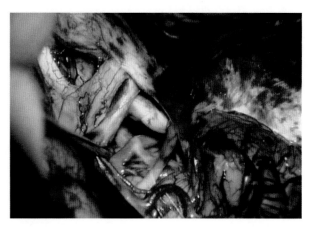

Fig. 16.23 The anterolateral route shows the interpeduncular cistern through the space between the carotid artery and the third nerve, exposing the basilar artery.

Moderators
Surgical Approaches to Basilar Apex Aneurysms
Duke Samson and Christopher S. Eddleman

Aneurysms of the basilar apex continue to pose one of the most difficult challenges to vascular neurosurgeons because of their deep, central location in the neuraxis and the eloquent environment of other critical vascular and nervous structures. Advances in microsurgical techniques have allowed greatly improved visualization of the basilar apex, and studies of these techniques report better patient outcomes. As more and more basilar apex aneurysms are treated with endovascular strategies, however, fewer and fewer are treated through microsurgical approaches. As a result, there is a diminishing supply of experienced vascular surgeons available to undertake such potentially complex surgical endeavors.

When microsurgery is appropriate, several considerations must be taken into account when approaching these vascular lesions. The two most important factors to consider are defining the lesion's characteristics and determining the desired surrounding anatomic environment. Together, these factors render a basilar apex aneurysm able to be safely managed through a microsurgical approach.

Characteristics of the Aneurysm

Successful microsurgical management of basilar apex aneurysms depends in large measure on certain favorable morphological characteristics (**Fig. 16.24**). The most obvious of these is a modest aneurysmal size. Large and giant aneurysms (> 15 mm diameter) pose significant problems in terms of obtaining proximal control and complete visualization of all afferent and efferent vessels. In addition, these larger lesions tend to have expansive necks, which frequently encompass one or both P1 origins, and often contain intra-aneurysmal thrombosis as well as intramural atheroma, all of which mandate aneurysm decompression before definitive clip ligation. Although the techniques of aneurysm decompression do not obviate the feasibility of microsurgical treatment, their use does complicate the operative procedure and significantly increase the risk of surgical morbidity.

In addition, the projection of the aneurysmal dome plays an important role in determining the ease and success of surgery. The most favorable projection of a basilar apex aneurysm is anteriorly, which allows visualization of the posterior projecting basilar perforating arteries critical to the vascular supply of the mesencephalon with minimal retraction of the aneurysmal sac. Basilar aneurysms that project posteriorly pose a significant amount of difficulty, especially when the surgeon uses more superior surgical approaches because of the necessity of displacing the dome anteriorly to visualize these vital perforators. It is an unpleasant fact of life that the degree of posterior angulation of the fundus seen intraoperatively is almost always greater

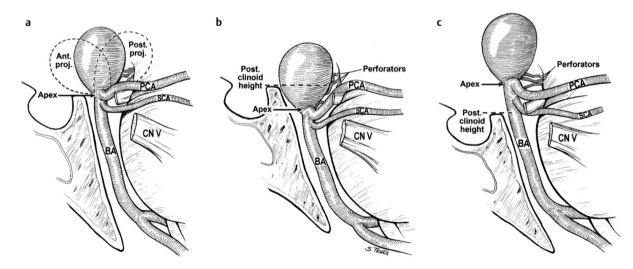

Fig. 16.24a–c The relationship of basilar apex aneurysms to the surrounding bony and neural anatomy. **(a)** A basilar apex aneurysm at the level of the posterior clinoid process. Ghost projections of anterior and posterior projecting aneurysms are also shown with respect to the posterior perforating arteries. **(b)** A low-lying aneurysm with respect to the posterior clinoid process. The posterior perforating arteries are often in close association with the aneurysmal dome. **(c)** A high-lying aneurysm with respect to the posterior clinoid process. BA, basilar artery; CNV, fifth cranial nerve; PCA, posterior cerebral artery; SCA, superior cerebellar artery.

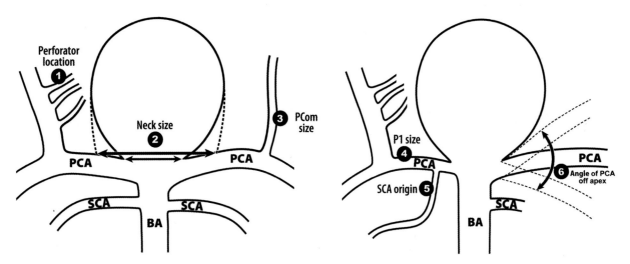

Fig. 16.25 Vascular considerations with respect to the surgical approaches to basilar apex aneurysms. *1*, visualization of the perforating arteries, whether emanating from the basilar apex, posterior communicating, or P1 segments, is extremely important, and sacrifice of these arteries is the primary contributor to postoperative morbidity. *2*, the surgeon must establish whether the aneurysmal neck incorporates the P1 origins. *3*, the size of the posterior communicating artery may determine whether it can be sacrificed. *4*, if the P1 segment is small and associated with a large posterior communicating artery, it may be sacrificed. *5*, the superior cerebellar arteries could emanate from the P1 segment, thus obstructing the surgically important views. *6*, acute angles of the PCAs may obstruct the view of the basilar apex, perforators, or contralateral vessels. BA, basilar artery; PCA, posterior cerebral artery; PCom, posterior communicating artery; SCA, superior cerebellar artery.

than is appreciated on the lateral angiographic images. Although it is rare, some basilar apex lesions can project laterally, especially in the presence of a tortuous basilar trunk, and these lesions should be approached from the side opposite the projection, so that the dome of the aneurysm does not obstruct the surgical corridor.

Finally, although not directly related to the aneurysm's morphology, the anatomic position of the aneurysmal neck as it relates to the posterior clinoid process has a significant effect on the choice of surgical approach. When the neck is at or superior to the posterior clinoid process, any of the microsurgical approaches suffices for visualizing the basilar apex. It is when the neck is below the posterior clinoid process that microsurgical approaches can be difficult, especially when the surgeon is not familiar or comfortable with drilling the posterior clinoid process or approaching the aneurysm from a more lateral position, for example, pretemporal or subtemporal.

Surrounding Vascular Anatomy

Although the basilar apex aneurysm is the primary focus of the microsurgical approach, one cannot completely evaluate which approach is best without first evaluating the surrounding vascular anatomy (**Fig. 16.25**). For example, very short internal carotid arteries limit the pterional access portal into the interpeduncular cistern. This restriction can sometimes be overcome by elective sacrifice of a small posterior communicating artery. Other cases may require dissection of the posterior wall of the aneurysm and the distal basilar trunk from between the origins of the posterior cerebral and superior cerebellar arteries. This dissection permits clip ligation of the aneurysmal neck through some modification of Drake's original "fenestrated clip."

The PCAs themselves may also emanate from the apex at extreme angles, for example, traveling along the dome of the aneurysm and obscuring the view of the contralateral vessels. This acute angle of the PCAs can be overcome with a fenestrated clip around the vessel. The superior cerebellar arteries may also be problematic if emanating from the PCA, obstructing the surgeon's view of the basilar apex. Obstruction of the posterior aspect of the basilar apex, however, may lead to inadvertent injury of the posterior thalamoperforating arteries. Drake and Simon were the first to notice that such injury is the overwhelming source of morbidity and mortality in these patients. Therefore, it is imperative that, regardless of the surgical approach selected, the surgeon must visually confirm that none of the small end arteries lie in the path of the posterior clip blade.

Surgical Principles

Microsurgical approaches to the basilar apex naturally require a thorough understanding of the aneurysm and the surrounding anatomy. It is only when these characteristics are known that one can then begin to consider the number of microsurgical approaches mentioned here. But no microsurgical approach should be undertaken without considering the many basic surgical principles that influence these potentially complex procedures. We now discuss how the four surgical approaches under consideration, in addition to the more classic subtemporal exposure, measure up when evaluated according to these basic terms.

Minimal Brain Tissue Retraction

Even in the setting of a relaxed brain, the anatomic location of the interpeduncular cistern necessitates the use of significant retraction of either one temporal lobe, one frontal lobe, or, more commonly, both lobes to expose the basilar apex. Focused resection of the temporal squama, zygoma, orbital roof, anterior clinoid process, and, on occasion, the posterior clinoid process, coupled with broad opening of the sylvian fissure and basal cisterns, can minimize this necessity, just as any degree of cerebral edema increases it. Although intraoperative measurements of the comparative extent of brain retraction vary, we believe the pretemporal approach probably routinely requires the least, followed in order by the cranio-orbital zygomatic, the classic pterional, the transcavernous, and the subtemporal exposures.

Access for Proximal Control

Without much question, the approach providing the earliest and most reliable access to the distal basilar artery at the level of the superior cerebellar origins is the classical subtemporal exposure pioneered by Drake and currently championed by his disciple, Juha Hernesniemi. This route of access is excellent regardless of the height of the basilar apex, its relationship to the clivus, or its laterality. The pretemporal exposure developed by de Oliveira offers the surgeon excellent exposure to a longer segment of the basilar artery, but at the cost of a much more extensive and lengthy bone removal, whereas the transcavernous approach of Krisht provides a somewhat more anterior view of the distal basilar artery than either of these two previous exposures through a more restricted access corridor. The cranio-orbital zygomatic exposure and its parent, the classic pterional approach, as detailed by Al-Mefty and Origitano and by Fox, offer the most limited exposure of the distal basilar artery, although both can be modified within the interpeduncular cistern to improve that access.

Visualization of the Distal Vasculature

As the surgical approach used becomes more lateral in its origin, an unimpeded view of the arteries of the basilar "quadrification" rapidly becomes more limited. Therefore, the transcavernous exposure provides the best *en face* exposure, with the cranio-orbital zygomatic and pterional exposures running a close second. The pretemporal route hampers the surgeon to some degree in visualizing the contralateral superior cerebellar arteries and the PCAs; this limitation remains one of the major drawbacks of the true subtemporal approach and was one of the major incitements to the development of the transsylvian exposures.

Visualizing the Perforators

Drake's remarkable experience with the subtemporal exposure, accumulated at the dawn of the microsurgical era, is striking testimony to the unparalleled exposure of the critical thalamoperforating arteries and the concomitant capability to spare these vessels at the time of clip placement that this exposure offers. This view is almost replicated in the pretemporal approach, whereas all three remaining operative corridors are more medially located and, as such, offer at best an imperfect view of the dorsal aspect of the basilar apex. This limitation mandates that surgeons using these exposures be prepared to displace the aneurysm anteriorly to first dissect the perforating arteries from the aneurysm and then to maintain the aneurysmal neck in that position during clip placement. Most surgeons achieve this end by the use of temporary basilar occlusion during the final stages of dissection and definitive clip placement.

Size of the Working Corridor

"Spacious" is not a term most surgeons associate with technical procedures within the confines of the interpeduncular cistern. These exposures are all narrow, deep, and restricted by important, fragile vascular and neural boundaries; they can be extended somewhat by mobilizing some of the cistern's contents, by focused bone resection at the margins of the cistern, or by incisions into the cavernous sinus, but even in the best of hands they remain quite limited. The two oldest approaches (the subtemporal and pterional) are the most constrained, whereas we believe the transcavernous, the pretemporal and the cranio-orbital zygomatic derivatives are at least potentially more capacious.

Conclusion

The patient presented here has a basilar apex aneurysm with a wide neck involving the bilateral PCAs. The projection of the aneurysm is mostly superior and the level of the apex appears to be at the level of the posterior clinoid process. All of these outstanding surgeons and authors certainly could deal with this aneurysm successfully using their own preferred approach, and Drake would doubtlessly have had the intact patient awake in the recovery room by 9:00 AM, assuming a 7:00 AM start. However, the surgical judgment and extensive operative experience that presage excellent results in the management of basilar apex aneurysms is rapidly becoming a quality in short supply. Despite the advanced surgical approaches discussed here, the "best" approach is always the one that offers the patient the best possible results with the least associated risk. Although elegant dissection techniques coupled with ingenious bone resections may provide unprecedented surgical views, the enhanced risk of potential morbidity and the protracted recovery period associated with such surgical tours de force should limit their performance to the recognized masters among us.

References

1. Fox JL. Atlas of Neurosurgical Anatomy. New York: Springer, 1989:165–200
2. Fox JL. Intracranial Aneurysms. New York: Springer, 1983:771–787, 1024–1069
3. Fox JL. Microsurgical exposure of vertebrobasilar aneurysms. In: Rand RW, ed. Microneurosurgery, 3rd ed. St. Louis: CV Mosby, 1985:589–599
4. Ito Z. Microsurgery of Cerebral Aneurysms. Amsterdam: Elsevier, 1985:180–201
5. Sugita K. Microneurosurgical Atlas. Berlin: Springer, 1985:62–81
6. Yasargil MG, Antic J, Laciga R, Jain KK, Hodosh RM, Smith RD. Microsurgical pterional approach to aneurysms of the basilar bifurcation. Surg Neurol 1976;6:83–91
7. Samson DS, Hodosh RM, Clark WK. Microsurgical evaluation of the pterional approach to aneurysms of the distal basilar circulation. Neurosurgery 1978;3:135–141
8. Wright DC, Wilson CB. Surgical treatment of basilar aneurysms. Neurosurgery 1979;5:325–333
9. Peerless SJ, Drake CG. Management of aneurysms of the posterior circulation. In: Youmans JR, ed. Neurological Surgery, 3rd ed. Philadelphia: WB Saunders, 1990:1764–1806
10. Sundt TM Jr. Surgical Techniques for Saccular and Giant Intracranial Aneurysms. Baltimore: Williams & Wilkins, 1990: 213–233
11. Al-Mefty O. Supraorbital-pterional approach to skull base lesions. Neurosurgery 1987;21:474–477
12. Drake CG. The surgical treatment of aneurysms of the basilar artery. J Neurosurg 1968;29:436–446
13. Origitano TC, Anderson DE, Tarassoli Y, Reichman OH, al-Mefty O. Skull base approaches to complex cerebral aneurysms. Surg Neurol 1993;40:339–346
14. Ikeda K, Yamashita J, Hashimoto M, Futami K. Orbitozygomatic temporopolar approach for a high basilar tip aneurysm associated with a short intracranial internal carotid artery: a new surgical approach. Neurosurgery 1991;28:105–110
15. Al-Mefty O. Operative Atlas of Meningiomas. Philadelphia: Lippincott-Raven, 1998
16. Bowles AP, Kinjo T, Al-Mefty O. Skull base approaches for posterior circulation aneurysms. Skull Base Surg 1995;5:251–260
17. Origitano TC, Al-Mefty O. Skull base approaches to the basilar bifurcation. In: Al-Mefty O, Origitano TC, Harkey H, eds. Controversies in Neurosurgery. New York: Thieme, 1996:163–166
18. Dolenc VV, Skrap M, Sustersic J, Skrbec M, Morina A. A transcavernous-transsellar approach to the basilar tip aneurysms. Br J Neurosurg 1987;1:251–259
19. Fujitsu K, Kuwabara T. Zygomatic approach for lesions in the interpeduncular cistern. J Neurosurg 1985;62:340–343
20. Sano K. Temporo-polar approach to aneurysms of the basilar artery at and around the distal bifurcation: technical note. Neurol Res 1980;2:361–367
21. Batjer HH, Samson DS. Causes of morbidity and mortality from surgery of aneurysms of the distal basilar artery. Neurosurgery 1989;25:904–915, discussion 915–916
22. Bavinzski G, Killer M, Gruber A, Reinprecht A, Gross CE, Richling B. Treatment of basilar artery bifurcation aneurysms by using Guglielmi detachable coils: a 6-year experience. J Neurosurg 1999;90:843–852
23. Halbach VV, Higashida RT, Dowd CF, et al. The efficacy of endosaccular aneurysm occlusion in alleviating neurological deficits produced by mass effect. J Neurosurg 1994;80:659–666

24. Hernesniemi J, Vapalahti M, Niskanen M, Kari A. Management outcome for vertebrobasilar artery aneurysms by early surgery. Neurosurgery 1992;31:857–861, discussion 861–862
25. Lawton MT. Basilar apex aneurysms: surgical results and perspectives from an initial experience. Neurosurgery 2002;50: 1–8, discussion 8–10
26. Rice BJ, Peerless SJ, Drake CG. Surgical treatment of unruptured aneurysms of the posterior circulation. J Neurosurg 1990;73: 165–173
27. Guglielmi G, Viñuela F, Duckwiler G, et al. Endovascular treatment of posterior circulation aneurysms by electrothrombosis using electrically detachable coils. J Neurosurg 1992;77:515–524
28. Lusseveld E, Brilstra EH, Nijssen PC, et al. Endovascular coiling versus neurosurgical clipping in patients with a ruptured basilar tip aneurysm. J Neurol Neurosurg Psychiatry 2002;73:591–593
29. Vallee JN, Aymard A, Vicaut E, Reis M, Merland JJ. Endovascular treatment of basilar tip aneurysms with Guglielmi detachable coils: predictors of immediate and long-term results with multivariate analysis 6-year experience. Radiology 2003;226: 867–879
30. Juvela S, Porras M, Heiskanen O. Natural history of unruptured intracranial aneurysms: a long-term follow-up study. J Neurosurg 1993;79:174–182
31. Juvela S, Porras M, Poussa K. Natural history of unruptured intracranial aneurysms: probability of and risk factors for aneurysm rupture. J Neurosurg 2000;93:379–387
32. Wiebers DO, Whisnant JP, Huston J III, et al; International Study of Unruptured Intracranial Aneurysms Investigators. Unruptured intracranial aneurysms: natural history, clinical outcome, and risks of surgical and endovascular treatment. Lancet 2003; 362:103–110
33. Day JD, Giannotta SL, Fukushima T. Extradural temporopolar approach to lesions of the upper basilar artery and infrachiasmatic region. J Neurosurg 1994;81:230–235
34. Drake CG, Peerless SJ, Hernesniemi J. Surgery of Vertebrobasilar Aneurysms: London, Ontario, Experience on 1767 Patients. Vienna: Springer, 1996
35. Hernesniemi J, Ishii K, Niemelä M, Kivipelto L, Fujiki M, Shen H. Subtemporal approach to basilar bifurcation aneurysms: advanced technique and clinical experience. Acta Neurochir Suppl (Wien) 2005;94:31–38
36. Inao S, Kuchiwaki H, Hirai N, Gonda T, Furuse M. Posterior communicating artery section during surgery for basilar tip aneurysm. Acta Neurochir (Wien) 1996;138:853–861
37. Nutik SL. Pterional craniotomy via a transcavernous approach for the treatment of low-lying distal basilar artery aneurysms. J Neurosurg 1998;89:921–926
38. Seoane E, Tedeschi H, de Oliveira E, Wen HT, Rhoton AL Jr. The pretemporal transcavernous approach to the interpeduncular and prepontine cisterns: microsurgical anatomy and technique application. Neurosurgery 2000;46:891–898, discussion 898–899
39. Sugita K, Kobayashi S, Shintani A, Mutsuga N. Microneurosurgery for aneurysms of the basilar artery. J Neurosurg 1979; 51:615–620
40. Tanaka Y, Kobayashi S, Sugita K, Gibo H, Kyoshima K, Nagasaki T. Characteristics of pterional routes to basilar bifurcation aneurysm. Neurosurgery 1995;36:533–538, discussion 538–540

41. Yaşargil MG. Microneurosurgery, vol. 2. New York: Thieme, 1984:232–295

42. Krisht AF, Krayenbühl N, Sercl D, Bikmaz K, Kadri PA. Results of microsurgical clipping of 50 high complexity basilar apex aneurysms. Neurosurgery 2007;60:242–250, discussion 250–252

43. Krisht AF, Kadri PA. Surgical clipping of complex basilar apex aneurysms: a strategy for successful outcome using the pretemporal transzygomatic transcavernous approach. Neurosurgery 2005;56(2, Suppl):261–273, discussion 261–273

44. Krisht AF, Bikmaz K, Kadri PAS, Partington S. Outcome of surgical clipping of 40 complex basilar aneurysms using the transcavernous route: paper 34. Neurosurgery 2006;58:407

45. Ono M, Ono M, Rhoton AL Jr, Barry M. Microsurgical anatomy of the region of the tentorial incisura. J Neurosurg 1984;60:365–399

46. Yaşargil MG. Basilar artery bifurcation aneurysms. In: Yaşargil MG, ed. Microneurosurgery, vol. 2. Stuttgart: Thieme, 1984:232–246

47. Drake CG. The treatment of aneurysms of the posterior circulation. Clin Neurosurg 1979;26:96–144

48. Chaddad Neto F, Ribas GC, Oliveira Ed. [The pterional craniotomy: step by step]. Arq Neuropsiquiatr 2007;65:101–106

49. De Oliveira E, Siqueira M, Tedeschi H, Peace DA. Surgical approaches for aneurysms of the basilar artery bifurcation. In: Matsushima T, ed. Surgical Anatomy for Microneurosurgery VI: Cerebral Aneurysms and Skull Base Lesions. Tokyo: Scientific Medical Publications, 1993:34–42

50. De Oliveira E, Tedeschi H, Siqueira MG, Peace DA. The pretemporal approach to the interpeduncular and petroclival regions. Acta Neurochir (Wien) 1995;136:204–211

51. Tedeschi H, De Oliveira E, Wen HT. Pretemporal approach to basilar bifurcation aneurysms. Tech Neurosurg 2000;6:191–199

52. Dorsch NW. Aid to exposure of the upper basilar artery: technical note. Neurosurgery 1988;23:790–791

Chapter 17

Treatment of an Arteriovenous Malformation in Eloquent Areas

Case

This 40-year-old otherwise healthy woman came to medical attention with recurrent episodes of numbness in her left hand. Digital subtraction angiography revealed a 1.5-cm right parietal arteriovenous malformation fed by distal branches of the middle cerebral artery with superficial drainage into the superior sagittal sinus. A T1-weighted axial magnetic resonance image with contrast confirmed that this lesion was within millimeters of, but posterior to, her primary somatosensory cortex.

Participants

Microsurgery for Small Arteriovenous Malformations: Bradley A. Gross and Rose Du

Gamma Knife Radiosurgery for Arteriovenous Malformations: Mark E. Linskey

Proton Beam Stereotactic Radiosurgery for Arteriovenous Malformations: Jay Loeffler and Pankaj K. Agarwalla

Moderators: The Treatment of Arteriovenous Malformations in Eloquent Areas: Ramsey Ashour and Jacques J. Morcos

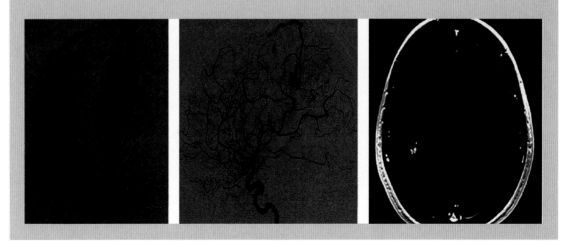

Microsurgery for Small Arteriovenous Malformations

Bradley A. Gross and Rose Du

Cerebral arteriovenous malformations (AVMs) are a considerable source of morbidity and mortality in neurosurgical patients, often as a consequence of hemorrhage but also as a result of debilitating seizures and neurologic deficits.[1–4] Management options include observation, microsurgical resection, radiosurgery, embolization (often adjunctive or palliative), or a combination of these approaches **(Table 17.1)**.

Observation is a consideration for large AVMs in eloquent locations (high grade), particularly if they are asymptomatic or discovered in older patients. Small AVMs (less than 3 cm), particularly if symptomatic or certainly if they have previously hemorrhaged, are ubiquitously considered for intervention. Microsurgical resection is the time-honored therapeutic modality in the treatment of AVMs, providing immediate and often definitive therapy. In reviewing the natural history, microsurgical, and radiosurgical results for small AVMs, we show that microsurgery should be considered first, unless the lesion is in a surgically inaccessible, eloquent location or the patient is medically unfit for surgery.

Natural History

Although most patients with AVMs come to attention because of hemorrhage, 20% present with seizures, with an annual development rate of de novo seizures of 1%.[1] Factors associated with a greater risk of epileptogenesis from AVMs include younger age, a cortical or temporal location (or both), and a larger size. Approximately 7 to 10% of patients with AVMs present with nonhemorrhagic focal neurologic deficits, in some cases attributable to local steal phenomena.[1–4]

Reviewing both modern and older natural history studies reveals a consistent overall annual hemorrhage rate of 2 to 4% for AVMs.[1–4] More recent reports have consistently shown an increased risk of hemorrhage among patients with a prior hemorrhage, with overall annual re-bleed rates of 3 to 7%.[2–4] Early re-bleed rates in the first year range

from 6% to as high as 15% in some studies.[3] Associated aneurysms, deep venous drainage, and a deep location were often associated with further elevated hemorrhage risks, independent of hemorrhagic presentation.[2–4] Although a small AVM size is not consistently noted among these studies, it has also been proposed as a risk factor for hemorrhage, potentially as a result of increased feeding artery pressures.[5]

Given the risk of rehemorrhage, we recommend treatment of all small AVMs that have bled. To potentially mitigate and prevent the progression of seizures or focal neurologic deficits, we also recommend the treatment of symptomatic small AVMs. Unruptured, asymptomatic small AVMs should also be treated given the lifetime risk of hemorrhage and the development of focal deficits or seizures, particularly in younger patients.

Microsurgery

Microsurgical resection of AVMs is the time-honored treatment modality that affords an immediate cure in the vast majority of patients. The associated risk is up-front, with outcomes generally improving as follow-up time accumulates. The Spetzler–Martin grading scale, used to predict surgical risk, underscores the importance of size as a factor influencing the difficulty of resection.[6] In essence, any small AVM would be deemed operable by this scheme given that all AVMs of less than 3 cm would receive a grade of I to III. Nevertheless, an AVM in an eloquent locale such as the motor cortex, internal capsule, or brainstem, without a corridor of access, regardless of size, may be deemed inoperable. In addition to anatomic corridors of access, a hematoma may provide access to an eloquent AVM and even facilitate dissection by separating the nidus from the brain. Thus, in addition to factors such as eloquence and deep venous drainage evaluated by the Spetzler–Martin scale, the AVM rupture status and the patient's neurologic status should be considered. Although both may redefine the significance of an AVM in an eloquent locale, a prior

Table 17.1   Management Options and Factors Favoring Each Approach

	Microsurgery With and Without Adjunctive Embolization	Radiosurgery	Observation
Age	Younger	Older	Older
Presentation	Previous hemorrhage Neurologic deficit Seizures	Asymptomatic	Asymptomatic
Angiography architecture	Associated aneurysm	Compact nidus	
Size or Spetzler–Martin grade	Small or low grade more favorable	Small	High grade
Location	Non-eloquent	Eloquent	Eloquent

Table 17.2 Surgical Series of Small Arteriovenous Malformations (AVMs)

Series	Patients	Obliteration	Permanent Morbidity	Mortality
Sisti et al (1993)[8]	67	63/67 (94%)	1/67 (1%)	0/67
Johnston and Johnston[a] (1996)[9]	71	67/71 (94%)	0/71	1/71 (1%)[b]
Schaller and Schramm (1997)[10]	62	61/62 (98%)	2/62 (3%)	0/62
Pikus et al (1998)[11]	19	19/19 (100%)	0/19	0/19
Pik and Morgan (2000)[12]	110	109/110 (99%)	3/110 (3%)	0/110
Lawton[c] (2003)[13]	35	35/35 (100%)	0/35	1/35 (3%)[d]

[a]All AVMs in this series were deep.

[b]The one mortality in this series was from pulmonary complications.

[c]All AVMs in this series were grade III—eloquent and with deep venous drainage.

[d]The one mortality in this series was from seemingly unrelated fulminant liver failure.

hemorrhage also indicates surgical intervention given the greater risk of rehemorrhage, particularly in the first year after rupture. On the other hand, an AVM with a significant perforator supply, a diffuse nidus, or both may be particularly more challenging from a surgical vantage point, in spite of the fact that these factors are not included in the Spetzler–Martin grading scale.[7]

Reviewing results from surgical series of small AVMs, we see exceedingly high obliteration rates (94–100%) with very limited surgical morbidity and mortality (0–3%) **(Table 17.2)**.[8–13] Lawton's[13] series reflects results from 35 grade III AVMs with only one death that was attributed to fulminant liver failure. In this series, Lawton illustrates that small grade III AVMs present the lowest surgical risk compared with moderate-sized (3–6 cm) AVMs with deep venous drainage or in an eloquent location. These exceptional results reinforce the fact that any small AVM, particularly if ruptured, should always be considered for microsurgical treatment first.

Radiosurgery

Although small AVM size is associated with greater rates of AVM obliteration,[14] the exceptional surgical results we illustrate in **Table 17.2** reinforce the fact that radiosurgery remains a secondary option for small AVMs, reserved for those deemed to be of high operative risk. This category essentially includes patients with small AVMs in eloquent locales without a reasonable corridor of surgical access.

In a group of 81 small AVMs treated with radiosurgery, the obliteration rate was 90%; however, nine patients (11%) suffered from AVM rupture after stereotactic radiosurgery (SRS), resulting in three deaths.[15] Five patients also suffered adverse radiation effects (6%). Although most SRS series do not stratify results according to the size of the AVM, the University of Pittsburgh group recently published its experience with SRS of 217 grade I or grade II AVMs (primarily small AVMs).[16] The overall obliteration rate was 58% at 3 years, 87% at 4 years, and 93% at 10 years. However the actual angiographically confirmed obliteration rates were

41% at 3 years, 66% at 4 years, and 83% at 10 years. Five patients (2%) suffered from transient radiation effects, two (1%) developed delayed cysts, and 13 (6%) suffered from hemorrhage after SRS. Six patients (3%) died of hemorrhage during the latency period.

These results compare unfavorably to those for surgery of small AVMs. An evaluation of radiosurgical results is further limited by the methods used to report obliteration and the fact that complications accrue with time. The importance of confirming the obliteration of AVMs after microsurgery leads to consistent reporting of formal, angiographically confirmed obliteration rates. On the other hand, many radiosurgical reports inflate obliteration rates by using magnetic resonance imaging (MRI) in lieu of formal angiography to confirm obliteration. In fact, even patients with complete angiographic obliteration after SRS have been known to have delayed rebleeding.[17]

In addition to delayed hemorrhage and adverse radiation effects after SRS, delayed cyst formation, arteriopathy, and even de novo pseudoaneurysm development may occur **(Fig. 17.1)**.[15–18] Debilitating radiation necrosis may even require surgical resection.[19] These events occur at overall rates proportional to the actual follow-up time. Unlike after successful microsurgical obliteration of AVMs, rupture after SRS is a cause of morbidity and mortality.[15–18]

Given the greater risk of re-rupture from ruptured AVMs, these AVMs should be managed through surgery unless they are embedded in eloquent tissue without any reasonably safe surgical corridor (e.g., the brainstem). Furthermore, associated aneurysms should be treated expeditiously and taken into account when considering SRS. In the report from the University of Pittsburgh team, the rate of bleeding of an AVM with an associated aneurysm after SRS was 28% at 5 years.[16]

Germane to the case at hand, seizure outcomes are generally better after surgery for AVMs as compared with SRS. In one study of 110 patients with epileptogenic AVMs, 81% of those undergoing surgery were free of disabling seizures at follow-up as opposed to only 43% of patients undergoing radiosurgery.[20] Furthermore, from a lifestyle perspective,

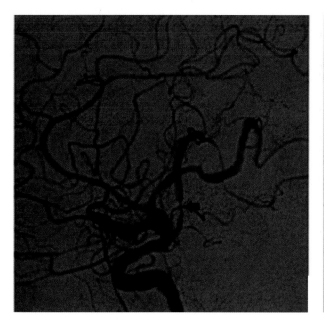
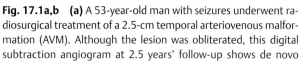

a

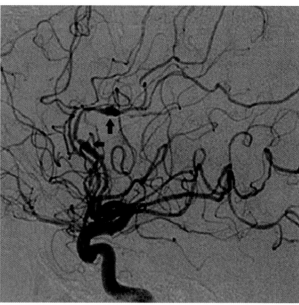

b

Fig. 17.1a,b **(a)** A 53-year-old man with seizures underwent radiosurgical treatment of a 2.5-cm temporal arteriovenous malformation (AVM). Although the lesion was obliterated, this digital subtraction angiogram at 2.5 years' follow-up shows de novo stenosis of a former middle cerebral feeding artery (*arrow*). **(b)** A 50-year-old man returned 14 years after radiosurgery for his callosal AVM with a devastating rupture of one of two de novo pericallosal pseudoaneurysms (*arrows*).

the ability to achieve an expedient cure of the AVM through microsurgery allows for the swifter alleviation of potentially debilitating seizures.

Case Discussion

Planning a strategy for AVMs requires a systematic approach that first evaluates their natural history followed by the potential treatment options and their attendant risks and benefits. The malignant natural history of ruptured AVMs warrants treatment. We strongly believe that surgery should be used to avoid the risk of hemorrhage in the latency period. Although unruptured AVMs have a relatively more benign natural history, they continue to present a risk of hemorrhage as well as morbidity from potential neurologic deficits or seizures. We believe that symptomatic small AVMs should be treated with microsurgery, given the attendant risk of hemorrhage and continued or even worsening morbidity. Surgical results are clearly superior to those of radiosurgery for small AVMs, except for lesions embedded in eloquent cortex without safe surgical access.

The ARUBA study (A Randomized Trial of Unruptured Brain AVMs) is a prospectively designed trial aimed at comparing observation with outcomes after surgery for unruptured AVMs.[21] The early pilot paper will likely show worse outcomes in the surgical group given the up-front, early risks that this cohort must undertake. With sufficient follow-up, morbidity and mortality from hemorrhage will accumulate and eventually outweigh the risks of surgery as early postoperative deficits improve. Unfortunately, ample follow-up will require years, and we hope the study does not conclude early because of the expected better early outcomes in the observed cohort.

The same concept applies to radiosurgery. As with observation, complications from radiosurgery accrue with time. The patient faces a cumulative, continued risk of hemorrhage, radiation necrosis, delayed cyst formation, and even arteriopathic complications with time (**Fig. 17.1**).[15–18] These complications are at the expense of a chance, rather than a guarantee, of obliteration. Although significantly greater obliteration rates after microsurgery as compared with radiosurgery are not a subject of debate, we strongly believe that the cumulative side effects of radiosurgery clearly outweigh the up-front risks of microsurgery for small AVMs, as long as they are surgically accessible.

Conclusion

We would offer microsurgery to the patient in this chapter's case presentation. Given her young age and her symptoms, microsurgery provides a definitive means of early cure, potentially alleviating her symptoms and eliminating her lifetime risk of hemorrhage. Radiosurgery would provide a lower chance of cure at the expense of a latency period of hemorrhage and delayed adverse radiation events.

Gamma Knife Radiosurgery for Arteriovenous Malformations

Mark E. Linskey

This case represents a technical challenge for any treatment approach as well as an excellent platform for philosophical discussion. At less than 3 cm in size (< 1.5 cm in size with 1.75 cm^3 in volume), with superficial venous drainage, and a location in a primary sensory strip, this lesion represents a Spetzler–Martin grade II AVM.[6] The patient's history suggests the possibility of simple partial sensory seizures for the mode of presentation. Neither the history nor MRI suggests any recent hemorrhage, which might potentially increase the short-term risk of AVM hemorrhage.[4,22] The images provided are limited, but there does not appear to be evidence of restricted venous outflow, an intranidal aneurysm, a draining varix, or a feeding artery aneurysm. The presence of any of these factors might be expected to increase the chances of the annual risk of rupture.[23–27]

According to actuarial data from the United States Social Security Administration in 2007, at age 40, this patient has a median life expectancy of an additional 44 years.[28] With an annual hemorrhage rate for unruptured AVMs of 1 to 2.2% per year,[29–31] this information translates into a generous lifetime risk estimate of AVM hemorrhage of 55%.[32] Given a general per-hemorrhage mortality risk of 10%, with another 10% risk of permanent major neurologic morbidity,[33] expectant observation with an acceptance of the consequences of the natural history, in our opinion, would not be a prudent recommendation.

Several validating microsurgical studies of the Spetzler–Martin grading system suggest a 36% chance of any deficit, a 0 to 6% chance of a permanent disabling deficit, and a less than 1% mortality rate for microsurgical resection of this lesion in very experienced cerebrovascular microsurgical hands.[6,34–36] There is evidence, however, that not all "eloquent" locations are equally eloquent when it comes to assessing the treatment risk. Precentral involvement is particularly susceptible to a permanent new deficit.[37] Although this AVM is immediately postcentral in location, its draining vein is the vein of Trolard, which provides the dominant venous drainage for the precentral gyrus and primary motor strip. Any interruption in this drainage runs some risk of venous infarction of the primary motor strip.

The lesion appears to have a single arterial feeder to a tight compact nidus, which potentially increases the chance of endovascular cure with complete and permanent obliteration of the nidus.[38–41] However, periprocedural risks remain heavily weighted toward primary motor strip morbidity from either the arterial or venous side, which would portend a potentially significant permanent neurologic deficit. Indeed, at present, curative embolization of AVMs remains somewhat problematic, with utility better proven for preparatory microsurgery or SRS.

Stereotactic radiosurgery is very feasible for this small AVM. Radiosurgery obliteration rates are dose-threshold dependent, with a predictive obliteration rate of more than 80% if 20 Gy or more can be delivered to the nidus margin.[42] This small AVM could certainly tolerate 20 Gy to the margin from a dose-volume toxicity standpoint.[42,43] Indeed, the predictive obliteration rate at 3 to 5 years is 90%.[16] The main risks of SRS are AVM hemorrhage during the latency period of 3 to 5 years and temporary, symptomatic, adverse radiation effects. The risk of hemorrhage during latency is 9%[32] (translating into a 0.9% mortality risk and an additional 0.9% risk of permanent neurologic morbidity[33]) over 5 years, plus those associated with a 10% risk of nonobliteration. The adverse radiation effects comprise a 20% risk of MRI-detectable signal change on the T2-weighted fluid-attenuated inversion recovery (FLAIR) images at 3 to 9 months after radiosurgery, of which less than 10% would be temporarily symptomatic. Assuming a 12-Gy volume of less than 5 cm^3, the chance of a new, permanent neurologic deficit can be predicted to be less than 1 to 2%.[43]

With all these considerations in mind, we recognize that microsurgical excision, an attempt at curative embolization, and SRS are all reasonable options for treatment based on the individual patient's view of the relative advantages and disadvantages and the patient's life goals and priorities. We would likely advise SRS as the preferred and recommended approach.

Stereotactic radiosurgery has been defined by the American Association of Neurological Surgeons, the Congress of Neurological Surgeons, and the American Society for Therapeutic Radiology and Oncology as typically "performed in a single session using a rigidly attached stereotactic guiding device, other immobilization technology and/or a stereotactic image guidance system, but can be performed in a limited number of sessions, up to a maximum of five."[44] For AVMs, SRS is optimally done in a single session. There are no good data to suggest multisession radiosurgery or fractionated radiotherapy to treat AVMs. Single-session radiosurgery can be done with any one of several different technologies:

- The gamma knife (Elekta AB, Stockholm, Sweden)
- The CyberKnife (Accuray, Inc., Sunnyvale, CA)
- The Novalis system (BrainLAB AG, Feldkirchen, Germany)
- The Varian Trilogy system (Varian Medical Systems, Inc., Palo Alto, CA)
- The X-knife (Integra Life Sciences, Radionics Division, Plainsboro, NJ)
- Charged particle devices (protons, helium, and carbon)

The gamma knife is a cobalt 60 (^{60}Co)-based system. The CyberKnife, the Novalis and Varian Trilogy systems, and the X-knife are linear accelerator-based, and charged particle systems require a cyclotron. As long as a minimum dose threshold is achieved, all SRS modalities have similar results. Certainly, gamma knife SRS has the largest portfolio of published evidence to support its use. Of the 1,145 articles documenting the use of radiosurgery for AVMs published in English and listed in the National Library of Medicine Medline database as of February 2012, 70.2% report the results of gamma knife SRS. Linear accelerator results account for 23.1% of publications (only 1.75% of publications involve the CyberKnife), whereas reports of the results of charged particle units account for 6.6% of peer-reviewed publications.

In our center, we prefer the Leksell Perfexion Gamma Unit (Elkta AB, Stockholm, Sweden) for SRS. In this chapter's presented case, we would use both catheter angiography and stereotactic MRI studies for targeting to eliminate veins from the target volume as well as optimize and limit the three-dimensional nidus definition. By limiting the nidus volume definition, we would minimize potential treatment morbidity from adverse radiation effects as well as maximize our safe minimal dose prescription. Multi-isocenter planning is the cornerstone for achieving three-dimensional conformality when treatment planning with gamma units. For this patient, we would anticipate a 90% chance of AVM obliteration 3 to 5 years after radiosurgery using our treatment strategy, with a 0.9% mortality risk and an additional 0.9% risk of permanent neurologic morbidity from hemorrhage during the latency interval. We would also expect a less than 1 to 2% risk of permanent neurologic morbidity related to the radiosurgery treatment.

Proton Beam Stereotactic Radiosurgery for Arteriovenous Malformations

Jay Loeffler and Pankaj K. Agarwalla

Procedure

Before discussing the specifics of this case, it would be useful to review how our institution, the Massachusetts General Hospital, carries out SRS using a proton beam. As described previously, patients first undergo insertion of three 1/16-inch surgical-grade stainless steel fiducial markers into the surface of the skull under local anesthesia.[45] During the same visit, custom dental fixation is made for a modified, relocatable Gill–Thomas–Cosman frame, and computed tomography (CT) scans are obtained and merged with previous images from MRI, CT angiography, or both, for radiosurgical planning for patients with an AVM. The target and nidus volumes are measured on the merged images, and custom-built brass apertures and range compensators are constructed. At the time of treatment, the patient wears the Gill–Thomas–Cosman frame and is placed into a calibrated robotic chair designed to move the patient and target into position for the immobile proton beam, which has the appropriate custom apertures and compensators for each convergent beam delivery. To calibrate this system, plain skull films are used to align the fiducial markers and match the preoperative imaging exactly **(Fig. 17.2)**.

For proton-beam SRS, treatments are done in one to two fractions with energy-degraded 160-MeV or 230-MeV beams at approximately 16 Gy (relative biological effectiveness) prescribed to a 90% isodose **(Fig. 17.3)**. For further history and details, see Bussière and colleagues[46] and Grusell and associates.[47] Although the details of the actual procedure for proton-beam SRS vary, the basic concepts of preoperative image planning and stereotactic localization and calibration at the time of treatment remain the same across institutions.

Although we are emphasizing proton-beam radiotherapy of AVMs in this discussion, it should be noted that much research on radiosurgery for AVMs has also been done with photons or other particles such as light ions. Hence, the studies cited here reflect a combined experience of SRS using protons, photons, or both. From an historical perspective, however, it is interesting to note that AVMs were one of the first neurosurgical conditions treated with proton-beam radiosurgery.[48–50]

Natural History

At present, there is some debate regarding the necessity of treating AVMs, particularly to prevent the morbidity and mortality associated with them, including seizures, hemorrhage, and neurologic deficits.[51] A thorough review of the natural history of AVMs is beyond the scope of this discussion, but current data suggest that previously unruptured AVMs have an annual hemorrhage rate ranging from 0.9 to 8%, according to one study,[3] with similar findings from other research.[2,52–55] Furthermore, several factors increase the baseline risk of hemorrhage, including a deep location, deep venous drainage, associated aneurysms, and previous hemorrhage.[2,27,30,54,55]

Although current research suggests that this patient's AVM has a lower annual risk of hemorrhage given her age,

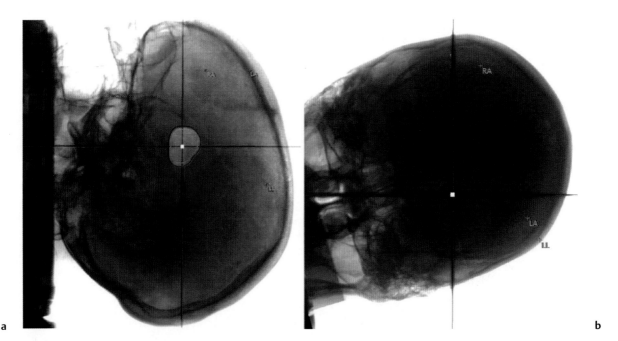

Fig. 17.2a,b   Plain skull films with fiducials marked as RA (right anterior), LA (left anterior), and LL (left lateral) in a patient with a midbrain AVM (*circled*). The patient is moved into position in a calibrated robotic chair to align the fiducial markers on these films with the predetermined plan. **(a)** Lateral view. **(b)** Oblique anterior view. (Courtesy of Marc Bussière.)

the AVM location, and its superficial drainage, we would still recommend treating this lesion, particularly because the patient is symptomatic with seizures and has a significant cumulative lifetime risk of hemorrhage.[32]

Treatment Options and the Case for Microsurgery

The options for treatment include microsurgical obliteration, endovascular occlusion, and radiosurgery. Because the role of endovascular therapy as a primary treatment modality versus adjunctive therapy to radiosurgery and mi-

crosurgery is still being studied and the data are sparse, we shall defer further discussion at this time.[56] In terms of surgery, several factors must be considered before offering surgical treatment. First and foremost, the goal of surgery is to improve the patient's outcome, either by preventing future complications such as hemorrhage, seizure, and neurologic deficits, or by addressing current clinical symptoms. One study in children showed a 4% recurrence rate of AVMs after surgical obliteration.[57] The consensus based on available data suggests that, in the proper hands of an experienced surgeon, obliteration rates can be very high, particularly for "low-risk" AVMs.[53,58] In terms of sei-

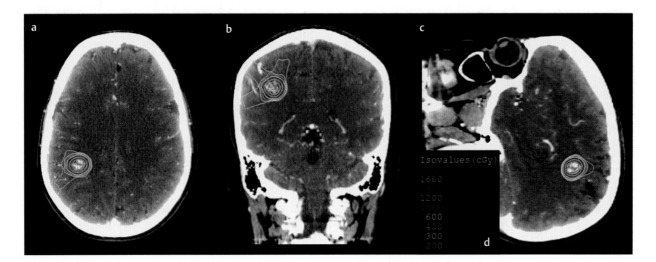

Fig. 17.3a–d   Axial **(a)**, coronal **(b)**, and sagittal **(c)** computed tomography (CT) images in a patient with a small right parietal AVM similar to that in the chapter's presented case. This patient was treated with 15 Gy (relative biological effectiveness) normalized to an 87% isodose line. **(d)** The legend for isodose values. (Courtesy of Marc Bussière.)

zure outcomes, our work at the Massachusetts General Hospital has shown surgery to be effective in obtaining Engel class I outcomes, although complete obliteration was more important than any specific treatment modality in predicting seizure outcome.[20]

For neurologic outcomes, however, the situation is more challenging because surgery can address baseline neurologic deficits but also has a significant risk of causing neurologic deficits. Therefore, any discussion of efficacy and outcomes necessitates a discussion of surgical risk. In 1986, Spetzler and Martin[6] published a landmark paper that risk-stratified AVMs according to size, location, and venous drainage. A Chinese group led by Shi and Chen also published a similar AVM grading schema in the same journal, but Spetzler and Martin's scale has withstood the test of time as the basic method of communicating surgical risk associated with AVMs.[59,60] The current patient's AVM would be considered Spetzler–Martin grade II (SM-II) given its size of 1.5 cm, superficial venous drainage, and adjacency to eloquent sensorimotor cortex. According to their original paper, this ranking would confer a 95% chance of no deficit after surgical resection, with the remaining 5% for a minor deficit.[6] In addition to the SM grade, factors that increase the surgical risk include the patient's age, a diffuse nidus morphology, and a deep perforating arterial supply.[7,61,62]

Since the original paper by Spetzler and Martin, further studies have emphasized that surgical risk from retrospective analysis of single-surgeon/single-institution case series might reflect a selection bias.[63] In fact, the surgical risk of 5% quoted for SM-II lesions might actually be as high as 9.5% in one study, based on the modified Rankin Scale as a more sensitive measure of outcome.[63] In one series by Hartmann and associates,[64] surgery for SM-II AVMs resulted in 36% of patients suffering from any type of neurologic deficit postoperatively. A series by Pik and Morgan[12] reflects excellent outcomes for patients with low-grade AVMs but also suffers from an acknowledged selection bias. Lawton and his group[61] have developed a supplementary scale to the Spetzler–Martin schema, which incorporates a ruptured presentation, the patient's age, and diffuseness of the nidus. Based on the Lawton scale, the surgical risk for our patient, given her age of 40 years, the lesion's unruptured presentation, and a presumed nondiffuse nidus, would be a 9.1% worse outcome as measured with the modified Rankin Scale score.[61] Risks of surgery are significant, even with low-grade lesions in eloquent areas, and the approach can require additional surgical techniques such as language and motor mapping and stereotaxy.[65,66]

The purpose of this discussion is not to show that surgical obliteration is the "wrong" option, but rather to emphasize why radiosurgery is an appropriate first step for treating this patient. Radiosurgery can offer high rates of obliteration with low morbidity, and the immediate procedural risk and cost of microsurgery are much higher than radiosurgery. Those arguing against radiosurgery point to several complications: failure to obliterate lesions, hemorrhage during the latency period, and neurologic deficits

from the effects of radiation. Although these risks are real, an appropriate understanding of how to choose patients for radiosurgery is critical and is discussed below.

Radiosurgery

Grading Scales

To frame the efficacy of radiosurgery as well as the risks, it is useful to review a new grading scale for radiosurgery developed by Pollock and Flickinger[67,68] to emphasize the important factors that affect obliteration rates as well as neurologic deficits after radiosurgery. In their modified and updated scale, an AVM score is assigned according to the following equation:

AVM Score = (0.1) (volume, mL) + (0.02) (age, years) + (0.5) (location: hemispheric, corpus callosum, cerebellar = 0; basal ganglia, thalamus, brainstem = 1)

With a mean follow-up of 70 months (range 3 to 200 months), patients with AVM scores of less than 1 had an 89% obliteration rate without new deficits. For those with a score of 1 to 1.5, the rate was similar (70%).[66] Higher scores, as expected, had lower obliteration rates. According to one study, factors that are associated with better outcomes (obliteration and limitation of any new neurologic deficit) include a smaller AVM volume, several draining veins, a younger age, and the location in the hemisphere.[69] In the same study, AVMs smaller than 4 cm³ had a nidus obliteration rate of 83%.[69] Obliteration rates ranging from 60 to 80% have been reported in similar studies, particularly for smaller AVMs (**Table 17.3**).[16,70–83]

Other groups have postulated relatively straightforward radiosurgery grading scales, such as that by Milker-Zabel and associates.[84] Their research independently shows that obliteration is related to the patient's age at treatment, the nidus volume, the maximum diameter, and the applied dose. Andrade-Souza and colleagues[85] randomly selected patients from their experience with linear accelerator radiosurgery for AVMs and found that, of those with a Pollock–Flickinger AVM score of less than 1, 91.7% had excellent outcomes, which were defined as complete obliteration and no neurologic deficit. The Pollock–Flickinger score has been further validated in other studies as well.[14,84–89] The AVM score developed by Pollock and Flickinger is a useful new tool to select patients and at present appears to be the new standard in discussing AVM radiosurgery.

Outcomes and Adverse Radiation Effects

In terms of neurologic and functional outcomes, Pollock and Brown[90] have shown that the modified Rankin Scale is an appropriate and sensitive measure of outcome after radiosurgery for AVMs. The modified Rankin Scale score has also been used as the outcome measure for microsurgery, making it an excellent standard for comparing outcomes among different modalities of treatment for

Table 17.3 Obliteration Rates from Selected Studies Emphasizing Small Superficial AVMs

Author	Year	Radiation	Follow-Up	Obliteration Rate
Kjellberg et al[49]	1983	Proton	2 years	20% complete obliteration, 56% had greater than 50% obliteration of variable AVMs
Steinberg et al[48]	1990	Helium-ion	3 years	100% obliteration for AVM < 4 cm^3, 95% for AVM 4–25 cm^3, and 70% for AVM > 25 cm^3
Steiner et al[70]	1992	Gamma knife	Unknown	81% complete obliteration for variable AVMs
Seifert et al[71]	1994	Proton	2 years	58.8% complete obliteration and 41.2% no change for AVM < 3 cm diameter; remaining AVM in series had no change
Pollock et al[69]	1998	Gamma knife	2 years	83% complete obliteration for AVM < 4 cm^3
Miyawaki et al[72]	1999	LINAC	3 years	67% obliteration for AVM < 4 cm^3, 58% for AVM 4–13.9 cm^3, and 22% for AVM ≥ 14 cm^3
Hadjipanayis et al[73]	2001	Gamma knife	Median 3 years	87% obliteration for AVM < 3 cm^3, 64% for AVM 3–10 cm^3, and 25% for AVM > 10 cm^3
Inoue and Ohye[74]	2002	Gamma knife	At least 1 year	92% obliteration for AVM < 4 cm^3, 77.8% for AVM 4–10 cm^3, and 36.4% for AVM > 10 cm^3
Pollock et al[75]	2003	Gamma knife	At least 2 years	73% complete obliteration for variable AVMs
Friedman et al[76]	2003	LINAC	3 years	87.9% obliteration for AVM < 1 cm^3, 62.0% for AVM 1–4 cm^3, 38.6% for AVM 4–10 cm^3, and 12.2% for AVM > 10 cm^3
Silander et al[77]	2004	Proton	3 years	70% complete to near-complete obliteration for AVM < 10 cm^3
Shin et al[78]	2004	Gamma knife	5 years	81.7–88.1% complete obliteration depending on neuroimaging criteria for variable AVMs
Vernimmen et al[79]	2005	Proton (2–3 fractions)	At least 4 years	67% obliteration for AVM < 14 cm^3 and 43% obliteration for AVM ≥ 14 cm^3
Liscák et al[80]	2007	Gamma knife	Median 2 years	92% obliteration rate for variable AVMs
Colombo et al[81]	2009	CyberKnife	3 years	81.2% obliteration rate for variable AVMs
Flores et al[82]	2011	LINAC	5 years	82.4% obliteration for AVMs < 3 cm diameter
Sun et al[83]	2011	Gamma knife and LINAC	Median 3.5 years	64% obliteration for variable AVMs
Kano et al[16]	2012	Gamma knife	4 years	87% obliteration for SM-I and SM-II AVMs

Abbreviations: LINAC, linear accelerator; SM, Spetzler–Martin grade.

AVMs, although further adoption of this measure is necessary.[61–63] Outcomes have also been measured in terms of obliteration and neurologic deficit, with an excellent outcome defined as complete obliteration and no neurologic deficit.[68] In one study, 11% of patients reported new or worsened neurologic symptoms,[83] but in a similar study 95% of patients remained neurologically stable or improved.[91]

In a series examining radiosurgery on a majority of patients with AVMs who had undergone previous treatment, 88% did not have neurologic decline after radiosurgery, but there was a significant association between the size of the AVM and deficits after radiosurgery.[89] Neurologic deficit after radiosurgery appears to be most related to the AVM volume and remains low across studies, particularly in subgroup analyses of smaller volume AVMs, a low Pollock–Flickinger AVM score, or both.[14,53,68,80,87] In terms of seizure

outcome specifically, Yang and associates[92] have shown improvement after radiosurgery, particularly in those patients with documented obliteration of the AVM, a fact that is relevant to this patient and her presenting symptoms of seizure.

Outside of neurologic complications, radiation itself can have an adverse effect on brain tissue, even without clinical manifestations. This effect can be seen as changes on MRI. Adverse radiation effects occur from occlusive hyperemia[93] or radiation damage itself to adjacent structures. Ganz and associates[94] showed that, for AVMs, there was a significant relationship between target volume and adverse radiation effects as measured by signal change on T2-weighted MRI. Hayhurst and coworkers[95] found that target volume greater than 4 cm^3 and a lack of prior hemorrhage were predictors of adverse radiation effects in their series. In the series by Kano and colleagues[16] examining SM-I and SM-II AVMs, 2.3% of patients developed temporary symptomatic adverse radiation effects, with 1% developing permanent delayed cysts. After repeated radiosurgery, 4.9% of patients in the study of variable AVMs by Stahl and associates[96] experienced adverse radiation effects. Our own group showed that, with proton-beam SRS specifically, the treatment dose and volumes were significant risk factors for radiation injury.[97] Although the risk of radiation injury is not insignificant, it is low, particularly for small, conformal radiation fields.[76,79,82] Should injury occur, however, surgical resection of any residual AVM and radiation injury can improve the clinical outcome.[19]

Hemorrhage

One of the major concerns and risks is hemorrhage during the latency period after radiosurgery but before complete obliteration of the lesion. Radiosurgery obliterates AVMs through progressive endothelial proliferation and occlusion of the AVM nidus over the course of years.[98–100] In a study by Parkhutik and colleagues,[98] AVMs that were not hemorrhagic at the time of presentation had a hemorrhage rate of 1.4% annually for the first 3 years followed by a 0.3% annual hemorrhage rate thereafter. The mean obliteration time was 37 months, which is consistent with a higher hemorrhage rate for the first 3 years when the majority of AVMs have not been completely obliterated. In their study looking only at SM-I and SM-II AVMs, Kano and coauthors[16] reported a 3.7% annual hemorrhage rate the first year after radiosurgery and a 0.3% annual hemorrhage rate for postoperative years 1 through 5. As expected, factors that lead to higher baseline AVM hemorrhage rates, such as an associated aneurysm, were found by these authors to lead to higher post-radiosurgery hemorrhage rates.[16] Similar rates were found by others.[80,83,101,102]

Decision Making

Turning to this chapter's case presentation and the treatment decision, there are several factors to consider. Based on modern risk assessment, the patient's surgical risk is as high as 9% for decline in the modified Rankin Scale score, a sensitive outcome measure. Although surgery would likely obliterate the lesion immediately and decrease her seizures, it would also likely leave a deficit. If we calculate the modified radiosurgery AVM score (the Pollock–Flickinger score) for the patient, however, we find that it is 0.98 if we assume the volume of the AVM to be approximated to that of a sphere with a 1.5-cm diameter. Her modified AVM score would be less than 1 and she would have a 90% chance of obliteration with no risk of decline in the modified Rankin Scale score.[68] Finally, if the AVM is not obliterated after the initial attempt at radiosurgery, it is safe to attempt a repeated treatment. Kano and associates[16] showed that repeated radiosurgery is effective, particularly for patients with smaller residual nidus volumes and no previ-

ous hemorrhage. Other studies have also shown that repeated radiosurgery is safe and effective with limited complications.[14,96,103] Some data also suggest that resection after radiosurgery is safe.[104]

Caveats

Any discussion of radiosurgery for an AVM must mention some caveats. First, there is significant variability among studies, not only in the type of radiation applied, but also in how obliteration and neurologic outcomes are determined. Because AVMs are not as common as other neurosurgical conditions, the published experience from a single institution often spans more than a decade, during which time significant advances have occurred in the delivery of radiosurgery and in the decision-making process. When comparing studies or reviewing the literature, one must account for these inherent limitations.

One of the most variable factors in radiosurgery is the applied dose, which is confounded by the types of radiation delivered (photons versus Bragg-peak particles including protons and light ions). A full discussion of dose is beyond the scope of this chapter, but it is important to realize that obliteration of AVMs after radiosurgery appears to relate to the radiation dose, particularly the marginal dose, and AVM volume, which are affected by the method of administering the radiation.[82–84,86,89,94,101,103,105] Here, particle radiosurgery can take advantage of the steep dose drop-off of the Bragg peak to give more conformal and higher target volume doses with fewer side effects from spillover into adjacent sites.[77,106] In addition, there is ongoing work on the role of fractionated radiotherapy versus radiosurgery for treating patients with AVMs.[45,107]

Conclusion

We strongly believe that the patient presented here would benefit from radiosurgery because it is safe and effective with a low chance of permanent neurologic deficit or radiation injury. Furthermore, the natural history of her lesion, based on current knowledge, does not put her at significant risk for hemorrhage during the latency period after radiosurgery. Her seizure symptoms should improve and ultimately, if radiosurgery fails to obliterate the lesion, microsurgery is a viable option without the patient having undertaken its risk upfront.

The debate among microsurgery, radiosurgery, and, increasingly, endovascular treatments for both small and large AVMs will only grow as our strategies become more advanced. With regard specifically to radiosurgery, improved protocols for radiation delivery as well as more standardized outcome measures and grading scales will improve the generalization of data. The treatment of patients with an AVM, however, is still limited by its relatively low prevalence, the lack of randomized data, and the variability of factors associated with AVMs.

Treatment of an Arteriovenous Malformation in Eloquent Areas

Ramsey Ashour and Jacques J. Morcos

To Treat or Not to Treat?

Although our understanding of the natural history of cerebral AVMs continues to evolve, high annual risks of hemorrhage, ranging from 2 to 4% per year, have been documented in numerous series.[1,22,30,31,52,54,55] In general, most patients warrant treatment for this reason. The threshold to intervene is lower in younger patients and in those with previously ruptured AVMs because these groups experience an increased cumulative lifetime risk of AVM hemorrhage.[1–4,32] Furthermore, patients with unruptured AVMs that cause seizures, focal neurologic deficits, or both, are more likely to be offered treatment to improve or control the offending symptoms, while also reducing the risk of AVM hemorrhage.

Unruptured AVMs may carry a lower hemorrhagic risk than ruptured ones.[1,3] Thus, the benefit of intervention for unruptured AVMs is an area of recent controversy. Stapf and colleagues[3] reported natural history data (mean follow-up of 829 days) obtained from a prospective database of 622 consecutive AVM patients evaluated at their center, the ARUBA study[51] sponsor site; they identified multiple risk factors predictive of hemorrhage, including the patient's increased age, a deep location, deep venous drainage, and a hemorrhagic presentation. In those patients with superficial, unruptured AVMs without deep venous drainage, similar to the patient described in this chapter, the hemorrhage rate over the study period was only 0.9% per year. Based in part on these data,[108] the ARUBA study,[51] which itself has raised controversy because of numerous concerns over its design,[109,110] was initiated (and is ongoing) as a randomized trial comparing observation versus intervention (surgery, radiosurgery, embolization, or all) for patients with unruptured AVMs. However, as pointed out by Cockroft and associates,[110] "it appears unlikely that any widely generalizable information will be obtained" from the ARUBA study because of its broad enrollment criteria, heterogeneous clinician and center experience, the variability in treatment modalities that are included, the inconsistent equipoise and associated selection bias, and an inadequate length of follow-up, among other factors. Because of predictably slow patient enrollment, the trial's initial 30-month recruitment period was extended to 60 months, and the initial target sample size of 800 patients was reduced to 400 patients.[51]

Most unruptured AVMs should be considered for treatment, particularly in younger patients who would otherwise be exposed to the substantial risk of AVM hemorrhage over several years without treatment. For example, in a 40-year-old woman with an unruptured, superficially lo-cated AVM without deep venous drainage, who is expected to live another 40 years, if we assume that (1) the risk of AVM hemorrhage stays constant at 0.9% per year and (2) the hemorrhagic risk for any given year behaves independently of the other years, then by the multiplicative law of probability, her lifetime risk of AVM hemorrhage would be calculated as 30%.[32] If instead we use the 4.3% per year hemorrhage risk in patients presenting with seizures, as reported by Ondra and colleagues,[52] the calculated risk of hemorrhage over 40 years increases to 83%. Of course, hemorrhagic risk does not behave independently from year to year and would certainly increase if the AVM hemorrhaged; however, even our most conservative estimate suggests that the risk of AVM hemorrhage over a 40-year period is substantial. Ultimately, the decision to treat a given AVM must be individualized to account for numerous unique patient-specific and lesion-specific factors and cannot be reduced to any single grading scheme or statistical calculation.

In the case presented, it is our position that the patient's young age (implying both a longer cumulative life at risk and a better propensity to recover from potential treatment-related injury), her symptomatic presentation, a Spetzler–Martin grade of II, and a compact nidus all collude to indicate treatment. Let's examine the various options.

How to Treat?

Irrespective of the treatment modality used, the AVM must be obliterated to reduce the risk of future hemorrhage; incomplete obliteration does not result in partial protection from,[48,111] and may even increase the risk of,[112] AVM hemorrhage. The more contentious issue is how best to achieve complete AVM obliteration with the lowest possible risk for a given patient. Should open surgery, radiosurgery, or embolization be offered? To cut, burn, or occlude? That is the question, among others, raised by the current case example and well addressed in the preceding sections.

Surgical Resection

Complete, angiographically confirmed surgical AVM resection immediately and durably eliminates the risk of future hemorrhage in adults, and is generally considered the most effective treatment with the longest track record for this purpose.[35,55] However, not all AVMs can be resected safely. In the past, some patients with large, complex, or small but deep-seated AVMs that today would be considered nonsurgical were operated on with significant morbidity, which was accepted as necessary to "defuse the bomb" in their heads. Fortunately, significant advances in the realms of radiosurgery and embolization have led to safer treatment pathways for some of these patients. Additionally, an increasingly balanced assessment of treatment risk against natural history has led to the recognition that certain AVMs should be followed or palliated rather than treated for cure, although some centers continue to push forward the frontier in this arena with multimodality treatment paradigms for even the most difficult lesions.[8,11,12,35,36,55,64]

Arteriovenous malformation surgical risk has been codified though incompletely addressed by numerous AVM grading schemes[6,61,62,115–118]; however, the Spetzler–Martin grade is the most widely used and takes into account AVM size, eloquent versus non-eloquent brain locations, and superficial versus deep venous drainage.[6] In their original paper, Spetzler and Martin[6] retrospectively applied the grading scheme to 100 consecutive patients who underwent complete AVM resection, and they were able to positively correlate the AVM grade with surgical morbidity. No patient with a low-grade AVM (I or II) experienced a major deficit. One of 21 patients with a grade II AVM (5%) experienced a minor deficit. In the follow-up prospective application of this grading scheme in 120 consecutive patients undergoing complete AVM resection, Hamilton and Spetzler[36] correlated an increasing AVM grade with new transient and permanent neurologic deficits and reported that no patient with lesions of grade I or grade II experienced a permanent neurologic deficit. They also analyzed the individual components of the grading system and found that the AVM size and the pattern of venous drainage were each statistically significant predictors of the development of permanent neurologic deficits after surgery. An eloquent location alone was a statistically significant predictor of early transient but not permanent neurologic deficits.

More recently, Lawton and associates[61] introduced a supplementary AVM grading scale to account for three additional important features not addressed in the Spetzler–Martin scheme: the patient's age, hemorrhagic versus nonhemorrhagic presentation, and a compact versus diffuse nidus. When applied to 300 consecutive surgically resected AVMs, this supplementary grading scale was a better predictor of the patient's neurologic outcome after surgery than was the Spetzler–Martin grade, and the strongest predictive ability was achieved by combining both systems.

As applied to the patient presented here, a 40-year-old woman with an unruptured AVM located in an eloquent area and with superficial venous drainage and a compact nidus measuring 1.5 cm, this lesion would be categorized as Spetzler–Martin grade II, supplemental grade III, with a combined grade (SM grade + supplemental grade) of V. Statistically, these scores predict a worsened neurologic outcome after surgery in 24.4%, 22.1%, and 21.1% of patients, respectively, according to the series by Lawton and colleagues.[61] These results stand in contrast to those previously reported by Heros and associates[35] and Hamilton

and Spetzler,[36] in which no permanent neurologic morbidity was reported in 98.7% and 100% of patients, respectively, undergoing resection of AVMs of SM grade I to II. One possible explanation for the discrepancy, among others, is that Table 5 in Lawton's paper, in which the correlates of outcome are analyzed, is based on only 73 patients.

Multiple series have suggested that small AVMs, even ones in eloquent areas, can be resected relatively safely in well-selected patients. For example, in a retrospective series of 100 consecutive surgically resected AVMs of less than 3 cm in size, Pik and Morgan[12] reported neurologic worsening in two of 46 patients (4.3%) with AVMs in eloquent areas. In another retrospective series of 67 surgically resected AVMs of less than 3 cm in size, Sisti and associates[8] reported permanent neurologic worsening in only one patient (1.5%); the proportion of AVMs in eloquent locations was not clearly specified but appears to have been at least 25%. In another retrospective series of 72 consecutive surgically resected AVMs, Pikus and coauthors[11] reported that, in the 19 patients with AVMs of less than 3 cm in size, no new postoperative neurologic deficits occurred. Finally, Lawton and associates[13] retrospectively analyzed technical and clinical results in 74 consecutively resected grade III AVMs and reported that, in the 35 patients with small lesions (< 3 cm) in eloquent areas with deep venous drainage, there were no new neurologic deficits after surgery, and there was one death secondary to fulminant liver failure of unknown cause, presumably unrelated to surgery. Small-sized grade III AVMs carried a lower overall surgical risk (2.9%) as compared with moderately sized (3–6 cm) lesions (7.1–14.8%).

Radiosurgery

Arteriovenous malformation obliteration after radiosurgery occurs in a delayed fashion through radiation-induced endothelial cell proliferation, progressive vessel wall thickening, and eventual luminal closure.[119–121] Although complete AVM obliteration rates reported after radiosurgery vary depending on the length of follow-up, the number of treatments attempted, the radiation dose used, and the imaging modality used (MRI versus cerebral angiography) to ascertain the final outcome, overall AVM obliteration rates ranging from 60 to 90% have been documented in numerous clinical series,[16,69–71,77,80,122] and both a smaller AVM size and a higher radiation dose correspond with better obliteration rates after radiosurgery. A larger volume treated, a higher radiation dose, and repeated radiosurgery are also associated with higher rates of adverse effects, including cerebral edema and direct radiation-induced neurologic injury.[16,94–96] On rare occasions, delayed rebleeding can occur even after complete angiographic obliteration is achieved.[17]

In a retrospective series of 217 grade I and II AVMs treated with radiosurgery as the primary therapy, Kano and colleagues[16] reported obliteration rates of 58%, 87%,

90%, and 93% at 3, 4, 5, and 10 years, respectively. The median follow-up after radiosurgery was 64 months, the median time until total obliteration (as seen on MRI) was 30 months, and factors associated with a higher rate of total obliteration on univariate analysis included a smaller target volume, a smaller maximum diameter, and a higher margin dose. Thirteen hemorrhages (6%) occurred after radiosurgery, resulting in six deaths (2.8%)

In another retrospective series of 300 consecutive radiosurgically treated AVMs, Liscák and associates[80] reported a 74% obliteration rate occurring at a median of 25 months after initial radiosurgery and a total obliteration rate of 92% after repeated radiosurgery in patients with persistent AVMs 3 years after the initial treatment. Smaller AVM volumes and higher radiation doses were correlated with a higher chance of AVM obliteration. The cumulative risk of new permanent neurologic morbidity related to radiosurgery was 3.4%. Nineteen patients (6.3%) experienced AVM hemorrhage after radiosurgery, and three (1%) died as a consequence.

The modified Pollock–Flickinger grading scale is a validated tool used to predict radiographic and neurologic outcome after AVM radiosurgery, and takes into account the patient's age, the AVM volume, and the AVM location.[68] In a series of 220 patients with radiosurgically treated AVMs, Pollock and Flickinger[68] reported a 75% overall AVM obliteration rate and found that lower AVM scores, as calculated with their formula, correlated with higher obliteration rates without neurologic deficits. Twenty-three patients (9%) experienced hemorrhage after radiosurgery, resulting in nine permanent neurologic deficits (4%) and eight deaths (3%).

As applied to the case described in this chapter, in a 40-year-old woman with a 1.5-cm parietal AVM, the modified Pollock–Flickinger score would be 0.98, which corresponds to an 89% chance of complete AVM obliteration without a new neurologic deficit after treatment.[68]

Embolization

Embolization is typically used as a preoperative adjunctive therapy to facilitate surgical resection by devascularizing the nidus or through targeted occlusion of deep arterial feeders that are not easily accessible at surgery (or both). Although it is an important tool, embolization must be used judiciously, as it carries its own unique risks. For example, Taylor and colleagues[123] reported a 6.5% permanent morbidity rate and a 1.2% mortality rate attributable to preoperative AVM embolization in 339 total procedures. We strongly believe that embolization of surgically accessible feeders is unnecessary and introduces the added risks of angiography and embolization, contrast agents, radiation exposure, and economic cost without significantly reducing the surgical risk. Additionally, embolization can be done to treat feeding artery aneurysms, typically in the setting of acute rupture, before later definitive therapy for

the AVM itself. Less commonly, partial embolization is used to decrease the size of an AVM nidus to make it amenable to subsequent radiosurgical treatment; however, the utility of this technique is not well established. Indeed, prior embolization has been reported to be a negative predictor of outcome after AVM radiosurgery.[69,124]

Embolization as a primary curative therapy has generally been limited to small lesions that are typically supplied by a single vascular territory with arterial feeders that are accessible through a microcatheter. The same factors that make an angiographic cure possible after embolization, however, tend to also increase the likelihood of a low-risk surgical cure, but unlike the surgical track record, the durability of AVM obliteration after embolization alone remains to be established. On the other hand, highly selected patients with small inoperable lesions and favorable angioarchitecture for embolization or those who have accessible lesions but contraindications that preclude surgery can be considered for embolization; however, such patients are typically offered radiosurgery, which is the tried-and-true option. Nonetheless, embolization offers the possibility of an immediate angiographic cure that, if durable, constitutes an obvious advantage over radiosurgery, which typically requires 2 to 5 years to effect obliteration, with no protection from hemorrhage during the latency period.

Onyx (ev3 Neurovascular, Irvine, CA) is now the liquid embolic agent of choice for AVM embolization. Compared with n-butyl cyanoacrylate, which was formerly the more widely used agent, Onyx carries less risk of microcatheter retention and can be injected slowly, in a more controlled fashion, to achieve deeper, diffuse AVM nidal penetration. As familiarity and experience with Onyx continue to accrue, the range of AVMs treated for cure with embolization will likely continue to expand. Although initial reports documented early obliteration rates with Onyx embolization ranging from 20 to 54%,[38,39,125,126] recent studies suggest that short-term curative embolization can be achieved in 94 to 96% of well-selected patients.[127,128] However, these are indeed highly selected patients and the results are nowhere close to general applicability. Long-term outcomes after curative AVM embolization remain unknown.

Seizure Outcome

The effect of AVM treatment on seizure outcome in patients presenting with seizures depends on a variety of factors reviewed elsewhere.[20] Previous studies have suggested that about half of AVM patients are rendered free of seizures after either open surgery[35] or radiosurgery[129]; however, more recent series have documented rates approaching 80%.[130,131]

In a series of 130 AVM patients with preoperative seizures who underwent surgical resection, 96% had a modified Engel class I outcome, characterized by freedom from seizures (80%) or only one postoperative seizure (16%) at a mean follow-up of 20.7 months.[130] In another series of 86

AVM patients with a history of seizures treated with radiosurgery, 76.7% were free of seizure at a mean follow-up of 89.8 months; 96.7% of patients in whom the AVM was obliterated remained free of seizure, whereas only 30.8% were free of seizures when the AVM was not completely obliterated.[131] In general, surgical resection and radiosurgery of AVMs appear to be comparable with regard to seizure outcome, and the patient described here has a good chance of complete freedom from seizure with either type of treatment, although this result would take longer to achieve with radiosurgery.

Discussion

Although we recognize that many practitioners would elect to follow this patient conservatively because her AVM is unruptured and in a so-called eloquent area, we would recommend treatment. She is young, the cumulative risk of rupture over the course of her expected lifetime is substantial even by conservative estimates, she has a better potential to recover from postoperative sequelae, and her AVM is small, superficial, compact (as opposed to diffuse) and situated posterior to the sensory cortex.

Not to belittle the use of "eloquence" as simplified and categorized by Spetzler and Martin, but it escapes no one that the concept has been oversimplified for the purpose of convenient categorization—hence its utility and limitations. All eloquent brain is not created equal. A small AVM in the sensory cortex can be treated with less risk than a small AVM in the brain stem or thalamus. On the other hand, we respect the fact that significant injury to the sensory cortex could also result in significant disability for the patient, including the disturbing alien hand syndrome. Radiosurgery is a reasonable option, which avoids the upfront risks of surgery with a high likelihood of complete AVM obliteration within 3 to 5 years. However, because there is no protection from hemorrhage during the latency period, because this continued risk of hemorrhage naturally carries more severe consequences when the AVM is situated within an eloquent location, and because there is the possibility of devastating, delayed, radiation-induced injury to the sensory cortex, a compelling argument can be made for surgical resection, if it can be done safely.

To this end, we would obtain a preoperative functional MRI scan with diffusion tensor imaging and fiber tractography to guide our resection, accepting the small risk of injury to the posterior sensory cortex. **Figure 17.4** illustrates these points in a similar patient we treated successfully through surgery, in whom the AVM directly abutted the anterior bank of the motor cortex. **Figure 17.5** illustrates the potentially devastating, and not so rare, consequences of radiosurgery in AVMs in eloquent areas, which necessitated surgical resection in another patient.

If radiosurgery were done up front in the sample case described here, with a 90% chance of complete obliteration in 3 to 5 years, what would be the next course of action for the 10% chance that obliteration was not achieved? Radiosurgery could be repeated, with an increased risk of adverse radiation effects (5%)[96] and with a continued hemorrhagic risk during the second latency period. On the other hand, previous radiosurgery has been reported to facilitate AVM resection while reducing surgical morbidity.[104] Both repeated radiosurgery and surgical resection are valid options in this scenario, and the same considerations apply.

Conclusion

Managing an AVM requires an understanding of its natural history, which must be balanced against the risks of treatment before reaching a well-informed decision. Even when armed with this understanding, experts in the field may have divergent opinions, as this and the preceding chapters illustrate. Every AVM and every patient is unique, and no single grading scheme or statistical calculation can completely dictate the appropriate strategy for a given case. In fact, the final treatment decision, in this practical world of ours, very much depends on the available resources and experience of the surgeon and center at which the patient is seen. Although it goes without saying that a multidisciplinary approach is laudable, ultimately, experienced neurosurgeons must strive to know the indications, efficacy, and complications of all potential treatment modalities, including surgery, radiosurgery, and embolization, in their own hands, in their own center, to counsel patients appropriately, especially in the face of controversy.

Multidisciplinary consultation works best when the learned opinions of the many contribute the necessary elements of experience that enrich the wisdom of the decision of the one and final decider. Such consultation, unfortunately, is misused all too often as a vehicle to abrogate individual responsibility and to diffuse, rather than consolidate, the sense of moral obligation to the patient. Treatment by committee works no better than having several people maneuver the steering wheel of one car. No single person will feel responsible for the crash. One leader and driver is indispensable. And, at the risk of preaching fiscal heresy and disregard for the "bottom line" of hospitals and physician practices, the ethical practitioner who recognizes that the best treatment may not be available at his or her own facility should refrain from resorting to the too commonly used strategy of prescribing "what is available at our center" rather than prescribing what is best for the patient at another center.

In the final analysis, if the patient discussed here were a patient of the senior moderator at the University of Miami, she would undergo surgical resection.

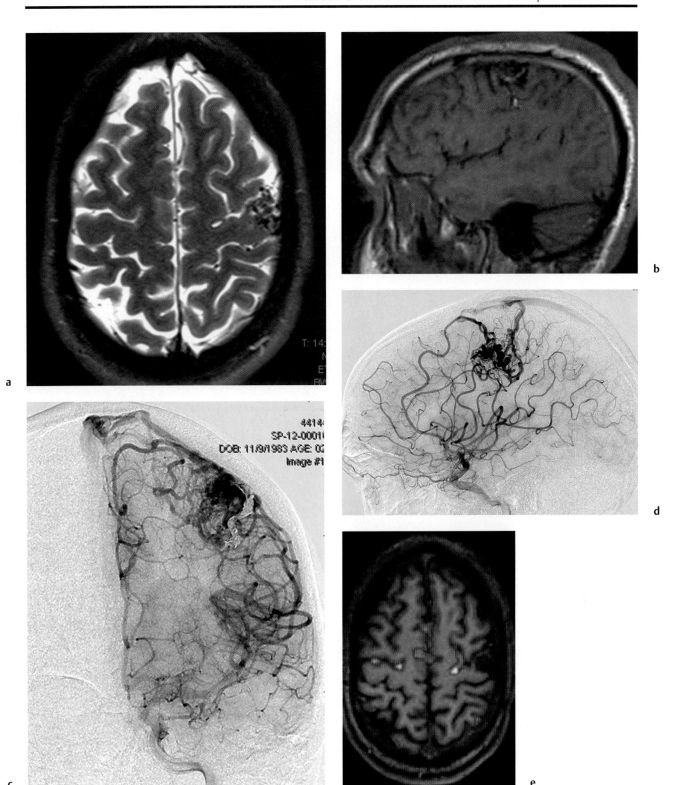

Fig. 17.4a–m A 22-year-old man presented with multiple jacksonian seizures involving the right arm. At another institution, he was diagnosed with an AVM of the left motor cortex and underwent partial Onyx embolization. No clear treatment goal was defined and the patient sought our opinion. The initial plain magnetic resonance imaging (MRI) scans of the brain—T2-weighted axial **(a)** and T1-weighted sagittal **(b)**—show a 2.4-cm nidus abutting and indenting the anterior bank of the left motor strip. A standard left internal carotid artery (LICA) angiogram—anterior-posterior **(c)** and lateral **(d)**—confirms the arterial supply through the branches of the anterior and middle cerebral branches, with a partial Onyx cast seen in the branches of the middle cerebral artery, as well as superficial venous drainage. The AVM was Spetzler–Martin grade II. **(e)** Functional MRI shows activation zones for right-hand motor function. (*continued on next page*)

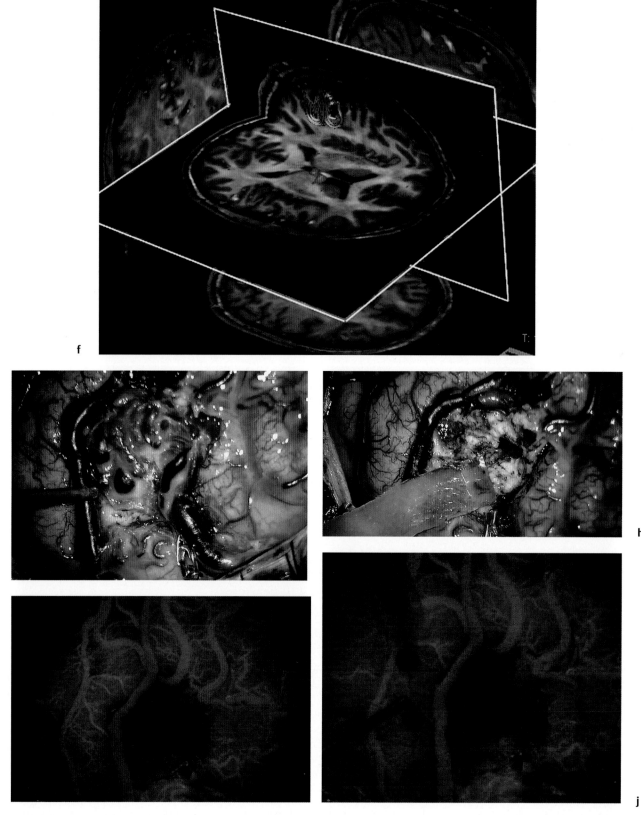

Fig. 17.4a–m (*continued*) **(f)** Diffusion tensor imaging (DTI) tractography well illustrates that the fibers immediately adjacent to the AVM may be transcortical U-fibers rather than the corticospinal tract. The decision was made to resect the lesion. **(g)** At surgery, the partial Onyx cast is well seen. Careful intraoperative corticography confirms the position of the motor strip immediately posterior to the vein. **(h)** A complete resection is achieved without changes in the motor evoked potentials or somatosensory evoked potentials. **(i)** Intraoperative indocyanine green videography confirms the total resection. **(j)** The subdural strip electrode is placed on the motor strip after resection to confirm the integrity of the motor pathway. The patient had no postoperative deficits whatsoever.

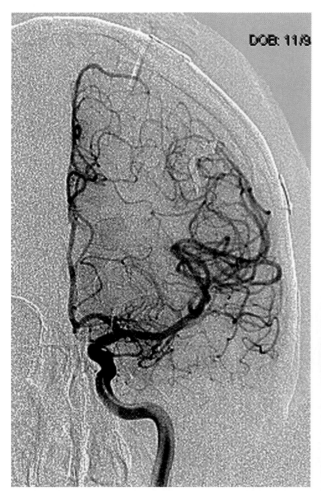

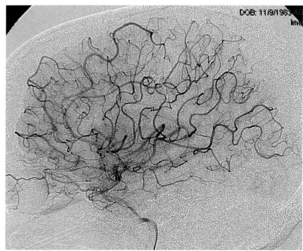

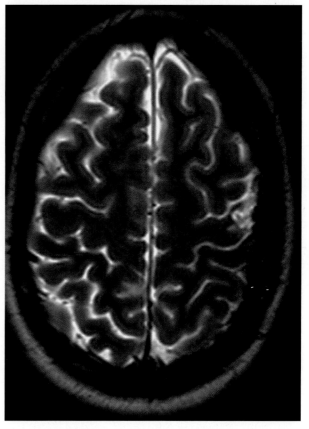

Fig. 17.4a–m (*continued*)   **(k,l)** Anterior-posterior and lateral angiograms on postoperative day 2 confirm the gross total resection. **(m)** The patient is cured of seizures as of his 6-month follow-up visit and his MRI is normal.

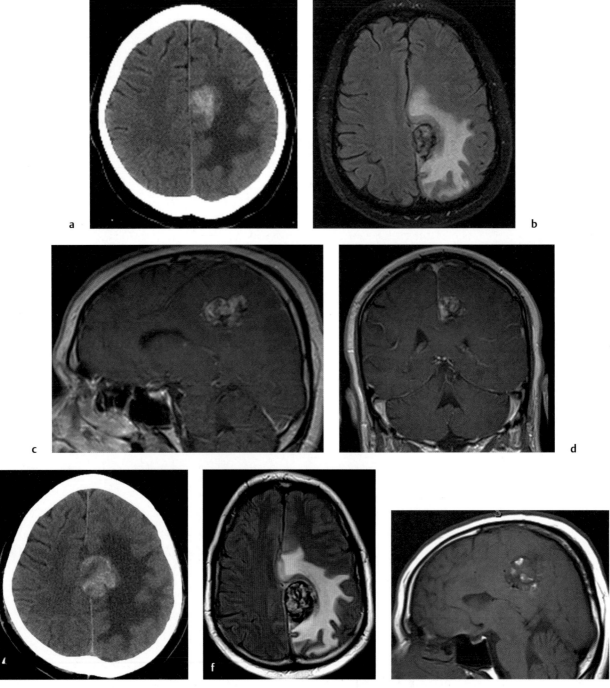

Fig. 17.5a–l This 38-year-old man presented to another institution with headaches. A small 1.8-cm AVM of the left paracentral lobule was diagnosed, and he underwent CyberKnife radiosurgery in three fractions. At around 14 months after treatment, he began to complain of weakness in his right foot, which progressed proximally. He was treated with steroids for 3 months before being referred to our institution. At his first evaluation with us, he had already deteriorated significantly. He was using a walker, was severely depressed with intense headaches, displayed cushingoid features, and was suffering from a multitude of steroid-induced ailments and dependence. The initial pretreatment MRI and an-

giograms were not available for review. The lesion was an AVM of the left paracentral lobule, with venous drainage to the superior sagittal gyrus, making it Spetzler–Martin grade II. **(a–d)** Images showing hemorrhagic changes, necrosis, and surrounding edema: **(a)** plain CT scan; **(b)** axial fluid-attenuated inversion recovery (FLAIR) MRI; **(c)** T1-weighted gadolinium-enhanced sagittal MRI; **(d)** T1-weighted gadolinium-enhanced coronal MRI, which coincided with the early onset of clinical and radiographic radiation necrosis at 14 months. **(e–g)** By 17 months after treatment, the changes were more marked, as if the radionecrosing AVM were behaving as an enlarging malignant tumor.

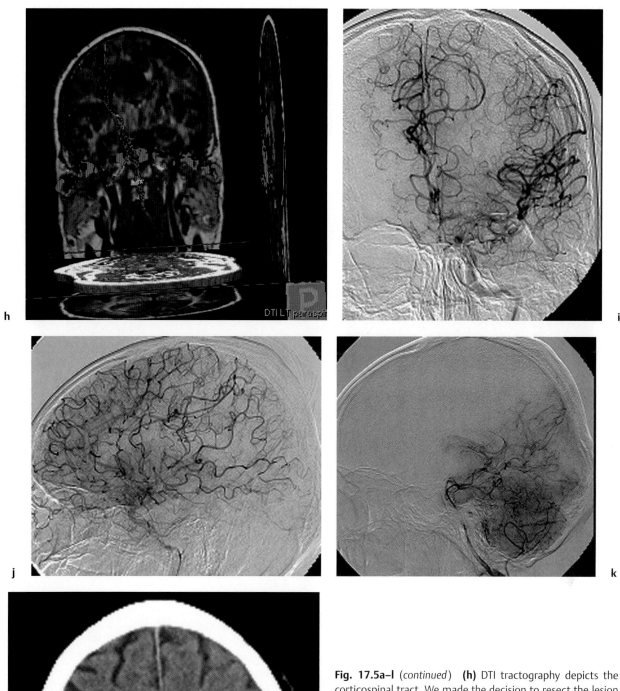

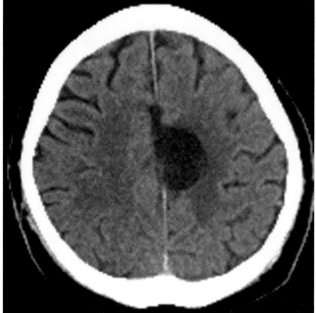

Fig. 17.5a–l (*continued*)   **(h)** DTI tractography depicts the corticospinal tract. We made the decision to resect the lesion in the face of clinical worsening. **(i–k)** At 17 months after CyberKnife treatment, angiography shows seeming obliteration of the nidus. Thus, to spare the injured ipsilateral left parasagittal motor cortex, the lesion was approached through a contralateral right-sided interhemispheric transfalcine access, with the expectation of encountering necrotic, easily resectable tissue. Unfortunately, the tissue was still bloody and functioned as if the AVM was still partially live. Thus, the surgery was aborted. Immediately after surgery, the patient suffered from severe paraparesis but slowly recovered to his preoperative state at 3 months. An ipsilateral interhemispheric approach was then performed and the lesion successfully resected. By 3 months after the resection, he had made a remarkable recovery, was independent, and off steroids. **(l)** CT scan showing marked resolution of the radionecrotic changes.

References

1. Crawford PM, West CR, Chadwick DW, Shaw MD. Arteriovenous malformations of the brain: natural history in unoperated patients. J Neurol Neurosurg Psychiatry 1986;49:1–10

2. da Costa L, Wallace MC, Ter Brugge KG, O'Kelly C, Willinsky RA, Tymianski M. The natural history and predictive features of hemorrhage from brain arteriovenous malformations. Stroke 2009;40:100–105

3. Stapf C, Mast H, Sciacca RR, et al. Predictors of hemorrhage in patients with untreated brain arteriovenous malformation. Neurology 2006;66:1350–1355

4. Yamada S, Takagi Y, Nozaki K, Kikuta K, Hashimoto N. Risk factors for subsequent hemorrhage in patients with cerebral arteriovenous malformations. J Neurosurg 2007;107:965–972

5. Spetzler RF, Hargraves RW, McCormick PW, Zabramski JM, Flom RA, Zimmerman RS. Relationship of perfusion pressure and size to risk of hemorrhage from arteriovenous malformations. J Neurosurg 1992;76:918–923

6. Spetzler RF, Martin NA. A proposed grading system for arteriovenous malformations. J Neurosurg 1986;65:476–483

7. Du R, Keyoung HM, Dowd CF, Young WL, Lawton MT. The effects of diffuseness and deep perforating artery supply on outcomes after microsurgical resection of brain arteriovenous malformations. Neurosurgery 2007;60:638–646, discussion 646–648

8. Sisti MB, Kader A, Stein BM. Microsurgery for 67 intracranial arteriovenous malformations less than 3 cm in diameter. J Neurosurg 1993;79:653–660

9. Johnston JL, Johnston IH. The surgical treatment of small deep intracranial arteriovenous malformations: a report of 85 cases. J Clin Neurosci 1996;3:338–345

10. Schaller C, Schramm J. Microsurgical results for small arteriovenous malformations accessible for radiosurgical or embolization treatment. Neurosurgery 1997;40:664–672, discussion 672–674

11. Pikus HJ, Beach ML, Harbaugh RE. Microsurgical treatment of arteriovenous malformations: analysis and comparison with stereotactic radiosurgery. J Neurosurg 1998;88:641–646

12. Pik JH, Morgan MK. Microsurgery for small arteriovenous malformations of the brain: results in 110 consecutive patients. Neurosurgery 2000;47:571–575, discussion 575–577

13. Lawton MT; UCSF Brain Arteriovenous Malformation Study Project. Spetzler-Martin grade III arteriovenous malformations: surgical results and a modification of the grading scale. Neurosurgery 2003;52:740–748, discussion 748–749

14. Raffa SJ, Chi YY, Bova FJ, Friedman WA. Validation of the radiosurgery-based arteriovenous malformation score in a large linear accelerator radiosurgery experience. J Neurosurg 2009; 111:832–839

15. Colombo F, Pozza F, Chierego G, Casentini L, De Luca G, Francescon P. Linear accelerator radiosurgery of cerebral arteriovenous malformations: an update. Neurosurgery 1994;34:14–20, discussion 20–21

16. Kano H, Lunsford LD, Flickinger JC, et al. Stereotactic radiosurgery for arteriovenous malformations, part 1: management of Spetzler-Martin grade I and II arteriovenous malformations. J Neurosurg 2012;116:11–20

17. Shin M, Kawahara N, Maruyama K, Tago M, Ueki K, Kirino T. Risk of hemorrhage from an arteriovenous malformation confirmed to have been obliterated on angiography after stereotactic radiosurgery. J Neurosurg 2005;102:842–846

18. Yamamoto M, Jimbo M, Hara M, Saito I, Mori K. Gamma knife radiosurgery for arteriovenous malformations: long-term follow-up results focusing on complications occurring more than 5 years after irradiation. Neurosurgery 1996;38:906–914

19. Massengale JL, Levy RP, Marcellus M, Moes G, Marks MP, Steinberg GK. Outcomes of surgery for resection of regions of symptomatic radiation injury after stereotactic radiosurgery for arteriovenous malformations. Neurosurgery 2006;59:553–560, discussion 553–560

20. Hoh BL, Chapman PH, Loeffler JS, Carter BS, Ogilvy CS. Results of multimodality treatment for 141 patients with brain arteriovenous malformations and seizures: factors associated with seizure incidence and seizure outcomes. Neurosurgery 2002; 51:303–309, discussion 309–311

21. Stapf C, Mohr JP, Choi JH, Hartmann A, Mast H. Invasive treatment of unruptured brain arteriovenous malformations is experimental therapy. Curr Opin Neurol 2006;19:63–68

22. Graf CJ, Perret GE, Torner JC. Bleeding from cerebral arteriovenous malformations as part of their natural history. J Neurosurg 1983;58:331–337

23. Stefani MA, Porter PJ, terBrugge KG, Montanera W, Willinsky RA, Wallace MC. Angioarchitectural factors present in brain arteriovenous malformations associated with hemorrhagic presentation. Stroke 2002;33:920–924

24. Willinsky R, Lasjaunias P, Terbrugge K, Pruvost P. Brain arteriovenous malformations: analysis of the angio-architecture in relationship to hemorrhage (based on 152 patients explored and/or treated at the Hôpital de Bicêtre between 1981 and 1986). J Neuroradiol 1988;15:225–237

25. Marks MP, Lane B, Steinberg GK, Chang PJ. Hemorrhage in intracerebral arteriovenous malformations: angiographic determinants. Radiology 1990;176:807–813

26. Turjman F, Massoud TF, Viñuela F, Sayre JW, Guglielmi G, Duckwiler G. Correlation of the angioarchitectural features of cerebral arteriovenous malformations with clinical presentation of hemorrhage. Neurosurgery 1995;37:856–860, discussion 860–862

27. Brown RD Jr, Wiebers DO, Forbes GS. Unruptured intracranial aneurysms and arteriovenous malformations: frequency of intracranial hemorrhage and relationship of lesions. J Neurosurg 1990;73:859–863

28. Social Security Administration. Retirement and survivors benefits. Life expectancy calculator. http://www.ssa.gov/oact/population/longevity.html

29. Kim H, McCulloch CE, Johnston SC, Lawton MT, Sidney S, Young WL. Comparison of 2 approaches for determining the natural history risk of brain arteriovenous malformation rupture. Am J Epidemiol 2010;171:1317–1322

30. Hernesniemi JA, Dashti R, Juvela S, Väärt K, Niemelä M, Laakso A. Natural history of brain arteriovenous malformations: a long-term follow-up study of risk of hemorrhage in 238 patients. Neurosurgery 2008;63:823–829, discussion 829–831

31. Brown RD Jr, Wiebers DO, Forbes G, et al. The natural history of unruptured intracranial arteriovenous malformations. J Neurosurg 1988;68:352–357

32. Kondziolka D, McLaughlin MR, Kestle JR. Simple risk predictions for arteriovenous malformation hemorrhage. Neurosurgery 1995;37:851–855

33. Fisher WS III. Therapy of AVMs: a decision analysis. Clin Neurosurg 1995;42:294–312

34. Hartmann A, Mast H, Mohr JP, et al. Morbidity of intracranial hemorrhage in patients with cerebral arteriovenous malformation. Stroke 1998;29:931–934

35. Heros RC, Korosue K, Diebold PM. Surgical excision of cerebral arteriovenous malformations: late results. Neurosurgery 1990; 26:570–577, discussion 577–578

36. Hamilton MG, Spetzler RF. The prospective application of a grading system for arteriovenous malformations. Neurosurgery 1994;34:2–6, discussion 6–7

37. Schaller C, Schramm J, Haun D. Significance of factors contributing to surgical complications and to late outcome after elective surgery of cerebral arteriovenous malformations. J Neurol Neurosurg Psychiatry 1998;65:547–554

38. Katsaridis V, Papagiannaki C, Aimar E. Curative embolization of cerebral arteriovenous malformations (AVMs) with Onyx in 101 patients. Neuroradiology 2008;50:589–597

39. Weber W, Kis B, Siekmann R, Kuehne D. Endovascular treatment of intracranial arteriovenous malformations with onyx: technical aspects. AJNR Am J Neuroradiol 2007;28:371–377

40. Mounayer C, Hammami N, Piotin M, et al. Nidal embolization of brain arteriovenous malformations using Onyx in 94 patients. AJNR Am J Neuroradiol 2007;28:518–523

41. Söderman M, Andersson T, Karlsson B, Wallace MC, Edner G. Management of patients with brain arteriovenous malformations. Eur J Radiol 2003;46:195–205

42. Karlsson B, Lindquist C, Steiner L. Prediction of obliteration after gamma knife surgery for cerebral arteriovenous malformations. Neurosurgery 1997;40:425–430, discussion 430–431

43. Flickinger JC, Kondziolka D, Lunsford LD, et al; Arteriovenous Malformation Radiosurgery Study Group. Development of a model to predict permanent symptomatic postradiosurgery injury for arteriovenous malformation patients. Int J Radiat Oncol Biol Phys 2000;46:1143–1148

44. Barnett GH, Linskey ME, Adler JR, et al; American Association of Neurological Surgeons; Congress of Neurological Surgeons Washington Committee Stereotactic Radiosurgery Task Force. Stereotactic radiosurgery—an organized neurosurgery-sanctioned definition. J Neurosurg 2007;106:1–5

45. Hattangadi JA, Chapman PH, Bussière MR, et al. Planned two-fraction proton beam stereotactic radiosurgery for high-risk inoperable cerebral arteriovenous malformations. Int J Radiat Oncol Biol Phys 2012;83:533–541

46. Bussière MR, Loeffler JS, Chapman PH, Cascio E, Shih HA. Proton radiosurgery. In: Winn HR, ed. Youmans' Neurological Surgery, vol. 3, 6th ed. Philadelphia: Elsevier Saunders, 2011:2616–2621

47. Grusell E, Montelius A, Russell KR, et al. Patient positioning for fractionated precision radiation treatment of targets in the head using fiducial markers. Radiother Oncol 1994;33:68–72

48. Steinberg GK, Fabrikant JI, Marks MP, et al. Stereotactic heavy-charged-particle Bragg-peak radiation for intracranial arteriovenous malformations. N Engl J Med 1990;323:96–101

49. Kjellberg RN, Hanamura T, Davis KR, Lyons SL, Adams RD. Bragg-peak proton-beam therapy for arteriovenous malformations of the brain. N Engl J Med 1983;309:269–274

50. Ogilvy CS. Radiation therapy for arteriovenous malformations: a review. Neurosurgery 1990;26:725–735

51. Mohr JP, Moskowitz AJ, Stapf C, et al. The ARUBA trial: current status, future hopes. Stroke 2010;41:e537–e540

52. Ondra SL, Troupp H, George ED, Schwab K. The natural history of symptomatic arteriovenous malformations of the brain: a 24-year follow-up assessment. J Neurosurg 1990;73:387–391

53. van Beijnum J, van der Worp HB, Buis DR, et al. Treatment of brain arteriovenous malformations: a systematic review and meta-analysis. JAMA 2011;306:2011–2019

54. Halim AX, Johnston SC, Singh V, et al. Longitudinal risk of intracranial hemorrhage in patients with arteriovenous malformation of the brain within a defined population. Stroke 2004;35:1697–1702

55. Mast H, Young WL, Koennecke HC, et al. Risk of spontaneous haemorrhage after diagnosis of cerebral arteriovenous malformation. Lancet 1997;350:1065–1068

56. Yashar P, Amar AP, Giannotta SL, et al. Cerebral arteriovenous malformations: issues of the interplay between stereotactic radiosurgery and endovascular surgical therapy. World Neurosurg 2011;75:638–647

57. Kader A, Goodrich JT, Sonstein WJ, Stein BM, Carmel PW, Michelsen WJ. Recurrent cerebral arteriovenous malformations after negative postoperative angiograms. J Neurosurg 1996;85:14–18

58. Davidson AS, Morgan MK. How safe is arteriovenous malformation surgery? A prospective, observational study of surgery as first-line treatment for brain arteriovenous malformations. Neurosurgery 2010;66:498–504, discussion 504–505

59. Davies JM, Kim H, Young WL, Lawton MT. Classification schemes for arteriovenous malformations. Neurosurg Clin N Am 2012; 23:43–53

60. Shi YQ, Chen XC. A proposed scheme for grading intracranial arteriovenous malformations. J Neurosurg 1986;65:484–489

61. Lawton MT, Kim H, McCulloch CE, Mikhak B, Young WL. A supplementary grading scale for selecting patients with brain arteriovenous malformations for surgery. Neurosurgery 2010; 66:702–713, discussion 713

62. Spears J, Terbrugge KG, Moosavian M, et al. A discriminative prediction model of neurological outcome for patients undergoing surgery of brain arteriovenous malformations. Stroke 2006;37:1457–1464

63. Morgan MK, Rochford AM, Tsahtsarlis A, Little N, Faulder KC. Surgical risks associated with the management of grade I and II brain arteriovenous malformations. Neurosurgery 2007;61(1, Suppl):417–422, discussion 422–424

64. Hartmann A, Stapf C, Hofmeister C, et al. Determinants of neurological outcome after surgery for brain arteriovenous malformation. Stroke 2000;31:2361–2364

65. Gabarrós A, Young WL, McDermott MW, Lawton MT. Language and motor mapping during resection of brain arteriovenous malformations: indications, feasibility, and utility. Neurosurgery 2011;68:744–752

66. Russell SM, Woo HH, Joseffer SS, Jafar JJ. Role of frameless stereotaxy in the surgical treatment of cerebral arteriovenous malformations: technique and outcomes in a controlled study of 44 consecutive patients. Neurosurgery 2002;51:1108–1116, discussion 1116–1118

67. Pollock BE, Flickinger JC. A proposed radiosurgery-based grading system for arteriovenous malformations. J Neurosurg 2002; 96:79–85

68. Pollock BE, Flickinger JC. Modification of the radiosurgery-based arteriovenous malformation grading system. Neurosurgery 2008;63:239–243, discussion 243

69. Pollock BE, Flickinger JC, Lunsford LD, Maitz A, Kondziolka D. Factors associated with successful arteriovenous malformation

radiosurgery. Neurosurgery 1998;42:1239–1244, discussion 1244–1247

70. Steiner L, Lindquist C, Adler JR, Torner JC, Alves W, Steiner M. Clinical outcome of radiosurgery for cerebral arteriovenous malformations. J Neurosurg 1992;77:1–8

71. Seifert V, Stolke D, Mehdorn HM, Hoffmann B. Clinical and radiological evaluation of long-term results of stereotactic proton beam radiosurgery in patients with cerebral arteriovenous malformations. J Neurosurg 1994;81:683–689

72. Miyawaki L, Dowd C, Wara W, et al. Five year results of LINAC radiosurgery for arteriovenous malformations: outcome for large AVMS. Int J Radiat Oncol Biol Phys 1999;44:1089–1106

73. Hadjipanayis CG, Levy EI, Niranjan A, et al. Stereotactic radiosurgery for motor cortex region arteriovenous malformations. Neurosurgery 2001;48:70–76, discussion 76–77

74. Inoue HK, Ohye C. Hemorrhage risks and obliteration rates of arteriovenous malformations after gamma knife radiosurgery. J Neurosurg 2002;97(5, Suppl):474–476

75. Pollock BE, Gorman DA, Coffey RJ. Patient outcomes after arteriovenous malformation radiosurgical management: results based on a 5- to 14-year follow-up study. Neurosurgery 2003;52:1291–1296, discussion 1296–1297

76. Friedman WA, Bova FJ, Bollampally S, Bradshaw P. Analysis of factors predictive of success or complications in arteriovenous malformation radiosurgery. Neurosurgery 2003;52:296–307, discussion 307–308

77. Silander H, Pellettieri L, Enblad P, et al. Fractionated, stereotactic proton beam treatment of cerebral arteriovenous malformations. Acta Neurol Scand 2004;109:85–90

78. Shin M, Maruyama K, Kurita H, et al. Analysis of nidus obliteration rates after gamma knife surgery for arteriovenous malformations based on long-term follow-up data: the University of Tokyo experience. J Neurosurg 2004;101:18–24

79. Vernimmen FJ, Slabbert JP, Wilson JA, Fredericks S, Melvill R. Stereotactic proton beam therapy for intracranial arteriovenous malformations. Int J Radiat Oncol Biol Phys 2005;62:44–52

80. Liscák R, Vladyka V, Simonová G, et al. Arteriovenous malformations after Leksell gamma knife radiosurgery: rate of obliteration and complications. Neurosurgery 2007;60:1005–1014, discussion 1015–1016

81. Colombo F, Cavedon C, Casentini L, Francescon P, Causin F, Pinna V. Early results of CyberKnife radiosurgery for arteriovenous malformations. J Neurosurg 2009;111:807–819

82. Flores GL, Sallabanda K, dos Santos MA, et al. Linac stereotactic radiosurgery for the treatment of small arteriovenous malformations: lower doses can be equally effective. Stereotact Funct Neurosurg 2011;89:338–345

83. Sun DQ, Carson KA, Raza SM, et al. The radiosurgical treatment of arteriovenous malformations: obliteration, morbidities, and performance status. Int J Radiat Oncol Biol Phys 2011;80:354–361

84. Milker-Zabel S, Kopp-Schneider A, Wiesbauer H, et al. Proposal for a new prognostic score for linac-based radiosurgery in cerebral arteriovenous malformations. Int J Radiat Oncol Biol Phys 2012;83:525–532

85. Andrade-Souza YM, Zadeh G, Ramani M, Scora D, Tsao MN, Schwartz ML. Testing the radiosurgery-based arteriovenous malformation score and the modified Spetzler-Martin grading system to predict radiosurgical outcome. J Neurosurg 2005;103:642–648

86. Wegner RE, Oysul K, Pollock BE, et al. A modified radiosurgery-based arteriovenous malformation grading scale and its correlation with outcomes. Int J Radiat Oncol Biol Phys 2011;79:1147–1150

87. Skjøth-Rasmussen J, Roed H, Ohlhues L, Jespersen B, Juhler M. Complications following linear accelerator based stereotactic radiation for cerebral arteriovenous malformations. Int J Radiat Oncol Biol Phys 2010;77:542–547

88. Moreno-Jimenez S, Celis MA, Larraga-Gutierrez JM, et al. Intracranial arteriovenous malformations treated with LINAC-based conformal radiosurgery: validation of the radiosurgery-based arteriovenous malformation score as a predictor of outcome. Neurol Res 2007;29:712–716

89. Murray G, Brau RH; Clinical Article. A 10-year experience of radiosurgical treatment for cerebral arteriovenous malformations: a perspective from a series with large malformations. Clinical article. J Neurosurg 2011;115:337–346

90. Pollock BE, Brown RD Jr. Use of the Modified Rankin Scale to assess outcome after arteriovenous malformation radiosurgery. Neurology 2006;67:1630–1634

91. Zabel A, Milker-Zabel S, Huber P, Schulz-Ertner D, Schlegel W, Debus J. Treatment outcome after linac-based radiosurgery in cerebral arteriovenous malformations: retrospective analysis of factors affecting obliteration. Radiother Oncol 2005;77:105–110

92. Yang SY, Paek SH, Kim DG, Chung HT. Quality of life after radiosurgery for cerebral arteriovenous malformation patients who present with seizure. Eur J Neurol 2012;19:984–991

93. Chapman PH, Ogilvy CS, Loeffler JS. The relationship between occlusive hyperemia and complications associated with the radiosurgical treatment of arteriovenous malformations: report of two cases. Neurosurgery 2004;55:228–233, discussion 233–234

94. Ganz JC, Reda WA, Abdelkarim K. Adverse radiation effects after gamma knife surgery in relation to dose and volume. Acta Neurochir (Wien) 2009;151:9–19

95. Hayhurst C, Monsalves E, van Prooijen M, et al. Pretreatment predictors of adverse radiation effects after radiosurgery for arteriovenous malformation. Int J Radiat Oncol Biol Phys 2012;82:803–808

96. Stahl JM, Chi YY, Friedman WA. Repeat radiosurgery for intracranial arteriovenous malformations. Neurosurgery 2012;70:150–154, discussion 154

97. Barker FG II, Butler WE, Lyons S, et al. Dose-volume prediction of radiation-related complications after proton beam radiosurgery for cerebral arteriovenous malformations. J Neurosurg 2003;99:254–263

98. Parkhutik V, Lago A, Tembl JI, et al. Postradiosurgery hemorrhage rates of arteriovenous malformations of the brain: influencing factors and evolution with time. Stroke 2012;43:1247–1252

99. Akakin A, Ozkan A, Akgun E, et al. Endovascular treatment increases but gamma knife radiosurgery decreases angiogenic activity of arteriovenous malformations: an in vivo experimental study using a rat cornea model. Neurosurgery 2010;66:121–129, discussion 129–130

100. Storer KP, Tu J, Stoodley MA, Smee RI. Expression of endothelial adhesion molecules after radiosurgery in an animal model of arteriovenous malformation. Neurosurgery 2010;67:976–983, discussion 983

101. Blamek S, Tarnawski R, Miszczyk L. Linac-based stereotactic radiosurgery for brain arteriovenous malformations. Clin Oncol (R Coll Radiol) 2011;23:525–531

102. Yen CP, Sheehan JP, Schwyzer L, Schlesinger D. Hemorrhage risk of cerebral arteriovenous malformations before and during the latency period after gamma knife radiosurgery. Stroke 2011;42:1691–1696

103. Hauswald H, Milker-Zabel S, Sterzing F, Schlegel W, Debus J, Zabel-du Bois A. Repeated linac-based radiosurgery in high-grade cerebral arteriovenous-malformations (AVM) Spetzler-Martin grade III to IV previously treated with radiosurgery. Radiother Oncol 2011;98:217–222

104. Sanchez-Mejia RO, McDermott MW, Tan J, Kim H, Young WL, Lawton MT. Radiosurgery facilitates resection of brain arteriovenous malformations and reduces surgical morbidity. Neurosurgery 2009;64:231–238, discussion 238–240

105. Chang JH, Chang JW, Park YG, Chung SS. Factors related to complete occlusion of arteriovenous malformations after gamma knife radiosurgery. J Neurosurg 2000;93(Suppl 3): 96–101

106. Andisheh B, Brahme A, Bitaraf MA, Mavroidis P, Lind BK. Clinical and radiobiological advantages of single-dose stereotactic light-ion radiation therapy for large intracranial arteriovenous malformations. Technical note. J Neurosurg 2009;111: 919–926

107. Vernimmen FJ, Slabbert JP. Assessment of the alpha/beta ratios for arteriovenous malformations, meningiomas, acoustic neuromas, and the optic chiasma. Int J Radiat Biol 2010; 86:486–498

108. Stapf C. The rationale behind "A Randomized Trial of Unruptured Brain AVMs" (ARUBA). Acta Neurochir Suppl (Wien) 2010;107:83–85

109. Mohr JP, Moskowitz AJ, Parides M, Stapf C, Young WL. Hull down on the horizon: A Randomized trial of Unruptured Brain Arteriovenous malformations (ARUBA) Trial. Stroke 2012; 43:1744–1745

110. Cockroft KM, Jayaraman MV, Amin-Hanjani S, Derdeyn CP, McDougall CG, Wilson JA. A perfect storm: how a randomized trial of unruptured brain arteriovenous malformations' (ARUBA's) trial design challenges notions of external validity. Stroke 2012;43:1979–1981

111. Heros RC, Korosue K. Radiation treatment of cerebral arteriovenous malformations. N Engl J Med 1990;323:127–129

112. Miyamoto S, Hashimoto N, Nagata I, et al. Posttreatment sequelae of palliatively treated cerebral arteriovenous malformations. Neurosurgery 2000;46:589–594, discussion 594–595

113. Chang SD, Marcellus ML, Marks MP, Levy RP, Do HM, Steinberg GK. Multimodality treatment of giant intracranial arteriovenous malformations. Neurosurgery 2007;61(1, Suppl): 432–442, discussion 442–444

114. Chang SD, Marcellus ML, Marks MP, Levy RP, Do HM, Steinberg GK. Multimodality treatment of giant intracranial arteriovenous malformations. Neurosurgery 2003;53:1–11, discussion 11–13

115. de Oliveira E, Tedeschi H, Raso J. Comprehensive management of arteriovenous malformations. Neurol Res 1998;20:673–683

116. Tamaki N, Ehara K, Lin TK, et al. Cerebral arteriovenous malformations: factors influencing the surgical difficulty and outcome. Neurosurgery 1991;29:856–861, discussion 861–863

117. Höllerhage HG. Cerebral arteriovenous malformations: factors influencing surgical difficulty and outcome. Neurosurgery 1992;31:604–605

118. Pertuiset B, Ancri D, Kinuta Y, et al. Classification of supratentorial arteriovenous malformations. A score system for evaluation of operability and surgical strategy based on an analysis of 66 cases. Acta Neurochir (Wien) 1991;110:6–16

119. Lunsford LD, Kondziolka D, Flickinger JC, et al. Stereotactic radiosurgery for arteriovenous malformations of the brain. J Neurosurg 1991;75:512–524

120. Fabrikant JI, Lyman JT, Hosobuchi Y. Stereotactic heavy-ion Bragg peak radiosurgery for intra-cranial vascular disorders: method for treatment of deep arteriovenous malformations. Br J Radiol 1984;57:479–490

121. Steiner L, Leksell L, Greitz T, Forster DM, Backlund EO. Stereotaxic radiosurgery for cerebral arteriovenous malformations. Report of a case. Acta Chir Scand 1972;138:459–464

122. Friedman WA, Bova FJ, Mendenhall WM. Linear accelerator radiosurgery for arteriovenous malformations: the relationship of size to outcome. J Neurosurg 1995;82:180–189

123. Taylor CL, Dutton K, Rappard G, et al. Complications of preoperative embolization of cerebral arteriovenous malformations. J Neurosurg 2004;100:810–812

124. Pollock BE, Kondziolka D, Lunsford LD, Bissonette D, Flickinger JC. Repeat stereotactic radiosurgery of arteriovenous malformations: factors associated with incomplete obliteration. Neurosurgery 1996;38:318–324

125. Panagiotopoulos V, Gizewski E, Asgari S, Regel J, Forsting M, Wanke I. Embolization of intracranial arteriovenous malformations with ethylene-vinyl alcohol copolymer (Onyx). AJNR Am J Neuroradiol 2009;30:99–106

126. Saatci I, Geyik S, Yavuz K, Cekirge HS. Endovascular treatment of brain arteriovenous malformations with prolonged intranidal Onyx injection technique: long-term results in 350 consecutive patients with completed endovascular treatment course. J Neurosurg 2011;115:78–88

127. Abud DG, Riva R, Nakiri GS, Padovani F, Khawaldeh M, Mounayer C. Treatment of brain arteriovenous malformations by double arterial catheterization with simultaneous injection of Onyx: retrospective series of 17 patients. AJNR Am J Neuroradiol 2011;32:152–158

128. van Rooij WJ, Jacobs S, Sluzewski M, van der Pol B, Beute GN, Sprengers ME. Curative embolization of brain arteriovenous malformations with onyx: patient selection, embolization technique, and results. AJNR Am J Neuroradiol 2012;33:1299–1304

129. Schäuble B, Cascino GD, Pollock BE, et al. Seizure outcomes after stereotactic radiosurgery for cerebral arteriovenous malformations. Neurology 2004;63:683–687

130. Englot DJ, Young WL, Han SJ, McCulloch CE, Chang EF, Lawton MT. Seizure predictors and control after microsurgical resection of supratentorial arteriovenous malformations in 440 patients. Neurosurgery 2012;71:572–580, discussion 580

131. Yang SY, Kim DG, Chung HT, Paek SH. Radiosurgery for unruptured cerebral arteriovenous malformations: long-term seizure outcome. Neurology 2012;78:1292–1298

Chapter 18

Management of Symptomatic Carotid Stenosis

Case

A 65-year-old patient in otherwise good health has symptomatic 80% carotid occlusion.

Participants

Stenting for Carotid Stenosis: Rabih G. Tawk, Adnan H. Siddiqui, Elad I. Levy, and L. Nelson Hopkins

Advocating Carotid Endarterectomy: Markus Bookland and Christopher M. Loftus

Moderators: Managing Symptomatic Carotid Stenosis: Endarterectomy vs. Stenting: Ning Lin, A. John Popp, and Kai U. Frerichs

Stenting for Carotid Stenosis

Rabih G. Tawk, Adnan H. Siddiqui, Elad I. Levy, and L. Nelson Hopkins

This case is an excellent illustration of the difficulties associated with the decision-making process for patients with carotid artery disease. For this otherwise healthy patient, four essential approaches are possible: no treatment, medical treatment, endovascular intervention with carotid artery stenting (CAS), and open surgery with carotid endarterectomy (CEA). At our center, we prefer to define the degree of stenosis on the basis of a diagnostic cerebral angiogram, the study that continues to represent the gold standard for the evaluation of carotid disease. The diagnostic angiogram elucidates several factors that are essential to the decision-making process for selecting the optimal treatment for a given patient. In addition to the severity of stenosis, several essential elements guide our decision before recommending a treatment modality in general and in particular for this patient who is in good health. In this section, we review key studies comparing CAS to CEA and outline the advantages and current and practical indications for CAS. Our perspective is that of neurosurgeons trained in both open and endovascular surgery, and we define carotid lesions primarily on the basis of findings on the diagnostic cerebral angiogram. Because this patient has a symptomatic lesion, treatment with either CAS or CEA would be superior to medical treatment. In the presented case, we would evaluate the lesion's characteristics and the patient's candidacy for both CAS and CEA before making a final recommendation for or against CAS.

Background

Carotid artery disease is implicated in approximately 25% of ischemic stroke cases.[1] With advancements in endovascular technology and techniques and increasing experience and expertise among surgeons, the role of CAS in stroke prevention has continued to evolve. Many treatment centers now consider CAS to be a first-line, less invasive therapeutic alternative to CEA for patients at high risk for surgical complications. Subsequent to the publication of the results of the North American Symptomatic Carotid Endarterectomy Trial (NASCET)[2] and European Carotid Surgery Trial (ECST),[3] in which the benefits of CEA over the best available medical therapy were demonstrated, the Carotid Revascularization Endarterectomy versus Stent Trial (CREST)[4] and the Stenting and Angioplasty with Protection in Patients at High Risk for Endarterectomy (SAPPHIRE) trial[5] affirmed that CAS is not inferior to CEA for certain subgroups of patients.

Although the precise role of CAS in primary and secondary stroke prevention has not been defined, data from multiple reports have demonstrated the efficacy of CAS for treating patients with carotid artery stenosis.[6–9] Conse-

quently, the safety and the widespread use of CAS have created a dilemma regarding which method of carotid revascularization to use in which population, particularly in patients considered at high risk for CEA, as defined by NASCET.[10] Because the NASCET analysis included a highly selected group of patients and excluded those at high risk for surgery (**Table 18.1**), several newer trials documented the efficacy of CAS in both high-risk and standard-risk patients and compared these results with those from well-established reports on CEA.[4,9–13] The SAPPHIRE[5,13] and the Carotid Revascularization Using Endarterectomy or Stenting Systems (CaRESS)[11] trials suggested that the stenting procedure is not inferior in short- and long-term follow-ups of mixed cohorts of symptomatic and asymptomatic patients. The 30-day outcomes of the Endarterectomy Versus Angioplasty in Patients with Symptomatic Severe Carotid Stenosis (EVA-3S) study,[14] the Stent-supported Percutaneous Angioplasty of the Carotid artery versus Endarterectomy (SPACE) study,[2,9,15] and the International Carotid Stenting Study (ICSS)[16] have been analyzed extensively. Although EVA-3S[14] and SPACE[12] failed to reach the prespecified margin for the noninferiority of CAS compared with CEA for 30-day outcomes, longer term follow-up of these studies showed low and similar rates of ipsilateral stroke at 2 and 4 years of follow-up, respectively, in both treatment groups.

Recently, CREST demonstrated that the risk of the composite primary outcome of stroke (myocardial infarction) or death during the 30-day periprocedural period or ipsilateral stroke within 4 years after randomization did not differ significantly between CAS and CEA among standard-risk patients with symptomatic or asymptomatic carotid stenosis.[4] The incidence of stroke during the periprocedural period was lower in the CEA group than in the CAS group, and the incidence of periprocedural myocardial infarction and cranial nerve palsy was lower in the CAS group. The countervailing effects in the periprocedural event rates resulted in similar rates of primary outcomes in the two groups. After the periprocedural period, the ipsilateral stroke rates in CREST were 2.0% with CAS and 2.4% with CEA (similar to the rates in the SPACE and EVA-3S trials), suggesting excellent durability for up to 4 years.

Selection of Treatment Modality: CAS vs. CEA

The carotid stenosis population represents a heterogeneous mixture of individuals with specific underlying medical comorbidities and specific lesion characteristics. According to our experience, no single treatment can serve all patients as one group.[17] Both CEA and CAS are effective treatment options, and we believe that the treating physician should

Table 18.1 Criteria of Exclusion from the North American Symptomatic Carotid Endarterectomy Trial (NASCET)[2]

The following criteria were used to exclude patients from the study:

1. Age 80 years or older
2. Mentally compromised or unwilling to give consent
3. Both carotid arteries and their intracranial branches could not be visualized
4. An intracranial lesion was more severe than the surgically accessible lesion
5. Failure of the kidney, liver, or lung, or a cancer was judged likely to cause death within 5 years
6. Cerebral infarction on either side that deprived the patient of all useful function in the affected territory
7. Symptoms that could be attributed to nonatherosclerotic disease (e.g., fibromuscular dysplasia, aneurysm, or tumor)
8. Cardiac valvular or rhythm disorder likely to be associated with cardioembolic symptoms
9. Previous ipsilateral carotid endarterectomy

The following criteria were used to determine that patients were temporarily ineligible*:

1. Uncontrolled hypertension, diabetes mellitus, or unstable angina pectoris
2. Myocardial infarction within the previous 6 months
3. Signs of progressive neurologic dysfunction
4. Contralateral carotid endarterectomy within the previous 4 months
5. Major surgical procedure within the previous 30 days

*These patients could become eligible if the disorder causing their temporary ineligibility resolved within 120 days after their qualifying cerebrovascular events.

be able to match every patient to the technique that is safer, while realizing the highlights and the pitfalls of the existing data on each. Although the results from major trials that compared CAS to CEA (CREST, SPACE, EVA-3S) are similar to a certain degree with respect to specific parameters, CAS is particularly attractive in certain subgroups of patients, especially those who were excluded from the NASCET[2,10] because of associated medical "high risk" and poor surgical candidacy. The high-risk features for CEA that were adopted as criteria for including participants in CAS registries and trials are listed in **Table 18.2**. Therefore, selection of either CAS or CEA is not only about a better or a more durable technique but also requires attention to the patient's age, medical comorbidities, lesion characteristics, and proximal vascular anatomy (with respect to endovascular access). Further, as stent design, delivery systems, and cerebral embolic protection devices continue to be refined, the long-term outcomes for CAS continue to improve and the procedural risks continue to decrease.

Advantages of CAS

In the absence of detailed guidelines that specify the use of CEA or CAS, patients should be offered an approach that is both individualized and lesion-specific. We consider CEA and CAS as complementary methods for specific patient populations and lesions, and the assignment of a technique is not dichotomized for one technique versus the other. Indeed, patients at high risk for CEA are often low risk for CAS and vice versa. This objective evaluation allows us to select the optimal treatment modality for each patient, as most would be better served with a specific modality. From a

technical standpoint, CAS is a minimally invasive procedure and does not require neck dissection to expose the carotid artery, which is challenging especially in patients after radiation therapy or surgery of the neck area. Exposure is also very challenging in patients with a short neck and a lengthy stenotic lesion. In addition, CAS avoids prolonged brain hypoperfusion because no occlusion of the carotid artery is required. In CEA, the internal carotid artery (ICA) is occluded during resection of the lesion; thus, we favor CAS especially in patients with contralateral occlusion. Further, CEA-associated complications—mainly, cranial nerve palsies—are avoided. Moreover, some patients request the less invasive endovascular CAS procedure; thus, patient preference drives the approach selected as well.

Carotid artery stenting is particularly advantageous in several subgroups of patients, especially those with a variety of medical comorbidities. Such patients are deemed at high risk and therefore considered poor surgical candidates, yet could be easily treated with CAS. Another subgroup that would benefit substantially from CAS is represented by patients harboring very high lesions located toward the skull base. The retraction and dissection required to expose high lesions is substantial, and such lesions are associated with a high risk of cranial nerve injuries (in 7.6 to 27% of patients).[10,18] Patients who have undergone previous neck surgery have scar tissue that obscures the neurovascular structures and places them at an increased risk of injury.[19] Restenosis, which occurs in 1.5 to 49% of endarterectomy patients,[20,21] constitutes another technical challenge for CEA. With increasing patient longevity, medical comorbidities are increasingly encountered and carotid disease recurs with greater frequency. CAS circumvents the need to

Table 18.2 High-Risk Features for Carotid Endarterectomy

1. A history of myocardial infarction within 30 days
2. Unstable angina with electrocardiographic changes
3. Angina with two-vessel coronary artery disease
4. New York Heart Association class 3–4 congestive heart failure
5. An ejection fraction < 30%
6. Chronic obstructive pulmonary disease with < 30% of predicted forced expiratory volume in 1 second (FEV_1)
7. Heart surgery required within 30 days
8. Vascular surgery required within 30 days
9. Age > 75 years
10. High cervical or intrathoracic stenosis
11. A previous ipsilateral carotid endarterectomy
12. A history of radical neck dissection or neck irradiation
13. Bilateral carotid artery stenosis, contralateral occlusion
14. A previous contralateral carotid endarterectomy with cranial nerve palsy
15. Immobility of the cervical spine
16. A crescendo of or recent transient ischemic attacks
17. Tandem stenosis
18. Intracranial hypoperfusion
19. Tracheostomy

operate through scarring and permits the treatment of lesions located at the proximal and distal ends of the endarterectomy sites, which are difficult to access surgically. Because the complication rate associated with a repeated CEA can be as high as 10.9%, CAS is likely safer than a second CEA in cases of recurrent stenoses.[19,22–24] Another setting in which CAS is particularly beneficial is for patients in whom lesions are caused by diseases other than atherosclerosis, such as radiation-induced stenosis and fibromuscular dysplasia. Radiation-induced stenoses tend to be longer than atherosclerotic lesions, often extending from the origin of the ICA to the skull base, and are usually composed of atheromatous debris and sclerotic tissue, which clearly complicates CEA.[25–27] Such patients have altered anatomic planes and a poor capacity to heal and, therefore, might be better served with CAS.[28,29] Further, patients who develop stenosis after radiation are also more likely to have undergone previous neck surgery, another factor that complicates CEA.

Carotid artery stenting also represents a superior treatment option in patients with symptomatic thrombus, in which the stent can plaster the thrombus against the vascular wall and prevent it from distal migration. Likewise, CEA is difficult in the setting of carotid dissection because of the typically distal location and long extension of these lesions compared with atherosclerotic stenosis. Open surgical treatment of carotid dissections is associated with a high complication rate and normally consists of proximal vessel ligation, direct repair, embolectomy, or bypass, because CEA is generally not recommended.[30,31] For these lesions, CAS represents a superior option[32–40] and is now the treatment of choice for symptomatic dissections not responding to anticoagulants.[32,41,42] Stenting can reapproximate an intimal flap against the wall and maintain patency of the lumen. Endovascular techniques also permit possible treatment of associated pseudoaneurysms. In the absence of guidelines for the management of ICA dissections, we recommend stenting for cases in which the patient experiences ischemic symptoms despite medical therapy, for cases involving radiographic progression of the lesion, and for cases in which the stenosis exceeds 80%.

Another scenario in which we favor CAS is for cases of contralateral ICA occlusion. Compared with patients with unilateral disease, CEA is associated with a higher rate of complications in patients with contralateral occlusion, and, according to the NASCET investigators, the 30-day risk of stroke and death approaches 14.3%.[2] This risk is likely attributable to the time needed for ICA clamping during CEA (NASCET median, 32 minutes) in patients with poor intracranial collateral circulation. We have found CAS particularly advantageous in this setting because CAS avoids prolonged ICA occlusion, which is typically limited to 5 to 15 seconds to inflate the angioplasty balloon.[43] Further, we typically perform CAS with the patient under conscious sedation with continuous neurologic evaluation. In these settings, clinically significant complications (such as embolization of plaque that can lead to stroke) may be managed or treated immediately through the existing proximal access route.

To date, CAS outcomes likely have been hindered by our limited knowledge of atherosclerotic lesions and inappropriate selection of patients. Currently, the need for CEA or CAS is dictated solely by the degree of lumen obstruction, and many centers use only Doppler imaging, which is operator-dependent, to assess the severity of the stenosis. Recently, it has been shown that the histology, morphology, and composition of carotid plaques play a major role in and seem to influence the outcomes of CAS to a greater degree than those of CEA.[44] Although angiography is poor in detecting the composition of atherosclerotic lesions, virtual histology, a new technology incorporated into intravascular ultrasound equipment, allows a histological characterization of plaques by creating a reproducible analysis of the radiofrequency and amplitude data of the ultrasound waves that cross different tissues. By characterizing the morphology, extension, and histology of the plaque, this technique provides important information to confirm the percentage of stenosis and judge its embolic potential, tailor the procedure, guide the choice of stent, and check stent apposition and complete coverage of vulnerable plaques. We have had a favorable experience with intravascular ultrasound during CAS,[45] and virtual histology intravascular ultrasound has the potential to further optimize patient and lesion selection criteria for CAS to improve procedure-related outcomes.[44]

Conclusion

In our opinion, carotid revascularization with CAS or CEA, performed by highly qualified surgeons with dual training, is safe and effective. When assessing patients with ICA stenosis, we consider the relative risks associated with CEA and CAS and their applicability to specific patient populations and lesion types. CAS continues to be particularly attractive for several groups of patients, especially those at increased risk for undergoing CEA (e.g., patients who were excluded from the NASCET). Our practice of open and endovascular surgery performed by neurosurgeons with dual training represents an attempt to increase safety and completeness in the management of neurovascular disorders, and perhaps this practice model will bridge the gap between open and endovascular subspecialties and pave the way for treatment of cerebrovascular disorders in the future.

Advocating Carotid Endarterectomy

Markus Bookland and Christopher M. Loftus

As a disease entity, carotid artery stenosis rarely presents without serious and compelling comorbidities. Such comorbidities must be factored into any treatment strategy for carotid artery stenosis and to evaluate the merit of medical treatment alone, endovascular treatment (namely CAS), and surgical reconstruction (namely CEA) in search of the optimal therapy for these patients. Illustrating the benefits of CEA, we present a 64-year-old patient with severe bilateral carotid artery stenosis.

This patient presented initially with a sudden onset of right-sided central facial palsy and upper extremity paresis. She had a history of peripheral vascular disease and severe congestive heart failure. A standard stroke workup uncovered a left internal capsule infarct and bilateral ca-

rotid artery stenoses (**Fig. 18.1**). The patient had not previously sought treatment for her constellation of medical problems and was therefore referred initially for medical optimization. Her primary medical providers recommended she begin aspirin therapy and undergo placement of a defibrillator, and they consulted with our department for treatment of her stenosis. A left CEA was recommended, and the patient agreed to the procedure after a full discussion of the risks and benefits.

Procedure

The preparation of the patient for CEA began with general endotracheal intubation, the placement of an arterial

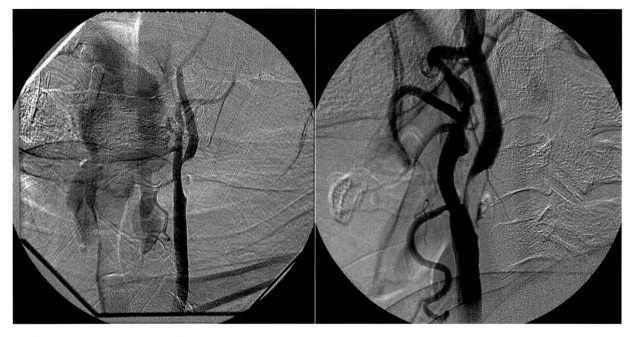

Fig. 18.1 Angiograms of the left and right common carotid arteries, respectively, showing more than 70% stenosis of the bifurcations.

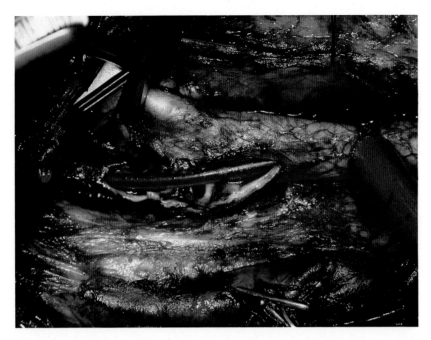

Fig. 18.2 The Loftus shunt can be seen bridging the arteriotomy from the common carotid artery to the internal carotid artery. The black stripe indicates the middle of the tubing and can be used to detect migration of the catheter.

line, and concurrent somatosensory evoked potential (SSEP) monitoring and electroencephalograph (EEG) for redundant electrophysiological monitoring during surgery. This preparation is consistent with our experimental protocol at Temple University School of Medicine.

After sterile preparation and draping, the patient's skin and subcutaneous tissues were dissected sharply down through the platysma, along the medial border of the sternocleidomastoid muscle. This dissection proceeded down until the common carotid artery (CCA) came into view. At this point, the anesthesiologist was instructed to administer 5,000 units of intravenous heparin. With the heparin given and with the CCA, ICA, and external carotid artery sufficiently exposed, a sterile marking pen was used to draw a line along the carotid, approximating the proposed arteriotomy.

Next, in preparation for cross-clamping the carotid vessels, we asked the EEG and SSEP technicians to obtain baseline readings. The ICA was occluded first, followed by the CCA, and finally the external carotid artery was closed. The arteriotomy was begun in the CCA with a No. 11 scalpel blade and followed with Potts angled scissors. The blue-marked arteriotomy line was followed from the CCA up to the bifurcation, and then up the ICA until normal vessel lumen was encountered.

Some small left-sided EEG/SSEP changes were noted upon clamping of the ICA; for this reason, a Loftus carotid endarterectomy shunt (Integra LifeSciences, Plainsboro, NJ) was carefully passed into the CCA and secured by pulling up on the silk tie surrounding the artery **(Fig. 18.2)**. A small Scanlan–Loftus custom ICA pinch clamp was used to secure the shunt after its passage into the distal ICA. With the plaque exposed and carotid blood flow controlled, a Freer

plaque dissector was then used to gently dissect the plaque away from the arterial wall.

Once the vessel wall was clean and smooth, we repaired the arteriotomy defect with a Hemashield patch graft, as is our routine. A running, nonlocking 6–0 Prolene suture (BV-1 needle) stitch was used to close the fitted patch to the arteriotomy walls **(Fig. 18.3)**. To remove the Loftus shunt, a small opening was temporarily left on the lateral CCA wall to retrieve the catheter.

With the arteriotomy fully repaired and the shunt removed, the de-clamping sequence began. A heparinized saline syringe with a blunt tip was inserted into a small lateral wall opening while the two stitches abutting the syringe were held tight. The vessel was filled with heparinized saline, while a surgeon's knot was thrown and laid down against the syringe. The final release of the arterial clamps then proceeded in the following sequence: first the external carotid artery, then the CCA, and, after a 10-second pause, the ICA.

Next, the retractors were removed and wound hemostasis was ensured by direct inspection. Carotid patency was once again confirmed with the handheld Doppler. A layered closure followed, including the carotid sheath, platysma, and skin. Subsequent to closure, the patient was awakened and extubated without complications; she was neurologically and hemodynamically stable.

A more extensive discussion of our recommended detailed surgical technique can be found in our carotid texts.[46–48]

CEA vs. CAS

Surgical intervention is the most highly effective treatment option for patients with carotid artery stenosis.[2] There is,

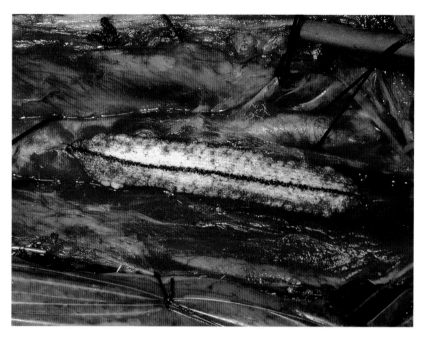

Fig. 18.3 The finished arteriotomy patch repair. The CCA, ICA, and external carotid artery have all been isolated with 0 silk ties. Toward the top of the image, the protected vagus nerve can be seen, and the hypoglossal nerve lies within a rubber loop just along the lateral edge of the figure.

however, a subset of high-risk patients with carotid artery stenosis and significant comorbidities, such as advanced age, poor cardiac function, and limited pulmonary reserve, that justifies consideration of alternative therapies. For this reason, some have advocated stenting (namely CAS) as a suitable alternative to CEA when dealing with complicated circumstances and frail patients.

The case presented above is an example of just such a patient. Her cardiac condition was complex, and the patient had been recommended for cardiac catheterization and defibrillator placement at some point in the perioperative period. Additionally, the patient had a significant oxygen requirement at baseline and suffered near constant dyspnea. Although we agree that these comorbidities warrant consideration of a stent, CAS, somewhat surprisingly, has simply not proved to be as effective or safe as surgical carotid reconstruction.

We have reviewed 11 reports of randomized controlled trials comparing CEA and CAS.[5,8,9,11,13,49–54] The results have varied, but they have universally failed to validate CAS as a superior treatment for carotid artery stenosis. In fact, several have found CAS to have a much higher risk of subacute cardiovascular events than does carotid surgery. In 1998, the Leicester trial, though limited by a small sample size, found a 45% increase in periprocedural cardiovascular events among CAS patients compared with CEA patients. In 2001, the WALLSTENT multicenter randomized controlled trials found an alarming rate of ipsilateral strokes and deaths among CAS patients (CAS 12.1% vs. CEA 3.6%).[52,54] Several randomized controlled trials have since attempted to reverse the stigma of 30-day and 1-year infarcts from carotid

stenting, but these have largely failed. The SAPPHIRE trial, released in 2004, stands as the lone exception. We note, however, that the trial included an enormous number of patients, nearly all receiving stents, who were treated outside of the trial, which always introduces the specter of a selection bias against surgery. In addition, the SAPPHIRE results that claim equipoise, unfortunately, have not been reproducible in subsequent, larger randomized controlled trials.[5,13]

In the absence of equipoise, then, for low-risk patients, CAS has been most strongly advocated for treating patients with carotid artery stenosis who have significant comorbidities. Elderly patients are often considered to be a high-risk group for whom CAS might be attractive. However, several prospective and retrospective studies have compared CEA and CAS in the elderly and found that age does not significantly alter the results. A review of 53 patients older than 70 years at the University of Iowa Hospital found no differences in CEA outcomes in these patients when compared with historic, younger controls.[55] Similarly, and alarmingly, a meta-analysis of eight CAS study groups and 33 CEA study groups that selected for patients over 80 years of age identified increased rates of postprocedural stroke among CAS patients, similar to those rates noted in past randomized controlled trials. No other differences were seen in periprocedural or long-term mortality and myocardial events in these studies.[56]

Some groups have recommended CAS rather than CEA for patients with unfavorable cervical anatomy, the so-called hostile neck. Patients with previous neck surgeries, high carotid bifurcations, irradiated cervical fields, or a nonextendable neck may be considered more efficaciously approached through an endovascular route. A case-controlled trial in 2009 addressed this question by prospectively pairing and following 154 CEA patients. In the final analysis, no difference in periprocedural ischemic events or mortality was noted.[57] Although a direct comparison between CAS and CEA patients with difficult anatomy has yet to be done, these initial data would give credence to the thought that the hostile neck has little bearing on CEA outcomes when a skilled surgeon performs the procedure.

Carotid artery stenting (with distal protective devices) has been an innovative new technique for the treatment of carotid stenosis, and no doubt has its place in the management of this disease. But the evidence to date is unequivocal and strongly favors surgical repair. No high-risk group yet stratified has shown improved results with CAS when compared with CEA, and in broader-based randomized controlled trials there has been consistent and reproducible evidence for a lower 30-day stroke and death rate for patients randomized to CEA. The results of the CREST trial, comparing endovascular and surgical treatment for non–high-risk carotid stenosis patients, are eagerly awaited as this chapter was being written. In the absence of novel data to support CAS, however, current evidence-based medicine continues to confirm the superiority of CEA over CAS for treating patients with carotid stenosis.

Managing Symptomatic Carotid Stenosis: Endarterectomy vs. Stenting

Ning Lin, A. John Popp, and Kai U. Frerichs

From the outset, it should be stated that the senior author of each of the above two sections (L.N.H. and C.M.L.) not only are thought leaders in their respective fields but also have extensive experience and have been involved with the evolution of the management paradigm for symptomatic carotid stenosis over the past three decades. Although we find little fault with what has been stated by either group of authors, we believe that the issues being explored may be much more nuanced than the "either/or" scenarios proposed by the two sections. These nuances form the substance of our discussion.

In essence, Bookland and Loftus advocate endarterectomy as superior to carotid stenting with lower periprocedural stroke and death rates, and they have highlighted the importance of the technical proficiency of the operating surgeon. Tawk and associates emphasize the benefit of carotid stenting in certain subsets of patients with symptomatic carotid stenosis, while taking an evolutionary view of the field by asserting the complementary nature of endarterectomy and stenting. In this section, we provide a review of the currently available literature on the treatment of symptomatic carotid stenosis and discuss the relative advantages and limitations of these two approaches.

Early Clinical Trials

Atherosclerotic stenosis of the carotid artery is an important cause of cerebral ischemia and is estimated to be responsible for up to 20% of all ischemic strokes.[51,58,59] The management of carotid bifurcation atherosclerosis as a source of stroke first received detailed conceptual and pathoanatomic attention from C. Miller Fisher in the early 1950s.[60] Thereafter, reports of successful surgical treatment of carotid bifurcation atherosclerosis followed.[61] Between 1950 and 1991, opinions about the utility of CEA fluctuated considerably due to conflicting findings regarding the risks, benefits, and proper indications for the procedure.[62–65] A series of randomized controlled clinical trials in the 1990s performed in North America[2,66] and Europe[67] unequivocally demonstrated that CEA combined with medical therapy is superior to medical therapy alone for stroke prevention in certain symptomatic patients with high-grade carotid stenosis. As a result of these trials, for nearly two decades CEA was established firmly as superior to the best medical treatment of the era for certain patients with symptomatic carotid stenosis.

Initially, the technique for endovascular treatment of carotid stenosis was balloon angioplasty, which was first introduced in 1980s.[68–70] Early, nonrandomized case series showed the potential benefits of an endovascular approach, including no surgical incision, a need for only local anesthesia, and a shorter length of stay, but there remained a substantial concern about the safety of the procedure.[52,68,71,72] One of the first randomized controlled trials, the Carotid and Vertebral Artery Transluminal Angioplasty Study (CAVATAS),[51] compared the results of carotid balloon angioplasty with or without stenting to endarterectomy in patients with symptomatic carotid stenosis (**Table 18.3**). This study showed that the 30-day stroke or death rate was similar in both groups (approximately 10%) and that minor complications such as cranial nerve palsies and wound complications occurred more frequently in the CEA group. Although the study highlighted the benefits of a minimally invasive approach, the periprocedural stroke/

Table 18.3 Major Randomized Controlled Clinical Trials Comparing Endarterectomy and Carotid Stenting for the Treatment of Symptomatic Carotid Stenosis

Study	Pub. Year	No. of Patients	Patient Population	Degree of Stenosis	Primary Endpoint	Follow-up Period	Cumulative Incidence of Adverse Events at 30 Days	Cumulative Incidence of Adverse Events at Latest Follow-Up	Conclusion
CAVATAS[51]	2001 2009	504	Symptomatic	> 50%	Stroke + death	5 years	10.0% in CAA/CAS, 9.9% in CEA (p = 0.98)	11.3% in CAA/CAS, 8.6% in CEA (p = NS)*	Similar risks and effectiveness for CAS/CAA and CEA
SAPPHIRE[5]	2004 2008	334	Symptomatic and asymptomatic, high risk	> 50%	Stroke + death + MI	3 years	4.7% CAS, 9.8% in CEA (p = 0.09)	24.6% in CAS versus 26.9% in CEA (p = 0.71)	CAS not inferior to CEA
EVA-3S[8]	2006 2008	527	Symptomatic	> 60%	Stroke + death	4 years	9.6% in CAS, 3.9% in CEA (p = 0.01)	11.1% in CAS, 6.2% in CEA (p = 0.03)	CAS more risky than CEA
SPACE[9]	2006 2008	1,200	Symptomatic	> 50%	Stroke + death	2 years	6.8% in CAS, 6.3% in CEA (p = 0.09)	9.5% in CAS, 8.8% in CEA (p = 0.62)	Failed to prove noninferiority of CAS versus CEA
ICSS[16]	2010	1,713	Symptomatic	> 50%	Stroke + death + MI	120 days	7.4% in CAS, 4.0% in CEA (p = 0.003)	8.5% in CAS, 5.2% in CEA (p = 0.006)	CAS more risky than CEA
CREST[4]	2010	2,502	Symptomatic and asymptomatic	> 50%	Stroke + death + MI	4 years	5.2% in CAS, 4.5% in CEA (p = 0.38)	7.2% in CAS, 6.8% in CEA (p = 0.51)	CAS equivalent to CEA

Abbreviations: CAA, carotid artery angioplasty; CAS, carotid angioplasty and stenting; CEA, carotid endarterectomy; MI, myocardial infarction; NS, not significant.

Trial names: CAVATAS, Carotid and Vertebral Artery Transluminal Angioplasty Study; SAPPHIRE, Stenting and Angioplasty with Protection in Patients at High Risk for Endarterectomy; EVA-3S, Endarterectomy versus Angioplasty in Patients with Symptomatic Severe Carotid Stenosis; SPACE, Stent-Protected Percutaneous Angioplasty of the Carotid versus Endarterectomy; ICSS, International Carotid Stenting Study; CREST, Carotid Revascularization Endarterectomy versus Stent Trial.

* Ipsilateral non-perioperative stroke rate at long-term follow-up.

death rate was high in both groups (10.0% for stenting vs. 9.9% for endarterectomy), and stenting was used only in 26% of the patients. Long-term results (median follow-up of 5 years) assessed by determining the rate of non-perioperative stroke (greater than 30 days after the procedure) did not differ between the CAS and CEA groups (1.4% vs. 1.1% per year, respectively),[73] but the study itself was not designed to detect a significant difference.

Since the completion of CAVATAS, carotid artery angioplasty and CAS largely replaced angioplasty alone, and distal embolic protection devices specifically engineered for stenting procedures have been introduced. Subsequently, European investigators have performed two randomized controlled trials comparing carotid stenting to endarterectomy (EVA-3S and SPACE)[8,9] and another trial was done in the U.S. in patients with high risks for open surgery (SAPPHIRE).[5] All three trials were designed to test the hypothesis that CAS was not inferior to CEA for treating high-grade carotid stenosis. The SAPPHIRE trial was the first large randomized study to use crush-resistant stents with an embolic protection device.[5] The trial recruited both symptomatic and asymptomatic patients with high surgical risks (e.g., significant cardiac disease, recurrent stenosis, age older than 80, etc.), and used a composite endpoint of death, stroke, or myocardial infarction within 30 days of intervention or death or ipsilateral stroke up to 1 year postprocedure to test its noninferiority hypothesis. The authors reported that the composite endpoint occurred less frequently in the CAS group (12.2% vs. 20.1%, p = 0.004 for noninferiority), and concluded that CAS with an embolic protection device was not inferior to CEA for high-risk patients with severe carotid stenosis. In a follow-up analysis, there was again no significant difference in the cumulative incidence of major cerebrovascular events between the two groups 3 years after intervention.[13]

Although SAPPHIRE included both symptomatic and asymptomatic patients, both European trials recruited only patients with symptomatic carotid stenosis. The EVA-3S study, conducted in France, was terminated prematurely for reasons of safety and futility after enrollment of 527 patients.[8] The authors reported a higher 30-day risk of stroke or death in the CAS group compared with the CEA group (9.6% vs. 3.9%, respectively, p = 0.01), and in a follow-up publication,[14] a higher cumulative probability of periprocedural stroke or death and nonprocedural ipsilateral stroke after 4 years in the CAS group was identified as well (11.1% vs. 6.2%, respectively, p = 0.03). In addition, most of the difference in cumulative outcome at 4 years could be accounted for by the higher incidence of periprocedural complications in the CAS group. The other European trial, SPACE, was conducted in Germany during the same time period.[9] This study randomized 1,200 patients and reported a similar 30-day risk of stroke or death in the CAS and the CEA groups (6.84% vs. 6.34%, respectively); however, it failed to prove noninferiority (p = 0.09), probably because of small differences in outcome and an insufficient number of patients. The long-term results showed that the

cumulative risk of ipsilateral stroke or death up to 2 years was again similar, but recurrent stenosis (> 70%) after initial treatment occurred more frequently in the CAS group (11.1%) than in the CEA group (4.6%).[12]

Although neither EVA-3S nor SPACE proved the noninferiority of CAS compared with CEA, the data suggested that the stroke risk after stenting was likely concentrated in the periprocedural period, and that the mid- to long-term recurrent stroke rate was low (approximately 1% per year) regardless of the treatment selected. Both studies were criticized for using a wide variety of stents and for including inexperienced neurointerventionists in the trial. Therefore, there was a strong demand for larger, more rigorously designed trials to further assess the risks and benefits of carotid stenting.

The Latest Clinical Trials

In 2010, the International Carotid Stenting Study (ICSS) trial closed enrollment and an interim safety analysis[16] was published. The study randomized 1,713 patients with symptomatic moderate-to-severe carotid stenosis (> 50%) in 50 centers, mostly in Europe. The investigators reported that, within 120 days of intervention, the incidence of stroke, death, or periprocedural myocardial infarction was 8.5% for the CAS group and 5.2% in the CEA group (p = 0.006). The individual risks of any stroke (7.7% vs. 4.1%, p = 0.002) or all-cause death (2.3% vs. 0.8%, p = 0.017) were both higher in the stenting group. Not surprisingly, the rate of cranial nerve and wound complications was lower in the CAS group. A subset of patients enrolled in the ICSS trial participated in an imaging study that required them to undergo magnetic resonance imaging before and after treatment. Almost three times more patients were found to have new diffusion-weighted-image bright, ischemic lesions on posttreatment scans in the CAS group than in the CEA group.[74] The ICSS authors concluded that stenting carried a higher periprocedural risk and that endarterectomy should remain the treatment of choice for patients with symptomatic severe carotid stenosis.

The CREST is the largest randomized controlled trial of these two approaches.[4] The study randomized 2,502 patients with symptomatic or asymptomatic carotid stenosis in 117 centers in the United States and Canada, and collected follow-up data for up to 4 years. The primary endpoint was again the composite of 30-day rates of stroke, myocardial infarction, or death or ipsilateral stroke occurring after the periprocedural period. The study found no statistical difference between the CAS and the CEA groups (7.2% vs. 6.8%, respectively, p = 0.51). The risk of periprocedural stroke or death was higher in the CAS group (4.4% vs. 2.3%, p = 0.005), whereas myocardial infarction occurred more frequently in the CEA group (1.1% vs. 2.3%, p = 0.03). When considering only the 1,321 symptomatic patients, the risk of periprocedural stroke or death was also higher in the CAS group (6.0% vs. 3.2%, p = 0.02). Nevertheless, if myocardial infarction was included in the cumulative endpoint, there was no significant difference between the CAS and CEA groups (6.7% vs. 5.4%, respectively, $p = 0.30$). The investigators concluded that, despite the higher periprocedural risk, carotid stenting could be a safe and effective alternative treatment for carotid stenosis if performed by sufficiently trained neurointerventionists.

The completion of these two large, multinational, randomized controlled trials fueled the latest debate about stenting versus endarterectomy. These most recent studies were well executed with overall low stroke rates in both CAS and CEA groups, which suggests many technical advancements and improvements in medical management since the publication of the NASCET.[2] Both trials reported a higher 30-day stroke rate in the stenting group. The rate of myocardial infarction reported in CREST was much higher than in the ICSS (42 cases, or 1.7% vs. eight cases, or 0.5%, respectively). This difference was likely due to different screening criteria for periprocedural cardiovascular events; although the CREST investigators routinely screened postoperative cardiac biomarkers, those of the ICSS evaluated only patients with cardiac symptoms. Including myocardial infarction in the composite primary endpoint was controversial and was different from earlier trials; nevertheless, the acceptably low stroke rate after stenting and its overall durability confirmed in CREST underlined the merit of CAS as a stroke-prevention procedure. Additional subgroup analyses and risk stratification will provide further insights into the proper patient selection and utilization of CAS.

The Relative Advantages and Disadvantages of Each Approach

When results from all clinical trials are considered (**Table 18.3**), several preliminary conclusions can be drawn. The periprocedural stroke rate for low- to medium-risk patients with symptomatic carotid stenosis appears to be higher with CAS than with CEA, a disadvantage that has been consistently demonstrated in four of the most recent randomized clinical trials (EVA-3S, SPACE, ICSS, CREST). In contrast, CEA seems to carry a higher risk of periprocedural myocardial infarction, especially in high-risk patients. These data should not be taken to suggest that the two forms of complication are equivalent; for example, CREST found that major and minor strokes had a significant impact on physical health at 1 year, whereas myocardial infarction did not.

On the other hand, there has been a marked improvement in outcomes from CAS since the first randomized, controlled trial, CAVATAS. The two most recent large studies (ICSS and CREST) reported outcomes after CAS similar to the postoperative results in NASCET.[2] Data from 2 to 4 years of follow-up also show that the additional stroke risk after stenting is mostly periprocedural, and CAS is as effective and durable as CEA for middle-term stroke prevention.[4,14] These results collectively suggest that CAS could be a reasonable choice for patients with symptomatic carotid stenosis (> 50%) who may not be considered for surgery or who prefer to avoid open procedures. This is not an inconsequential observation, because it has been reported in other surgical specialties that patients, in general, choose less invasive treatments,[75–77] and such a mindset likely exists in patients with symptomatic carotid stenosis.

Patients with coexisting conditions, such as severe cardiac or pulmonary disease, prior neck radiation, or recurrent carotid stenosis that could potentially increase surgical risks, were excluded from most of the large clinical trials. Although the results from SAPPHIRE indicate the noninferiority of CAS compared with CEA in treating high-risk patients, the study included both symptomatic and asymptomatic patients. Additional investigation is necessary to further establish risk-and-benefit profiles for symptomatic patients with concurrent medical comorbidities, because multiple studies after NASCET have shown that the most frequent inappropriate indication for endarterectomy is high comorbidity,[78] and that patients with increased comorbidities have a higher perioperative risk of stroke and death.[78–81] In addition, despite the strong advocacy of Bookland and Loftus for using CEA in patients with recurrent stenosis or prior neck radiation, CEA is certainly more technically difficult in such settings. Carotid stenting may provide a less invasive and safer alternative for patients with these unfavorable preoperative risk profiles.

Provider and Institution Volume and the Lessons of Clinical Trials

The most recent randomized clinical trials have similar inclusion/exclusion criteria, and have focused on medium-risk patients with moderate-to-severe symptomatic carotid stenosis. The standardization of the trial design has made it possible to apply the study results to most patients with symptomatic carotid stenosis in the general population who fit the inclusion criteria of the studies. Those with high surgical risks, on the other hand, were not included in these trials. In addition to this caveat, practitioner expertise may be a challenging facet of the overall ability to generalize the recently conducted trials. When studying evolving technology or cutting-edge techniques, an important aspect of trial design is to ensure a common, high level of experience and expertise in the study investigators. Hence, CREST used a rigorous credentialing process for all interventionists in the trial to ensure sufficient endovascular expertise in carotid stent placement, which was only loosely regulated in other studies. However, the practitioner profiles of those involved in the trial are not likely representative of the wider community of neurosurgeons, vascular surgeons, and neurointerventionists. Additional studies are therefore needed before the results of CREST can be applied to the general population. A similar phenomenon was observed after NASCET and the Asymptomatic Carotid Artery Stenosis (ACAS) study legitimized and popularized endarterectomy for both symptomatic and asymptomatic patients with severe carotid stenosis. Multiple subsequent population-based studies showed that the outcome after CEA was closely associated with provider and hospital volume.[82–84]

Future Investigations

Although carotid endarterectomy is a mature procedure that has been practiced and perfected for almost half a century, carotid stenting is still in the developmental period. Better stent design and more effective embolic protection technology are crucial areas of future investigations. For example, the currently available distal embolic protection devices were not uniformly shown to reduce the risk of periprocedural stroke,[74,85] and one study using Doppler ultrasonography reported that continued distal emboli could be detected throughout the stenting procedure, despite placement of an embolic protection device.[86] A newer technology for proximal embolic protection has recently been introduced. It simulates the antegrade and retrograde blood-flow cessation achieved during CEA (common and external carotid clamping) with balloon occlusion of the common and external carotid artery before traversing the stenotic lesions.[87] This device has been used in Europe, and a recently completed pivotal trial in the U.S. reported the periprocedural risk of stroke and myocardial infarction to be 2.7%,[87] lower than that reported in CREST and ICSS.

Additional investigation is also needed to establish demographic and clinical parameters associated with complications after CAS stenting for better risk stratification and patient selection. A recent subgroup analysis of the EVA-3S trial, focusing on the anatomic and technical factors, found that increased ICA to CCA angulation (> 60 degrees), left-sided CAS, and target stenotic lesions longer than 10 mm were associated with higher periprocedural stroke or death after CAS.[85] In addition, both CREST[74] and a recent meta-analysis[88] of pooled data from ICSS, EVA-3S, and SPACE reported that age was an important predictor of periprocedural stroke after carotid stenting. Older patients (> 70 years) were found to have a significantly higher risk compared with younger patients, most likely because of increased vascular tortuosity and the overall atherosclerotic

burden that increases with age. These results need to be confirmed to refine the proper indications for carotid stenting.

There has been a growing demand to reassess the relative benefit of any form of intervention compared with the best available medical management for carotid stenosis; this may require a clinical trial that features a treatment arm of aggressive medical therapy alone versus intervention. Given the convincing results from NASCET and ECST and the substantial risk reduction provided through surgery, such a study is unlikely to be conducted on symptomatic patients with carotid stenosis. However, several recent investigations suggest that the overall stroke risk from asymptomatic carotid stenosis, especially in women, is low if the patient is under maximum medical management.[89,90] Some stroke neurologists recommend revascularization for patients with asymptomatic carotid stenosis only if carotid ultrasonography shows plaque echolucency[91] or transcranial Doppler detects microembolic events.[91,92] A three-arm randomized controlled trial in asymptomatic patients, SPACE II, is ongoing and the results are anticipated in a few years.[93]

Conclusion

We believe that endarterectomy and stenting are complementary, rather than competing, treatments for symptomatic carotid stenosis. As an evolving procedure, CAS is undergoing the same process of technical refinement and analysis that endarterectomy did several decades ago. Ultimately, it is important that clinicians neither dismiss stenting as an inferior choice compared with surgery nor claim that stenting, at its current technical state, is a suitable choice for all patients with carotid stenosis. A close collaboration between open and endovascular surgeons and additional bioengineering as well as clinical research should be pursued to provide improved benefits to patients with symptomatic carotid stenosis.

References

1. Zhu CZ, Norris JW. Role of carotid stenosis in ischemic stroke. Stroke 1990;21:1131–1134
2. North American Symptomatic Carotid Endarterectomy Trial Collaborators. Beneficial effect of carotid endarterectomy in symptomatic patients with high-grade carotid stenosis. N Engl J Med 1991;325:445–453
3. Randomised Trial of Endarterectomy for Recently Symptomatic Carotid Stenosis. Randomised trial of endarterectomy for recently symptomatic carotid stenosis: final results of the MRC European Carotid Surgery Trial (ECST). Lancet 1998;351:1379–1387
4. Brott TG, Hobson RW II, Howard G, et al; CREST Investigators. Stenting versus endarterectomy for treatment of carotid-artery stenosis. N Engl J Med 2010;363:11–23
5. Yadav JS, Wholey MH, Kuntz RE, et al; Stenting and Angioplasty with Protection in Patients at High Risk for Endarterectomy Investigators. Protected carotid-artery stenting versus endarterectomy in high-risk patients. N Engl J Med 2004;351:1493–1501

6. Featherstone RL, Brown MM, Coward LJ; ICSS Investigators. International carotid stenting study: protocol for a randomised clinical trial comparing carotid stenting with endarterectomy in symptomatic carotid artery stenosis. Cerebrovasc Dis 2004;18:69–74
7. Hobson RW II. Update on the Carotid Revascularization Endarterectomy versus Stent Trial (CREST) protocol. J Am Coll Surg 2002;194(1, Suppl):S9–S14
8. Mas JL, Chatellier G, Beyssen B, et al; EVA-3S Investigators. Endarterectomy versus stenting in patients with symptomatic severe carotid stenosis. N Engl J Med 2006;355:1660–1671
9. Ringleb PA, Allenberg J, Brückmann H, et al; SPACE Collaborative Group. 30 day results from the SPACE trial of stent-protected angioplasty versus carotid endarterectomy in symptomatic patients: a randomised non-inferiority trial. Lancet 2006;368:1239–1247
10. North American Symptomatic Carotid Endarterectomy Trial. Methods, patient characteristics, and progress. Stroke 1991;22:711–720

11. CARESS Steering Committee. Carotid Revascularization using Endarterectomy or Stenting Systems (CARESS): phase I clinical trial. J Endovasc Ther 2003;10:1021–1030

12. Eckstein HH, Ringleb P, Allenberg JR, et al. Results of the Stent-Protected Angioplasty versus Carotid Endarterectomy (SPACE) study to treat symptomatic stenoses at 2 years: a multinational, prospective, randomised trial. Lancet Neurol 2008; 7:893–902

13. Gurm HS, Yadav JS, Fayad P, et al; SAPPHIRE Investigators. Long-term results of carotid stenting versus endarterectomy in high-risk patients. N Engl J Med 2008;358:1572–1579

14. Mas JL, Trinquart L, Leys D, et al; EVA-3S investigators. Endarterectomy Versus Angioplasty in Patients with Symptomatic Severe Carotid Stenosis (EVA-3S) trial: results up to 4 years from a randomised, multicentre trial. Lancet Neurol 2008;7: 885–892

15. Stingele R, Berger J, Alfke K, et al; SPACE investigators. Clinical and angiographic risk factors for stroke and death within 30 days after carotid endarterectomy and stent-protected angioplasty: a subanalysis of the SPACE study. Lancet Neurol 2008; 7:216–222

16. Ederle J, Dobson J, Featherstone RL, et al; International Carotid Stenting Study investigators. Carotid artery stenting compared with endarterectomy in patients with symptomatic carotid stenosis (International Carotid Stenting Study): an interim analysis of a randomised controlled trial. Lancet 2010;375: 985–997

17. Ecker RD, Lau T, Levy EI, Hopkins LN. Thirty-day morbidity and mortality rates for carotid artery intervention by surgeons who perform both carotid endarterectomy and carotid artery angioplasty and stent placement. J Neurosurg 2007;106:217–221

18. Yadav JS, Roubin GS, Iyer S, et al. Elective stenting of the extracranial carotid arteries. Circulation 1997;95:376–381

19. Callow AD. Recurrent stenosis after carotid endarterectomy. Arch Surg 1982;117:1082–1085

20. Hobson RW II, Goldstein JE, Jamil Z, et al. Carotid restenosis: operative and endovascular management. J Vasc Surg 1999;29: 228–235, discussion 235–238

21. Diethrich EB, Gordon MH, Lopez-Galarza LA, Rodriguez-Lopez JA, Casses F. Intraluminal Palmaz stent implantation for treatment of recurrent carotid artery occlusive disease: a plan for the future. J Interv Cardiol 1995;8:213–218

22. Das MB, Hertzer NR, Ratliff NB, O'Hara PJ, Beven EG. Recurrent carotid stenosis. A five-year series of 65 reoperations. Ann Surg 1985;202:28–35

23. Lanzino G, Mericle RA, Lopes DK, Wakhloo AK, Guterman LR, Hopkins LN. Percutaneous transluminal angioplasty and stent placement for recurrent carotid artery stenosis. J Neurosurg 1999;90:688–694

24. Rothwell PM, Slattery J, Warlow CP. A systematic review of the risks of stroke and death due to endarterectomy for symptomatic carotid stenosis. Stroke 1996;27:260–265

25. Ahuja A, Blatt GL, Guterman LR, Hopkins LN. Angioplasty for symptomatic radiation-induced extracranial carotid artery stenosis: case report. Neurosurgery 1995;36:399–403

26. Mellière D, Becquemin JP, Berrahal D, Desgranges P, Cavillon A. Management of radiation-induced occlusive arterial disease: a reassessment. J Cardiovasc Surg (Torino) 1997;38:261–269

27. Rockman CB, Riles TS, Fisher FS, Adelman MA, Lamparello PJ. The surgical management of carotid artery stenosis in patients with previous neck irradiation. Am J Surg 1996;172:191–195

28. Albuquerque FC, Teitelbaum GP, Larsen DW, Giannotta SL. Carotid endarterectomy compared with angioplasty and stenting: the status of the debate. Neurosurg Focus 1998;5:e2

29. Teitelbaum GP, Lefkowitz MA, Giannotta SL. Carotid angioplasty and stenting in high-risk patients. Surg Neurol 1998;50: 300–311, discussion 311–312

30. Müller BT, Luther B, Hort W, Neumann-Haefelin T, Aulich A, Sandmann W. Surgical treatment of 50 carotid dissections: indications and results. J Vasc Surg 2000;31:980–988

31. Schievink WI, Piepgras DG, McCaffrey TV, Mokri B. Surgical treatment of extracranial internal carotid artery dissecting aneurysms. Neurosurgery 1994;35:809–815, discussion 815–816

32. Bejjani GK, Monsein LH, Laird JR, Satler LF, Starnes BW, Aulisi EF. Treatment of symptomatic cervical carotid dissections with endovascular stents. Neurosurgery 1999;44:755–760, discussion 760–761

33. Coric D, Wilson JA, Regan JD, Bell DA. Primary stenting of the extracranial internal carotid artery in a patient with multiple cervical dissections: technical case report. Neurosurgery 1998; 43:956–959

34. Crawley F, Brown MM, Clifton AG. Angioplasty and stenting in the carotid and vertebral arteries. Postgrad Med J 1998;74: 7–10

35. Dorros G, Cohn JM, Palmer LE. Stent deployment resolves a petrous carotid artery angioplasty dissection. AJNR Am J Neuroradiol 1998;19:392–394

36. Griewing B, Brassel F, Schminke U, Kessler C. Angioplasty and stenting in carotid artery dissection. Eur Neurol 1998;40:175–176

37. Hong MK, Satler LF, Gallino R, Leon MB. Intravascular stenting as a definitive treatment of spontaneous carotid artery dissection. Am J Cardiol 1997;79:538

38. Horowitz MB, Miller G III, Meyer Y, Carstens G III, Purdy PD. Use of intravascular stents in the treatment of internal carotid and extracranial vertebral artery pseudoaneurysms. AJNR Am J Neuroradiol 1996;17:693–696

39. Hurst RW, Haskal ZJ, Zager E, Bagley LJ, Flamm ES. Endovascular stent treatment of cervical internal carotid artery aneurysms with parent vessel preservation. Surg Neurol 1998;50:313–317, discussion 317

40. Perez-Cruet MJ, Patwardhan RV, Mawad ME, Rose JE. Treatment of dissecting pseudoaneurysm of the cervical internal carotid artery using a wall stent and detachable coils: case report. Neurosurgery 1997;40:622–625, discussion 625–626

41. Bush RL, Lin PH, Dodson TF, Dion JE, Lumsden AB. Endoluminal stent placement and coil embolization for the management of carotid artery pseudoaneurysms. J Endovasc Ther 2001;8: 53–61

42. Malek AM, Higashida RT, Phatouros CC, et al. Endovascular management of extracranial carotid artery dissection achieved using stent angioplasty. AJNR Am J Neuroradiol 2000;21:1280–1292

43. Mericle RA, Kim SH, Lanzino G, et al. Carotid artery angioplasty and use of stents in high-risk patients with contralateral occlusions. J Neurosurg 1999;90:1031–1036

44. Inglese L, Fantoni C, Sardana V. Can IVUS-virtual histology improve outcomes of percutaneous carotid treatment? J Cardiovasc Surg (Torino) 2009;50:735–744

45. Wehman JC, Holmes DR Jr, Ecker RD, et al. Intravascular ultrasound identification of intraluminal embolic plaque material

during carotid angioplasty with stenting. Catheter Cardiovasc Interv 2006;68:853–857

46. Loftus CM. Carotid Endarterectomy: Principles and Technique. St. Louis: Quality Medical Publishing, 1995

47. Loftus CM, Kresowik TF, Eds. Carotid Artery Surgery. New York: Thieme, 1999

48. Loftus CM. Carotid Artery Surgery: Principles and Technique, 2nd ed. New York: Informa Publishing, 2006

49. Halliday A, Mansfield A, Marro J, et al; MRC Asymptomatic Carotid Surgery Trial (ACST) Collaborative Group. Prevention of disabling and fatal strokes by successful carotid endarterectomy in patients without recent neurological symptoms: randomised controlled trial. Lancet 2004;363:1491–1502

50. Halliday AW, Thomas D, Mansfield A; Steering Committee. The Asymptomatic Carotid Surgery Trial (ACST). Rationale and design. Eur J Vasc Surg 1994;8:703–710

51. CAVATAS Investigators. Endovascular versus surgical treatment in patients with carotid stenosis in the Carotid and Vertebral Artery Transluminal Angioplasty Study (CAVATAS): a randomised trial. Lancet 2001;357:1729–1737

52. Naylor AR, Bolia A, Abbott RJ, et al. Randomized study of carotid angioplasty and stenting versus carotid endarterectomy: a stopped trial. J Vasc Surg 1998;28:326–334

53. Brooks WH, McClure RR, Jones MR, Coleman TC, Breathitt L. Carotid angioplasty and stenting versus carotid endarterectomy: randomized trial in a community hospital. J Am Coll Cardiol 2001;38:1589–1595

54. Alberts MJ, McCann R, Smith TP, et al. A Randomized trial of carotid stenting versus endarterectomy in patients with symptomatic carotid stenosis: study design. J Neurovasc Dis. 1997;2: 228–234

55. Loftus CM, Biller J, Godersky JC, Adams HP, Yamada T, Edwards PS. Carotid endarterectomy in symptomatic elderly patients. Neurosurgery 1988;22:676–680

56. Usman AA, Tang GL, Eskandari MK. Metaanalysis of procedural stroke and death among octogenarians: carotid stenting versus carotid endarterectomy. J Am Coll Surg 2009;208:1124–1131

57. Frego M, Bridda A, Ruffolo C, Scarpa M, Polese L, Bianchera G. The hostile neck does not increase the risk of carotid endarterectomy. J Vasc Surg 2009;50:40–47

58. Perkins WJ, Lanzino G, Brott TG. Carotid stenting vs endarterectomy: new results in perspective. Mayo Clin Proc 2010;85: 1101–1108

59. Petty GW, Brown RD Jr, Whisnant JP, Sicks JD, O'Fallon WM, Wiebers DO. Ischemic stroke subtypes: a population-based study of incidence and risk factors. Stroke 1999;30:2513–2516

60. Estol CJ. Dr. C. Miller Fisher and the history of carotid artery disease. Stroke 1996;27:559–566

61. Eastcott HH, Pickering GW, Rob CG. Reconstruction of internal carotid artery in a patient with intermittent attacks of hemiplegia. Lancet 1954;267:994–996

62. Muuronen A. Outcome of surgical treatment of 110 patients with transient ischemic attack. Stroke 1984;15:959–964

63. Warlow C. Carotid endarterectomy: does it work? Stroke 1984; 15:1068–1076

64. Winslow CM, Solomon DH, Chassin MR, Kosecoff J, Merrick NJ, Brook RH. The appropriateness of carotid endarterectomy. N Engl J Med 1988;318:721–727

65. Tu JV, Hannan EL, Anderson GM, et al. The fall and rise of carotid endarterectomy in the United States and Canada. N Engl J Med 1998;339:1441–1447

66. Mayberg MR, Wilson SE, Yatsu F, et al. Carotid endarterectomy and prevention of cerebral ischemia in symptomatic carotid stenosis. Veterans Affairs Cooperative Studies Program 309 Trialist Group. JAMA 1991;266:3289–3294

67. MRC European Carotid Surgery Trial: interim results for symptomatic patients with severe (70–99%) or with mild (0–29%) carotid stenosis. European Carotid Surgery Trialists' Collaborative Group. Lancet 1991;337:1235–1243

68. Naylor AR, London NJ, Bell PR. Carotid endarterectomy versus carotid angioplasty. Lancet 1997;349:203–204

69. Brown MM. Balloon angioplasty for cerebrovascular disease. Neurol Res 1992;14(2, Suppl):159–163

70. Brown MM, Butler P, Gibbs J, Swash M, Waterston J. Feasibility of percutaneous transluminal angioplasty for carotid artery stenosis. J Neurol Neurosurg Psychiatry 1990;53:238–243

71. Brown MM, Clifton A, Taylor RS. Concern about safety of carotid angioplasty. Stroke 1996;27:1435–1436

72. Beebe HG, Archie JP, Baker WH, et al. Concern about safety of carotid angioplasty. Stroke 1996;27:197–198

73. Ederle J, Bonati LH, Dobson J, et al; CAVATAS Investigators. Endovascular treatment with angioplasty or stenting versus endarterectomy in patients with carotid artery stenosis in the Carotid and Vertebral Artery Transluminal Angioplasty Study (CAVATAS): long-term follow-up of a randomised trial. Lancet Neurol 2009;8:898–907

74. Bonati LH, Jongen LM, Haller S, et al; ICSS-MRI study group. New ischaemic brain lesions on MRI after stenting or endarterectomy for symptomatic carotid stenosis: a substudy of the International Carotid Stenting Study (ICSS). Lancet Neurol 2010; 9:353–362

75. Archer SB, Sims MM, Giklich R, et al. Outcomes assessment and minimally invasive surgery: historical perspective and future directions. Surg Endosc 2000;14:883–890

76. Peterson CY, Ramamoorthy S, Andrews B, Horgan S, Talamini M, Chock A. Women's positive perception of transvaginal NOTES surgery. Surg Endosc 2009;23:1770–1774

77. Dorr LD, Thomas D, Long WT, Polatin PB, Sirianni LE. Psychologic reasons for patients preferring minimally invasive total hip arthroplasty. Clin Orthop Relat Res 2007;458:94–100

78. Halm EA, Chassin MR, Tuhrim S, et al. Revisiting the appropriateness of carotid endarterectomy. Stroke 2003;34:1464–1471

79. Estes JM, Guadagnoli E, Wolf R, LoGerfo FW, Whittemore AD. The impact of cardiac comorbidity after carotid endarterectomy. J Vasc Surg 1998;28:577–584

80. Karp HR, Flanders WD, Shipp CC, Taylor B, Martin D. Carotid endarterectomy among Medicare beneficiaries: a statewide evaluation of appropriateness and outcome. Stroke 1998;29: 46–52

81. Tu JV, Wang H, Bowyer B, Green L, Fang J, Kucey D; Participants in the Ontario Carotid Endarterectomy Registry. Risk factors for death or stroke after carotid endarterectomy: observations from the Ontario Carotid Endarterectomy Registry. Stroke 2003;34: 2568–2573

82. Wennberg DE, Lucas FL, Birkmeyer JD, Bredenberg CE, Fisher ES. Variation in carotid endarterectomy mortality in the Medicare population: trial hospitals, volume, and patient characteristics. JAMA 1998;279:1278–1281

83. Hannan EL, Popp AJ, Tranmer B, Fuestel P, Waldman J, Shah D. Relationship between provider volume and mortality for carotid endarterectomies in New York state. Stroke 1998;29: 2292–2297

84. Cebul RD, Snow RJ, Pine R, Hertzer NR, Norris DG. Indications, outcomes, and provider volumes for carotid endarterectomy. JAMA 1998;279:1282–1287

85. Naggara O, Touzé E, Beyssen B, et al; EVA-3S Investigators. Anatomical and technical factors associated with stroke or death during carotid angioplasty and stenting: results from the endarterectomy versus angioplasty in patients with symptomatic severe carotid stenosis (EVA-3S) trial and systematic review. Stroke 2011;42:380–388

86. Schmidt A, Diederich KW, Scheinert S, et al. Effect of two different neuroprotection systems on microembolization during carotid artery stenting. J Am Coll Cardiol 2004;44:1966–1969

87. Ansel GM, Hopkins LN, Jaff MR, et al; Investigators for the ARMOUR Pivotal Trial. Safety and effectiveness of the INVATEC MO.MA proximal cerebral protection device during carotid artery stenting: results from the ARMOUR pivotal trial. Catheter Cardiovasc Interv 2010;76:1–8

88. Bonati LH, Dobson J, Algra A, et al; Carotid Stenting Trialists' Collaboration. Short-term outcome after stenting versus endarterectomy for symptomatic carotid stenosis: a preplanned meta-analysis of individual patient data. Lancet 2010;376: 1062–1073

89. Marquardt L, Geraghty OC, Mehta Z, Rothwell PM. Low risk of ipsilateral stroke in patients with asymptomatic carotid stenosis on best medical treatment: a prospective, population-based study. Stroke 2010;41:e11–e17

90. Markus HS, King A, Shipley M, et al. Asymptomatic embolisation for prediction of stroke in the Asymptomatic Carotid Emboli Study (ACES): a prospective observational study. Lancet Neurol 2010;9:663–671

91. Topakian R, King A, Kwon SU, Schaafsma A, Shipley M, Markus HS; ACES Investigators. Ultrasonic plaque echolucency and emboli signals predict stroke in asymptomatic carotid stenosis. Neurology 2011;77:751–758

92. Spence JD, Coates V, Li H, et al. Effects of intensive medical therapy on microemboli and cardiovascular risk in asymptomatic carotid stenosis. Arch Neurol 2010;67:180–186

93. Reiff T, Stingele R, Eckstein HH, et al; SPACE2-Study Group. Stent-protected angioplasty in asymptomatic carotid artery stenosis vs. endarterectomy: SPACE2 - a three-arm randomised-controlled clinical trial. Int J Stroke 2009;4:294–299

Chapter 19

Treatment of Patients with Trigeminal Neuralgia

Case

A 65-year-old woman had typical V_2-V_3 trigeminal neuralgia that became unresponsive to medical treatment. Magnetic resonance imaging of the head is normal, and the patient is in good health.

Participants

Balloon Compression Rhizotomy for Trigeminal Neuralgia: Jeffrey A. Brown

Microvascular Decompression for Trigeminal Neuralgia: Peter J. Jannetta

Radiofrequency Rhizotomy for Trigeminal Neuralgia: G. Robert Nugent

Stereotactic Radiosurgery for Trigeminal Neuralgia: Stephen J. Monteith and Jason P. Sheehan

Moderator: Treatment of Patientts with Trigeminal Neuralgia: G. Robert Nugent

Balloon Compression Rhizotomy for Trigeminal Neuralgia

Jeffrey A. Brown

More than a dozen years have passed since the first volume of *Controversies in Neurosurgery* raised the issue of treatment of trigeminal neuralgia (TN). At the time, I recommended percutaneous trigeminal nerve balloon compression. But now I suggest that treatment depends on a number of factors. In this section, I outline why and for which circumstances I recommend this procedure. I also explain the circumstances for which I do not recommend this procedure as my first choice.

I co-chair the TNA–Facial Pain Association (formerly the Trigeminal Neuralgia Association), which serves as an advocate for patients with TN and related facial pain conditions by providing information, encouraging research, and offering support. My mission is to serve as a balanced source of information for each patient, tailored to that patient's personal needs. In this role, I am not an advocate of any single surgical treatment for TN. Ideally, a neurosurgeon with knowledge of a wide range of medical and surgical options should evaluate the patient described in this chapter's case presentation.

Must medical management always precede any surgical option? When can we conclude that medical management has failed? One should increase the dose of carbamazepine when it is used to treat facial pain, for example, until pain relief or an average maximum maintenance dose of 600 mg daily is achieved. Too rapid an increase can cause lethargy, leading patients to assume that they have a drug intolerance. Nearly all patients taking carbamazepine report that it reduces their ability to concentrate, to think, and to react.[1] Doses of carbamazepine greater than 600 mg per day increase the risk of bone marrow suppression in addition to cognitive depression. Patients taking other anticonvulsant medications may reach tolerance levels because of metabolic issues. High-dose treatment with oxcarbazepine often causes hyponatremia. I do not recommend multiple drug regimens. When a single anticonvulsant drug ceases to be effective in alleviating classic TN pain, it is unlikely that additional drugs will succeed without causing cognitive deficits. Furthermore, some patients may not tolerate any anticonvulsant therapy and need to proceed to surgical treatment.

Is a 65-year-old woman too old to undergo microvascular decompression (MVD)? Current thinking suggests evaluating the relative medical condition of the patient rather than the absolute age. For example, a 63-year-old woman with a previous stroke associated with atrial fibrillation who is also on chronic anticoagulation therapy is at significant risk if she undergoes an MVD, or even balloon compression. The mean age at treatment in my series of patients who underwent balloon compression is 68 years. Anticoagulation is a significant issue in patients prone to TN. Balloon compression, radiofrequency thermal rhizotomy, and MVD require a temporary discontinuation of anticoagulation. Other comorbidities may increase the risk of MVD. However, patients in their seventh decade of life may still be reasonable candidates for MVD, especially given their overall greater longevity.

The advantage of MVD is that the likelihood of recurrence requiring another surgical procedure and the risk of associated postoperative numbness are lower than those seen with ablative procedures. Older patients have larger subarachnoid spaces and require less cerebellar retraction to expose the trigeminal nerve. Technically, these circumstances simplify the surgery. However, the increased comorbidity in older patients may increase the morbidity of MVD in older patients. Because of the reduced compliance of the brain in older patients, there may be an increased risk of postoperative subdural hemorrhage and headache from pneumocephalus. No surgical series has shown these outcomes, however.[2,3] Indeed, the evidence suggests that there is no increased morbidity in elderly patients undergoing MVD.

One of the advantages of balloon compression over radiosurgery, with either the CyberKnife or the gamma knife, is that, in most situations, the pain is relieved immediately after surgery. In some situations, when compression is mild and the pain severe, the pain is not relieved for several days. With MVD, pain relief is also immediate, although there is no clear explanation for that immediate relief. Biopsies of the trigeminal nerve from the site adjacent to the compressive vessel show demyelinization.[4] How this causes pain, and how removing a source of pulsating compression leads immediately to pain relief, is unknown.

Is there an economic advantage to performing a percutaneous procedure? Balloon compression is an outpatient or overnight-stay procedure, whereas the length of stay after MVD is about 3 days. The length of stay is the most significant economic force increasing health care costs. If one assumes only a single procedure, then balloon compression is significantly less expensive. The recurrence risk with balloon compression, however, is 25% in 3 to 5 years. For MVD, the risk is 15% after 15 years. If one assumes an additional 25% recurrence rate every 5 years with balloon compression, and that such recurrence leads to a second surgery, and that the cost of MVD is three times more than that of balloon compression (because of the length of stay), then the two procedures are approximately equal in total cost after 15 years. Other factors, such as the cost of additional medications needed after recurrence, might further equalize the costs involved. The economic analysis is more complex than this, however. The present-day cost of a single operation may be less than the future costs of repeated balloon compressions. This point only serves to equalize the overall costs of the two operations.

In a letter to me in 1993, William Sweet stated the fundamental argument in favor of balloon compression: "I can't accept treatment for a nonfatal disease which is accompanied by consistent mortality or major disability even though rare, as in the case with microvascular decompression."

There is a flaw in this logic, however. Balloon compression also has an associated mortality rate and a risk of major disability. The risk is lower than with MVD, but present nonetheless. There have been deaths associated with balloon compression.

What about the numbness associated with balloon compression? The incidence of bothersome numbness after compression in my series of patients is 6%.[5] MVD can cause numbness, for example, because of nerve manipulation or heat transfer during bipolar coagulation of a vein. In the informed consent process, patients are essentially asked to weigh the benefit from the reduced risk of major morbidity or mortality of balloon compression against the discomfort that results from persistent facial numbness, even though mild. This is a form of behavioral economic decision making. Patients are weighing the value of initial pain relief, without the additional pain and risk of MVD, against their future risks of recurrent pain or need for surgery. In choosing between balloon compression and MVD, as "altruistic" neurosurgeons, we are evaluating personal, emotional, economic, immediate, and future health concerns.[6]

Several scenarios would lead me to recommend balloon compression for this patient as my first choice. I carry out thin-cut magnetic resonance imaging (MRI) scans in my office as a part of the patient's initial evaluation. The absence of an obvious vessel associated with the trigeminal nerve may lead me to recommend an ablative procedure. If the patient's pain is unremitting and he or she is unable to wait for the effects of radiosurgery, then I would recommend balloon compression. Pain relief is usually immediate. If the

pain is in the first division, then balloon compression may be safer than thermal rhizotomy. Balloon compression selectively preserves the unmyelinated fibers that mediate the corneal reflex, which limits the likelihood of corneal anesthesia and visual loss when compared with thermal rhizotomy.[7] If the patient, because of cognitive issues, cannot cooperate with the surgeon to evaluate the site of stimulation or the extent of sensory loss intraoperatively, as is done with thermal rhizotomy, then balloon compression is easier. In general, balloon compression is easier to perform than thermal rhizotomy because it does not require the patient to be awake during the procedure. If the patient has already undergone MVD and reexploration, then I may recommend balloon compression as the next procedure. Reexploration after MVD is reasonable, especially if there is a vascular association shown on thin-cut MRI scans. Patients may not be able to tolerate the thought of another decompression. Balloon compression is reasonable in such a situation.

The technique of percutaneous balloon compression has been well described in previous publications[5] (**Fig. 19.1**). An important issue to consider is the necessity of continuing anticoagulation. Warfarin, clopidogrel, and aspirin must be stopped before the patient undergoes balloon compression, and anticoagulation is restarted soon after surgery. Determining when to restart anticoagulation is based on how many times it was necessary to reposition the cannula or balloon during surgery and whether there is blood seen on postoperative computed tomography (CT) images.

Are there any situations in which balloon compression is contraindicated? The patient with multiple sclerosis and bilateral TN presents some difficulty. Here, the function of the contralateral pterygoid muscle is important. Bilateral pterygoid muscle weakness will make it difficult for the patient to chew, but this weakness usually resolves within

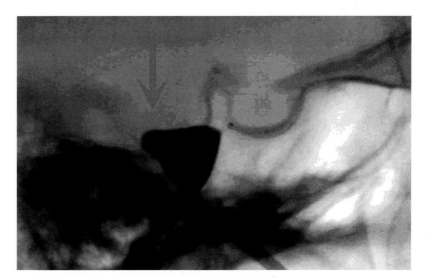

Fig. 19.1 The lateral image intensifier view shows the correct "pear shape" (*arrow*) of the balloon when properly inflated with its tip positioned at the entrance to Meckel's cave. If this pear shape does not appear, there will not likely be adequate compression pressure to injure the large myelinated fibers of the trigeminal nerve.

a month. Some patients cannot tolerate any lip or tongue numbness. For example, a professional musician who plays a woodwind or brass instrument could have difficulty with such sensory loss. More important, however, is the safety of discontinuing anticoagulation.

Despite these issues, balloon compression is a simple outpatient procedure with low morbidity that remains a mainstay in the treatment of patients with the debilitating pain of TN. It is an option for every patient considering a surgical procedure to treat this neuropathic pain.

Microvascular Decompression for Trigeminal Neuralgia

Peter J. Jannetta

Before surgeons found a way to apply the binocular surgical microscope to the operative treatment of TN, the treatment consisted of deliberate injury to the trigeminal nerve. Historically, the nerve was sectioned or the peripheral branches or ganglion injected with absolute alcohol. The object of the therapy was to replace one symptom, pain, with another, numbness.

In the winter of 1965–1966, I developed a microsurgical procedure based on a clarification of the trigeminal nerve anatomy partly described by Dandy. At the first operation, performed with the assistance of John Alksne, the superior cerebellar artery was seen to pulsate into and compress the nerve. I said, "That's the cause of the trigeminal neuralgia." My lack of understanding of the process of acceptance was naive. But young and naive people see and do new things, partly because they do not understand that something cannot be done.

In *The Structure of Scientific Revolutions*, Thomas Kuhn[8] clearly organized the sequence of thoughts in the trials and assumption of new ideas. He was the first to describe the paradigm shift, and he clarified the sequence elegantly. His book should be read by anyone doing new work in science or medicine. It generally takes 20 years or more for a new paradigm to be developed and accepted. This time lag occurs as we wait for the old guard, to whom the new ideas are anathema, to retire or die. The younger generation accepts the new paradigm as more profound and acceptable than the old system of thought. But the better the new idea, the longer it may take for acceptance.

The concept of vascular compression of the cranial nerves and of treatment with MVD went through this annealing process before general acceptance. It can now be safely said that, in many or most centers throughout the world, MVD is the treatment of choice for TN. And yet, several areas of controversy remain. The following questions are, in a sense, secondary and perhaps problem-solving areas, or "normal science" as Kuhn described it:

Is TN always caused by blood vessels? Almost always. The exception is that many patients with TN due to multiple sclerosis have a causative blood vessel in addition to the sclerotic plaque in the root entry zone. The major question is *not*, "Is there a causative vessel here or not?" but rather, "Am I good enough to find *all* the causative vessels?"

Can the offending blood vessels be seen on a scan? We obtain MRI scans not to see the offending blood vessel(s) but to rule out congenital abnormalities such as a Chiari I malformation, to find arteriovenous malformations, to see arterial aneurysms, and to identify dolichoectatic arteries. Even with advanced scanning techniques, the offending vessel is often missed. We frequently see a larger artery apparently compressing the nerve but find that a smaller artery, arteriole, vein, or venule is the true cause. It is less than smart to think that a blood vessel is not present and causing TN just because one cannot see it on MRI. The eye is a much better monitor than a scan.

Is the size of the blood vessel important? No, no, and no.

Are there subtle vascular compressions in TN that the surgeon should understand? Yes. An artery or vein under the ala of the cerebellum can be the only vessel or can contribute to the TN. Cerebellar support by a retractor can move a blood vessel off the nerve, as can the drainage of spinal fluid. I have seen four patients with a large vein inside the portio major, completely unexpectedly. A distal crossing vein, which may be hidden under a bony enostosis in dolichocephalic patients, may be missed. I occasionally see patients who have had a "negative exploration" at a prior operation have this vein.

Should neurophysiological monitoring be performed intraoperatively? I use it. Although this operation can be done without it, I prefer it and not just for teaching purposes. The use of auditory evoked potential monitoring helps ordinary people like me to perform the MVD with a clean and safe technique. MVD without monitoring may be admirable to some, but I do not admire it. To extrapolate this thinking, one can do a vascular decompression of a nerve without magnification but not very well. Surgical progress implies that the difficult becomes common and the extraordinary, ordinary.

What local care is necessary postoperatively? I do not send patients to the intensive care unit. It is unnecessary.

The patients are comfortable in a bed on a regular ward and are ready for discharge the next day. I hardly ever have to readmit a patient to the hospital.

Are there age restrictions regarding eligibility for MVD? In general, no. Young children are usually misdiagnosed, even by pediatric neurosurgeons. Our youngest patient suffered the onset of typical TN at age 7 months. We saw him at age 22 months, undernourished, undersized, underdiagnosed, and being fed through a gastrostomy tube. Elderly patients generally tolerate MVD well. The rule is, Do they have a 5-year estimated survival? Can they well tolerate 2 hours of general anesthesia? It is not chronology but general health that helps us make the decision regarding MVD.

What TN syndromes can be treated with MVD? Typical TN is considered below. Here I discuss the variations. TN can become "atypical" for several reasons. The first is medication. Carbamazepine, the best of the anti-TN drugs, may relieve lancinating pain, but a background continuous pain, usually burning in character, may persist. More medication may stop the persistent pain. Other drugs may also do this but much less frequently. TN of long duration may convert from typical lancinating pain to constant burning pain (modified TN). Those patients who never had lancinating pain do not fare as well after MVD, and nothing else helps them. We can relieve the pain in 40 or 50% of these patients.

Is there a clinicopathological relationship in TN? Yes. But it is not as clear as in the facial nerve (hemifacial spasm) or the auditory nerve (vertigo, disequilibrium, tinnitus, and hearing loss). In general, the clinicopathological relationships in TN are as follows:

- Rostral compression, most frequently by the superior cerebellar artery, causes V_3 TN.
- Lateral compression, by a downward and upward looping superior cerebellar artery or by a bridging vein, most likely an aberrant trigeminal vein, especially in young women, causes V_2 pain.
- Caudal compression, most frequently in elderly men who are heavy cigarette smokers, causes isolated V_1 pain. An advancing length of a superior cerebellar artery loop seems to be responsible for the spread of pain up the face from V_3 to include V_2 and all divisions.
- Distal compression of the motor-proprioceptive fascicles, usually by the superior cerebellar artery, causes constant pain, usually burning in character. As this portion of the nerve is stretched by the artery, hyperactive autonomic dysfunction may frequently occur. Over an extended period, mild numbness becomes more prominent in the area of pain.

The technique and results of a retromastoid craniectomy and MVD have been well described,[9,10] and the article by McLaughlin and colleagues[10] may be the best overview of these techniques. The retromastoid incision, 3 to 5 cm in length, must be placed posterior enough so that a good

angle of sight into the cerebellopontine angle is achieved. The craniotomy is placed high and lateral at the junction of the transverse and sigmoid sinuses. The opening in the dura mater, either curvilinear or with a T into the corner, must allow exposure at the junction of the sinuses. The entire trigeminal nerve must be exposed and inspected. Both arteries and veins may move out of position away from the nerve because of the drainage of spinal fluid or retractor displacement of the cerebellum.

The great majority of vascular blood vessels compressing the trigeminal nerve are overt and easily seen, whereas 5 to 10% are subtle. Many overt cases also have a secondary subtle cause, and these must always be appreciated. A vein or artery under the ala of the cerebellum, a very distal crossing vein, and a venule or arteriole must all be evaluated and treated. Pontine surface veins may be the cause of TN, more frequently in women than in men. Regrettably, these pontine surface veins are prone to recollateralizing after they have been coagulated and divided. This may occur as early as 6 weeks postoperatively. An early recurrence of TN is most likely due to the recollateralization of surface veins. Because the veins frequently lie under the pia mater instead of truly in the subarachnoid space, elevation and decompression using soft implants is tedious and difficult to perform without disrupting the integrity of the vessel wall. We try to save these veins in every case and this has reduced the early recurrence rate significantly. We do cranioplasties using titanium mesh secured in place with self-driving screws. This technique has decreased the incidence of chronic headaches, usually seen in 15 to 20% of patients with preoperative posterior fossa/cerebellopontine angle involvement, to virtually zero.

How do patients react to MVD for TN postoperatively? If their TN is gone, they feel better than they did preoperatively just as soon as they are over the acute effects of anesthesia. They are usually ready for discharge on the first postoperative day. If they do not feel well, they are hospitalized for another day. If they develop a severe headache, a CT scan is done to rule out a blood clot or cerebellar swelling (very rare). Once the obstruction is cleared, a lumbar puncture is done with a small needle. Any pressure above 100 cm H_2O is dropped halfway to 100. The patients are given one dose of dexamethasone (10 mg) parenterally. They almost universally feel well very rapidly.

What are the principles of postoperative care? If patients have traveled to our center from a distant locale, we see them on the fifth postoperative day before allowing them to return home. Medications are decreased rapidly starting immediately after surgery, except for carbamazepine. To prevent withdrawal symptoms, this drug must be slowly decreased over a 10-day period after an initial decrease to a small maintenance dose of 600 to 800 mg per day. During the postoperative visit, we check for any hearing loss, most of which is mild, due to fluid in the middle ear, and accompanied by a sense of fullness in the ear. This may take 5 or 6 weeks to dissipate. The patients are told to call us if they have any problems, to let us know if they move or change their phone number, and to e-mail or send a card with a status report at Christmas. They are reminded that the trip home will probably tire them out and that this is normal. They are told that they can gradually increase their activity to normal over a 6-week period. They need to work up a sweat to the point of fatigue, and the best way to do this is by walking vigorously, *a la* Harry Truman.

Radiofrequency Rhizotomy for Trigeminal Neuralgia

G. Robert Nugent

The pain of TN is so severe that many patients are satisfied with any treatment offered, provided pain relief is the outcome. The surgeon's predilection and experience, however, often color the process of informed consent and predetermine the patient's choice of therapeutic options. Naturally, a neurosurgeon experienced in microneurosugery of the posterior fossa might strongly recommend the surgically challenging MVD to the patient presented in this chapter.

Currently, the MVD procedure is considered the treatment of choice for TN because it stops the pain without the trade-off of numbness in the face. The second option is one of the treatments aimed at inflicting some damage (at best minimal) to the ganglion or retrogasserian rootlets to eliminate the pain. These include radiofrequency (RF) thermocoagulation, glycerol infusion, or balloon compression. The third treatment option is the currently popular gamma knife radiosurgery procedure.

The Radiofrequency Technique: A Method

Here I present a case in favor of RF treatment, which argues that most surgeons misuse this technique by making the face too numb, believing that this is necessary to ensure a good result. This is a self-defeating practice and often leads to the patient's dissatisfaction because of annoying dysesthesias in the face. Many surgeons do not realize that only a minimal sensory deficit is necessary for lasting relief from the pain. Only the RF technique, when properly performed, permits control of both the location and extent of the deficit produced. The aim is to produce a mild degree of numbness in the face with which the patient can be comfortable. The key word here is *comfortable.*

The indications for the RF procedure are similar to those for other procedures aimed at creating some injury to the trigeminal nerve. Patients must have true or classic TN because this procedure is definitely contraindicated in other, atypical types of facial pain. Differentiating TN from other types of pain should not be a problem because true TN is one of the classic syndromes in all of clinical medicine. Patients with true TN have pain that is usually refractory to medical management or they suffer from intolerable side effects of such therapy. Those who have had a satisfactory result from a peripheral block may opt for more permanent numbness. Furthermore, some patients will not choose an intracranial operation with its remote, but not insignificant, risk of complications. Finally, some patients simply opt for a more benign, less time-consuming, and less expensive form of treatment.

Preliminary Considerations

The informed consent form for the RF treatment must specify the possibility of annoying dysesthesias in the face, the worst of which is anesthesia dolorosa; recurrence of the pain, requiring a second treatment; and the very remote and unlikely possibility of visual impairment from inadvertent corneal anesthesia. Anesthetic safeguards must be in place to prevent intracranial hemorrhage from the occasional reflex hypertensive bursts that may occur when the foramen ovale is penetrated.

I have argued that the RF technique allows much more control of the extent and location of the lesion than other destructive techniques. This control is achieved through the use of a small, angled electrode of 0.4 mm **(Fig. 19.2)**. Because lesions behind the gasserian ganglion are virtually painless, or at least the pain is tolerable, lesions with this small electrode can be made while the patient is awake. It is thermal lesions in the ganglion and distal divisions of the nerve that are intolerably painful. Of great importance, therefore, is creating the lesion with its sensory deficit while the patient is fully awake, permitting constant online monitoring of the sensory deficit being produced and at the same time protecting corneal sensation. By making small incremental lesions, it is possible to "creep up" on a moderate sensory deficit.

I do not use the larger temperature monitoring electrode that is popular with many because its heat reaches the ganglion and the resulting pain requires that the patient be anesthetized. Furthermore, the required final temperature varies tremendously depending on where within the retrogasserian rootlets the electrode tip lies. The lesion develops at a lower temperature if the electrode lands ide-

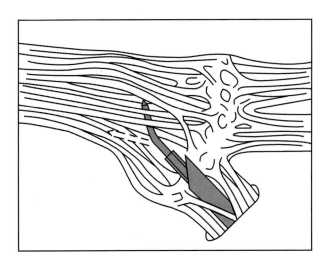

Fig. 19.2 This small electrode enables lesions to be made behind the ganglion where the thermocoagulation is painless. The electrode permits online evaluation of the location and the extent of sensory deficit while the lesion is being made. The angle of the electrode introduces another parameter for localization in the rootlets in addition to the mere depth of penetration.

ally in those rootlets. Sweet and Wepsic[11] note that "the necessary final electrode temperatures varied through an amazing range from 47° to 108°C," and Siegfried[12] states that the temperature at the tip of the electrode and the intensity of current show no consistent direct relationship. Relying on temperature may lead to a lesion that is too dense. Therefore, I am convinced that online monitoring of the awake patient while the lesion is being made is far more important than temperature monitoring.

The surgeon can prevent the spread of current into the first division of the nerve by stopping the process when the patient has a decreased blink response to eyelash stimulation. Monitoring the blink response is also important while making lesions in the second division because, for reasons unexplained, the first division fibers seem to be more sensitive to heat, and a lesion may be made in the first division with no associated eye or forehead pain or discomfort. Consequently, it is possible to destroy the first division rootlets without the surgeon or patient being aware of what is happening. With proper technique, corneal anesthesia can be kept to an incidence of 3 to 4%. In our last several hundred procedures, the rate of corneal anesthesia has been 2%. Of patients with first-division pain (the pain is always triggered by touching the eyebrow or hairline), 90% have been treated satisfactorily, with only partially diminished corneal sensation. The technique is described in detail elsewhere.[13] The RF technique can indeed be indicated for the treatment of first division pain.

Results

Experience with the RF procedure convinces one that most patients with TN are glad to accept a "comfortable" degree

of facial numbness to be rid of the pain and the medication. In our series of 1,456 patients, 6% found the numbness "annoying," but 53% of those patients who found the dysesthesias annoying also rated the overall results of the procedure as good to excellent. In our series, 0.7% of patients described the annoying facial sensations as moderate to severe, 3% described them as severe, and 0.4% described them as intolerable.[13] The proof that this is a satisfactory treatment, however, is that most patients experiencing a recurrence immediately request another RF treatment, and many of my new patients come from referrals from satisfied patients.

Microvascular Decompression vs. Radiofrequency

Recurrence

The recurrence rate after the RF procedure should be 25 to 30%. Our 10-year recurrence rate is 27%, which could be lower if we elected to make more dense sensory deficits. The reported recurrence or failure rate for MVD in selected series is as follows: 47% over 8.5 years,[14] 29%,[15] 28%,[16] 29%,[17] and 30%.[9] The recurrence rates, therefore, are similar for the RF and MVD treatments. But a comparison should not be made on the basis of recurrence because this is not a critical issue with RF. If the pain recurs, the procedure is simply done over again.

Deafness

In various series, the incidence of deafness on the side of the MVD surgery was 8%,[15] 7.6%,[16] 4%,[18] and 7%.[19] As other investigators have pointed out,[18] this loss of hearing is not related to the experience of the surgeon. One author with extensive experience using the MVD operation has stated that a 3% incidence of hearing loss is to be expected.[20] Those with vast experience using the MVD approach will have a lower rate. The online monitoring of hearing is controversial and not endorsed by all.

In 1977, Apfelbaum compared his patients' satisfaction with the MVD operation and RF ablation and found a preference for MVD. A total of 18% of his patients would not have another radiofrequency procedure performed.[21] But this finding is not surprising because 15% of his RF patients had a severe degree of numbness, 13% had corneal anesthesia, and 11% had anesthesia dolorosa or annoying dysesthesias. This finding merely tells us that, like others performing the RF technique, he was making the face far too numb. No wonder the patients did not like the RF operation. The procedure itself should not be blamed by those inflicting unwanted and unnecessary sensory deficits.

Vascular compression of the trigeminal nerve is the cause of TN in many if not most patients, but the argument that MVD has the advantage of treating the disease means little to the patient who only wants pain relief.

Glycerol vs. Radiofrequency

A major problem with glycerol treatment is that, although it is neurotoxic, it is not neurotoxic enough to provide lasting pain relief. The failure or recurrence rate in some series is reported to be as high as 57%, 72%, and even 90%.[9,13–24] Paradoxically, however, glycerol may occasionally produce dense and unwanted sensory deficits, including anesthesia dolorosa (4.7% of patients[24]), anesthesia and keratitis (3.1%[22]), facial anesthesia (7%[25]), and analgesia (8%[26]). In several series, corneal anesthesia occurred in 4%,[24] 7%,[25] 5%,[27] and 14%[28] of patients. Corneal anesthesia occurred in 3.5% of our patients, but this was early in our experience when more dense sensory deficits were intentionally the end point.

Because of the gliosis and scarring from the first glycerol injection, repeated injections often lead to more severe sensory deficits, 50% after a second injection, and 70% after a third.[19–31] They are also more severe in patients who have had a prior nonglycerol treatment.[23,24,32]

This approach is uncontrolled because the surgeon cannot be certain of the outcome after injecting glycerol into the trigeminal cistern. The RF procedure offers a much more controlled and predictable treatment than injecting glycerol into the cistern to see what happens. Both the patient and the neurosurgeon should be prepared for some surprises when glycerol is used.

Balloon Compression vs. Radiofrequency

The overall results with balloon compression relate generally to how long and to what pressure the balloon is inflated, and there is a considerable difference of opinion with this approach. Annoying dysesthesias can occur in as many as 12% of patients if the balloon remains inflated for long periods of time,[33] and, as with glycerol, facial numbness is more marked after a repeated balloon compression.[34] There is nothing magic about balloon compression. This technique is merely another method of injuring the trigeminal nerve but, as with glycerol and gamma knife treatment, the location and degree of sensory deficit cannot be controlled as well as with RF.

Gamma Knife vs. Radiofrequency

Many problems related to gamma knife treatment stem from the variables in the reports of its results. These include variations in the dose (although 85 Gy seems close to the best), and variation in the following items: the recurrence rate (18 to 25%), the output factors and isocenters used, the definitions of "good" or "excellent" results, the time at which postoperative results are tabulated, and the site and length of the nerve treated.[35] At this date, the emerging consensus is that the most successful gamma knife treatment, like the glycerol treatment, produces a mild degree of sensory deficit in the face.[36] But the gamma knife treatment cannot control or predict the amount, if any, of sensory deficit produced, as can be done with RF. As yet, the gamma knife technique has not been standardized to the extent that a minimal amount of numbness can be consistently produced. In other words, you don't know what you are going to get.

Conclusion

I believe that surgeons who prefer other therapeutic approaches never learned to perform the RF procedure properly and generally create too much sensory deficit. Those who have developed skill and experience with the technique share the conviction that it is an excellent treatment. I disagree with those who believe that RF offers a cure only at the expense of an unacceptable trade-off of permanent numbness in the face.[37] Those treated with RF are generally among the most grateful and appreciative patients a neurosurgeon has the pleasure of treating. A properly performed RF procedure offers a simple, quick, safe, and economical way of relieving the worst pain that patients can suffer.

Stereotactic Radiosurgery for Trigeminal Neuralgia

Stephen J. Monteith and Jason P. Sheehan

The History of Radiosurgery for Trigeminal Neuralgia

From the inception of radiosurgery, Lars Leksell realized its potential to treat pain, and he initially used an orthovoltage stereotactic technique to treat patients with TN, with some relief of symptoms.[38] It was some 20 years later that the gamma knife was developed and used for gamma thalamotomies in patients with tremor or intractable pain. But the use of the gamma knife for patients with TN fell out of favor in the 1970s and 1980s due to difficulties in localizing the gasserian ganglion with X-rays alone. Thus, radiosurgery for TN was replaced with new pain-modulating drugs and minimally invasive percutaneous techniques. With the development of high-resolution MRI, however, the trigeminal nerve was easily visualized, and interest in gamma knife radiosurgery for TN was rekindled.

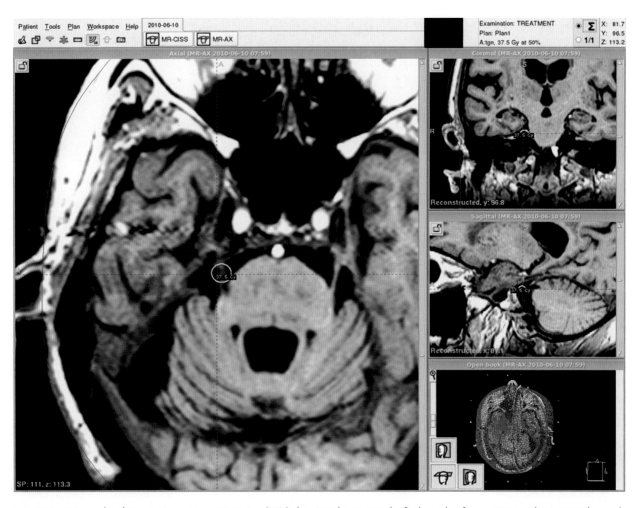

Fig. 19.3 T1-weighted magnetic resonance imaging (MRI) showing the gamma knife dose plan for a patient with trigeminal neuralgia. The nerve is targeted with a single 4-mm isocenter. The yellow circle represents the 50% isodose line.

Targeting

The first step in targeting for radiosurgery is obtaining adequate images to visualize the trigeminal nerve and the nerve root entry zone. Typically, MRI is done with at least a 1.5-tesla system. Critical structures are identified with T1-weighted, T2-weighted, and fast spin-echo sequences **(Fig. 19.3)**. Constructive interference in steady state (CISS) sequences can also help delineate the trigeminal nerve, particularly after previous neurosurgery **(Fig. 19.4)**. Axial sequences are most important, but coronal images may identify the nerve. Gadolinium administration and three-dimensional reconstructions can also be done to help identify the target. CT with or without cisternography can be used in patients who cannot undergo MRI scanning (for example, those with a pacemaker).

Once the trigeminal nerve is identified, the surgeon must be cognizant of variations in the patient's anatomy. Longer cisternal segments may allow for a minimal dose to the brainstem or eliminate the need for blocking or beam shaping. The converse is true with shorter cisternal segments, and the resultant dose to the brainstem may

be higher. Compensatory measures, such as adjusting the gamma angle of 110 degrees, may be taken to align the isocenter with the axis of the trigeminal nerve, thereby minimizing the dose to adjacent structures.

Once the nerve is clearly delineated, a target must be chosen. Controversy surrounds whether the nerve should be targeted more proximally or distally.[39,40] The rate of pain relief appears to be higher when the target is closer to the brainstem, but the trade-off is a higher rate of complications when the brainstem receives a higher dose. Dose selection has also been an area of debate. Typically, doses of 70 to 85 Gy are used **(Table 19.1)**,[40–62] and rates of pain control increase when higher doses reach the brainstem. However, doses greater than 90 Gy have been associated with an unacceptable rate of complications; therefore, the dose should be kept below this level. Impingement on the trigeminal nerve by an adjacent vascular structure has long been postulated as the pathophysiological mechanism in TN. But a recent study has shown that patients with vascular impingement seen on MRI were more likely to improve if the radiosurgical target was closer to the site of neurovascular contact.[63]

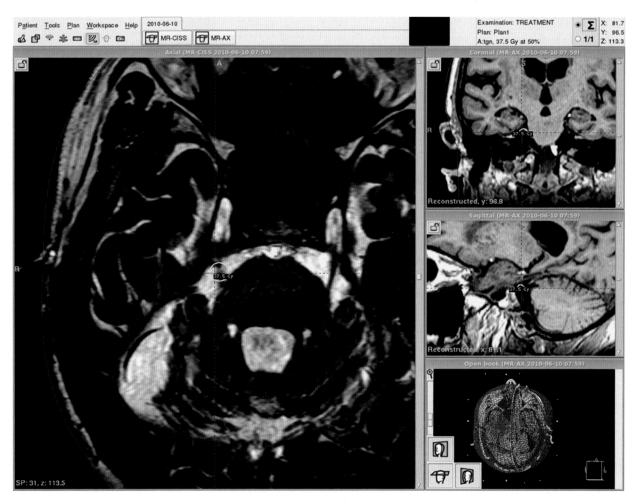

Fig. 19.4 The constructive interference in steady state (CISS) sequence MRI clearly delineates the cisternal segment of the trigeminal nerve. CISS sequencing can be particularly helpful in patients with prior surgery of the affected trigeminal nerve.

Rationale and the Factors Related to Successful Treatment

Radiosurgery is often used as a salvage treatment for patients in whom minimally invasive percutaneous treatments or MVD have failed. However, patients treated with radiosurgery in whom MVD has failed may have higher rates of recurrence, with some studies reporting 60% of treated patients maintaining complete pain relief at 1 year, dropping to 33% at 5 years.[60] In addition, Régis and colleagues[40] reported that the chance of pain relief at 1 year for patients who did not have previous surgery was 88%, compared with 82%, 80%, and 75% in patients with one, two, or three prior surgical interventions, respectively. Kondziolka and associates[41] similarly found that a higher number of prior procedures was a predictor of poor long-term results after radiosurgery.

The presence of atypical facial pain is also a negative prognostic factor.[41] Maesawa and coworkers[60] found that 44% of patients with atypical pain improved compared with 84% of patients with typical pain. Reports of age as a predictor of treatment success have been mixed. Pollock and colleagues[59] found that a younger age was favorable.

The series by Régis and associates,[40] however, found that patients younger than 60 years fared worse (56% were pain free compared with 91% of older patients).

Results and Follow-Up

Patients should be followed up clinically at 3- to 6-month intervals and with MRI scans at 6 to 12 months after radiosurgery. MRI and clinical examination are necessary to detect recurrent disease as well as radiation-induced complications. Clinical examination of the trigeminal nerve should be done carefully, as nerve function can be helpful in predicting patient outcome. Some mild degree of facial sensory loss is associated with the pain relief after radiosurgery. Similarly, patients with trigeminal deficits are more likely to have excellent pain relief, compared with those with normal nerve function after radiosurgery.[41,59]

Although MVD remains the treatment of choice for TN, gamma knife surgery may be appropriate for patients who are unable or unwilling to undergo open surgery. A summary of results from current series in the literature is presented in **Table 19.1**. The highest rate of pain control was achieved by Régis and colleagues,[40] in which 97% of patients

Table 19.1 Summary of Contemporary Radiosurgery Series for Trigeminal Neuralgia

Authors/ Year	Number of Patients	Mean Age/ Median Age	Device	Median Dose/Range (Gy)	Median Time to Complete Pain Relief (Range)	Previous Surgery (%)	Pain-Free or Good Result (%)	Treatment Failure (%)	Recurrence (%)	Repeat Radiosurgery (%)	Mean/Median Follow-Up— Months (range)	Facial Numbness (%)
Kondziolka et al, 2010[41]	503	NA/72	Gamma knife	80 (60–90)	1 month (1 day to 1 year)	43	89 (1 year)	29	43	18	NA/24 (3–156)	11
Villavicencio et al, 2008[42]	95	70/NA	CyberKnife	75 (50–86.4)	14 days (0.3–180)	37	67	33	31	18	NA/60 (12–96)	20
Fountas et al, 2007[43]	106	72/NA	Gamma knife	80/85 (70–85)	50/53 showed response within the first 4 weeks	46	90	10	60 had excellent results at 5 years	Not stated	12/NA (36+)	4
Longhi et al, 2007[44]	160	63/NA	Gamma knife	85 (mean) (75–95)	45 days	43	90	10	18	Not stated	NA/12 (1–60)	0
Pusztaszeri et al, 2007[45]	17	71/NA	LINAC	50–56	1 month (2 weeks to 6 months)	59	70	30	29	Not stated	24/22 (12–46)	47
Régis et al, 2006[40]	100	68/NA	Gamma knife	85 (70–90)	10 days (0–25 weeks)	42	83	17	34	10	NA/19 (2–96)	9
Lim et al, 2005[46]	41	68	CyberKnife	78 (71.4 to 86.3)	7 days (< 24 hour to 4 months)	32	93 at 24 hours to 4 months, 78 at 11 months	7	16	4	12 (1–40)	11
McNatt et al, 2005[47]	49	68/NA	Gamma knife	80 for all	Mean 5.5 weeks	21	61	39	23	Not stated	22/23 (5–55)	29
Richards et al, 2005[48]	28	74	LINAC	80	1 month	54	75	14	46	Not stated	NA/14 (3–31)	18
Sheehan et al, 2005[49]	136	68	Gamma knife	80 (50–90)	24 days (1–180)	54	90 at 1 year, 70 at 3 years	10	24	Not stated	11/NA (6–22)	51
Urgosik et al, 2005[50]	107	NA/75	Gamma knife	80 (70–80)	3 months (1 day–13 months)	60	96	4	25	6	44/49 (12–70)	29
Brisman, 2004[51]	293	68/70	Gamma knife	75 (104 pts) 76.8 (189 pts)	NA	43	68	8	24	Not stated	NA/8	6
Chen et al, 2004[52]	32	NA/67	LINAC	85–90 (repeat dose of 60)	42 days	31	78	13	Not stated	13	NA/30 (8–66)	7

(continued on next page)

Table 19.1 (Continued)

Authors/Year	Number of Patients	Mean Age/Median Age	Device	Median Dose/Range (Gy)	Median Time to Complete Pain Relief (Range)	Previous Surgery (%)	Pain-Free or Good Result (%)	Treatment Failure (%)	Recurrence (%)	Repeat Radiosurgery (%)	Mean/Median Follow-Up—Months (range)	Facial Numbness (%)
Frighetto et al, 2004[53]	22	70/NA	LINAC	90 (75–90)	Mean 2.7 months (0–12 months)	0	95	5	24	Not stated	37/NA (6–144)	3
Massager et al, 2004[54]	47	NA/69	Gamma knife	90/90	NA	38	75	25	8	6	16/NA (6–42)	43
Shaya et al, 2004[55]	40	64/NA	Gamma knife	80 (mean) (70–90)	Mean 25 weeks	25	70 at 14 months' median follow-up	30	30	4	NA/18 (8–52)	32
Goss et al, 2003[56]	25	NA/65	LINAC	90 for all	60 days (0–365)	32	68 at last follow-up; initially, 100 had good or excellent results	32 at last follow-up; initially, 100 had good or excellent results	32 at 4–13 months	11	NA/26 (1–48)	8
Petit et al, 2003[57]	112	NA/64	Gamma knife	75 (70–80)	21 days (0–168)	31	75	23	29 after a median of 8.5 months	19	NA/24 (6–78)	8
Kondziolka et al, 2002[58]	220	70/NA	Gamma knife	80 (60–90)	2 months (81.6% within 6 months)	61	86	25	14	5	14(3–30)	17
Pollock et al, 2002[59]	117	68/NA	Gamma knife	80 (70–90)	21 days (1–140)	58	75	14	23	0	NA/12 (3–28)	14
Maesawa et al, 2001[60]	220	NA/70	Gamma knife	80 (60–90)	2 months (up to 33 months)	61	86 at 1 year	21	14	6	16 (6–42)	4
Nicol et al, 2000[61]	42	61/NA	Gamma knife	90 for all	Not stated	29	95	5	5	18 with previous gamma knife; repeats not stated	34/36 (12–72)	16
Rogers et al, 2000[62]	54	NA/67	Gamma knife	70–80	63 days (1–253)	46	89	11	21	Not stated	NA/12 (3–28)	9

Abbreviation: LINAC, linear accelerator; NA, not available; pts, patients.

Note: Although each series presents results in a different fashion, every effort has been made to summarize that data appropriately to allow a direct comparison of results.

had an excellent or good response at their last follow-up. Typically, there is a delay of several weeks before pain is relieved. Fountas and associates[43] reported a response within 3 weeks, and Pollock and coworkers[59] within 2 weeks. However, a latent response has been reported up to 8 weeks after surgery. This delay must be kept in mind when counseling patients about their options for treatment, especially for patients suffering a severe acute attack.

In the series from the University of Virginia, 151 cases of TN were treated with the gamma knife and had appropriate follow-up. The chosen target was 2 to 4 mm anterior to the entry of the trigeminal nerve into the pons. The procedure was done twice in 14 patients and three times in one patient. Of the 151 patients, 122 had typical TN. The maximum dose delivered to the target ranged from 50 to 90 Gy. The mean time to pain relief was 24 days, but this time period was highly variable (1–180 days). Twelve patients (9%) developed new facial numbness as a result of treatment. Of the total group, 90%, 77%, and 70% of patients had some improvement in pain at a follow-up of 1, 2, and 3 years, respectively. At the same time points, respectively, 47%, 45%, and 34% of patients were completely pain-free without medication.[49]

Complications

Potential complications of stereotactic radiosurgery include changes in brain parenchyma (both reversible and irreversible), radiation-induced neoplasia, and vascular injury. The surgeon should also be vigilant for facial numbness and anesthesia dolorosa. Rates of new trigeminal dysfunction range from 6 to 66% **(Table 19.1)**. The study by Pollock and associates[59] found that 54% of patients treated with 90 Gy developed facial numbness compared with 15% of patients treated with 70 Gy. Anesthesia dolorosa and an absent corneal reflex are reported only rarely. Some authors have noted an increased risk of facial numbness after repeated gamma knife radiosurgery,[64,65] whereas others have not shown any difference.[66]

Recurrence and Retreatment

Recurrence rates after radiosurgery for TN range from 5 to 46% **(Table 19.1)**. If a patient's pain recurs, it may be reasonable to offer retreatment with radiosurgery. Two groups of authors found that patients who had initial success where likely to benefit from repeated treatment.[59,60] A longer duration of effect after initial treatment may also predict a greater chance of improvement with retreatment. The target for retreatment remains an area of controversy. Shetter and colleagues[65] and Pollock and associates[59] report using a 4-mm collimator shot targeted in the trigeminal nerve at its juncture with the brain stem. In contrast, Hasegawa and associates[64] use a single 4-mm collimator anterior to the portion of the trigeminal nerve targeted in the previous treatment, so that a greater length of nerve is treated without increasing the total dose to the brainstem.

Patients undergoing retreatment are less likely to have enough pain relief to completely discontinue pain medications. Reasons for this outcome may include factors specific to the patient, more severe disease, or more conservative dosimetry in treatment planning.

Rationale for Choosing Radiosurgery or Surgery

Microvascular decompression remains the gold-standard treatment for patients with TN. Barker and colleagues[9] reported complete pain relief in 70% of patients who underwent MVD, with a follow-up of 10 years. The follow-up period for the radiosurgical series is not so long; therefore, a direct comparison is difficult. Pollock and associates[59] reported a 67% rate of complete pain relief at 1 and 3 years, whereas Maesawa and coworkers[60] observed a 70% rate of complete pain relief at 9 months and 5 years.

Clearly, the major disadvantages of radiosurgical treatment are the rate of recurrence and the delay in onset of pain relief. Until long-term follow-up is available, MVD should remain the first line of treatment for patients who can and are willing to undergo the operation because of the durability of its treatment effect. For those unwilling or unable to tolerate the open operation, radiosurgery is an appropriate alternative to percutaneous techniques. Surgical risk after initial MVD is significantly higher. For this reason, patients who have recurrent symptoms after initial MVD may also be considered candidates for radiosurgery. However, both the patient and the physician should be aware that radiosurgery after previous treatment will have a lesser chance of long-term success than an initial treatment.

Stereotactic radiosurgery was introduced as a minimally invasive alternative for patients with TN. For the patient described in this chapter's case presentation, stereotactic radiosurgery is a very appealing treatment approach. The operative risks associated with her age and the absence of neural impingement noted on MRI make MVD less attractive. If the patient can be given medications to make the neuralgia tolerable, the immediate relief afforded by percutaneous ablative procedures is not required. Moreover, such ablative approaches inherently have more up-front risks than radiosurgery and often obscure the neuroanatomy, making targeting more difficult should a subsequent stereotactic radiosurgery be required.

Radiosurgery has a high likelihood of ending or significantly relieving pain, and a radiosurgically induced decrease in pain is not necessarily accompanied by diminished sensation. Overall, this procedure has the safest side-effect profile of all neurosurgical options, and the ease of repeated application should the pain recur is attractive to patients and clinicians. Furthermore, radiosurgery does not burn bridges that would preclude other neurosurgical procedures from being done if radiosurgery simply did not work. As such, stereotactic radiosurgery is the recommended initial neurosurgical approach for this 65-year-old woman with medically refractory TN.

Conclusion

Microvascular decompression remains the gold-standard treatment for TN. Radiosurgery should be considered an option for patients who are not candidates for MVD, or in whom MVD has failed. Patients with typical facial pain are more likely to achieve remission compared with those with atypical pain. Target selection and dose remain topics of debate among neurosurgeons. Follow-up with MRI and clinical examination is necessary to detect recurrent disease as well as radiation-induced complications.

Moderator

Treatment of Patients with Trigeminal Neuralgia

G. Robert Nugent

Things We Think We Are Sure About Regarding Trigeminal Neuralgia and Its Treatment

The first thing we think we know is that surgery should be reserved only for those whose pain becomes refractory to medication. But what answer do we have for patients who ask, "Why did you put me on that medication for all those years that cost so much, upset my stomach, and made me goofy, when you could have done the surgery that cured me earlier?"

The MVD procedure is considered the treatment of choice because it treats the cause of the pain and produces no numbness in the face. But are there some surgeons who prefer this operation because it is technically more challenging, more of a "fun" operation, and also generates a more handsome income than the more minor procedures? It is generally accepted that MVD is indeed the treatment of choice, but not everyone is a candidate, so other options become important and necessary.

If microvascular compression of the nerve is the cause of the pain, why are spontaneous remissions early on so common? And, how come even Jannetta has a 30% recurrence rate at 10 years? The inert foreign body is still there on the nerve. Jannetta believes that recurrence is most often due to the recanalization of veins around the nerve, but, in the experience of many, veins are far less a cause of compression than arteries.

Things That We Are Not Sure About

For the gamma knife treatment, the correct dosage, the ideal target site (more proximal or distal), the best isocenter, and so on, vary from series to series with no uniform or standardized policy that emerges as a sound guideline. The discussion by Monteith and Sheehan in their section nicely reviews the wide discrepancy in techniques and results reported in the literature so far. Similarly, the reported results of radiofrequency ablation vary tremendously from series to series because of the different techniques used and the different attitudes about how much numbness is required for a cure. Many clinicians do not appreciate that less numbness is better than more.

What is the cause of TN when no vascular compression is found? Confounding the cause is the observation that there is a familial incidence of TN in which the pain is bilateral in 18 to 20% of patients, tends to involve the same side and same division in the same family, and the onset is earlier, averaging 44.4 years.[67] Something strange is going on here.

I am impressed that the overall recurrence or failure rate for all surgical or ablative treatments seems to hover around 30%. Is there some bio-anatomic underlying defect in the myelin or other factors in these patients, perhaps inherited, that ultimately leads to failure? Do surgical procedures only temporarily influence a complex set of factors involved in causing the disease? And what do we do when we find no vascular compression of the nerve? Some elect to section part of the nerve. Others injure the nerve by pinching it with forceps or rubbing it with an applicator stick.

Things That I Think I Am Sure About

The best long-term results with any of the ablative procedures, and the gamma knife treatment is one of them,[37] occur when a minimal sensory deficit is produced in the trigger area. This being the case, the ideal treatment should be the creation of this sensory deficit. The gamma knife, glycerol infusion, and balloon compression procedures are unable to do this in a controlled fashion. With each, the nerve as a whole is unselectively treated in a hopeful fashion. The result is always in doubt, and unwanted sensory deficits always a possibility. This is in contrast to radiofrequency ablation where, with a small, angled electrode placed in the retrogasserian rootlets behind the ganglion, the lesion can be made while the patient is awake, enabling constant online monitoring of the location and extent of the sensory deficit being produced. With multiple small, incremental lesions, one can creep up on a minimal deficit with which the patient is comfortable. What is the end point? It is the loss of a one-point light touch of a corner of facial tissue but appreciation of the drag of the tissue. At this point, there is some decrease in pinprick but not analgesia.[68] This approach produces lasting relief of the pain and a very satisfied patient. Watching the blink reflex in the awake patient while the lesion is made allows safe treatment of first-division pain and triggering, which is always through touching the eyebrow or hairline.

In the whole spectrum of TN, there is a small number of patients, perhaps 5%, in whom cure is most difficult to achieve regardless of the kind and number of treatments used. These patients must be recognized and included when looking at any long-term results. TN in patients with multiple sclerosis is most difficult to cure and the usual techniques should be altered to allow the creation of dense sensory deficits, or early recurrence is assured. In my opinion, all treatments of atypical pain should be excluded from TN treatment series. Inclusion does nothing but cloud and distort the issue. It is an unrelated disease process in most cases.

In the final analysis, however, there are several ways to skin the TN cat. Even when the recurrence rate is as high as 50%, the other 50% of patients have been cured. One does what one does best. As in other areas, there is nothing like experience.

References

1. Hessen E, Lossius MI, Reinvang I, Gjerstad L. Influence of major antiepileptic drugs on attention, reaction time, and speed of information processing: results from a randomized, double-blind, placebo-controlled withdrawal study of seizure-free epilepsy patients receiving monotherapy. Epilepsia 2006;47:2038–2045
2. Broggi G, Ferroli P, Franzini A, Servello D, Dones I. Microvascular decompression for trigeminal neuralgia: comments on a series of 250 cases, including 10 patients with multiple sclerosis. J Neurol Neurosurg Psychiatry 2000;68:59–64
3. Berk C, Honey CR. Microvascular decompression for trigeminal neuralgia in patients over 65 years of age. Br J Neurosurg 2001;15:76–77
4. Devor M, Govrin-Lippmann R, Rappaport ZH. Mechanism of trigeminal neuralgia: an ultrastructural analysis of trigeminal root specimens obtained during microvascular decompression surgery. J Neurosurg 2002;96:532–543
5. Brown JA, Pilitsis JG. Percutaneous balloon compression for the treatment of trigeminal neuralgia: results in 56 patients based on balloon compression pressure monitoring. Neurosurg Focus 2005;18:E10
6. Stewart S. Can behavioral economics save us from ourselves? University of Chicago Magazine 2005;97:3
7. Brown JA, Hoeflinger B, Long PB, et al. Axon and ganglion cell injury in rabbits after percutaneous trigeminal balloon compression. Neurosurgery 1996;38:993–1003, discussion 1003–1004
8. Kuhn TSS. The Structure of Scientific Revolutions. Chicago: University of Chicago Press, 1962
9. Barker FG II, Jannetta PJ, Bissonette DJ, Larkins MV, Jho HD. The long-term outcome of microvascular decompression for trigeminal neuralgia. N Engl J Med 1996;334:1077–1083
10. McLaughlin MR, Jannetta PJ, Clyde BL, Subach BR, Comey CH, Resnick DK. Microvascular decompression of cranial nerves: lessons learned after 4400 operations. J Neurosurg 1999;90:1–8
11. Sweet WH, Wepsic JG. Controlled thermocoagulation of trigeminal ganglion and rootlets for differential destruction of pain fibers. 1. Trigeminal neuralgia. J Neurosurg 1974;40:143–156
12. Siegfried J. Percutaneous controlled thermocoagulation of gasserian ganglion in trigeminal neuralgia experience with 1000 cases. In: Samii M, Jannetta PJ, eds. The Cranial Nerves: Anatomy, Pathology, Pathophysiology, Diagnosis, Treatment. Berlin: Springer-Verlag, 1985:322–330
13. Nugent GR. Surgical treatment: radiofrequency gangliolysis and rhizotomy. In: Fromm GH, Sessle BJ, eds. Trigeminal Neuralgia: Current Concepts Regarding Pathogenesis and Treatment. London: Heinemann, 1990:159–184
14. Burchiel KJ, Clarke H, Haglund M, Loeser JD. Long-term efficacy of microvascular decompression in trigeminal neuralgia. J Neurosurg 1988;69:35–38
15. Piatt JH Jr, Wilkins RH. Treatment of tic douloureux and hemifacial spasm by posterior fossa exploration: therapeutic implications of various neurovascular relationships. Neurosurgery 1984;14:462–471
16. Breeze R, Ignelzi RJ. Microvascular decompression for trigeminal neuralgia. Results with special reference to the late recurrence rate. J Neurosurg 1982;57:487–490
17. Ferguson GG, Brett DC, Peerless SJ, Barr HW, Girvin JP. Trigeminal neuralgia: a comparison of the results of percutaneous rhizotomy and microvascular decompression. Can J Neurol Sci 1981;8:207–214
18. Bederson JB, Wilson CB. Evaluation of microvascular decompression and partial sensory rhizotomy in 252 cases of trigeminal neuralgia. J Neurosurg 1989;71:359–367
19. Kolluri S, Heros RC. Microvascular decompression for trigeminal neuralgia. A five-year follow-up study. Surg Neurol 1984;22:235–240
20. Apfelbaum RI. A comparison of percutaneous radiofrequency trigeminal neurolysis and microvascular decompression of the trigeminal nerve for the treatment of tic douloureux. Neurosurgery 1977;1:16–21
21. Apfelbaum RI. Advantages and disadvantages of various techniques to treat trigeminal neuralgia. In: Rovit RL, Murali R, Jannetta PJ, eds. Trigeminal Neuralgia. Baltimore: Williams & Wilkins, 1990:239–250
22. Fraioli B, Esposito V, Guidetti B, Cruccu G, Manfredi M. Treatment of trigeminal neuralgia by thermocoagulation, glycerolization, and percutaneous compression of the gasserian ganglion and/or retrogasserian rootlets: long-term results and therapeutic protocol. Neurosurgery 1989;24:239–245
23. Fujimaki T, Fukushima T, Miyazaki S. Percutaneous retrogasserian glycerol injection in the management of trigeminal neuralgia: long-term follow-up results. J Neurosurg 1990;73:212–216

24. Saini SS. Retrogasserian anhydrous glycerol injection therapy in trigeminal neuralgia: observations in 552 patients. J Neurol Neurosurg Psychiatry 1987;50:1536–1538

25. Burchiel KJ. Percutaneous retrogasserian glycerol rhizolysis in the management of trigeminal neuralgia. J Neurosurg 1988;69:361–366

26. Young RF. Stereotaxic procedures for facial pain. In: Apuzzo MLJ, ed. Brain Surgery: Complication Avoidance and Management. New York: Churchill Livingstone, 1993:2097–2113

27. Dieckmann G, Bockermann V, Heyer C, Henning J, Roesen M. Five-and-a-half years' experience with percutaneous retrogasserian glycerol rhizotomy in treatment of trigeminal neuralgia. Appl Neurophysiol 1987;50:401–413

28. Sweet WH. Treatment of trigeminal neuralgia by percutaneous rhizotomy. In: Youmans JR, ed. Neurological Surgery. Philadelphia: WB Saunders, 1990

29. Lunsford LD. Percutaneous retrogasserian glycerol rhizotomy. In: Rovit RL, Murali R, Jannetta PJ, eds. Trigeminal Neuralgia. Baltimore: Williams & Wilkins, 1990:145–164

30. Rappaport ZH, Gomori JM. Recurrent trigeminal cistern glycerol injections for tic douloureux. Acta Neurochir (Wien) 1988;90:31–34

31. Waltz TA, Dalessio DJ, Copeland B, Abbott G. Percutaneous injection of glycerol for the treatment of trigeminal neuralgia. Clin J Pain 1989;5:195–198

32. Sahni KS, Pieper DR, Anderson R, Baldwin NG. Relation of hypesthesia to the outcome of glycerol rhizolysis for trigeminal neuralgia. J Neurosurg 1990;72:55–58

33. Belber CJ, Rak RA. Balloon compression rhizolysis in the surgical management of trigeminal neuralgia. Neurosurgery 1987;20:908–913

34. Lobato RD, Rivas JJ, Sarabia R, Lamas E. Percutaneous microcompression of the gasserian ganglion for trigeminal neuralgia. J Neurosurg 1990;72:546–553

35. Tawk RG, Duffy-Fronckowiak M, Scott BE, et al. Stereotactic gamma knife surgery for trigeminal neuralgia: detailed analysis of treatment response. J Neurosurg 2005;102:442–449

36. Pollock BE. Radiosurgery for trigeminal neuralgia: is sensory disturbance required for pain relief? J Neurosurg 2006;105(Suppl):103–106

37. Taarnhøj P. Decompression of the posterior trigeminal root in trigeminal neuralgia. A 30-year follow-up review. J Neurosurg 1982;57:14–17

38. Leksell L. The stereotaxic method and radiosurgery of the brain. Acta Chir Scand 1951;102:316–319

39. Kondziolka D, Lunsford LD, Flickinger JC, et al. Stereotactic radiosurgery for trigeminal neuralgia: a multiinstitutional study using the gamma unit. J Neurosurg 1996;84:940–945

40. Régis J, Metellus P, Hayashi M, Roussel P, Donnet A, Bille-Turc F. Prospective controlled trial of gamma knife surgery for essential trigeminal neuralgia. J Neurosurg 2006;104:913–924

41. Kondziolka D, Zorro O, Lobato-Polo J, et al. Gamma knife stereotactic radiosurgery for idiopathic trigeminal neuralgia. J Neurosurg 2010;112:758–765

42. Villavicencio AT, Lim M, Burneikiene S, et al. CyberKnife radiosurgery for trigeminal neuralgia treatment: a preliminary multicenter experience. Neurosurgery 2008;62:647–655, discussion 647–655

43. Fountas KN, Smith JR, Lee GP, Jenkins PD, Cantrell RR, Sheils WC. Gamma knife stereotactic radiosurgical treatment of idiopathic trigeminal neuralgia: long-term outcome and complications. Neurosurg Focus 2007;23:E8

44. Longhi M, Rizzo P, Nicolato A, Foroni R, Reggio M, Gerosa M. Gamma knife radiosurgery for trigeminal neuralgia: results and potentially predictive parameters—part I: Idiopathic trigeminal neuralgia. Neurosurgery 2007;61:1254–1260, discussion 1260–1261

45. Pusztaszeri M, Villemure JG, Regli L, Do HP, Pica A. Radiosurgery for trigeminal neuralgia using a linear accelerator with BrainLab system: report on initial experience in Lausanne, Switzerland. Swiss Med Wkly 2007;137:682–686

46. Lim M, Villavicencio AT, Burneikiene S, et al. CyberKnife radiosurgery for idiopathic trigeminal neuralgia. Neurosurg Focus 2005;18:E9

47. McNatt SA, Yu C, Giannotta SL, Zee CS, Apuzzo ML, Petrovich Z. Gamma knife radiosurgery for trigeminal neuralgia. Neurosurgery 2005;56:1295–1301, discussion 1301–1303

48. Richards GM, Bradley KA, Tomé WA, Bentzen SM, Resnick DK, Mehta MP. Linear accelerator radiosurgery for trigeminal neuralgia. Neurosurgery 2005;57:1193–1200, discussion 1193–1200

49. Sheehan J, Pan HC, Stroila M, Steiner L. Gamma knife surgery for trigeminal neuralgia: outcomes and prognostic factors. J Neurosurg 2005;102:434–441

50. Urgosik D, Liscak R, Novotny J Jr, Vymazal J, Vladyka V. Treatment of essential trigeminal neuralgia with gamma knife surgery. J Neurosurg 2005;102(Suppl):29–33

51. Brisman R. Gamma knife surgery with a dose of 75 to 76.8 gray for trigeminal neuralgia. J Neurosurg 2004;100:848–854

52. Chen JC, Girvigian M, Greathouse H, Miller M, Rahimian J. Treatment of trigeminal neuralgia with linear accelerator radiosurgery: initial results. J Neurosurg 2004;101(Suppl 3):346–350

53. Frighetto L, De Salles AA, Smith ZA, Goss B, Selch M, Solberg T. Noninvasive linear accelerator radiosurgery as the primary treatment for trigeminal neuralgia. Neurology 2004;62:660–662

54. Massager N, Lorenzoni J, Devriendt D, Desmedt F, Brotchi J, Levivier M. Gamma knife surgery for idiopathic trigeminal neuralgia performed using a far-anterior cisternal target and a high dose of radiation. J Neurosurg 2004;100:597–605

55. Shaya M, Jawahar A, Caldito G, Sin A, Willis BK, Nanda A. Gamma knife radiosurgery for trigeminal neuralgia: a study of predictors of success, efficacy, safety, and outcome at LSUHSC. Surg Neurol 2004;61:529–534, discussion 534–535

56. Goss BW, Frighetto L, DeSalles AA, Smith Z, Solberg T, Selch M. Linear accelerator radiosurgery using 90 gray for essential trigeminal neuralgia: results and dose volume histogram analysis. Neurosurgery 2003;53:823–828, discussion 828–830

57. Petit JH, Herman JM, Nagda S, DiBiase SJ, Chin LS. Radiosurgical treatment of trigeminal neuralgia: evaluating quality of life and treatment outcomes. Int J Radiat Oncol Biol Phys 2003;56:1147–1153

58. Kondziolka D, Lunsford LD, Flickinger JC. Stereotactic radiosurgery for the treatment of trigeminal neuralgia. Clin J Pain 2002;18:42–47

59. Pollock BE, Phuong LK, Gorman DA, Foote RL, Stafford SL. Stereotactic radiosurgery for idiopathic trigeminal neuralgia. J Neurosurg 2002;97:347–353

60. Maesawa S, Salame C, Flickinger JC, Pirris S, Kondziolka D, Lunsford LD. Clinical outcomes after stereotactic radiosurgery for idiopathic trigeminal neuralgia. J Neurosurg 2001;94:14–20

61. Nicol B, Regine WF, Courtney C, Meigooni A, Sanders M, Young B. Gamma knife radiosurgery using 90 Gy for trigeminal neuralgia. J Neurosurg 2000;93(Suppl 3):152–154

62. Rogers CL, Shetter AG, Fiedler JA, Smith KA, Han PP, Speiser BL. Gamma knife radiosurgery for trigeminal neuralgia: the initial experience of the Barrow Neurological Institute. Int J Radiat Oncol Biol Phys 2000;47:1013–1019

63. Sheehan JP, Ray DK, Monteith S, et al. Gamma knife radiosurgery for trigeminal neuralgia: the impact of magnetic resonance imaging-detected vascular impingement of the affected nerve. J Neurosurg 2010;113:53–58

64. Hasegawa T, Kondziolka D, Spiro R, Flickinger JC, Lunsford LD. Repeat radiosurgery for refractory trigeminal neuralgia. Neurosurgery 2002;50:494–500, discussion 500–502

65. Shetter AG, Rogers CL, Ponce F, Fiedler JA, Smith K, Speiser BL. Gamma knife radiosurgery for recurrent trigeminal neuralgia. J Neurosurg 2002;97(5, Suppl):536–538

66. Herman JM, Petit JH, Amin P, Kwok Y, Dutta PR, Chin LS. Repeat gamma knife radiosurgery for refractory or recurrent trigeminal neuralgia: treatment outcomes and quality-of-life assessment. Int J Radiat Oncol Biol Phys 2004;59:112–116

67. Kirkpatrick DB. Familial trigeminal neuralgia: case report. Neurosurgery 1989;24:758–761

68. Nugent GR. Percutaneous techniques for trigeminal neuralgia. In: Kaye AH, Black P, eds. Operative Neurosurgery. London: Churchill Livingstone, 1999:1615–1633

Chapter 20

Treatment of Intractable Facial Pain

Case

A 50-year-old man underwent resection of a petroclival meningioma. Three months after surgery, he began to have facial pain that was persistent and increasing, associated with dysesthesia, and intractable to all forms of medical treatment.

Participants

Percutaneous Descending Trigeminal Tractotomy–Nucleotomy for Intractable Facial Pain: *Yucel Kanpolat*

Central Neurostimulation for Intractable Neuropathic Facial Pain: Esmiralda Yeremeyeva, Chima Oluigbo, and Ali Rezai

Moderator: Treatment of Intractable Facial Pain: Kim J. Burchiel

Percutaneous Descending Trigeminal Tractotomy–Nucleotomy for Intractable Facial Pain

Yucel Kanpolat

In the 1996 edition of *Controversies in Neurosurgery*, three great masters of neurologic surgery—Schvarcz,[1] Burchiel,[2] and Gybels[3]—provided some unique recommendations for a patient with neuropathic pain after the removal of a petroclival meningioma. With my 40 years' experience in medical pain practice, I would emphasize the following points regarding this problematic case:

1. Drugs usually fail to resolve neuropathic pain; nevertheless, I still recommend antidepressants or gabapentin for such patients.

2. Peripheral lesions are usually contraindicated and worsen the neuropathic pain; thus, they are useless.
3. The efficacy of stimulation is unsatisfactory.
4. Tractotomy-nucleotomy is preferable for such patients as a first step. If it is only partially effective, a nucleus caudalis dorsal root entry zone (DREZ) lesion can be created as a final stage.

The practice of central lesioning of the trigeminal tract, which contains the fibers of the fifth, seventh, ninth, and tenth nerves of pain areas, was initiated by Sjöqvist[4] in 1938

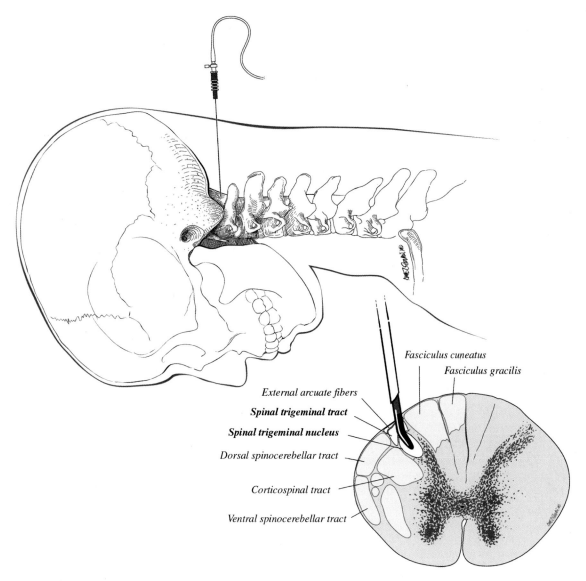

Fasciculus cuneatus

Fasciculus gracilis

External arcuate fibers

Spinal trigeminal tract

Spinal trigeminal nucleus

Dorsal spinocerebellar tract

Corticospinal tract

Ventral spinocerebellar tract

Fig. 20.1   Schematic drawing of the percutaneous puncture of the occiput-C1 level 6 to 8 mm lateral from the midline, and the target-electrode relationship and main anatomic structures in the percutaneous tractotomy-nucleotomy.

and designated as *trigeminal tractotomy*. The procedure was done as open surgery. In 1970, Hitchcock[5] described a stereotactic percutaneous trigeminal tractotomy, and in 1972, Crue and colleagues[6] published their description of radiofrequency trigeminal tractotomy. In view of the lesioning of the oral pole of the nucleus caudalis, the procedure was termed *trigeminal nucleotomy* by Schvarcz (personal communication, 1993).[7,8] Sindou[9] performed lesioning of the substantia gelatinosa and named the procedure *selective posterior rhizotomy*. Nashold and associates[10,11] used the procedure with radiofrequency electrodes and named it the DREZ operation. In 1987, Bernard and colleagues[12] described the procedure as nucleus caudalis DREZ lesions. I began to use computed tomography (CT) imaging in the practice of destructive pain procedures and CT guidance for lesioning of the trigeminal tract and nucleus.[13–17] Over a period of 23 years (1988–2011), I performed 95 trigeminal tractotomy-nucleotomy procedures in 80 patients and 13 nucleus caudalis DREZ operations in some special pain cases.[17] Tractotomy-nucleotomy was used as a special method for understanding the benefit of the nucleus caudalis DREZ operation. In 12 of the 13 patients undergoing the nucleus caudalis DREZ procedure, trigeminal tractotomy-nucleotomy was effective, but not sufficiently so, and I decided to carry out a nucleus caudalis DREZ operation in these patients.[17]

Although Schvarcz used the term *trigeminal nucleotomy*, as noted above, I believe the term *tracto-nucleotomy* is more appropriate, and it has been used by many authors. In the brainstem, the spinal trigeminal nucleus is in close proximity to the descending trigeminal nucleus. We know that lesioning of the system affects not only the oral pole of the trigeminal nucleus but also the descending trigeminal tract. For this reason, the term *trigeminal tracto-nucleotomy* is more accurate.

The procedure is done with the patient lying face down, and a posterior approach is preferred (**Fig. 20.1**). The target is located at the occiput-C1 level. The needle or cannula is inserted either freehand or stereotactically 6 to 8 mm from the midline at the occiput-C1 level. The neck is flexed and the target is one third of the lateral part of the ipsilateral upper spinal cord. The depth of the electrode is planned according to the diametral measurements of the spinal cord in this region, 3 to 3.5 mm from the posterior surface of the spinal cord. This method has been described previously.[13–17] The first part of the procedure entails localization of the needle electrode system morphologically; after the morphology is determined, the physiological part of the procedure becomes crucial (**Fig. 20.2**). The lesion side is chosen through stimulation, with the first branch of the trigeminal nerve at the most distant point anteriorly and the seventh, ninth, and tenth nerves at the most distant point posteriorly. Stimulation and impedance measurement are mandatory at this point. Impedance is usually more than 1,000 Ohm and the stimulation parameters are started from the lowest level: 2 to 5 Hz, 0.03 to 1 V. The procedure is painful, and patients sometimes cannot tolerate the high standard-frequency electrical stimulation.

The final stage of the procedure is lesioning. The surgeon must remember that lesioning of the nucleus caudalis or descending trigeminal tract is painful. As the patient cannot tolerate high standard lesions, Schvarcz recommended that I elevate the caudal extent of the curved electrode tip in an upward and downward motion. However, I have been unable to use the technique because of my own lack of sufficient experience in this regard.

Over the past 23 years, I have performed 95 procedures in 80 patients. Most of them had craniofacial cancer pain, atypical facial pain, and glossopharyngeal, geniculate, and vagal neuralgias. Definitive diagnoses included 17 patients with craniofacial cancer pain, 15 with atypical facial pain, four with geniculate neuralgia, and 17 with glossopharyngeal neuralgia. The rest of the patients had mixed pain and were not given one definitive final diagnosis. In this group, there was only one neuropathic pain problem immediately after the removal of a petroclival neurofibroma from the cerebellopontine angle. The diagnosis was neuropathic pain, and the procedure was not effective.

As a last choice, we performed 13 nucleus caudalis DREZ operations. In 12 of them, the tractotomy-nucleotomy was effective. Based on this result, we can state that, if the tractotomy-nucleotomy is effective, there is hope that the nucleus caudalis DREZ lesion will be even more effective. I consider the tractotomy-nucleotomy as my first-line destructive procedure in this neuropathic central pain condition. If the procedure is only partially effective, I can use nucleus caudalis DREZ lesioning for further efficacy.

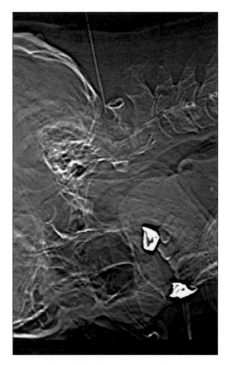

Fig. 20.2a–c The percutaneous approach to the occiput-C1 level in the trigeminal tracto-nucleotomy. **(a)** Lateral scanogram of the procedure. (*continued on next page*)

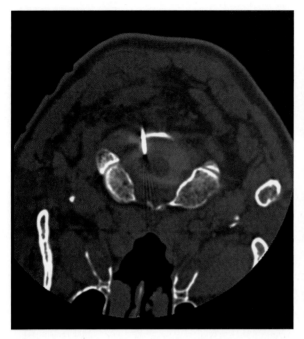
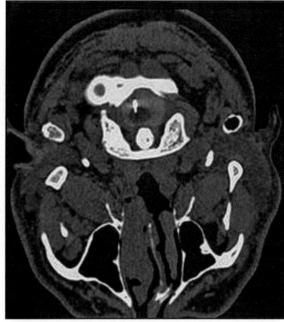

b

c

Fig. 20.2a–c (*continued*) **(b)** Final position of the cannula. **(c)** Final position of the electrode.

The presented case represents the most problematic type of patient in neurosurgical practice, and there is no standard algorithm for treatment decisions. Based on my personal experience, I recommend tractotomy-nucleotomy for such patients. If it is only partially effective, as a final procedure I would recommend a nucleus caudalis DREZ lesion.

Central Neurostimulation for Intractable Neuropathic Facial Pain

Esmiralda Yeremeyeva, Chima Oluigbo, and Ali Rezai

Chronic neuropathic pain has a significant impact on the quality of life of 70 million Americans.[18] The economic burden of chronic pain is reflected in health care costs, missed work days, and high unemployment rates. Patients with chronic neuropathic pain experience a substantially lower health-related quality of life than the general population.[19]

Chronic neuropathic pain is mainly characterized by a constant pain often accompanied by amplified responses to both noxious and nonnoxious stimuli. It results from a lesion anywhere in the afferent nociceptive pathways. Associated symptoms may be negative (hypoesthesia, hypoalgesia) or positive (sensitivity to cold or heat, hyperalgesia, paresthesias, allodynia).[20]

Pain to the face can be referred, but most pain sensation is through the trigeminal nerve, which provides the sensory innervations to the face.[21] The causes of intractable neuropathic facial pain are numerous—tumors, the herpes virus (shingles), malignant or benign neoplasms, multiple

sclerosis, infections, sarcoidosis, orofacial surgery—or they may be idiopathic. In contrast to trigeminal neuralgia, neuropathic facial pain is continuous, burning, or aching, although there are some fluctuations in the severity. Because the sources of pain can be various or even unknown, it is particularly hard to treat this pain with medication.

According to Burchiel's[22] new classification of facial pain, classic trigeminal neuropathic pain (TNP) is a consequence of an accidental injury to the trigeminal nerve, for example, from trauma or surgery. Deafferentation facial pain results from intentional injury to the nerve through ablative procedures, with the goal of treating trigeminal neuralgia or neuropathy. Other types are trigeminal postherpetic neuralgia in a dermatomal distribution, facial pain from multiple sclerosis, and atypical facial pain, which is secondary to a somatoform pain disorder.[22]

Various mechanisms may be responsible for the development of chronic neuropathic pain and its accompanying negative and positive symptoms. Wallerian degeneration and its consequent surrounding inflammation upregulate receptors for neurotrophic factors and cytokines, thus increasing the excitability of the primary sensory neurons. This phenomenon creates an exaggerated response to the peripheral stimulus and manifestations of allodynia and mechanical hypersensitivity. Another effect of peripheral nerve injury is the development of new contacts between the sensory neurons and the sympathetic nervous system. This development has been shown in two investigations in which α_2-subtype receptors, which are normally present on dorsal root ganglion sensory neurons, were increased in models of peripheral nerve injury.[23,24] The connectivity of sensory afferents may also be abnormal because of novel synapse formation in the dorsal horn.[25]

Opioid medications are generally not effective for treating patients with chronic neuropathic pain, and there have been relatively few new alternatives, such as antiepileptics and antidepressants. Clinical trials show that pharmacotherapy in clinical practice offers only 40 to 50% symptomatic pain relief and no changes in the pathophysiology of the disease.[26]

Surgical Intervention

Several neuromodulation surgical options, such as central and peripheral stimulation, exist. In this section we focus on two central neurostimulation modalities used to treat neuropathic facial pain: motor cortex stimulation (MCS) and deep brain stimulation (DBS). The general surgical approach in patients with chronic neuropathic pain must be done by a multidisciplinary team that includes a pain specialist, who assesses the patient first and ultimately exhausts all the medical options; a neuropsychologist, who determines if there is significant cognitive impairment and active psychiatric issues; and a neurosurgeon. A social support system is imperative in caring for these patients postoperatively as well.

Motor Cortex Stimulation

Background

In 1991, Tsubokawa and colleagues[27] attempted to stimulate the sensory and motor cortex as components of the somatosensory pathway and noted efficacy from stimulation of the motor cortex. In their cat model, stimulation of the motor cortex completely and persistently inhibited the burst hyperactivity of thalamic neurons. They theorized that thalamic pain syndromes can be addressed through chronic stimulation of the motor cortex. They proceeded to stimulate 12 patients with medically refractory central deafferentation pain and achieved a 67% rate of a lasting decrease in pain.[28] In 1993, Meyerson and colleagues[29] treated their patients with motor cortex stimulation (MCS) and noted that all patients with TNP had significant lessening of their pain. In the past 15 years, there has been rising interest in this modality of pain treatment, as demonstrated by

Fontaine and associates[30] in their review of 244 MCS studies of chronic neuropathic pain (1991–2006). Despite this growing interest, the exact mechanism of action is still unknown. Positron emission tomography studies of patients undergoing MCS implicate the thalamus as the key structure mediating functional MCS effects.[31,32] One hypothesis derived from functional studies is that descending axons activated by MCS from the motor and pre-motor cortices in turn activate thalamic nuclei, which cycle with other pain-related structures receiving afferent pain perception, such as the medial thalamus, anterior cingulate cortex, and upper brain stem.[31,32] Another hypothesis points to an increase in the secretion of endogenous opioids triggered by chronic MCS.[33]

Motor cortex stimulation is mainly used to treat central thalamic pain, TNP,[30] and, less so, peripheral neuropathic pain. Other indications reported in the literature include phantom limb pain, brachial plexus avulsion, spinal cord injury, post-herpetic neuralgia, and peripheral nerve lesions, including nerve root or nerve trunk pain related to previously excised tumors.[34-39]

Surgical Technique

Recording a detailed history of the patient is imperative to confirm the diagnosis, and a neuropsychological evaluation must be done to determine the presence of ongoing uncontrolled depression, anxiety disorders, substance abuse, or other major psychological issues, which must be addressed and stabilized before surgery. The patient should understand that a trial period of several days with the electrodes is required. A positive response must be at least a 50% reduction in pain; if the pain is not reduced during the trial, the electrodes are removed without further consideration of MCS. The general sequence of events is preoperative localization of the motor cortex, intraoperative electrophysiological mapping of the face area of the motor cortex, implantation of the MCS electrodes followed by an externalized MCS trial, and then internalization of the system after a successful trial.

The face area of the motor cortex can be localized through a fusion of preoperative images with the neuronavigation system, which enables anatomic localization of the motor cortex. Functional magnetic resonance imaging (MRI) and transcranial magnetic stimulation may also be used (**Fig. 20.3**). Electrodes may be placed through bur holes or a small craniotomy. A craniotomy may allow a more accurate intraoperative electrophysiological evaluation. The procedure is done with the patient either under general endotracheal anesthesia or, in some centers, awake under monitored anesthesia care. Paralytic agents are not used, as they block the electromyographic responses used for electrical cortical mapping. The patient's head is fixed with a three-pin headholder to eliminate motion and to allow the use of the frameless navigation system. The outline of the precentral gyrus is projected onto the scalp with preoperative imaging fused with the neuronavigation system, and the incision is centered over this region. We prefer a 4-cm craniotomy, which is large enough to allow the epidural placement of a 4 × 4 electrode grid. The 16-electrode testing grid is then placed in the epidural space (**Fig. 20.4**).

Intraoperative electrophysiological testing allows confirmation of the previously obtained position of the central sulcus and localizes the motor cortex through stimulation. First, the site and orientation of the central sulcus is identified based on the N20-P20 wave shift (phase reversal) obtained during recording of somatosensory evoked potentials (**Fig. 20.5**). Then the cortex anterior to the central sulcus is stimulated through the electrode grid, while the surgeon looks for motor contractions in the facial muscles. Commonly used muscles are the orbicularis oris, orbicularis oculi, and masseter. The position of the stimulating electrodes that produced motor contractions at the lowest threshold is marked on the dura with a pen. This position defines the optimal site for MCS. A cold solution should be immediately available for irrigation of the motor cortex in case of a seizure induced by the stimulation.

Two 2-plate paddle electrode arrays (or one 4-plate array) are then placed in the epidural space in the previously determined optimal position and are oriented perpendicularly to the central sulcus and sutured to the dura (**Fig. 20.6**). Leads are tunneled externally and connected to an external pulse generator to test the efficacy of stimulation over several days. During the trial, the stimulation amplitude is set at a value of 80% of the threshold for motor

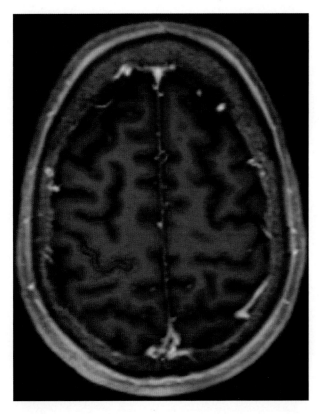

Fig. 20.3 A high-resolution preoperative magnetic resonance image is used to identify the central sulcus (*red line*), which follows a classic "Ω" pattern.

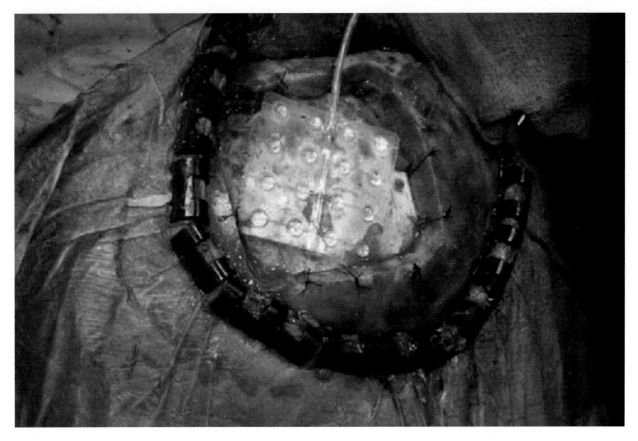

Fig. 20.4 The 16-electrode testing grid is placed into a 4-cm craniotomy in the epidural space to carry out neurophysiological testing.

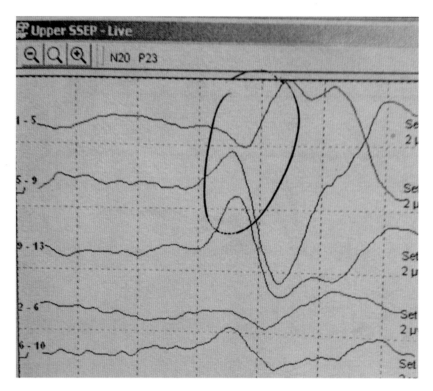

Fig. 20.5 An N20-P20 wave shift (phase reversal) is shown with a positive sensory wave and a negative motor wave.

contraction. Typical stimulation parameters are amplitudes of 1 to 3 V, a frequency of 40 Hz, and a pulse width of 90 microseconds. A trial is considered successful if patients experience pain relief of at least 50% with stimulation.

During the internalization, the scalp flap is partially reopened to expose the MCS electrode lead that was coiled under the galea during the first procedure. This lead is then connected to a new extension wire that is tunneled under the skin and connected to an implantable pulse generator,

which is typically placed in a subcutaneous or subfascial pocket created in the infraclavicular region **(Fig. 20.7)**.

Outcome after Motor Cortex Stimulation

Reviewing outcomes for the past 15 years, Fontaine and associates[40] reported that 57.6% of patients had "good" postoperative pain relief (defined in various studies as pain relief ≥ 40% or ≥ 50%), whereas 30% of patients had a ≥ 70%

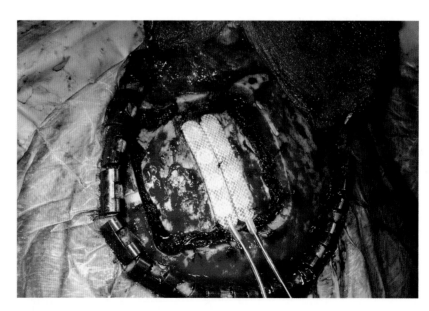

Fig. 20.6 Two 2-plate paddle electrode arrays are placed in the epidural space over the facial area of the motor cortex. They are oriented perpendicularly to the central sulcus and sutured to the dura.

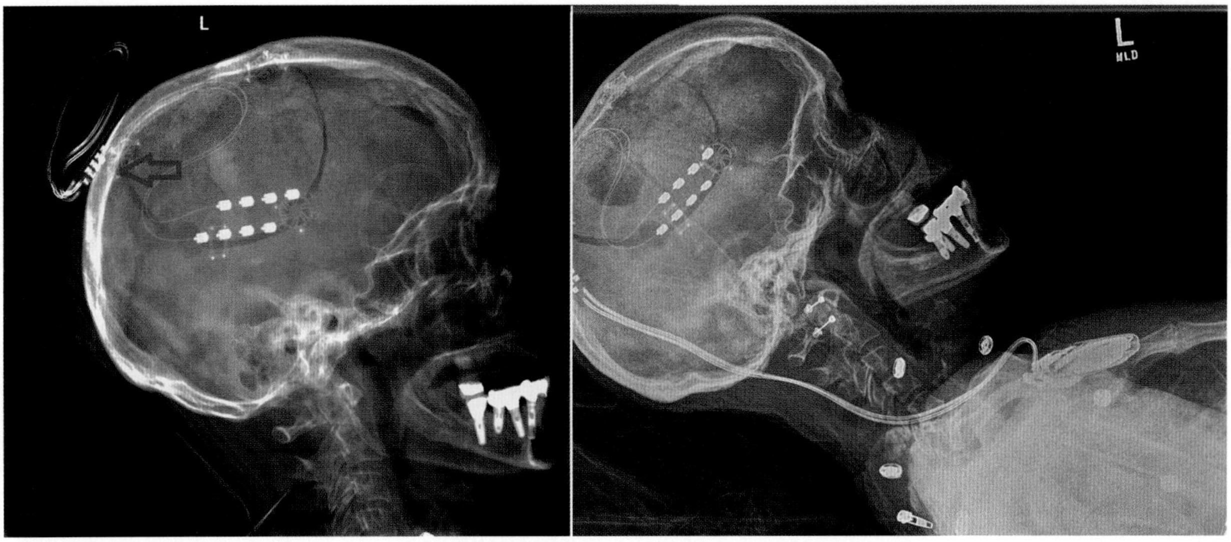

a   b

Fig. 20.7a,b For the trial, the leads are coupled to the temporary extensions at the distal connector site (**a**, *red arrow*). The
temporary extensions are kept under the galea proximally, and
the distal parts are tunneled out under the scalp. During permanent implantation (**b**), the temporary leads are disconnected and
removed, and the permanent extensions are tunneled down to
the infraclavicular region to be connected to the pulse generator.

reduction of pain. In the 152 patients who had a follow-up
of longer than 1 year, 45.4% had a "good postoperative outcome." Again, outcomes were best in patients with facial
neuropathic pain. A randomized double-blinded trial by
García-Larrea and colleagues[31] reported a pain reduction of
40% or more at 1 year in all eight patients who received an
implant with MCS. The most notable surgical risks are epidural hematoma, infection, and intraoperative seizures.
Neither permanent neurologic deficit or injury after stimulator placement nor the development of chronic seizures
has been reported.[41] Overall, the literature recommends
MCS as an effective and safe treatment of medically refractory neuropathic facial pain in very well-selected patients.

Deep Brain Stimulation

Background

Deep brain stimulation (DBS) has been a surgical option for
chronic pain long before its popularization as a treatment
for movement disorders.[42–44] The two main targets are the
sensory thalamic nuclei and periventricular/periaqueductal
gray (PVG/PAG) matter. In general, neuropathic facial pain
responds best to the stimulation of the ventroposterome-
dial (VPM) thalamic nuclei, rather than the PVG/PAG.[45,46]
Other targets include the medial lemniscus, internal capsule, and thalamic posterior nucleus ovalis.[45] Sometimes,
for mixed nociceptive (i.e., facial allodynia) and neuropathic
symptoms, both VPM and PVG/PAG are used. As with MCS,
the mechanism of action is not well understood. In a primate model, spinothalamic tract neurons were strongly
inhibited through the stimulation of either the ipsilateral
or contralateral sensory thalamus.[47] On positron emission
tomography scans, sustained activation of the anterior

cingulate cortex, which receives nociceptive input from the
thalamus, was observed during DBS.[48]

Surgical Procedure

This procedure is done in a similar fashion to DBS for movement disorders.[49] As with the MCS, however, a similar preoperative multidisciplinary approach and a several-day trial
period with pain relief of 50% is required for permanent
implantation.

For unilateral facial pain, the contralateral thalamus is
approached. Either frameless or framed systems may be
used for stereotactic localization. At our institution, we use
the Leksell stereotactic head frame. The coordinates for
VPM are chosen within the Talairach space, 1 to 2 mm
below the anterior-posterior commissural line, 10 to 11 mm
lateral to the wall of the third ventricle, and 2 to 3 mm
anterior to the posterior commissure. The patient is kept
under monitored anesthesia care and is awake during the
microelectrode recording and stimulation. During the recording, light touch and deep pressure are tested on the
contralateral face and body to define the somatotopy. Once
the target is reached, micro- or macrostimulation is used to
determine the coverage of the pain area and any side effects. Multiple tracks may be needed. Satisfactory placement provides stimulation that is tolerable at usual settings
(see below) and covers the face without effects spreading
to the body. Electrodes are connected to extensions and
tunneled for an external trial, which usually lasts 5 to 7
days in an inpatient setting. Stimulation is tested in a range
of amplitude of 2 to 3 V, a pulse width of 100 to 200 microseconds, and a frequency of 25 to 75 Hz, respectively. If the
patient's overall pain relief is more than 50%, the DBS sys-

tem is permanently implanted in similar fashion to the MCS system.

Outcome After Deep Brain Stimulation for Chronic Neuropathic Pain

In terms of outcome, a meta-analysis by Levy and colleagues[45] showed that 50% of patients had long-term successful pain relief. When the sensory thalamic nucleus was targeted for neuropathic pain, a long-term success rate of 56% was achieved. In a more recent meta-analysis, Bittar and associates[50] broke down the results according to the site of pain. Four patients with trigeminal neuropathy, one with atypical facial pain, and 28 with anesthesia dolorosa had successful pain relief of 100%, 100%, and 47%, respectively. The most dreaded complication of DBS is hemorrhage, which occurred in between 1.9% and 4.1% of patients in the series of Bittar and colleagues, but permanent neurologic deficit from such bleeding is rare. The incidence of infectious complications from DBS ranges from 3.3 to 13.3%. No correlation was found between the time the electrode was externalized and the occurrence of infection.[45]

Emerging Options for Deep Brain Stimulation for Pain

These brain targets for central neurostimulation involve the conscious processing of nociception. Functional MRI has furthered our knowledge about cortical-subcortical circuits a great deal. It has been shown that the dorsolateral prefrontal cortex, the anterior cingulate cortex, and the anterior and posterior insula are involved in the actual awareness and emotional processing of pain.[51] In a placebo analgesia model, the dorsolateral prefrontal cortex was shown to influence the dorsal anterior cingulate cortex.[52] Zaki and colleagues[53] noted that the anterior cingulate cortex and the anterior insula are engaged in patients both while experiencing their own pain and while watching other people experience pain. The anterior cingulate cortex in turn influences the nucleus accumbens,[54] which may be involved in an analgesic response to chronic pain.[55] These cortical and subcortical structures may serve as adjunct targets for neurostimulation for chronic facial pain in the future.

Conclusion

Both MCS and DBS are safe surgical options for the treatment of intractable neuropathic facial pain. The ventromedial nucleus of the thalamus is the preferred site for DBS for this type of pain. The careful selection of patients by a multidisciplinary team is mandatory, and a surgical trial is required to ensure the success of these interventions. An evolving knowledge of the neurocircuitry involved in chronic pain may allow us to refine and personalize the treatment strategies for patients with chronic TNP in the future.

Moderator
Treatment of Intractable Facial Pain
Kim J. Burchiel

Al-Mefty has again challenged us with one of the most daunting problems in neurologic surgery. This patient must have suffered an incidental trigeminal nerve injury consequent to his resective surgery. The attendant deafferentation has produced what would be categorized as TNP.

Yucel Kanpolat, widely regarded as the world's authority on this topic, has contributed a succinct assessment of his experience with similar cases. I find that his recommendations concerning the medical intractability of this pain, and the general observation that antidepressants and gabapentin must be on the list of agents that have been tested, ring completely true. I also agree that further peripheral deafferentation would be both ineffective and potentially dangerous; the pain can be made worse. My experience also echoes his, in that peripheral electrical stimulation is of little benefit. Kanpolat concludes that CT-guided trigeminal tractotomy-nucleotomy (TR-NC) would be his first choice for this patient. If the results of this procedure are encouraging, the patient could also go on to an open "caudalis DREZ" or, more properly, open trigeminal nucleotractotomy.

Kanpolat states that the one patient he did perform TR-NC on, who had the diagnosis of TNP after the removal of a petroclival neurofibroma from the cerebellopontine angle, had unsatisfactory pain relief. In his hands, TR-NC was used in 21 patients with "atypical facial pain" and adequate pain relief was achieved in 91%.[16] Further, four of five patients with failed trigeminal neuralgia were also effectively treated with TR-NC. These are impressive results, but not clearly relevant to the present case. My conclusion is that, after appropriate informed consent is obtained, a TR-NC done by a skilled practitioner of that procedure could be recommended, with the caveats that outcome data for this particular condition are not available, and essentially no one in the world has experience with this procedure comparable to that of Kanpolat.

Yeremeyeva, Oluigbo, and Rezai were assigned the task of describing the roles of DBS and MCS in this case. Their introduction of the topic of TNP is on target, to the point, and scholarly.

In my opinion, TNP outcome data for MCS remain problematic. Naturally, the scientific literature reflects a bias for positive results, and this seems to be a pernicious problem in the area of neuromodulation for pain. Although it has been in use now for more than 20 years, MCS still represents the most recent potential innovation in surgical pain control that I am aware of. Tsubokawa and colleagues[27,28] originally introduced this procedure as an alternative to DBS for treating patients with thalamic pain. Meyerson and associates[29] identified TNP as a particularly attractive target for the procedure, and it is on this condition that most attention on MCS has focused in the intervening years.

Yeremeyeva, Oluigbo, and Rezai cite several encouraging articles from respected centers and investigators[45,50,56] about the role of MCS for treating neuropathic pain. These positive findings are counterbalanced by reports from other institutions, where the results of MCS for TNP have not been uniformly good. For example, an industry-sponsored European study of MCS to treat facial (trigeminal) and central poststroke deafferentation pain was closed by the sponsor because of slow enrollment. Only 24 patients out of a planned 104 were enrolled and underwent implantation in 2 years. Seven of these 24 patients (29%) withdrew or were discontinued from the study after lead implantation but before randomization to a sham procedure or active MCS because of a lack of efficacy during either the trial stimulation or early on in their therapeutic course. Eleven patients were randomized and completed a blinded one-way crossover MCS (on to off, or off to on; 4 weeks' duration each). Of these 11 patients, none expressed a preference for the MCS "on" condition regardless of the on-off sequence to which they were randomized.[57]

The results of DBS for TNP must likewise be viewed with some skepticism. In a structured review of the DBS literature, Coffey[58] concluded: "Deep brain stimulation has not

been shown to produce effective long-term pain relief." This review was later reprised and amplified in a recent textbook chapter. In that review, Coffey and associates[57] concluded that late results of DBS for pain are not substantiated by results 6 to 24 months after implantation, and no reviewed study achieved the 50% success threshold typically applied to this literature. All of the studies analyzed showed substantial problems with both data gathering and analysis.

As is the case for MCS, the evidence that DBS would be effective in the patient presented here is weak. Further confounding the treatment of our patient, at least in the United States, is the fact that neither MCS nor DBS is approved by the Food and Drug Administration for the indication of pain control. The Medicare program does not authorize MCS or DBS, and, as a result, the procedures are rarely done in patients on Medicare. Most major insurance companies have followed suit and do not approve this therapy. As a consequence, both MCS and DBS for pain are only sporadically done in the United States, making it very difficult to obtain consistent or contemporaneous case series at most institutions.

Conclusion

At this point, it is difficult to enthusiastically recommend any surgical intervention for this patient solely for the purpose of alleviating his TNP. TR-NC might be considered, but supportive data are not available, and finding a neurosurgeon to perform the procedure would be very difficult. The data that MCS or DBS might work for this patient is not compelling, but both of these procedures have the advantage of "testability." A trial of neurostimulation (MCS or DBS) could be undertaken, if the patient's insurance coverage would allow it.

This case emphasizes the difficulties we encounter with neuropathic pain in general. There are no specific analgesic agents available, and the evidence that surgery might work is entirely from personal case series (class III) or anecdotal. In my own practice, this patient would likely be treated nonsurgically in the context of a multidisciplinary pain center.

References

1. Schvarcz JR. Descending trigeminal nucleotomy for dysesthetic facial pain. In: Al-Mefty O, Origitano TC, Harkey HL, eds. Controversies in Neurosurgery. New York: Thieme, 1996:351–353
2. Burchiel KJ. Deep brain stimulation for facial pain. In: Al-Mefty O, Origitano TC, Harkey HL, eds. Controversies in Neurosurgery. New York: Thieme, 1996:353–354
3. Gybels JM. Treatment of facial pain: descending trigeminal nucleotomy vs. deep brain stimulation. In: Al-Mefty O, Origitano TC, Harkey HL, eds. Controversies in Neurosurgery. New York: Thieme, 1996:355–356
4. Sjöqvist O. Studies on pain conduction in the trigeminal nerve. A contribution to the surgical treatment of facial pain. Acta Psychiatr Neurol Scand, Suppl 1938;17:93–122
5. Hitchcock E. Stereotactic trigeminal tractotomy. Ann Clin Res 1970;2:131–135
6. Crue BL, Carregal EJ, Felsööry A. Percutaneous stereotactic radiofrequency trigeminal tractotomy with neurophysiological recordings. Confin Neurol 1972;34:389–397
7. Schvarcz JR. Stereotactic trigeminal tractotomy. Confin Neurol 1975;37:73–77
8. Schvarcz JR. Postherpetic craniofacial dysaesthesiae: their management by stereotaxic trigeminal nucleotomy. Acta Neurochir (Wien) 1977;38:65–72
9. Sindou M. Etude de la Junction Radiculo-Medullaire Posterieure: La Radicellotomie Posterieure Selective dans la Chirurgie de la Douleur [thesis]. Lyon, 1972

10. Nashold BS Jr, Urban B, Zorub DS. Phantom pain relief by focal destruction of the substantia gelatinosa of Rolando. In: Albe-Fessard DG, Bonica JJ, Liebeskind JC, eds. Advances in Pain Research and Therapy, vol. 1. New York: Raven Press, 1978: 959–963

11. Nashold BS Jr, el-Naggar A, Mawaffak Abdulhak M, Ovelmen-Levitt J, Cosman E. Trigeminal nucleus caudalis dorsal root entry zone: a new surgical approach. Stereotact Funct Neurosurg 1992;59:45–51

12. Bernard EJ Jr, Nashold BS Jr, Caputi F, Moossy JJ. Nucleus caudalis DREZ lesions for facial pain. Br J Neurosurg 1987;1:81–91

13. Kanpolat Y, Deda H, Akyar S, Cağlar S, Bilgiç S. CT-guided trigeminal tractotomy. Acta Neurochir (Wien) 1989;100:112–114

14. Kanpolat Y, Akyar S, Cağlar S. Diametral measurements of the upper spinal cord for stereotactic pain procedures: experimental and clinical study. Surg Neurol 1995;43:478–482, discussion 482–483

15. Kanpolat Y, Savas A, Cağlar S, Aydın V, Tascioglu AB, Akyar S. Computed tomography-guided percutaneous trigeminal tractotomy-nucleotomy. Tech Neurosurg 1999;5:244–251

16. Kanpolat Y, Kahiloğulları G, Uğur HÇ, Elhan AH. CT-guided percutaneous trigeminal tractotomy-nucleotomy (TR-NC): a technical report. Oper Neurosurg Suppl. 2008;1:ONS147–ONS155

17. Kanpolat Y, Tuna H, Bozkurt M, Elhan AH. The spinal and nucleus caudalis DREZ operations for chronic pain—technical report. Oper Neurosurg Suppl. 2008;1:ONS235–ONS244

18. Disability and Chronic Illness Behavior Committee on Pain. Pain and Disability: Clinical, Behavioral, and Public Policy Perspectives. Washington, DC: National Academies Press, 1987.

19. Doth AH, Hansson PT, Jensen MP, Taylor RS. The burden of neuropathic pain: a systematic review and meta-analysis of health utilities. Pain 2010;149:338–344

20. Baron R, Binder A, Wasner G. Neuropathic pain: diagnosis, pathophysiological mechanisms, and treatment. Lancet Neurol 2010;9:807–819

21. Larrier D, Lee A. Anatomy of headache and facial pain. Otolaryngol Clin North Am 2003;36:1041–1053, v

22. Burchiel KJ. A new classification for facial pain. Neurosurgery 2003;53:1164–1166, discussion 1166–1167

23. Gold MS, Dastmalchi S, Levine JD. Alpha 2-adrenergic receptor subtypes in rat dorsal root and superior cervical ganglion neurons. Pain 1997;69:179–190

24. Birder LA, Perl ER. Expression of alpha2-adrenergic receptors in rat primary afferent neurones after peripheral nerve injury or inflammation. J Physiol 1999;515(Pt 2):533–542

25. Shortland P, Woolf CJ. Chronic peripheral nerve section results in a rearrangement of the central axonal arborizations of axotomized A beta primary afferent neurons in the rat spinal cord. J Comp Neurol 1993;330:65–82

26. Backonja MM, Irving G, Argoff C. Rational multidrug therapy in the treatment of neuropathic pain. Curr Pain Headache Rep 2006;10:34–38

27. Tsubokawa T, Katayama Y, Yamamoto T, Hirayama T, Koyama S. Treatment of thalamic pain by chronic motor cortex stimulation. Pacing Clin Electrophysiol 1991;14:131–134

28. Tsubokawa T, Katayama Y, Yamamoto T, Hirayama T, Koyama S. Chronic motor cortex stimulation for the treatment of central pain. Acta Neurochir Suppl (Wien) 1991;52:137–139

29. Meyerson BA, Lindblom U, Linderoth B, Lind G, Herregodts P. Motor cortex stimulation as treatment of trigeminal neuropathic pain. Acta Neurochir Suppl (Wien) 1993;58:150–153

30. Fontaine D, Hamani C, Lozano A. Efficacy and safety of motor cortex stimulation for chronic neuropathic pain: critical review of the literature. J Neurosurg 2009;110:251–256

31. García-Larrea L, Peyron R, Mertens P, et al. Electrical stimulation of motor cortex for pain control: a combined PET-scan and electrophysiological study. Pain 1999;83:259–273

32. García-Larrea L, Peyron R, Mertens P, Laurent B, Mauguière F, Sindou M. Functional imaging and neurophysiological assessment of spinal and brain therapeutic modulation in humans. Arch Med Res 2000;31:248–257

33. García-Larrea L, Maarrawi J, Peyron R, et al. On the relation between sensory deafferentation, pain and thalamic activity in Wallenberg's syndrome: a PET-scan study before and after motor cortex stimulation. Eur J Pain 2006;10:677–688

34. Nguyen JP, Lefaucheur JP, Decq P, et al. Chronic motor cortex stimulation in the treatment of central and neuropathic pain. Correlations between clinical, electrophysiological and anatomical data. Pain 1999;82:245–251

35. Saitoh Y, Shibata M, Sanada Y, Mashimo T. Motor cortex stimulation for phantom limb pain. Lancet 1999;353:212

36. Smith H, Joint C, Schlugman D, Nandi D, Stein JF, Aziz TZ. Motor cortex stimulation for neuropathic pain. Neurosurg Focus 2001; 11:E2

37. Sol JC, Casaux J, Roux FE, et al. Chronic motor cortex stimulation for phantom limb pain: correlations between pain relief and functional imaging studies. Stereotact Funct Neurosurg 2001; 77:172–176

38. Son UC, Kim MC, Moon DE, Kang JK. Motor cortex stimulation in a patient with intractable complex regional pain syndrome type II with hemibody involvement. Case report. J Neurosurg 2003;98:175–179

39. Tani N, Saitoh Y, Hirata M, Kato A, Yoshimine T. Bilateral cortical stimulation for deafferentation pain after spinal cord injury. Case report. J Neurosurg 2004;101:687–689

40. Fontaine D, Bruneto JL, El Fakir H, Paquis P, Lanteri-Minet M. Short-term restoration of facial sensory loss by motor cortex stimulation in peripheral post-traumatic neuropathic pain. J Headache Pain 2009;10:203–206

41. Stadler JA III, Ellens DJ, Rosenow JM. Deep brain stimulation and motor cortical stimulation for neuropathic pain. Curr Pain Headache Rep 2011;15:8–13

42. Young RF, Kroening R, Fulton W, Feldman RA, Chambi I. Electrical stimulation of the brain in treatment of chronic pain. Experience over 5 years. J Neurosurg 1985;62:389–396

43. Mazars GJ. Intermittent stimulation of nucleus ventralis posterolateralis for intractable pain. Surg Neurol 1975;4:93–95

44. Richardson DE, Akil H. Long term results of periventricular gray self-stimulation. Neurosurgery 1977;1:199–202

45. Levy RM, Lamb S, Adams JE. Treatment of chronic pain by deep brain stimulation: long term follow-up and review of the literature. Neurosurgery 1987;21:885–893

46. Owen SL, Green AL, Nandi DD, Bittar RG, Wang S, Aziz TZ. Deep brain stimulation for neuropathic pain. Acta Neurochir Suppl (Wien) 2007;97(Pt 2):111–116

47. Gerhart KD, Yezierski RP, Fang ZR, Willis WD. Inhibition of primate spinothalamic tract neurons by stimulation in ventral posterior lateral (VPLc) thalamic nucleus: possible mechanisms. J Neurophysiol 1983;49:406–423

48. Davis KD, Taub E, Duffner F, et al. Activation of the anterior cingulate cortex by thalamic stimulation in patients with chronic pain: a positron emission tomography study. J Neurosurg 2000; 92:64–69

49. Rezai AR, Machado AG, Deogaonkar M, Azmi H, Kubu C, Boulis NM. Surgery for movement disorders. Neurosurgery 2008; 62(Suppl 2):809–838, discussion 838–839

50. Bittar RG, Kar-Purkayastha I, Owen SL, et al. Deep brain stimulation for pain relief: a meta-analysis. J Clin Neurosci 2005; 12:515–519

51. Brooks JC, Zambreanu L, Godinez A, Craig AD, Tracey I. Somatotopic organisation of the human insula to painful heat studied with high resolution functional imaging. Neuroimage 2005;27: 201–209

52. Craggs JG, Price DD, Verne GN, Perlstein WM, Robinson MM. Functional brain interactions that serve cognitive-affective processing during pain and placebo analgesia. Neuroimage 2007; 38:720–729

53. Zaki J, Ochsner KN, Hanelin J, Wager TD, Mackey SC. Different circuits for different pain: patterns of functional connectivity reveal distinct networks for processing pain in self and others. Soc Neurosci 2007;2:276–291

54. Haber SN, Kim KS, Mailly P, Calzavara R. Reward-related cortical inputs define a large striatal region in primates that interface with associative cortical connections, providing a substrate for incentive-based learning. J Neurosci 2006;26:8368–8376

55. Baliki MN, Geha PY, Fields HL, Apkarian AV. Predicting value of pain and analgesia: nucleus accumbens response to noxious stimuli changes in the presence of chronic pain. Neuron 2010; 66:149–160

56. Levy R, Deer TR, Henderson J. Intracranial neurostimulation for pain control: a review. Pain Physician 2010;13:157–165

57. Coffey RJ, Hamani C, Lozano AM. Evidence base: neurostimulation for pain. In: Winn HR, ed. Youmans' Neurological Surgery, 6th ed. Philadelphia: Elsevier, 2011:1809–1820

58. Coffey RJ. Deep brain stimulation for chronic pain: results of two multicenter trials and a structured review. Pain Med 2001; 2:183–192

Chapter 21

Deep Brain Stimulation: Frame vs. Frameless Stereotactic Treatment

Case

A 65-year-old man came to medical attention with long-standing Parkinson's disease that is intractable to medication. He also has bradykinesia and minor tremor. A subthalamic nucleus target is chosen for deep brain stimulation.

Participants

Deep Brain Stimulation: The Frameless Technique: Daryoush Tavanaiepour and Kathryn L. Holloway

The Frame-Based Approach to Subthalamic Nucleus Deep Brain Stimulation: Tejas Sankar and Andres M. Lozano

Moderator: Frame-Based vs. Frameless: Is It the Question?: Alim Louis Benabid

Deep Brain Stimulation: The Frameless Technique

Daryoush Tavanaiepour and Kathryn L. Holloway

In 1906, Clarke and Horsley[1] described the first stereotactic apparatus used for animals and coined the term *stereotaxic* from the Greek word *stereo* meaning "three dimensional" and *taxic* meaning "an arrangement."[2] It was not until 1947, however, that Spiegel and colleagues[3] introduced the first human stereotactic frame for neurosurgical procedures. Since then, there have been multiple modifications of the stereotactic frame, starting with Talairach and Riechert devices and culminating in the two most commonly used frames: the arc-based Cosman-Roberts-Wells system (CRW) system and Leksell frames.[2,4–7] The stereotactic frame has been the gold standard apparatus for functional neurosurgical interventions such as lesioning or deep brain stimulation (DBS) procedures for decades.[8–10]

However, there are some limitations to the stereotactic frame. It is a relatively heavy device with restrictive features requiring fixation to the operating table. This can be especially problematic in patients with moderate to severe Parkinson's disease undergoing DBS. At most institutions, patients are kept off their medications for Parkinson's disease the night before surgery, and the stereotactic frame is placed the morning of the operation. The operative day is long, with preoperative imaging and DBS trajectory planning done on the same day, and the patient may encounter difficulties tolerating the heavy, bulky stereotactic frame after stopping medication. Furthermore, during the procedure, the frame is attached to the operating table, which can be uncomfortable and restrict the awake patient. From the physician's perspective, the frame can prevent adequate assessment of the patient's facial features (to examine for stimulation-induced side effects) or the observation of intraoperative stimulation efficacy in patients with axial tremor or dystonia.[11,12] It also complicates management of the patient's airway. In addition, placement of the stereotactic frame and patient positioning can be challenging in patients with large head diameters, cervical or thoracic kyphosis, or claustrophobia.

With the development of advanced neuronavigation technology, it became possible to perform neurosurgery without the conventional stereotactic frame, and accurate localization of intracranial targets without the use of stereotactic frames has become commonplace.[13,14] For procedures such as tumor resection, in which real-time feedback regarding intracranial position is helpful, image-guided surgical systems have effectively replaced stereotactic frames. Nonetheless, trajectory-based procedures, such as DBS for movement disorders, are still extensively done with a stereotactic frame[15] because extreme accuracy is required for DBS surgery, as it relates directly to clinical efficacy.[16–19] The benefit of real-time positional feedback is less important than the accurate delivery of the DBS lead to a well-defined target. Skin fiducial markers, as traditionally used

in frameless localization, do not provide sufficient accuracy. Also, instrument holders for biopsy or other applications are not sufficiently rigid to meet the demands of true stereotactic accuracy.[20] In addition, DBS procedures require a stable platform for examining the brain with microelectrode recording and stimulation over many hours and through multiple parallel trajectories. Therefore, there was a need to develop a frameless stereotactic system specifically for DBS with accuracy and reliability equivalent to the traditional stereotactic frame but with the benefits of a frameless system.

Currently, there are two frameless stereotactic systems designed specifically for DBS surgery: the STarFix (FHC, Inc., Bowdoin, ME) and the Nexframe (Medtronic, Inc., Minneapolis, MN). The STarFix system incorporates the planned trajectory into a custom-built miniature platform (surgical targeting fixture), which is attached to bone fiducial markers. Therefore, it is specific to the individual patient and procedure. A few days before surgery, the patient undergoes imaging and placement of bone fiducials. The planned trajectory and images are submitted to the company, which builds a custom device in a relatively short time (typically 3 days) with a rapid-prototyping technology. Akin to the general principles of the traditional stereotactic frame, the custom-built platform is created by translating the image space to the patient's physical space through the bone fiducials. Furthermore, the target coordinates are referenced from the bone fiducial. Thus, the bone fiducials serve as both imaging reference points and anchors to attach the platform to the patient. This custom-built frame is sometimes referred to as a miniature frame. On the day of surgery, the completed custom-built device is attached to the patient through the previously placed bone fiducials and serves as a trajectory guide. The technical details of the STarFix system have been described previously.[12,21–25]

A description of the Nexframe stereotactic procedure as it is performed at our institution is outlined below. The emphasis is on the finer technical aspects, which we believe maximize the Nexframe system's clinical accuracy. Other aspects of the procedure, such as intraoperative microelectrode recording and stimulation testing, are not discussed.

The Nexframe Stereotactic Technique

The Nexframe system has been developed specifically to provide a high degree of targeting stability and accuracy during frameless DBS procedures. It depends on the surgeon's skill rather than on the manufacturer's quality control; it also allows the surgeon to explore more than one target at a time. The Nexframe is a skull-mounted platform linked with the Medtronic stealth neuronavigation system to provide real-time adjustment of the trajectory. The procedure is divided into two phases: preoperative and intraoperative.

Phase 1: Preoperative Planning

A few days before the surgery, preoperative imaging and bone fiducial placement are performed in an outpatient setting. We obtain a volumetric T1-weighted magnetic resonance imaging (MRI) scan with contrast to pinpoint the precise location of the intended target. The trajectory can be planned on this image at any time before the procedure. The bone fiducials are placed with sterile technique; after the administration of local anesthesia, a stab incision is made and the fiducial is inserted with a power screwdriver. The use of a power screwdriver is essential for a secure purchase of the fiducial, which will hold without loosening over several days. The fiducials are placed circumferentially around the top of the patient's head and forehead to ensure that the predicted 1-mm accuracy of the neuronavigation sphere completely encompasses the head (**Figs. 21.1, 21.2**). Fiducials are not placed on the side of the head, where the patient is likely to dislodge them during sleep. Attention is also given to placing the fiducials away from the planned incision.

A 0.5- to 1-mm computed tomography (CT) scan without contrast is obtained after the fiducials are placed. Next, the MRI and CT studies are loaded and merged on the Stealth

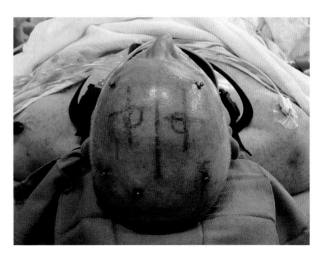

Fig. 21.1 The placement of bone fiducial markers.

neuronavigation workstation, with the CT scan as the reference image to carefully identify the center of each fiducial (**Fig. 21.3**).

Phase 2: Intraoperative Technique

On the day of surgery, the patient does not require any further imaging or other procedures and is taken directly to the operating room. The patient is placed on a comfortable,

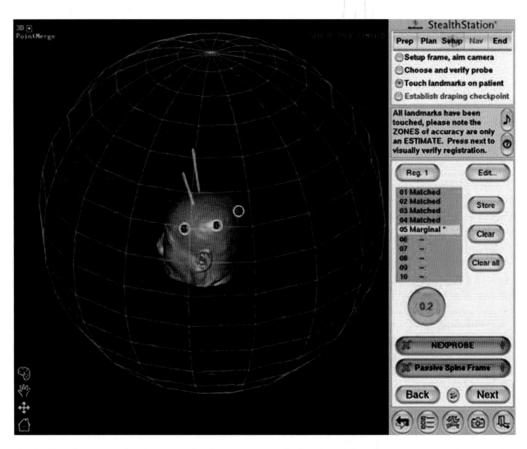

Fig. 21.2 The predicted 1-mm error sphere completely encompasses the head, and the registration error is less than 0.5 mm.

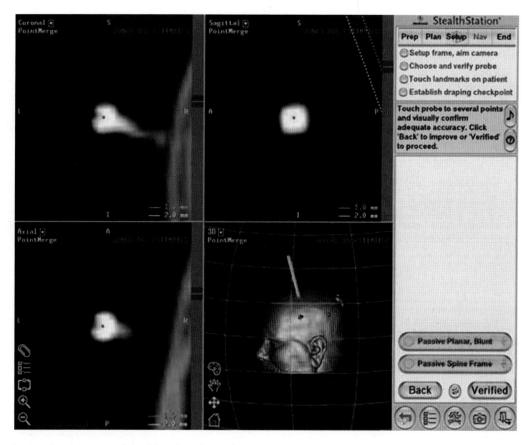

Fig. 21.3 Registering the center of the fiducial on the workstation.

noninvasive headrest with a cervical collar restraint (Passive Head Rest, Medtronic) (**Figs. 21.1, 21.4, 21.5**). The collar is kept on only during the incision and bur-hole placement, while the patient is sedated and more likely to move unexpectedly. The patient is prepared and draped with a transparent drape, which facilitates interaction with the patient, the operating room staff, and the anesthesiology and neurology team (**Fig. 21.6**). We also ensure that the drape encompasses all the fiducials so that they can be registered under sterile conditions (**Fig. 21.7**). The bur hole is made with a self-stopping cranial perforator and is widened laterally, as there is a tendency for the cannula to enter on the lateral edge of the bur hole (**Fig. 21.8**). The Stimloc device is then attached to the skull, followed by the Nexframe base, which is secured to the skull with the

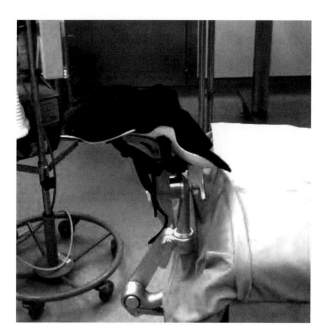

Fig. 21.4 The noninvasive headrest.

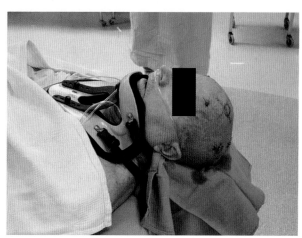

Fig. 21.5 The patient's position.

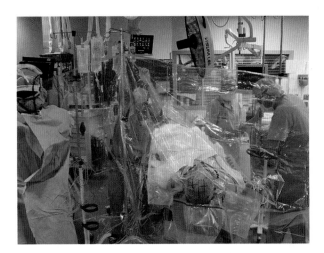

Fig. 21.6 The transparent drape.

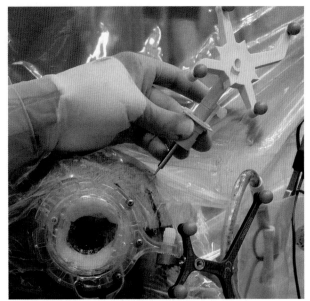

Fig. 21.7 The reference arc is attached to the Nexframe base and fiducial are registered with the Nexprobe.

powered screwdriver to ensure stability **(Fig. 21.9)**. If the target is the globus pallidus, a 1- to 2-mm thick Silastic sheet is placed under the lateral side of the Nexframe base, before attachment, to make alignment easier. The attachment of the Nexframe system is verified by ensuring that the Nexframe base and head move as one unit. The reference arc is then attached to the platform **(Fig. 21.7)**.

During registration, we ensure that the geometry error for both the Nexprobe and reference arc is less than 0.2 mm **(Fig. 21.10)** by adjusting the neuronavigation camera into optimal range, moving the operating room lights off the field, and verifying that the spheres are snapped on properly and are clean. When we register the fiducials, the Nexprobe is placed in-axis with the fiducial, and the geometry error is verified again to be less than 0.2 mm **(Figs. 21.7, 21.10)**. Once registration is completed, the accuracy is verified by ensuring that the predicted 1-mm error sphere completely encompasses the entire head and that the registration error is less than 0.7 mm **(Fig. 21.2)**. More importantly, we assess the accuracy of the registration by touching

several of the fiducials to verify that they are precisely located.

Next, the dura is opened and any vessels in the path of the trajectory are coagulated and sharply divided. To prevent a cerebrospinal fluid leak and subsequent brain shift, which could reduce the accuracy during the procedure, the bur hole is sealed with a combination of Gelfoam and dural sealant. The alignment tower is then attached to the platform, aligned to the target through the neuronavigation system, and locked in placed. Next, the tower is secured to the platform **(Fig. 21.11)**. The next stage, which employs the Ben-Gun (Schaerer-Mayfield, Lyon, France), entails the placement of one to five cannulas; we have found that accuracy is improved with cannulas that extend to 10 mm above the target in comparison to shorter cannulas. The

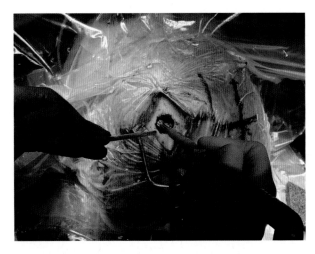

Fig. 21.8 The bur hole created by the self-stopping cranial perforator is extended laterally.

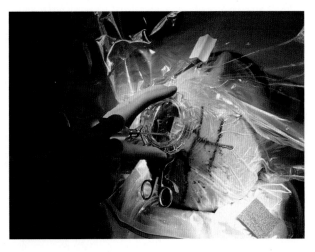

Fig. 21.9 Placement of the Nexframe base. Screws are initially placed with a power screwdriver and then tightened by hand.

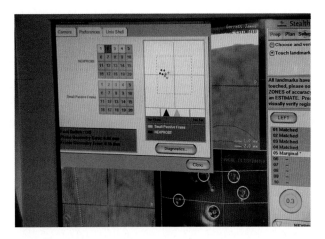

Fig. 21.10 During registration, we ensure that the geometry error for both the Nexprobe and reference arc is less that 0.2 mm.

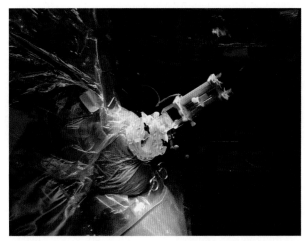

Fig. 21.11 The complete Nexframe system has been assembled.

rest of the procedure involves selecting the optimal track, by using microelectrode recording and macrostimulation, to assess for side effects and efficacy. The DBS lead is secured with the Stimloc and marked with a pen at the immediate junction of the DBS lead and the Stimloc. This mark provides visual confirmation that the lead has not moved during disassembly and is much more efficient than using repeated fluoroscopic images.

Comparison of the STarFix and Nexframe Systems

Both the STarFix and Nexframe systems have the advantages of the frameless technology, but there are some differences; the main one is the method by which the trajectory alignment is done. The trajectory alignment of the STarFix system is based on traditional stereotactic frame principles and is set by the manufacturer, which can theoretically lead to error, but a group describing its recent experience with 263 patients has not encountered this problem.[12] Furthermore, because the trajectory is set by the manufacturer, it does not allow for the flexibility to change the planned target. In contrast, the Nexframe system uses an optical tracking system for trajectory alignment during surgery, which allows for a change in the planned target. However, the system relies heavily on precise intraoperative registration and manual alignment of the trajectory. Another difference between the systems is that the STarFix system allows for simultaneous bilateral microelectrode recording, stimulation testing, and DBS placement, whereas the Nexframe system requires bilateral DBS placement to be done sequentially.

Accuracy of the Frameless and Frame Stereotactic Systems

Deep brain stimulation for Parkinson's disease requires extreme accuracy, as it directly relates to efficacy.[16–19] For example, the subthalamic nucleus (STN) is approximately 6 × 4 × 5 mm, and a DBS lead placement error of 3 to 4 mm can alter the outcome.[26,27] The accuracy of stereotactic frames and frameless systems has been well studied in in vitro phantom experiments. The mean accuracy of the CRW and Leksell frames has been shown to be 1.7 ± 0.1 mm and 1.8 ± 0.11 mm, respectively.[28] The mean accuracy for the Nexframe and STarFix systems has been measured to be 1.25 ± 0.6 mm and 0.42 ± 0.15 mm, respectively.[21,29]

Although the traditional frame-based stereotactic system has been used since the late 1940s, it was not until 2002 that the accuracy of the frame-based system in a clinical setting was established.[30] Such clinical studies require a marker for actual target localization, with an internal (anterior commissure–posterior commissure [AC-PC]) or external (frame) reference system on the postoperative scan to compare expected with actual target locations. Alternatively, this process can be accomplished with image fusion, which is a relatively recent development. Starr and colleagues[30] carefully assessed the postoperative coordinates of 76 STN DBS electrodes that had been placed with a Leksell frame. They found a mean deviation of 3.15 mm from the expected target location. Subsequently, similar results have also been reported by other groups.[31,32] The University of California–Los Angeles group evaluated the discrepancy between expected and actual targets in 217 DBS cases. There was a mean vector error of 2.9 mm (range 0.1–6.44 mm) for the ventral intermediate nucleus, 2.3 mm (range 0–7.61 mm) for STN, and 2.2 mm (range 0.03–4.5 mm) for targets in the globus pallidus.[31] O'Leary and colleagues[32] analyzed intraoperative radiographic data on 109 microelectrode tracks and found a 2.1-mm discrepancy between the theoretical microelectrode target and the values obtained from intraoperative fluoroscopic images. Schrader and associates[27] assessed the electrode location in six patients who had the Zamorano-Dujovny stereotactic ring. The calculated vector error from their data was 2.64 mm for the left side and 3.04 mm for the right side. Hamid and coworkers[33] examined the pre- and postoperative MRI scans to define the accuracy of lead placement in STN DBS for 16 patients who had the Leksell stereotactic frame; the calculated vector error was 3.02 mm.

In 2005, the clinical accuracy of the Nexframe system was investigated by Holloway and associates.[34] This multicenter study compared the accuracy of the Nexframe with the previously published data of frame-based clinical accuracy by Starr and colleagues.[30] A total of 47 electrodes were implanted in 38 patients. The target nucleus was the ventral intermediate (VIM) in 16 patients, the STN in 29, and the globus pallidus pars interna (GPI) in two patients. Vector errors were analyzed in the same manner as in the frame-based study by Starr and colleagues by comparing the difference between the expected target and the actual lead location. Analysis revealed a vector error of 3.15 mm for the Nexframe, which was the same as the vector error of the frame as reported by Starr and colleagues. A follow-up publication from a single institution further investigated the clinical accuracy of the Nexframe and frame-based systems.[35] Ninety patients underwent placement of 139 DBS leads with the CRW frame ($n = 70$) or the Nexframe system ($n = 69$). The final DBS location was identified on a postoperative CT fused to the preoperative CT and MRI scans. The vector error between the CRW frame (2.65 mm) and the frameless (2.78 mm) system did not differ ($p = 0.69$). The vector error for both systems declined with time, as the vector error of the last 20 implants was 1.99 mm for the CRW frame and 2.04 mm for the Nexframe. This decline was attributed to subtle changes in surgical techniques and experience. Another interesting finding from this study was the predictability of the vector error for the frameless system, with a proclivity toward the medial, posterior, and inferior directions, whereas the frame-based system did not have a predictable direction of error. The clinical accuracy of the STarFix system has also been examined recently by Konrad and colleagues.[12] A total of 263 patients who underwent 284 DBS implantations with the STarFix system were analyzed. The final DBS lead location was calculated using postoperative CT scans. The mean vector error was found to be 1.99 mm (standard deviation: 0.9).

Bjartmarz and Rehncrona[36] directly compared the frameless and framed approaches in a single operation. In bilateral procedures during a single surgical session, one side was implanted with the Nexframe approach while the other side was implanted with a Leksell G frame. The preoperative planning image was based on a volumetric, 1-mm slice thickness, T1-weighted MRI study. Unlike the preceding studies, the DBS lead position was not assessed with a CT or MRI scan but rather with a two-dimensional X-ray image using the reference frame of the Leksell system. This method heavily favors the frame, as the ground truth is defined as the stereotactic coordinates in the Leksell space. With this method, the frame vector error was 1.2 ± 0.6 mm and the frameless error was 2.5 ± 1.4 mm ($p < 0.05$). It is unclear what the error would have been

with the more commonly used method of postoperative imaging with CT or MRI studies, and there were other limitations to their frameless technique.[37] Despite showing a difference in clinical accuracy between the frame and frameless techniques, however, the clinical outcome was similar at follow-up regardless of the stereotactic technique.

Clinical studies show a greater error for both frame and frameless systems, as compared with phantom experiments. The increased error seen in the clinical situation is expected for several reasons, including weight bearing by the frame, mobility of the brain within the cranial cavity, loss of cerebrospinal fluid with subsequent brain shift, inaccuracies of localization introduced by selection of the lead tip and the AC-PC coordinates on postoperative imaging, and deviations of the microelectrode or DBS as it passes through the brain substance. Rohlfing and associates[38] found a decrease in the accuracy of stereotactic frames because of torque introduced by the effect of weight bearing on the frame. They assessed the effects of the mechanical loading of the frame and a change in patient position on localization error within the clinical situation. They chose to compare scans obtained while the patient was prone and supine, maximizing the adverse effect of linear mechanical loading. CT scans were obtained in 14 patients placed in the Brown-Roberts-Wells frame while supine and then prone, and the registration transformations were compared. The mean error was 0.97 ± 0.38 mm, but the registration error was greater than 1.5 mm in eight of 14 patients. The authors noted that the errors from positioning and mechanical loading were additive with other sources of error.

There are numerous pitfalls in attempting to measure postoperative lead locations accurately. First among these is the difficulty in locating the precise center and depth of the lead as it relates to the intended target. Both magnetic susceptibility artifact (on MRI) and beam-hardening artifact (on CT scans) conceal the lead and require estimation or interpolation of the electrode position. Papavassiliou and associates[39] evaluated DBS lead locations in eight cases by using both CT and MRI studies. They found differences between the two techniques ranging from 2.4 to 2.6 mm; the mean of these signed values was 0.1 to 0.3 mm and was not significant. Furthermore, because the last contact of a Medtronic DBS lead lies 1.5 mm from the actual tip of the electrode, determining its location on either modality can be difficult. Because the DBS trajectory is not perpendicular to the AC–PC plane, an error in localizing the electrode tip can lead to errors not only in z (depth) but also in the x and y directions, depending on the approach angle. Even if the lead position can be accurately determined on postoperative imaging, relating this position to the intended target requires a translation method such as image fusion or coordinate transfer, each of which has potential inaccuracies.

An additional category of error can relate directly to errors in lead placement. Some examples include deflection of the lead during implantation, slippage of the lead during anchoring, and various inaccuracies in stereotactic localization, which have been described elsewhere.[28,29,38,40] The direct measurement of localization errors in phantom studies eliminates the step of translating postoperative imaging to preoperative targeting, which may contribute to the relatively decreased accuracy noted in clinical studies compared with phantom studies.

In addition to studies that have focused on phantom and clinical accuracy of the frameless technique, two recent studies have compared the long-term clinical outcome between the frameless and frame-based techniques.[41,42] The DBS Study Group analyzed the 1-year clinical outcome for patients with Parkinson's undergoing STN DBS with the frameless technique.[15] There were 31 patients, 28 with bilateral and three with unilateral lead placements. The Unified Parkinson's Disease Rating Scale (UPDRS) was assessed at 6 and 12 months. All patients underwent DBS implantation with the Nexframe system. The mean improvement in UPDRS scores at 1 year was 58% with a mean reduction of medication of 50%. This level of clinical improvement is comparable to published frame-based clinical outcomes of 52 to 55%.[43,44] In a similar study, Tai and colleagues[42] directly compared the clinical outcome of patients with Parkinson's undergoing STN DBS with frameless and frame-based techniques. A total of 24 patients were enrolled, 12 who underwent the frameless (Nexframe) technique, and 12 who had the frame-based (CRW) technique. At 1-year follow-up, the mean UPDRS improvement for the frameless (60.9%) and frame-based (56.9%) group was similar ($p = 0.81$).

Conclusion

The frameless stereotactic system has been shown to be equivalent to the gold-standard frame-based system in experimental and clinical accuracy studies, as well as in clinical outcome studies. According to our experience and that of other published reports,[12,23,34–36,41,42] several advantages related to the use of the frameless system have been noted. Patients are much less apprehensive about fiducial marker placement than the application of a stereotactic frame. The ability to apply the fiducial markers one or more days before surgery allows imaging and planning to be separated from the procedure, decreasing operating room time and enhancing the patient's comfort because of the shorter periods spent without medication. Without rigid fixation to the operating table, patients are allowed greater mobility and seem better able to tolerate lengthy procedures. Intraoperative examination of the patient is easier without the bulky frame. As with any new device or procedure, however, the frameless system has a learning curve and requires attention to detail.[35] We believe that the frameless stereotactic system is a safe, accurate, and effective technique and provides a viable alternative to the frame-based system.

The Frame-Based Approach to Subthalamic Nucleus Deep Brain Stimulation

Tejas Sankar and Andres M. Lozano

Parkinson's disease (PD) is a progressive neurologic disorder, associated with the death of dopaminergic cells in the substantia nigra, but additionally with widespread effects across the entire central nervous system. Medical therapy for PD in the form of dopaminergic medications—most notably L-dopa—emerged in the 1960s[45] and has shown unquestioned efficacy in reducing the severity of the cardinal motor symptoms of the disease. Unfortunately, a large proportion of PD patients become disabled within 5 to 10 years despite medical therapy because of the limitations of dopaminergic medications, including the predictable "wearing off" of drug effect over the course of a day, more unpredictable "on-off" motor fluctuations, and disabling involuntary movements now recognized as L-dopa–induced dyskinesias.[46,47] In these patients, treatment with DBS may be a suitable option.[48] Strong evidence now exists from randomized controlled trials supporting DBS as superior to best medical management for patients with moderate to severe PD.[49–51] More than 80,000 DBS insertion procedures have been performed since the early 1990s, with an ongoing accrual of 8,000 to 10,000 patients annually.[52] Bilateral placement of DBS electrodes into the STN has emerged as the most common procedure worldwide, and is typically done with frame-based stereotaxy and MRI-based target selection, complemented by intraoperative electrophysiological guidance with microelectrode recording. This section focuses on our frame-based approach to STN DBS, which we discuss in the context of the patient in this chapter's case presentation.

Case Analysis

From the case description presented, a 65-year-old patient has been offered and has consented to STN DBS therapy.

Before proceeding with the neurosurgical implantation of DBS electrodes, however, it is worthwhile to ask whether he is an appropriate candidate for this therapy altogether. Patient selection is critical to successful long-term outcomes in DBS; by some estimates up to 30% of DBS failures may be ascribed to inappropriate indications for surgery.[53] At our center, the decision to offer DBS surgery to a given patient is based on a detailed and individualized analysis of several clinical factors. Central to this process is a multidisciplinary team composed of movement disorder neurologists, psychiatrists, and neuropsychologists, with the operating neurosurgeon being the ultimate arbiter.

The ideal candidate who is likely to benefit substantially from STN DBS is one suffering from moderate to advanced PD complicated by motor fluctuations, disabling dyskinesias, or tremor despite optimized drug therapy.[52,54] It is important to exclude patients with atypical parkinsonism or Parkinson plus syndromes such as progressive supranuclear palsy and multisystem atrophy, because these patients derive less benefit from DBS.[55] Similarly, patients with a preponderance of axial disturbances such as postural instability or gait disturbance[56,57] or prominent dysarthrophonia[58] do not typically experience improvement in these symptoms with STN DBS. Additionally, the ideal candidate is also one whose cardinal motor symptoms of PD are responsive to L-dopa.[44,59] At our center, all prospective patients undergo a formal L-dopa challenge, on which we require at least a 30% improvement in the UPDRS-III score. There is evidence that younger patients are more likely to do better with DBS,[49,60,61] and although we do not have an absolute age cutoff, we are extremely cautious about offering surgery to patients older than 75 years. Moreover, advanced age correlates with the presence of dementia or cognitive impairment, both of which are exclusion criteria for STN DBS.[62] As a rule, all patients in our practice undergo formal neuropsychological and cognitive testing before being considered for DBS. Finally, patients with unstable psychiatric conditions, particularly depression or impulsivity, must have their medication optimized before surgery because of the potential for deterioration in their psychiatric symptoms after STN DBS.[61,63–65] We frequently consider alternate DBS targets—most commonly the internal segment of the globus pallidus—in patients with a significant psychiatric history who would otherwise be good surgical candidates.

General medical fitness for surgery is also an important criterion.[61] Conditions such as hypertension, coronary artery disease, and diabetes should be optimized medically before surgery, and the patient should understand that these conditions may increase their surgical risk. Antiplatelet or anticoagulant medications should be withdrawn in advance of surgery and will require special management in the perioperative period.[66]

Assuming the 65-year-old man in this case meets these stringent criteria, frame-based stereotactic surgery for DBS electrode implantation into the STN can be offered as a viable option and undertaken once consent is obtained.

Surgical Approach and Technique

Several articles have described the various techniques used during the implantation of DBS systems.[66–69] Neurosurgeons typically select their preferred techniques based on their training and experience and institutional resources.[52] We highlight here some key points that we have used in our STN DBS procedures.

We insert electrodes for STN DBS in conscious patients, with minimal or no sedation, in the off-medication state. In this way, we can maximize the quality of electrophysiological information obtained during intraoperative microelectrode recording, and test the leads intraoperatively to determine their efficacy against PD symptoms and adverse effects, with the ultimate aim of optimizing electrode placement.

In our view, frame-based stereotaxy is the standard for accurate delivery of the DBS electrode to the target. We place the head frame (Leksell G, Elekta, Atlanta, GA) on the morning of surgery with the patient seated on a chair. The frame is placed by the principal surgeon and an assistant, who maintains the base ring of the frame in line with the AC-PC plane, which is roughly approximated by the canthomeatal line.[66] We liberally infiltrate the scalp at the pin sites with local anesthetic (1:1 mixture of 0.25% bupivacaine and 1% lidocaine with epinephrine). We take care to carefully estimate the optimal pin length to prevent readjustments or replacements. Orthogonal pins are tightened simultaneously.

Once the frame is in place, the patient is taken to the MRI scanner for preoperative imaging. We obtain a T1-weighted volumetric scan of the entire brain, as well as T2-weighted axial and coronal scans through the region of the STN. In total, the acquisition of all MRI sequences takes about 20 minutes. The patient is then taken to the operating room and prepared for surgery by the nursing and anesthesia team, while the neurosurgical team proceeds with anatomic planning on the recently acquired images. We use a combination of direct and indirect techniques to select the STN target on standard surgical planning software (FrameLink, Medtronic). Entry points and trajectories are also determined with navigation software. All target coordinates as well as frame arc and ring angles are verified independently by at least two different members of the neurosurgical team.

In the operating room, the patient is placed in the supine position with the knees flexed and the head elevated so that the operating table takes on the shape of a reclining chair. Care is taken to ensure that the patient's neck is in a comfortable position before affixing the head frame to the operating table. Draping is done is such a way as to allow access to the patient's face, arms, and legs. The scalp is liberally infiltrated with local anesthetic near the coronal suture. We prefer a single Souttar transverse skin incision extending to either side of the midline for bilateral procedures. Standard techniques are used to drill the bur holes, open the dura, and insert the cannula for the microelectrode to an offset 10 mm above the target.

Microelectrode recording is used in conjunction with clinical testing to ensure that the predetermined trajectory traverses at least a 5-mm segment of STN with kinesthetic-responsive units. Although the microelectrode recording data usually confirm the appropriate location of the MRI target within the motor territory of the STN, in roughly one of three patients the imaging target is suboptimal. Accordingly, an adjustment of 2 or 3 mm in the medial/lateral or anterior/posterior plane is usually required, although in some rare cases the error is greater. Because of this, we do not hesitate to record from additional trajectories as needed.

Once a satisfactory final trajectory has been determined and any target modifications have been made, the DBS electrode is introduced into the cannula and advanced to the target under fluoroscopic guidance. Test macrostimulation through the DBS electrode is then done with an external screener, employing typical therapeutic stimulation parameters (e.g., 130 Hz frequency, 1–5 V amplitude, 90 μs pulse width). This should confirm beneficial effects for tremor, rigidity, and bradykinesia without adverse stimulation-related side effects, including motor phenomena (contralateral contractions or dysarthria), ipsilateral ocular adduction, or uncomfortable paresthesias, corresponding to electrode positions that are too lateral, medial, or posterior, respectively.[66,70]

Finally, the DBS electrode is fixed in place with a standard lead fixation system under fluoroscopy, and the entire procedure is repeated on the contralateral side. Postoperative MRI to verify correct electrode placement is standard practice at our center **(Fig. 21.12)**, and we usually implant the pulse generator under general anesthesia a few days after the electrodes are inserted.

Our Preference for the Frame-Based Approach

The stereotactic frame has been a mainstay of functional neurosurgery since its development. Virtually all neurosurgeons who do modern DBS implantation procedures were trained to do so with strictly frame-based techniques, which have ultimately proven their worth with a stellar record of safety and efficacy. Frameless stereotaxy has gradually become more popular in general neurosurgical practice over the past two decades,[71] and is now the technique of choice in most centers for preoperative craniotomy planning, intraoperative neuronavigation, and to obtain stereotactic biopsies of intracranial mass lesions. It is only very recently, however, that frameless techniques have been used for functional work, in which the ultimate aim of correct electrode position places a premium on superb accuracy, which was long thought to be unattainable without a rigid head frame. Nevertheless, frameless approaches to DBS surgery are now increasingly in vogue be-

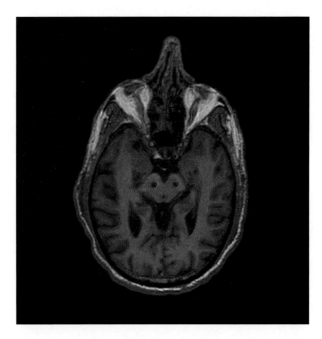

Fig. 21.12 Axial T1-weighted postoperative magnetic resonance imaging (MRI) showing deep brain stimulation (DBS) electrodes positioned bilaterally within the subthalamic nucleus.

cause of the widespread perception that they are minimally invasive.[72]

A few published reports directly compare the accuracy of frame-based to frameless approaches to DBS surgery.[34–36,41,42,73,74] These reports largely suggest that, for surgeons who have obtained sufficient experience with frameless techniques, the accuracy is comparable between the approaches. Although some may use such data to argue for a widespread transition to frameless surgery, we believe there are compelling reasons to stick with the frame-based approach that has served so many PD patients so well.

Perhaps the most important factor in favor of the traditional approach is its universal familiarity among functional neurosurgeons. The learning curve necessary to become proficient with the frameless approach is hard to justify in busy functional neurosurgery centers such as our own, in which hundreds of DBS procedures are done every year. The investment of capital, effort, and additional surgical time during the learning phase also seem particularly difficult to absorb when no data convincingly demonstrate the superiority of frameless techniques. In addition, several potential technical pitfalls are associated with the frameless approach. Chief among these is the lack of rigid head fixation, which can become a serious problem for tremulous patients—such as the 65-year-old patient described in this case—whose head may move significantly during drilling of the skull or while a probe is in the brain.[71] In our experience, the disadvantage of having a patient's head immobilized by a frame is more than outweighed by the confidence gained from knowing that unintended patient movements cannot jeopardize the procedure. Moreover, any adverse effects on patient comfort can be minimized by appropriately positioning the patient's neck at the beginning of the case and adjusting the neck position as needed during surgery.

Additional pitfalls in the frameless approach concern the placement of fiducial markers. These must be placed carefully to ensure that they do not translate, are not coplanar, and do not interfere with the headrest. Some authors even advocate placing five or more fiducials for redundancy.[71] Usually, fiducials are placed well before the day of surgery, meaning that patients must contend with the inconvenience of having structures attached to the head for up to several days. Contrast this with the placement of four pins in standard locations for a typical stereotactic frame, which are applied and removed on the day of surgery. Skull-based fiducial markers further introduce the possibility of error in fiducial registration, during which care must be taken to make sure that the center of each fiducial is identified precisely.[34,71] Frequently, re-registration may be required during adjustments to the target and trajectory. By comparison, target adjustments with a Cartesian-based frame are simple and do not require any additional calculations or reverifications. Another inconvenience is that fiducial registration requires the use of intraoperative neuronavigation and its associated camera hardware, which can further clutter an already crowded operating room. Finally, current frameless trajectory guide systems require constant verification of the rigidity of the guide, and must be removed and reattached to the contralateral side of the skull during bilateral procedures.

Naturally, some patients are apprehensive about frame placement and may believe that the placement of fiducial markers would be less painful and that the greater freedom of movement during surgery afforded by a frameless approach represents a considerable advantage. Similarly, the advantage of decoupling stereotactic imaging from the surgical procedure with the frameless approach[71] may shorten and thereby improve the patient's experience on the day of surgery. In our experience, these theoretical advantages may be overstated. In particular, we have found that patients tolerate stereotactic MRI acquisition in the head frame very well; those patients whom we suspect may experience discomfort during an MRI scan are usually offered the option of undergoing a rapid stereotactic CT scan on the morning of surgery, which can be fused to a preoperative MRI scan for planning.

Expected Outcomes and Possible Complications from Frame-Based Subthalamic Nucleus Deep Brain Stimulation

For this 65-year-old man with longstanding PD characterized by bradykinesia and minor tremor, there are good data to suggest that bilateral STN DBS will produce lasting improvements in his overall motor symptoms as well as in the severity of his parkinsonian tremor.[10,75–78] These motor improvements could possibly be sustained for up to 10 years or more after surgery.[79] Bilateral STN DBS should allow a reduction in the patient's overall L-dopa dose on the order of 22 to 70%, with a concomitant mean reduction in L-dopa–induced dyskinesias of 46.4 to 80%.[80] Nonetheless, we would expect the PD pathology to continue progressing despite surgery, accompanied by a worsening of L-dopa–resistant symptoms, including freezing of gait, postural instability, and cognitive decline.[52,81,82]

According to a recent review of key DBS-related issues by an expert panel, there is significant variability in the reported rate of surgical complications.[52] The dreaded complication of DBS surgery, namely symptomatic intracranial hemorrhage, was reported to occur in less than 2% of patients in most centers, which is in keeping with our experience. Hardware-related complications include infection, electrode misplacement or migration, lead fractures, or skin erosion. These are considerably more common than hemorrhage but exact risks are difficult to quantify in the absence of standardized reporting.[83–85] Nevertheless, the overall rate of hardware-related complications is likely decreasing over time because of technological improvements.[52]

Conclusion

Deep brain stimulation of the STN is the best treatment option for suitable medically refractory patients with moderate to severe PD, such as the patient presented in this case. As technology and experience evolve, the trend toward frameless systems supplemented by intraoperative real-time imaging will likely continue. For now, the bilateral insertion of DBS electrodes into the STN with a frame-based approach remains the procedure of choice among functional neurosurgeons.

Moderator

Frame-Based vs. Frameless: Is It the Question?

Alim Louis Benabid

The two opposite opinions presented here are brilliantly defended by their advocates, each group stressing the merits of the method they represent. At the end of this exercise, however, the question is: So what? What actually justifies this controversy? Aren't we just the victims of word abuses or of definitions summarized by expressions such as "frame-based" or "frameless," which lead us to war, when there might be finally no reason to go there? This is often the case when we go to war!

What do these two methods have in common? Do they have really serious differences? Do they have more advantages than drawbacks or vice versa? What are "frame-based" and "frameless"?

Frame-Based and Frameless Systems Share Several Features

Both systems are firmly secured to the head and hold accessories used to introduce a probe. Both rely on imaging techniques (MRI, fluoroscopy, CT) alone or combined, both are associated with microelectrode recording and stimulation, both call for multiple (simultaneous or subsequent) trajectories with or without a Ben-Gun, both can be adapted to preoperative planning and used with or without anesthesia, both allow bilateral procedures, either staged or in one session, and both have precision of around 2 to 3 mm with a standard deviation of 50%. These factors are barely significantly different, taking into account that no gold-standard method for comparison has been designed as a true reference, given the fact that, in all studies, the methodologies were slightly different.

In addition, every specific aspect is comparable or differs based on several invalid arguments. In all cases, there is a frame, made of a piece of equipment that creates a physical, solid link or bond between the head of the patient (actually, his brain) and tools or probes. These are designed to be introduced in a manner blinded to the surgeon's eyes, toward a target, which is expected to be reached with the highest precision. This precision is the ultimate quality expected from a procedure and, therefore, from the tools and methods used to achieve it.

All frames are fixed to the skull with pins or screws, or bolted with a circular opening, and are equally invasive. The criterion of minimal invasiveness is therefore no longer valid, particularly when one considers the additional fiducial markers, which for stereotaxy can no longer be adhesive landmarks on the skin or the scalp. The only difference is the weight of the device, frameless systems often being lighter, but within the frame-based category, some frames (Leksell) are much lighter than others (Talairach, CRW,

etc.). However, the recent sophisticated frameless systems, when equipped with supports for microrecording as well as motorized microdrives, are not weightless and exert a torque on the head of the patient, who does not feel so free and light.

What is invasive is the introduction of electrodes, regardless of the frame.

Differences Between Frames

There are some differences between frames, which are not always mentioned. The cost is not the same; it is higher in frameless systems because of the purchase of the equipment for each procedure. In addition to the frame, some accessories are disposable, without any real reason, even considering infection issues. This is mostly driven by some companies on the pretext of safer procedures and the desire of the patients. In some countries, this added cost is circumvented by the insurance reimbursement, but in other countries, where this is not the case, this cost makes a significant difference in the balance of advantages and disadvantages. I agree with this statement by Sankar and Lozano: "The learning curve necessary to become proficient with the frameless approach is hard to justify in busy functional neurosurgery centers such as [those] in which hundreds of DBS procedures are done every year." Indirect consequences in the operating room are also to be considered and are minimized with the frame-based approach.

Repositioning the Frame

Repositioning the frame is an important factor that may help manage the treatment by splitting the surgical procedure into several steps. Repositioning of the patient is not a feature specific to frame-based or frameless systems. This step can be realized with repositionable frames, which have already been developed. This is what I have done for 20 years with conventional frames, bone-fixed fiducials, screws, and so on.

What About Hybrid Systems?

Neither team of authors mentions robotic stereotactic arms, which are currently available on the market through at least two companies and which will be progressively used more often. Will it be a new controversy: robotic vs. not robotic? In which category should they be placed? In my own practice, I have been using the same method for 25 years, with the only difference being that MRI has been introduced lately. In all cases, the patient's head is held in a classic frame solidly mounted on a stand, and the probes are introduced by a tool-holding robotic arm playing the role of a goniometer. Should we say I am doing frameless surgery, as the tool-holding machinery is remotely connected to the head by the floor platform holding both frame and robotized arm? Or am I doing frame-based surgery, as I used to hold the head with a stereotactic frame playing the sole role of a sugar tong? I don't know. And actually, do we care? What is important is that the evolution of our system was motivated by the quest for increasingly efficient and precise procedures, progressively gathering features belonging to various devices.

Issues Independent of the Frame

Some important (or less important) issues are independent of the type of frame. Practitioners are still determining the quality of the procedure and their precision, which should be solved by all users.

The brain shift often mentioned has nothing to do with the frame but depends solely on the opening of the dura. A large number of neurosurgeons still open the dura to observe the cortex at the entry point and coagulate the cortical vessels to prevent bleeding. This approach is actually insufficient as the most dangerous vessels are in the sulci, invisible to the surgeon's eye, and opening the dura just allows a large amount of cerebrospinal fluid to escape and be replaced by air. The vascular risk can be better avoided through careful planning from the entry point, checking possible collisions with arteries and veins all along the trajectory of the probe by using neuronavigation based on MRI or CT studies with contrast medium. Piercing the dura under these circumstances can therefore be done safely and suppresses the leakage of cerebrospinal fluid, thereby preventing brain shift.

Precise targeting is the ultimate goal of stereotactic procedures. These two teams of authors report globally equivalent precision data, in vitro as well as in vivo. The care taken by the surgical team to achieve this precision is more important than which frame system is used. It depends on the neuronavigation software, which is compatible with all frames, in combination with microelectrode recording, intraoperative stimulation, and careful clinical evaluation of the beneficial or adverse effects. Determining the exact position of an electrode contact is a real challenge, and is responsible for more inaccuracy than the method used to position the electrode. Accuracy is defined by the distance between intended and actual targets, and it is measured through different methods. Such measurement is easier in vitro than in vivo, where measurement is indirect, and also includes additional causes of error, which are related not to the frame (deviation of the probe in the tissue and during penetration of the dura, using a guide tube, slippage of the lead during anchoring, etc.) but to various extra procedures and how they are executed.

Magnetic resonance imaging and CT are the only methods to provide x, y, and z coordinates relative to the same references, but they strongly depend on radiological artifacts, which in turn depend on the equipment and on the parameters used. Conventional X-rays are the most precise tools but are not available in all operating rooms and require strict reproducibility of the placement of the head (which is easier in frame-based situations, but still can be achieved with frameless devices) as well as correction of the parallax errors (from long distance setups or software corrections).

Magnetic resonance imaging compatibility is not a major issue today. The frame-based system (such as the Talairach) used to be incompatible with MRI, but there was no need for this at that time. The current versions of the CRW and Leksell systems are MRI compatible, as are the majority of frameless systems.

Claustrophobia happens, but not so often, and relates more to the CT or MRI gantries than to the type of head fixation.

Toward a Unified Stereotactic Methodology

Systems will eventually converge into an optimal compromise, similar to what happened with airplanes, which now share almost the same configuration of hull, wings, and engines. Currently, all companies are designing accessories and devices to provide smart solutions that decrease the differences, with each system adapting the advances of the others to improve the efficiency, precision, and ease of use. This tends to create better tools and procedures globally, and, in the long run, the consequence is that stereotactic procedures become more refined, to the benefit of the patient, and maybe more than to the benefit of the surgeon. (The frameless system is supposed to be easier to place, and allows a faster procedure with less risk, for example.) The future will bring more and more improvements that will become compatible with all types of systems (such as the Ben-Gun or more complex tools), as well as systems specifically for DBS that are accurate and reliable and combine the benefits of frame-based and frameless systems. For instance, one company has designed a smart platform that allows an X-Y correction of trajectories, which could be adapted to any type of frame-based system. Finally, frameless systems always have a frame of some sort. Thus, one could say, "stereotaxy is frame-based or is not stereotaxic." We should stop talking about frameless versus frame-based, and talk about innovative modifications of the stereotactic method, asking what they bring to the patient.

These two teams of authors show that both methods have advantages and drawbacks, and the drawbacks can be addressed through specially developed procedures. So this is not really the question of doing the procedure with or without a frame, which is addressed, but about how each team manages to solve problems with smart accessories or devices available from the various companies that are often meant to compensate for the drawbacks of a given system, either frame-based or frameless. The only valid comparison could be done by having two series of randomized patients treated by the same group using the same methods of imaging, microelectrode recording, and clinical testing, and comparing the results on the basis of clinical improvement (the conditions of which are themselves far from being consensual at this point). Our opinion is that we can save this effort and instead concentrate on defining the requirements a stereotactic method should fulfill, more than on how they are fulfilled. These requirements should include the following criteria:

- Reliability of head placement
- Reliability of spatial measurements
- Reliability and reproducibility of electrode placement and fixation
- Compatibility with most recent imaging techniques, particularly for intraoperative controls
- Compatibility with measurement methods, particularly electrophysiology

In addition, we need to develop standards of use, to be checked, taught, and transmitted to the users' community, in particular making sure that the apparent ease of the stereotactic method does not induce in young neurosurgeons the feeling that this procedure is better tolerated and that fewer precautions are necessary.

References

1. Clarke RH, Horsley V. On a method of investigating the deep ganglia and tracts of the central nervous system (cerebellum). BMJ 1906;2:1799–1800
2. Gildenberg PL. Principles of stereotaxis and instruments. In: DeSalles AAF, Goetsch SJ, eds. Stereotactic Surgery and Radiosurgery. Madison, WI: Medical Physics, 1993:17
3. Spiegel EA, Wycis HT, Marks M, Lee AJ. Stereotaxic apparatus for operations on the human brain. Science 1947;106:349–350
4. Leksell L. A stereotaxic apparatus for intracerebral surgery. Acta Chir Scand 1949;99:229–233
5. Hécaen H, Talairach T, David M, Dell M. Mémories originaux: coagulations limitées du thalamus dans les algies du syndrome thalamique. Rev Neurol (Paris) 1949;81:917–931
6. Riechert T, Wolff M. [A new stereotactic instrument for intracranial placement of electrodes.] Arch Psychiatr Nervenkr. Z Gesamte Neurol Psychiatr 1951;186:225–230
7. Gabriel EM, Nashold BS. Historical development of stereotactic frames. In: Gildenberg PL, Tasker RR, eds. Textbook of Stereotactic and Functional Neurosurgery. New York: McGraw-Hill, 1997:20
8. Benabid AL, Pollak P, Gervason C, et al. Long-term suppression of tremor by chronic stimulation of the ventral intermediate thalamic nucleus. Lancet 1991;337:403–406
9. Rehncrona S, Johnels B, Widner H, Törnqvist AL, Hariz M, Sydow O. Long-term efficacy of thalamic deep brain stimulation for tremor: double-blind assessments. Mov Disord 2003;18:163–170
10. Rodriguez-Oroz MC, Obeso JA, Lang AE, et al. Bilateral deep brain stimulation in Parkinson's disease: a multicentre study with 4 years follow-up. Brain 2005;128(Pt 10):2240–2249
11. Gorgulho AA, Shields DC, Malkasian D, Behnke E, Desalles AA. Stereotactic coordinates associated with facial musculature contraction during high-frequency stimulation of the subthalamic nucleus. J Neurosurg 2009;110:1317–1321
12. Konrad PE, Neimat JS, Yu H, et al. Customized, miniature rapid-prototype stereotactic frames for use in deep brain stimulator surgery: initial clinical methodology and experience from 263 patients from 2002 to 2008. Stereotact Funct Neurosurg 2011; 89:34–41
13. Benardete EA, Leonard MA, Weiner HL. Comparison of frameless stereotactic systems: accuracy, precision, and applications. Neurosurgery 2001;49:1409–1415, discussion 1415–1416
14. Kitchen ND, Lemieux L, Thomas DG. Accuracy in frame-based and frameless stereotaxy. Stereotact Funct Neurosurg 1993; 61:195–206
15. Ondo WG, Bronte-Stewart H; DBS Study Group. The North American survey of placement and adjustment strategies for deep brain stimulation. Stereotact Funct Neurosurg 2005;83:142–147
16. Anheim M, Batir A, Fraix V, et al. Improvement in Parkinson disease by subthalamic nucleus stimulation based on electrode placement: effects of reimplantation. Arch Neurol 2008;65:612–616
17. Ellis TM, Foote KD, Fernandez HH, et al. Reoperation for suboptimal outcomes after deep brain stimulation surgery. Neurosurgery 2008;63:754–760, discussion 760–761
18. McClelland S III, Ford B, Senatus PB, et al. Subthalamic stimulation for Parkinson disease: determination of electrode location necessary for clinical efficacy. Neurosurg Focus 2005;19:E12
19. Richardson RM, Ostrem JL, Starr PA. Surgical repositioning of misplaced subthalamic electrodes in Parkinson's disease: location of effective and ineffective leads. Stereotact Funct Neurosurg 2009;87:297–303
20. Woerdeman PA, Willems PW, Noordmans HJ, Tulleken CA, van der Sprenkel JW. Application accuracy in frameless image-guided neurosurgery: a comparison study of three patient-to-image registration methods. J Neurosurg 2007;106:1012–1016
21. Balachandran R, Mitchell JE, Dawant BM, Fitzpatrick JM. Accuracy evaluation of microTargeting Platforms for deep-brain stimulation using virtual targets. IEEE Trans Biomed Eng 2009; 56:37–44
22. Fitzpatrick JM, Konrad PE, Nickele C, Cetinkaya E, Kao C. Accuracy of customized miniature stereotactic platforms. Stereotact Funct Neurosurg 2005;83:25–31
23. D'Haese PF, Pallavaram S, Konrad PE, Neimat J, Fitzpatrick JM, Dawant BM. Clinical accuracy of a customized stereotactic platform for deep brain stimulation after accounting for brain shift. Stereotact Funct Neurosurg 2010;88:81–87
24. D'Haese PF, Cetinkaya E, Konrad PE, Kao C, Dawant BM. Computer-aided placement of deep brain stimulators: from planning to intraoperative guidance. IEEE Trans Med Imaging 2005; 24:1469–1478
25. Smith AP, Bakay RA. Frameless deep brain stimulation using intraoperative O-arm technology. Clinical article. J Neurosurg 2011;115:301–309

26. Richter EO, Hoque T, Halliday W, Lozano AM, Saint-Cyr JA. Determining the position and size of the subthalamic nucleus based on magnetic resonance imaging results in patients with advanced Parkinson disease. J Neurosurg 2004;100:541–546

27. Schrader B, Hamel W, Weinert D, Mehdorn HM. Documentation of electrode localization. Mov Disord 2002;17(Suppl 3):S167–S174

28. Maciunas RJ, Galloway RL Jr, Latimer JW. The application accuracy of stereotactic frames. Neurosurgery 1994;35:682–694, discussion 694–695

29. Henderson JM, Holloway KL, Gaede SE, Rosenow JM. The application accuracy of a skull-mounted trajectory guide system for image-guided functional neurosurgery. Comput Aided Surg 2004;9:155–160

30. Starr PA, Christine CW, Theodosopoulos PV, et al. Implantation of deep brain stimulators into the subthalamic nucleus: technical approach and magnetic resonance imaging-verified lead locations. J Neurosurg 2002;97:370–387

31. Patwardhan R.V., Behnke E.J., Krahl S., DeSalles A.A.F. Off-target measurements in deep brain stimulation: how much off target and why? American Association of Neurological Surgeons Meeting, May 3, 2004, Article ID 19710 (abstract)

32. O'Leary ST, Yoshida K, Arzbaecher J, Bakay RA. How accurate is accurate? Intraoperative radiographic measurement of microelectrode and DBS lead location. American Association of Neurological Surgeons Meeting, May 3, 2004, Article ID 19645 (abstract)

33. Hamid NA, Mitchell RD, Mocroft P, Westby GW, Milner J, Pall H. Targeting the subthalamic nucleus for deep brain stimulation: technical approach and fusion of pre- and postoperative MR images to define accuracy of lead placement. J Neurol Neurosurg Psychiatry 2005;76:409–414

34. Holloway KL, Gaede SE, Starr PA, Rosenow JM, Ramakrishnan V, Henderson JM. Frameless stereotaxy using bone fiducial markers for deep brain stimulation. J Neurosurg 2005;103:404–413

35. Kelman C, Ramakrishnan V, Davies A, Holloway K. Analysis of stereotactic accuracy of the Cosman-Robert-Wells frame and Nexframe frameless systems in deep brain stimulation surgery. Stereotact Funct Neurosurg 2010;88:288–295

36. Bjartmarz H, Rehncrona S. Comparison of accuracy and precision between frame-based and frameless stereotactic navigation for deep brain stimulation electrode implantation. Stereotact Funct Neurosurg 2007;85:235–242

37. Henderson JM, Holloway KL. Achieving optimal accuracy in frameless functional neurosurgical procedures. Stereotact Funct Neurosurg 2008;86:332–333

38. Rohlfing T, Maurer CR Jr, Dean D, Maciunas RJ. Effect of changing patient position from supine to prone on the accuracy of a Brown-Roberts-Wells stereotactic head frame system. Neurosurgery 2003;52:610–618, discussion 617–618

39. Papavassiliou E, Rau G, Heath S, et al. Thalamic deep brain stimulation for essential tremor: relation of lead location to outcome. Neurosurgery 2004;54:1120–1129, discussion 1129–1130

40. Romanelli P, Heit G, Hill BC, Kraus A, Hastie T, Brontë-Stewart HM. Microelectrode recording revealing a somatotopic body map in the subthalamic nucleus in humans with Parkinson disease. J Neurosurg 2004;100:611–618

41. Brontë-Stewart H, Louie S, Batya S, Henderson JM. Clinical motor outcome of bilateral subthalamic nucleus deep-brain stimulation for Parkinson's disease using image-guided frameless stereotaxy. Neurosurgery 2010;67:1088–1093, discussion 1093

42. Tai CH, Wu RM, Lin CH, et al. Deep brain stimulation therapy for Parkinson's disease using frameless stereotaxy: comparison with frame-based surgery. Eur J Neurol 2010;17:1377–1385

43. Weaver F, Follett K, Hur K, Ippolito D, Stern M. Deep brain stimulation in Parkinson disease: a metaanalysis of patient outcomes. J Neurosurg 2005;103:956–967

44. Kleiner-Fisman G, Herzog J, Fisman DN, et al. Subthalamic nucleus deep brain stimulation: summary and meta-analysis of outcomes. Mov Disord 2006;21(Suppl 14):S290–S304

45. Cotzias GC, Papavasiliou PS, Gellene R. Modification of Parkinsonism—chronic treatment with L-dopa. N Engl J Med 1969;280:337–345

46. Müller T, Russ H. Levodopa, motor fluctuations and dyskinesia in Parkinson's disease. Expert Opin Pharmacother 2006;7:1715–1730

47. Rascol O, Brooks DJ, Korczyn AD, De Deyn PP, Clarke CE, Lang AEA. A five-year study of the incidence of dyskinesia in patients with early Parkinson's disease who were treated with ropinirole or levodopa. 056 Study Group. N Engl J Med 2000;342:1484–1491

48. Sankar T, Lozano AM. Surgical approach to L-dopa-induced dyskinesias. Int Rev Neurobiol 2011;98:151–171

49. Weaver FM, Follett K, Stern M, et al; CSP 468 Study Group. Bilateral deep brain stimulation vs best medical therapy for patients with advanced Parkinson disease: a randomized controlled trial. JAMA 2009;301:63–73

50. Deuschl G, Schade-Brittinger C, Krack P, et al; German Parkinson Study Group, Neurostimulation Section. A randomized trial of deep-brain stimulation for Parkinson's disease. N Engl J Med 2006;355:896–908

51. Williams A, Gill S, Varma T, et al; PD SURG Collaborative Group. Deep brain stimulation plus best medical therapy versus best medical therapy alone for advanced Parkinson's disease (PD SURG trial): a randomised, open-label trial. Lancet Neurol 2010;9:581–591

52. Bronstein JM, Tagliati M, Alterman RL, et al. Deep brain stimulation for Parkinson disease: an expert consensus and review of key issues. Arch Neurol 2011;68:165

53. Okun MS, Tagliati M, Pourfar M, et al. Management of referred deep brain stimulation failures: a retrospective analysis from 2 movement disorders centers. Arch Neurol 2005;62:1250–1255

54. Morgante L, Morgante F, Moro E, et al. How many parkinsonian patients are suitable candidates for deep brain stimulation of subthalamic nucleus? Results of a questionnaire. Parkinsonism Relat Disord 2007;13:528–531

55. Shih LC, Tarsy D. Deep brain stimulation for the treatment of atypical parkinsonism. Mov Disord 2007;22:2149–2155

56. Bötzel K, Kraft E. Strategies for treatment of gait and posture associated deficits in movement disorders: the impact of deep brain stimulation. Restor Neurol Neurosci 2010;28:115–122

57. Johnsen EL, Mogensen PH, Sunde NA, Østergaard K. Improved asymmetry of gait in Parkinson's disease with DBS: gait and postural instability in Parkinson's disease treated with bilateral deep brain stimulation in the subthalamic nucleus. Mov Disord 2009;24:590–597

58. Klostermann F, Ehlen F, Vesper J, et al. Effects of subthalamic deep brain stimulation on dysarthrophonia in Parkinson's disease. J Neurol Neurosurg Psychiatry 2008;79:522–529

59. Charles PD, Van Blercom N, Krack P, et al. Predictors of effective bilateral subthalamic nucleus stimulation for PD. Neurology 2002;59:932–934

60. Ory-Magne F, Brefel-Courbon C, Simonetta-Moreau M, et al. Does ageing influence deep brain stimulation outcomes in Parkinson's disease? Mov Disord 2007;22:1457–1463

61. Lang AE, Houeto JL, Krack P, et al. Deep brain stimulation: preoperative issues. Mov Disord 2006;21(Suppl 14):S171–S196

62. Saint-Cyr JA, Trépanier LL, Kumar R, Lozano AM, Lang AE. Neuropsychological consequences of chronic bilateral stimulation of the subthalamic nucleus in Parkinson's disease. Brain 2000;123(Pt 10):2091–2108

63. Voon V, Krack P, Lang AE, et al. A multicentre study on suicide outcomes following subthalamic stimulation for Parkinson's disease. Brain 2008;131(Pt 10):2720–2728

64. Follett KA, Weaver FM, Stern M, et al; CSP 468 Study Group. Pallidal versus subthalamic deep-brain stimulation for Parkinson's disease. N Engl J Med 2010;362:2077–2091

65. Okun MS, Fernandez HH, Wu SS, et al. Cognition and mood in Parkinson's disease in subthalamic nucleus versus globus pallidus interna deep brain stimulation: the COMPARE trial. Ann Neurol 2009;65:586–595

66. Kopell BH, Machado A, Rezai AR. Chronic subthalamic nucleus stimulation for Parkinson disease. In: Starr PA, Barbaro NM, Larson PS, eds. Neurosurgical Operative Atlas: Functional Neurosurgery, 2nd ed. New York: Thieme, 2008:177–187

67. Sierens DK, Kutz S, Pilitsis JG, Bakay RAE. Stereotactic surgery with microelectrode recordings. In: Bakay RAE, ed. Movement Disorder Surgery: The Essentials. New York: Thieme, 2009: 83–114

68. Sakas DE, Kouyialis AT, Boviatsis EJ, Panourias IG, Stathis P, Tagaris G. Technical aspects and considerations of deep brain stimulation surgery for movement disorders. Acta Neurochir Suppl (Wien) 2007;97(Pt 2):163–170

69. Schuurman PR, Bosch DA. Surgical considerations in movement disorders: deep brain stimulation, ablation and transplantation. Acta Neurochir Suppl (Wien) 2007;97(Pt 2):119–125

70. Abosch A, Kapur S, Lang AE, et al. Stimulation of the subthalamic nucleus in Parkinson's disease does not produce striatal dopamine release. Neurosurgery 2003;53:1095–1102, discussion 1102–1105

71. Henderson JM. Frameless functional stereotactic approaches. In: Bakay RAE, ed. Movement Disorder Surgery: The Essentials. New York: Thieme, 2008:140–152

72. Larson PS. Minimally invasive surgery for movement disorders. Neurosurg Clin N Am 2010;21:691–698, vii

73. Fukaya C, Sumi K, Otaka T, et al. Nexframe frameless stereotaxy with multitract microrecording: accuracy evaluated by frame-based stereotactic X-ray. Stereotact Funct Neurosurg 2010;88: 163–168

74. Henderson JM. Frameless localization for functional neurosurgical procedures: a preliminary accuracy study. Stereotact Funct Neurosurg 2004;82:135–141

75. Rodriguez-Oroz MC, Zamarbide I, Guridi J, Palmero MR, Obeso JA. Efficacy of deep brain stimulation of the subthalamic nucleus in Parkinson's disease 4 years after surgery: double blind and open label evaluation. J Neurol Neurosurg Psychiatry 2004; 75:1382–1385

76. Schüpbach WM, Chastan N, Welter ML, et al. Stimulation of the subthalamic nucleus in Parkinson's disease: a 5 year follow up. J Neurol Neurosurg Psychiatry 2005;76:1640–1644

77. Krack P, Batir A, Van Blercom N, et al. Five-year follow-up of bilateral stimulation of the subthalamic nucleus in advanced Parkinson's disease. N Engl J Med 2003;349:1925–1934

78. Gervais-Bernard H, Xie-Brustolin J, Mertens P, et al. Bilateral subthalamic nucleus stimulation in advanced Parkinson's disease: five year follow-up. J Neurol 2009;256:225–233

79. Moro E, Lozano AM, Pollak P, et al. Long-term results of a multicenter study on subthalamic and pallidal stimulation in Parkinson's disease. Mov Disord 2010;25:578–586

80. Guridi J, Obeso JA, Rodriguez-Oroz MC, Lozano AA, Manrique M. L-dopa-induced dyskinesia and stereotactic surgery for Parkinson's disease. Neurosurgery 2008;62:311–323, discussion 323–325

81. Devos D, Defebvre L, Bordet R. Dopaminergic and non-dopaminergic pharmacological hypotheses for gait disorders in Parkinson's disease. Fundam Clin Pharmacol 2010;24:407–421

82. Merola A, Zibetti M, Angrisano S, et al. Parkinson's disease progression at 30 years: a study of subthalamic deep brain-stimulated patients. Brain 2011;134(Pt 7):2074–2084

83. Videnovic A, Metman LV. Deep brain stimulation for Parkinson's disease: prevalence of adverse events and need for standardized reporting. Mov Disord 2008;23:343–349

84. Blomstedt P, Hariz MI. Hardware-related complications of deep brain stimulation: a ten year experience. Acta Neurochir (Wien) 2005;147:1061–1064, discussion 1064

85. Hamani C, Lozano AM. Hardware-related complications of deep brain stimulation: a review of the published literature. Stereotact Funct Neurosurg 2006;84:248–251

Chapter 22

The Application of Artificial Discs

Case

A 40-year-old man, who is a smoker, has C7 radiculopathy that did not respond to medical treatment, and a large, soft single disc.

Participants

Advocating Against Artificial Cervical Discs: Rasha Germain and Volker K.H. Sonntag

Application of Artificial Cervical Discs: Ricardo B.V. Fontes and Vincent C. Traynelis

Posterior Discectomy for Soft Disc Herniation: Miguel A. Arraez

Moderator: The Puzzling Development of Artificial Cervical Disc Arthroplasty: A. El Khamlichi

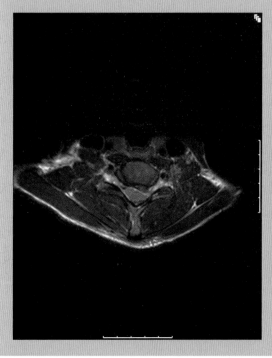
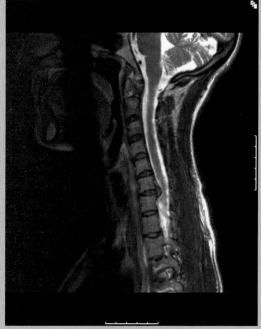

Advocating Against Artificial Cervical Discs

Rasha Germain and Volker K.H. Sonntag

Anterior cervical discectomy and fusion is the most common surgical procedure used and has proven successful in the treatment of symptoms caused by degenerative cervical disc disease. First described by Smith and Robinson in the 1950s and modified over the years, this procedure remains the gold standard for the treatment of disc herniation, foraminal and spinal stenosis, and axial discogenic pain. Excellent clinical and radiographic outcomes are obtained in 85 to 95% of patients. Despite these good outcomes, however, long-term studies of patients after discectomy and fusion have shown that as many as 25% of patients may develop recurrent radicular symptoms from adjacent segment degeneration. Furthermore, surgical intervention for symptomatic adjacent-level disease has been reported in as many as 2.9% of patients annually after fusion.[1] Finally, although it is not clinically correlated, radiographic evidence of adjacent-level disease has been reported in as many as 92% of fusion-treated patients 5 years after surgery.[2]

The cause of adjacent-level disease after fusion is debated. It may be the result of an altered biomechanical environment or due to the natural history of the degenerative process.[3] The effects of cervical fusion on spinal biomechanics have been heavily studied. Intradiscal pressures increase significantly during flexion at both superior and inferior adjacent levels.[4] Kinematic studies show increases in mobility and angular displacement at adjacent levels, both near and remote, after fusion.[5,6] Nonetheless, no direct clinical correlation with these biomechanical findings has been established. Whether the progression of cervical disease can be halted by maintaining preoperative kinematics is still unknown.

The development of nonfusion spinal devices for use in cervical arthroplasty has been driven by the hope that maintaining motion may decrease the incidence of adjacent-level disease. Over the past 10 years, technology in the realm of cervical arthroplasty has evolved and improved, with various design revisions and the establishment of clear indications for arthroplasty. The many device designs and their kinematic characteristics must be considered when selecting the appropriate device for implantation.[7]

Most arthroplasty devices have single-gliding or double-gliding interfaces, including ball-and-socket and saddle designs, which allow rotation and translation around an axis of rotation. To protect the facet joints from abnormal stresses, an implant must have an axis of rotation that is near-physiological. In some implants the axis of rotation is fixed, and in others it is mobile. These devices also may be semiconstrained or unconstrained, in which case they rely on surrounding soft tissues to provide restraint in the extremes of range of motion. Maintaining the posterior longitudinal ligament enhances stability, and resection of this ligament has been associated with hypermobility at the

index level and implant failure. Unconstrained devices allow translation and diminish stress at articulating surfaces, although they may subject the facet joints to greater stress. Unconstrained devices with a mobile axis of rotation are more forgiving of small errors in placement; fixed axis-of-rotation devices require more precise placement. Constrained devices achieve greater stability but transmit greater stresses to articulating surfaces and require stronger fixation.

The Prestige (Medtronic Sofamor Danek, Memphis, TN), ProDisc-C (Synthes, Paoli, PA), and porous coated motion (PCM) (Cervitech, Rockaway, NJ) are semiconstrained devices, whereas the Bryan disc (Medtronic Sofamor Danek) is unconstrained. Both the Bryan and Prestige discs have mobile centers of rotation, in contrast to the fixed centers of rotation of ProDisc-C and PCM devices. Thus, aside from general procedural considerations with the placement of a prosthesis, there are concerns about which device will best serve the patient.

Clinical trials in Europe, Canada, the United States, Australia, and China have sought to determine the safety and short-term efficacy of several of the available cervical discs. Many studies have focused on the Bryan disc, ProDisc-C, and Prestige.[8-10] Early surgical results appeared promising, with most reported complications related to the learning curve associated with device implantation. Early and 24-month clinical results appeared promising as well, with good postoperative ratings of patient satisfaction, an improved neck disability index, improved neck and arm pain scores, and an earlier return to activity as compared with traditional anterior cervical discectomy and fusion.[11-13]

Nonetheless, longer follow-up has raised several concerns that merit further investigation. First, it is difficult to assess the accuracy of clinical outcomes obtained through patient surveys. Within the noninferiority studies conducted in the U.S., a primary determinant of "success" has been more than a 15-point improvement in the neck disability index, a survey outcome measure that each patient completes during follow-up. When a new device becomes available, patients' enthusiasm for the "improved" technology is a well-known phenomenon. Patients who complete follow-up assessment forms are likely to express an inherent bias, especially if they are dissatisfied about not receiving the "new technology." Studies done with patients randomized at surgery, with both the patient and examiner blinded during follow-up to the treatment received, will help resolve this issue.

Second, the purpose of cervical arthroplasty has been to maintain the patient's preoperative level of functional spinal unit-motion parameters, including range of motion, translation, and center of rotation. Although most short-term studies document near-physiological motion after cervical arthroplasty, the magnitude of prothesis motion has been noted to decrease with time. Kinematically, therefore, several devices become equivalent to a fusion over time. In 2008, Sasso and Best[14] reported that, at 24 months, more flexion and extension motion was retained in the group of patients undergoing Bryan disc replacement than in those receiving plates at the index level (6.7 degrees vs. 0.6 degrees, respectively). During flexion and extension, however, the range of motion both above and below the operative level was not significantly different between the groups of patients. Likewise, at the 12-month follow-up, the increase in anterior/posterior translation initially noted at 6 months at the level above fusion in patients receiving plates was not significantly different from that of the disc replacement group. Longer follow-up is needed to determine whether disc replacement preserves preoperative kinematics at the levels adjacent to fusion, or whether the trend will continue toward loss of motion even with arthroplasty.

Heterotopic ossification, both anteriorly and posteriorly, resulting in fusion across the implant level has also been reported. McAfee and colleagues[15] proposed a classification scheme to study heterotopic ossification in the lumbar spine, and Mehren and associates[16] adapted the scheme for heterotopic ossification in the cervical spine (**Table 22.1**). In a prospective study of 54 patients (77 total implanted prostheses, ProDisc-C, Synthes), only 33.8% of patients showed no signs of heterotopic ossification at 1 year. Ossification of grade 2 to 3 was present in 49.4% of patients, and 10.4% of the patients had heterotopic ossification that restricted their range of motion. Spontaneous fusion of the treated segment was noted in 9.1% of cases. Furthermore, the rate of heterotopic ossification was significantly higher in multilevel cases compared with single-level cases. Goffin and colleagues[17] measured the range of motion of 139 implanted Bryan cervical discs at 1 year. The range of motion of 18 discs (12.9%) was less than 2 degrees, and further evaluation with computed tomography (CT) showed evidence of anterolateral paravertebral ossification. With a 3-year follow-up, Sola and coworkers[18] found evidence of heterotopic ossification in 16 of 21 patients with implanted Bryan discs (76.2%), missing motion in 10 (47.6%), and definite fusion in six patients (28.6%). The ossification appeared anteriorly in all of these patients. In the U.S., current investigational device-exemption study designs include a 2-week course of postoperative nonsteroidal antiinflammatory drugs, which, in orthopedic surgeries, have been shown to inhibit ossification when administered early in the postoperative period. The outcomes of long-term studies of this issue will be interesting.

Recently, several papers have addressed the issue of changes to sagittal cervical alignment after disc replacement. In 2004, Pickett and colleagues[19] reported that preoperative alignment worsened in all 14 of their patients who underwent implantation of a Bryan disc, with a mean change in end-plate angle of –3.8 degrees, and a mean change in functional spinal unit angle of –6 degrees. Simi-

Table 22.1 Grades of Heterotopic Ossification in Cervical Arthroplasty

Grade	Extent of Heterotrophic Ossification
0	None present
I	Detectable in adjacent soft tissues, but not within the confines of the intervertebral disc space
II	Present between end plates, with possible effect on prosthesis motion
III	Present with bridging osteophytes; restricting, but still permitting motion
IV	Causing fusion across the treated level

Source: Modified from McAfee PC, Cunningham BW, Devine J, Williams E, Yu-Yahiro J. Classification of heterotopic ossification (HO) in artificial disk replacement. J Spinal Disord Tech 2003;16:384–389; and Mehren C, Suchomel P, Grochulla F, et al. Heterotopic ossification in total cervical artificial disc replacement. Spine 2006;31:2802–2806.

larly, Johnson and associates[20] reported that, of 10 patients undergoing single-level arthroplasty, 80% developed endplate kyphosis through the prosthesis, with a mean loss of 4.7 degrees of lordosis. The overall loss of lordosis (C2-C7) was –2.7 degrees, which was not statistically significant. Fong and coworkers[21] reported that 9 of their 10 patients undergoing single-level arthroplasty developed kyphosis through the operative level, with a mean change of –9 degrees. No significant change in overall cervical alignment was detected. In a larger study by Sears and associates,[22] both the median loss in functional spinal unit lordosis and the median development of prosthesis shell kyphosis was 2 degrees. The mean overall loss in cervical lordosis (C2-C7) was 4 degrees. None of the changes in sagittal alignment were clinically correlated in any of the studies. Pickett and colleagues,[23] however, described one patient with marked segmental kyphosis after cervical arthroplasty who underwent revision surgery 8 months later to correct the deformity. His symptoms resolved 12 months after the second surgery.

Many studies have focused on the effect of fusion on the sagittal alignment of the cervical spine, and the development of kyphosis may prove to be clinically important in the development of adjacent-level disease and symptoms of pain. Kawakami and associates[24] found that the risk of axial symptoms after cervical fusion was significantly related to cervical kyphosis and loss of vertebral body height at the fused segment. In addition, one factor found to promote degenerative change in the levels adjacent to a fusion was kyphotic change across the fused segment and overall loss of cervical lordosis.[25] As yet, no single surgical or clinical factor appears directly responsible for the development of postoperative kyphosis after cervical arthroplasty. The issue merits further investigation if indeed kyphotic change is associated with progression of disease.

Finally, preservation of motion through nonfusion technology introduces the possibility of same-level degeneration, a problem not typically encountered after solid fusion. Same-level degeneration may involve the intervertebral disc, facet joints, or ligamentum flavum. Because segmental motion is preserved, progressive facet arthrosis leading to joint hypertrophy is a concern.[26] Exclusion criteria for cervical arthroplasty include facet arthrosis at the affected level.

Furthermore, imaging after cervical arthroplasty is problematic. Magnetic resonance imaging (MRI) is the standard modality for evaluating patients both before and after surgery. Despite promising early clinical results, reoperation at the index level after cervical arthroplasty has been reported, and imaging is necessary in the event of suspected device failure or in patients with new neurologic symptoms.[27] Due to image artifact after disc replacement, it may be more difficult to determine the presence of same- or adjacent-level disease. The clarity of MRIs was analyzed by comparing four available devices.[27] Both Bryan and Prestige LP devices enabled satisfactory visualization of the spinal canal, exit foramina, and both adjacent levels. However, the quality of MRIs deteriorated significantly at both index and adjacent levels with the ProDisc-C and PCM devices. The relatively high metal content of the devices also produced artifact on CT scans. Thus, after initial flexion/extension plain films have been obtained, further evaluation of the implant position and range of motion would require CT myelography.

More years of follow-up are needed before the role of cervical arthroplasty in the treatment of degenerative cervical disc disease can be determined. If the goals are to maintain segment motion and to offset the progression of adjacent-level disease, the focus must be on demonstrating that cervical arthroplasty meets these demands. Few reports on the long-term outcomes of cervical artificial discs are available, but some trends are developing. With 3 years of follow-up, Sola and associates[18] reported anterior ossification in 16 of 21 operated levels (76.2%), missing motion in 47.6%, and definite fusion in 28.6%. We have noted the progression of adjacent-level disease in patients after cervical arthroplasty (**Figs. 22.1, 22.2, 22.3**).

The experience with lumbar disc replacement has provided clues and ideas about how to avoid pitfalls with patient selection and device construction. Likewise, long-term studies with lumbar devices may provide clues about the future of cervical arthroplasty. With a 17-year follow-up, Putzier and associates[28] reported a spontaneous fusion rate of 60% with lumbar disc replacement. Bertagnoli and Schönmayr[29] reported a 5% incidence of adjacent-level degeneration with a 2-year follow-up, whereas Huang and colleagues[30] reported a 24% incidence with a 9-year follow-up.

Until long-term information about implanted cervical devices is available, our expectations and patient selection criteria should remain conservative. The device should be offered only to patients who stringently meet the determined criteria. Furthermore, the potential for progressive adjacent-level disease must be recognized, irrespective of the surgical technique employed.

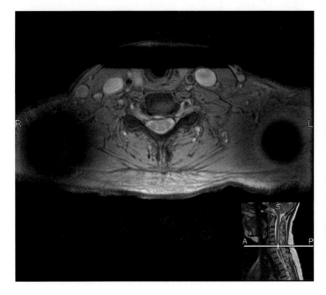

a

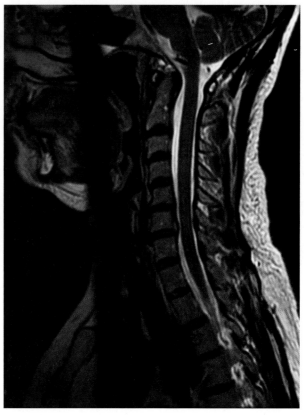

b

Fig. 22.1a,b   Preoperative axial **(a)** and sagittal **(b)** T2-weighted magnetic resonance imaging (MRI) scans showing a C6/7 herniated disc with right foraminal stenosis. The patient had suffered from persistent right-arm pain consistent with a right C7 radiculopathy for 2 years, and conservative treatment had failed. (Courtesy of the Barrow Neurological Institute.)

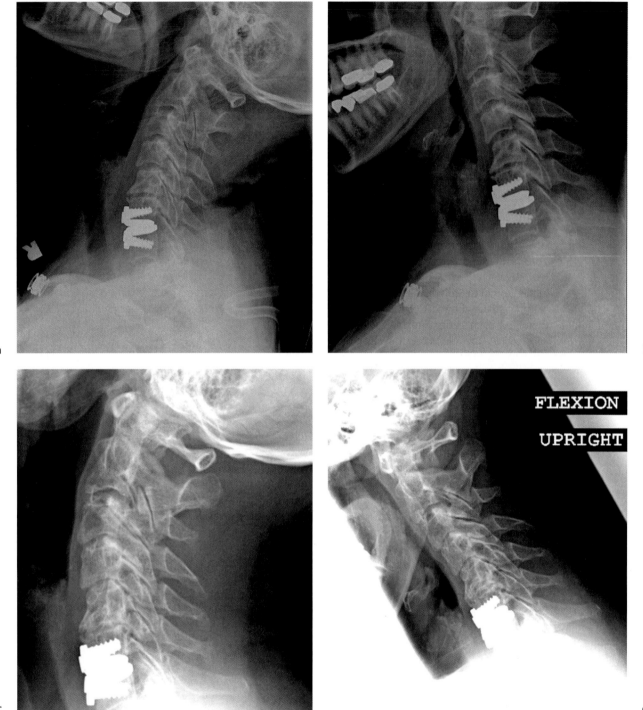

a

b

c

d

Fig. 22.2a–d Lateral view extension **(a,c)** and flexion **(b,d)** radiographs from the day of surgery **(a,b)** and 1 year later **(c,d)**. After undergoing placement of a Prestige artificial disc at C6/7, the patient still suffered the original pain and had new pain in the right arm. Note the loss of height at the superior adjacent level C5/6 and the loss of lordosis. (Courtesy of the Barrow Neurological Institute.)

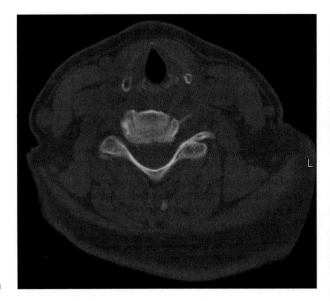

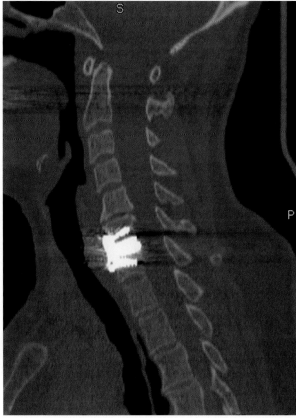

Fig. 22.3a,b Axial **(a)** and sagittal **(b)** computed tomography (CT) scan images obtained 15 months after surgery show evidence of adjacent-level loss of height at C5/6 and right foraminal narrowing consistent with the patient's new and worsened symptoms of right arm pain. (Courtesy of the Barrow Neurological Institute.)

Application of Artificial Cervical Discs

Ricardo B.V. Fontes and Vincent C. Traynelis

Several operative approaches are available to treat the cervical radiculopathy from this patient's disc herniation. We believe that cervical arthroplasty represents the best treatment strategy in such a relatively young individual who presents with single-level symptomatic disease with normal alignment and relatively little spondylosis. In this section, we present the evidence supporting this opinion.

Posterior Discectomy

Posterior cervical decompression promptly relieves radicular symptoms, and fusion is not required. Unfortunately, the durable efficacy of this treatment option has yet to be defined in any scientifically valid study. Experienced surgeons have published descriptions and analyses of the procedure and a critique of the most significant works follows. Scoville and colleagues[31] presented 208 cases with long-term follow-up, but the review is seriously flawed because of selection bias. The reported experience represents only 13% of the total group of patients treated with a posterior

cervical discectomy over the time of the study, and no information is provided to explain how the study group was chosen. Therefore, the findings from such a highly selected group cannot be expected to represent the overall outcomes of this procedure. Murphey and associates[32] treated 648 patients over a 34-year period but chose to report the outcomes of only 380 cases. Similar to the work of Scoville and colleagues, the reasons for limiting the review to a small subset of the total experience are unclear. These authors do not provide any information concerning the duration of follow-up, and data regarding axial neck pain and the need for additional surgery are not included. These shortcomings completely negate the reported findings.

Henderson and colleagues[33] performed a retrospective review of 846 consecutive patients with a mean follow-up of 146 weeks. Radicular symptoms recurred in 172 patients (20.3%) and a second procedure was required in 103 patients (12.2%). The average time between the two operations (169 weeks) was greater than the mean length of follow-up for the entire series, which led the authors to speculate that "the long-term recurrence rate might well be higher than indicated." Furthermore, in the course of the study, 32 patients (3.8%) were ultimately treated with an anterior cervical fusion.

Kumar and associates[34] addressed the outcome after cervical foraminotomy for radiculopathy due to osteophytic nerve-root compression, and the records of 89 consecutive patients were retrospectively reviewed. Although the mean postoperative follow-up was only 8.6 months, further surgery for recurrent root symptoms was required in 6.7% of patients, which represents a relatively high failure rate over such a short time. Clarke and coworkers[35] retrospectively reviewed 303 patients treated with a posterior cervical foraminotomy. In this group, 20% had less than 3 months of follow-up and 30% had less than 1 year of follow-up. The main interest of this study was to assess adjacent-segment disease after posterior discectomy, but the poor follow-up does not allow for a valid assessment of that problem.

All of these papers represent the best data available. Unfortunately, the selection process and short follow-up introduces significant bias, and none of the studies employed validated outcome measures. Axial neck pain and return to work were not included in the reviews. The best long-term study suggests that this procedure is associated with a rela-

tively high failure rate.[33] In summary, although posterior cervical discectomy may have excellent short- and long-term results, there are no data to support this conclusion.

Anterior Fusion and Arthroplasty

Anterior cervical discectomy and fusion (ACDF) enables direct neural decompression and reconstruction of the anterior spinal column. The overall outcomes of ACDF have been reported in numerous retrospective studies, and data have accumulated from prospective investigations. The best data were acquired in the arthroplasty trials, which compared single-level cervical arthroplasty to an instrumented anterior fusion. Each of these studies is reviewed in the following paragraphs.

In 2007, the results of a randomized trial comparing single-level arthroplasty with the metal-on-metal unconstrained Prestige cervical disk system (investigational) to an instrumented ACDF (control) were published[36] (**Fig. 22.4**). The 32-center study enrolled a total of 541 patients (276 arthroplasty, 265 ACDF), and 80% of the patients treated with arthroplasty and 75% of those treated with ACDF completed clinical and radiographic follow-up at the end of 2 years. The mean operative time was 90 minutes, and the

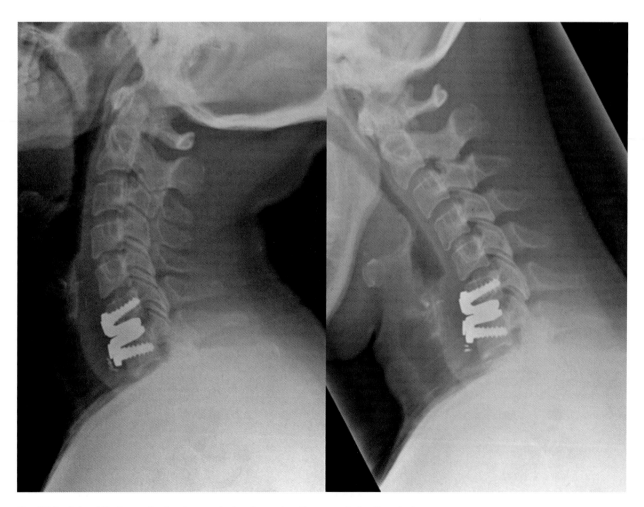

Fig. 22.4 Lateral flexion and extension cervical radiographs after a cervical arthroplasty.

average hospitalization was 1 day for both groups. The need for secondary surgical procedures (revisions, supplemental fixation, and hardware removal) in the ACDF group was 8.7%, which was statistically greater than that of the arthroplasty group (1.8%). Additionally, second surgeries at the adjacent levels were also more common in the ACDF group, with 11 procedures as opposed to three in the arthroplasty group. The incidence of adverse events was statistically similar in both treatment arms (arthroplasty 6.2%, ACDF 4.2%). Clinical outcome measures included the Neck Disability Index (NDI), the Short Form questionnaire (SF-36), neck and arm pain numeric rating scales, and neurologic and work status. Although great improvement was seen in both treatment groups compared with the patients' preoperative state, there were some discrepancies between the cohorts. The arthroplasty group showed higher rates of NDI improvement at all postoperative intervals compared with the ACDF group, achieving statistical significance at 3 months. The arthroplasty group had statistically favorable neck pain scores at 12 months compared with the ACDF group. Neurologic success was higher in the investigational group (92.8%) compared with the control group (84.3%) at the 2-year point. Patients undergoing arthroplasty returned to work 16 days sooner than those undergoing ACDF. The Prestige implant maintained segmental sagittal angular motion averaging more than 7 degrees at the 2-year follow-up.

The results of the semiconstrained metal-on-high-molecular-polyethylene ProDisc-C were published in 2009.[37] This study involved 13 centers at which 209 patients were enrolled. The investigational group consisted of 103 patients who underwent single-level arthroplasty with ProDisc-C, and the control group included 106 patients treated with an instrumented ACDF. Of these patients, 98% of the investigational group and 94.8% of the control group completed the 24-month follow-up period. The average intraoperative times for the investigational and control groups were 107.2 and 98.7 minutes, respectively. Blood loss and total hospitalization times were similar. The NDI scores improved tremendously after treatment with both modalities. Visual Analogue Score pain scores and the physical and mental components of the SF-36 showed statistically significant improvement compared with preoperative levels, but there was no difference between the two groups. Patient satisfaction was higher at all time points in patients undergoing reconstruction with an arthroplasty. Secondary surgical procedures occurred at a rate of 1.9% in the ProDisc-C group and 8.5% in the fusion group, similar to the results of the Prestige study. Device success (defined as no revision, removal, or reoperation) was 98.1% in the ProDisc-C group compared with 91.5% in the fusion group, which represented a statistically significant difference. The decline in narcotic and muscle relaxant use in the investigational group was statistically significant at 24 months. The ProDisc-C disc replacement successfully maintained motion throughout the study.

The study results for the Bryan cervical disc were also published in 2009.[13] There were 30 investigational sites and the study randomized 242 individuals into the arthroplasty group and 221 into the ACDF group. Of these, 230 patients in the arthroplasty group and 194 patients in the ACDF group completed 2-year follow-up. As with the other studies, blood loss and operative and hospitalization times were similar between the treatment groups. Patients receiving an artificial disc did significantly better in terms of NDI improvement and neck pain scores than those treated with arthrodesis. Overall, 1.7% of patients in the investigation group and 3.4% of patients in the control group suffered implant-related serious adverse events. At the end of the follow-up, 2.5% of patients receiving a Bryan disc replacement and 3.6% of patients treated with an instrumented arthrodesis required a second operation at the index level. Preoperatively, the affected levels in the arthroplasty group had an average of 6.5 degrees of flexion/extension motion, which increased to 8.1 degrees at the final follow-up. Before surgery, 65% of the patients in both groups were working. The overall return to work significantly favored the investigational group (48 vs. 61 days).

Further cost analyses add an interesting dimension to the debate. Bhadra and associates[38] studied the direct costs of four different surgical techniques to treat cervical radiculopathy. Arthroplasty yielded the second-lowest cost, second only to intervertebral allograft-only ACDF (without a plate). Recently, a health-economic assessment of cervical disc arthroplasty compared with allograft fusion showed that arthroplasty was associated with an average total savings of $6,978 per patient at 2 years after surgery. The cost difference was due to the lower reoperation rate and shorter return-to-work time of the arthroplasty group.[39]

Single-level ACDF does not alter global cervical motion, but there is increasing evidence that it alters biomechanical factors at adjacent levels, which may increase the risk of a patient developing adjacent-segment disease.[40–43] Even if the incidence of symptomatic adjacent-segment disease after arthroplasty is equal to that seen with arthrodesis, we believe that preserving motion alone is an important goal. Although a single-level fusion does not have an impact on global cervical motion, the same is not true once multilevel fusions are necessary. Every segment that maintains normal physiological motion increases the potential for the patient to resume a fully active life.

Conclusion

Cervical arthroplasty is one of the most carefully studied and documented spinal procedures. It has been shown to be safe and effective and it preserves normal segmental motion. It is associated with a higher return-to-work rate and more rapid normalization of NDI and analogue pain scores than is ACDF. It appears to be associated with a decreased need for further surgery over the 2-year study periods, and it has an economic advantage over ACDF. For these reasons, we believe that arthroplasty is the best treatment alternative for this patient.

Posterior Discectomy for Soft Disc Herniation

Miguel A. Arraez

A herniated disc is the most common indication for surgery in patients with disorders of the cervical spine. The posterior approach was developed in the 1930s and 1940s, but its obvious limitation in treating purely ventral herniated discs led to the use of the anterior approach. The posterior approach includes decompression techniques for patients with myelopathy as well as a posterolateral approach (laminoforaminotomy) for purely lateral root compression. This latter approach, which has been clearly encouraged in recent decades by the development of techniques for surgical field magnification, is the subject of this section.

Patient Selection

Patient selection through clinical and neuroradiological evaluation is of paramount importance for this approach. Only patients with cervical radiculopathy are candidates for the posterolateral approach, and those patients with concomitant spinal cord compression (myelopathy, myeloradiculopathy, or both) must be excluded. The neurologic examination can be complemented with a neurophysiological study to confirm the extent and severity of radicular involvement.

Pathophysiologically, root compression can be due to pure posterolateral disc herniation or to osseous root compression from foraminal stenosis. In patients with radicular involvement from a herniated disc, an MRI study can show the disc herniation as well as certain details of surgical in-

terest, such as the site of the disc material in relation to the common posterior ligament and the foramen (**Fig. 22.5**). The most satisfactory surgical results can be obtained in patients who have radicular symptoms from pure disc herniation with posterolateral extrusion. In these patients, the symptoms are usually of sudden onset. The other group of patients who can benefit from this approach present with root pain in relation to the phenomena of osteophytosis of the uncovertebral processes or adjacent facets, constituting a clear foraminal stenosis. In these patients, a CT scan with bone algorithm is clearly indicated. This scan enables the surgeon to analyze the osseous anatomy of the foramen and suggests the degree of decompression and facetectomy needed (**Fig. 22.6**).

Surgical Technique

The procedure is performed with the patient under general anesthesia and in either a sitting position or a prone decubitus position. I prefer the sitting position, as the surgical field more easily remains bloodless, and it allows for some contralateral tilt, which contributes to a certain degree of aperture of the involved interlaminar space. A needle situated in the interspinous region permits radioscopic localization of the space. A skin incision of just a few centimeters is followed by sectioning of the subcutaneous plane and fascia, with subperiosteal dissection and unilateral separation of the paraspinal musculature. The use of a tubular or

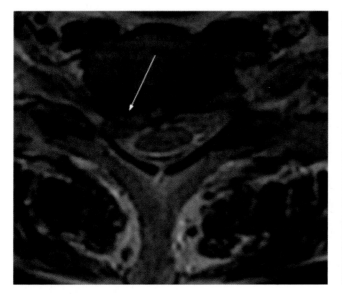
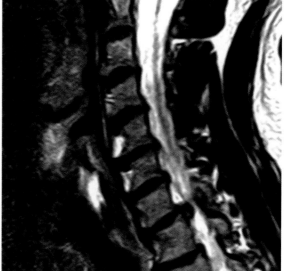

a   b

Fig. 22.5a,b **(a)** An MRI scan of a 45-year-old patient with an abrupt onset of right arm pain. The image shows a right herniated disc at C6-C7. Some fragments extrude through the posterior longitudinal ligament (*white arrow*) and compress the C7 root, a very good indication for the posterolateral laminoforaminotomy approach. **(b)** Sagittal view. The sequestered disc is completely out of the intervertebral space and behind the vertebral body.

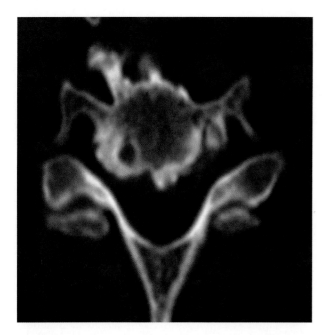

Fig. 22.6 A CT scan of a 63-year-old patient with right brachialgia from involvement of the C8 root. The posterolateral approach is useful to treat nerve root compression from foraminal stenosis. The scan with a bone algorithm shows marked degenerative changes and spondylotic foraminal stenosis. This bone algorithm is of great help to ascertain the extent of facetectomy needed to decompress the nerve root.

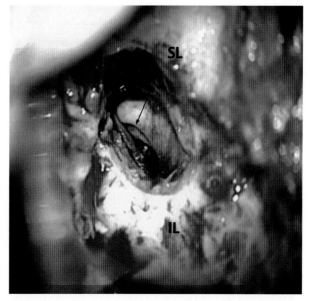

Fig. 22.7 Surgical view after disc removal through a left posterolateral micro-laminoforaminotomy approach. The foraminal region is exposed. The white arrow indicates the root, which has already been divided into sensory (superior and posterior) and motor (inferior and anterior) aspects before it enters the foramen. A minimal facetectomy was done. F, superior facet; IL, inferior lamina; SL, superior lamina.

autostatic retractor exposes the laminas and joint processes. The advantages of tubular retractors include less blood loss, less postoperative pain, and a shorter hospital stay.[44] Magnification is vitally important, either with microsurgery or endoscopy.

A high-speed drill or 2-mm Kerrison rongeur can be used to widen the interlaminar distance and expose the yellow ligament, which is poorly consistent. Depending on the individual patient, some degree of facetectomy may be necessary, more often in cases of foraminal stenosis. The affected dura mater and root are exposed, but sometimes an epidural tissue wraps the neural elements like a sleeve and may hinder their identification. The root can be separated into its motor and sensory components before exiting through the foramen (**Fig. 22.7**).

Epidural venous bleeding can occur, though it ceases easily through compression with cottonoids. Examination maneuvers (with a nerve hook or Penfield dissector) are usually done to mobilize the nerve root, but with a certain risk to its integrity. The circular movements and traction used with the nerve hook permit approximation to the surgical field of extruded fragments lodged between the dura mater and the posterior common vertebral ligament, as well as fragments extruded but anterior to this ligament (that sometimes require blunt penetration for disc removal). In any case, a discectomy at the level of the intervertebral space (nonextruded fragments) should not be exhaustive. It is worth noting that broad-based centrolateral hernia-

tion is not a good indication for this technique; neither, of course, is central disc herniation or any form of myelopathy.

When the compression involves bone, some degree of facetectomy is necessary, but this facetectomy should not surpass 30 to 50% of the joint as there may be a degree of postoperative instability and pain. Some anatomic studies show that exposing the root may be satisfactory with drilling of no more than 15%.[45] The resection of uncovertebral osteophytosis is usually dangerous for the root and should be avoided as much as possible. After adequate root decompression and confirmed hemostasis, the planes of the fascia, subcutaneous tissue and skin are closed. Patients do not normally require cervical immobilization, and can be discharged from the hospital after 24 to 48 hours. Excellent descriptions of this surgical procedure have been published by Zeidman and Ducker.[46,47]

Discussion

The choice of approach for patients with degenerative cervical disorders has been a constant controversy in the neurosurgical literature. Use of the anterior cervical approach is usually followed by intersomatic fusion and is associated with some potential risks: pain and infection at the graft donor site, graft or plate malposition, penetration of the mediastinal viscera, and arterial and cervical nerve lesions. Cervical immobilization is necessary after the surgery. When various levels are approached, the degree of limited cervical mobility after arthrodesis of various segments is a clear disadvantage. Adjacent-level degenerative changes and disease have been widely reported after anterior fusion. Although the current techniques for arthroplasty (an alternative for arthrodesis) avoid postoperative immobilization, they have not yet shown that long-term cervical motility is preserved or adjacent-level disease prevented.[48]

The approach through a posterior laminoforaminotomy does not require fusion or postoperative orthesis, as it preserves the anatomy and function of most of the affected disc and therefore eliminates any concern about degeneration of the adjacent segments. It also permits the examination and treatment of various adjacent levels simultaneously. Furthermore, the morbidity is somewhat lower than that of the anterior approach.[49]

The results of the posterolateral approach via laminoforaminotomy show improvement of the radicular symptoms in 85 to 97% of patients.[33,34,50–52] Zeidman and Ducker[46] reported improvement in pain and motor involvement in 97% and 98% of 172 patients, respectively. Patients with spondylotic foraminal stenosis have the same rate of improvement, but postoperative neck pain can be as high as 23%.[53] A constant finding in all studies is the high rate of functional recovery and return to normal activities,[33] and several studies report similar overall results when the procedure is undertaken with endoscopy rather than microsurgery.[54–57] A herniation relapse at the site of the operation is very uncommon.[33] A systematic review of the laminoforaminotomy technique according to evidence-based medicine concluded that posterior laminoforaminotomy "is an effective treatment for cervical radiculopathy" (evidence class III and strength of recommendation D).[58]

The morbidity of this approach is low. The most frequent complication is the appearance of postoperative dysesthesias. Postoperative radicular motor involvement is very unusual and often transitory. It is important to avoid excessive root traction and appropriately identify its motor component, which may be in one single sheath beside the sensory root or in an independent anteroinferior sheath. Another possible complication is a dural tear (less than 1%), which rarely leads to a frank cutaneous cerebrospinal fluid fistula. The appearance of neck pain may be due to an excessive facetectomy.

Conclusion

The posterolateral approach via micro-laminoforaminotomy is an excellent technique to treat patients with cervical radiculopathy from disc herniation or foraminal stenosis with no associated myelopathy. The technique avoids the need for intersomatic fusion, is highly effective to treat the pain, and has a low rate of complications. The clinical-radiological selection of the patient is crucial for this approach.

Moderator

The Puzzling Development of Artificial Cervical Disc Arthroplasty

A. El Khamlichi

Cervical radiculopathy caused by a herniated intervertebral disc is frequent in our daily neurosurgical practice. After conservative treatment fails, the nerve roots can be successfully decompressed through either anterior or posterior approaches. The main indications for a posterior laminoforaminotomy are lateral soft disc herniation and foraminal stenosis.[1,36,54,55,59,60] The ACDF is indicated for central and paracentral disc herniation with radial osteophytes and uncovertebral joint spears.[61–63] The ACDF, introduced by Smith and Robinson in 1958 and widely disseminated by Cloward, is considered today to be one of the most successful cervical spine procedures to treat patients with cervical radiculopathy. Its goals are to ensure decompression of neural structures, permanently stabilize the segments, and preserve the cervical disc height by replacing the removed disc with several grafting techniques.[63–66]

In spite of the high success rate of ACDF, several articles over the past 15 years emphasize that fusion increases the stress on adjacent segments and contributes to degeneration at these adjacent segments, which can lead over the years to symptomatic adjacent-level disease and a need for new surgery in some patients (3 to 25% at 10 years of follow-up).[1,37,42,67] This criticism of ACDF resulted in the development of the artificial cervical disc prosthesis to replace the removed disc (cervical arthroplasty). Theoretically, the artificial disc was designed to take the place of the normal intervertebral disc, with the aim of producing physiological motion while acting as a shock-absorber for the spine. Ideally, the disc prosthesis preserves motion at the operated level and prevents degeneration and symptomatic adjacent-level disease. Although the first report of cervical disc replacement in the medical literature came from Africa in 1964,[68] cervical arthroplasty was mainly developed over the past 10 years. Today, despite the large number of artificial discs already implanted in many patients and the several randomized trials comparing one-level cervical arthroplasty to one-level ACDF, the clinical relevance of disc arthroplasty has not yet been determined, and a great debate has been engaged between those who are in favor of and those who are against cervical arthroplasty.

Arguments Against Artificial Cervical Discs

Perhaps the greatest argument against the use of artificial cervical discs is their technical insufficiency. The mechanical characteristics of the discs available on the market today do not yet allow motion of the operated segment with respect to the physiological motion of the cervical spine so as not to harm other structures (facet joints, discs, vertebrae, ligaments, and muscles). In other words, the device that can best serve the patient has not yet been manufactured.

Although many clinical trials have reported good postoperative satisfaction by patients and promising results at short-term follow-up (6–12 months), long-term evaluation has revealed several problems that need more investigation. First, the results of randomized studies should be based not only on the patients' surveys but on both the patients' and examiners' blind appreciation during the follow-up. Second, although short-term studies document good motion after cervical arthroplasty, long-term follow-up has shown that the magnitude of this movement decreases with time. In addition, the range of motion seems to differ significantly above and below the operated level both in patients with arthroplasty and those undergoing fusion. Third, progressive ossification of the implanted disc, which has already been reported at the lumbar level, can also occur at the cervical level, and can result in fusion across the implant with definite loss of motion in more than half of patients after 3 years. Fourth, the long-term risk of kyphosis after cervical fusion and its role in the development of adjacent-level disease has been well documented in several studies. The loss of vertebral body height at the fused segment is known to be the main factor leading to these changes. Arthroplasty, with its preservation of motion of the artificial disc, was supposed to prevent such changes in the cervical spinal element. Unfortunately, as several studies demonstrated, kyphosis can also occur after disc replacement with degenerative changes at the adjacent levels. In addition, because of the nonphysiological segmental motion, these degenerative changes may involve facet joints and the ligamentum flavum. Nonsurgical and clinical factors have yet to be recognized as responsible for kyphosis and its consequences on arthroplasty.

The imaging quality after cervical arthroplasty also remains problematic, with artifacts degrading the quality of both MRI and CT scans. But these imaging techniques are often needed to assess the results of surgery or for patients with postoperative clinical symptoms.

Lastly, long-term experience with lumbar disc replacement has shown a high rate of spontaneous fusion and adjacent-level degeneration. These findings should be taken into consideration while we await the long-term evaluation of cervical disc replacement.

Arguments in Favor of Artificial Cervical Discs

The first point in support of the use of artificial cervical discs is that posterior discectomy has no durable efficacy, and there are no scientifically valid studies to evaluate the long-term results of this technique. Thus, it cannot replace the anterior approach.

Several randomized trials comparing single-level cervical arthroplasty with ACDF have shown better results with arthroplasty. In 2007, the 32-center study of 541 patients (276 arthroplasties with the unconstrained Prestige cervical disc and 265 ACDF) reported a greater need for a second surgery at the operated level or adjacent levels in patients undergoing ACDF than in those having arthroplasty, with slightly better results for neck pain and a return to work in the arthroplasty group.[36] A cumulative study of 13 sites involving 209 patients (103 arthroplasties with the unconstrained ProDisc and 106 ACDF) has also shown a higher rate of second surgery in the ACDF group compared with those undergoing arthroplasty.[37] This study also documented that the disc maintains motion at 2 years' follow-up. The 30-center study in 2009, involving 463 patients (242 arthroplasties with the Bryan disc and 221 ACDF) has shown better clinical results in patients undergoing arthroplasty than ACDF, with secondary surgery in 2.5% of those undergoing arthroplasty and 3.6% for the ACDF group. In a financial analysis of both techniques, two studies found that arthroplasty has a lower cost than ACDF.

Bridging the Gap Between Opinions

An analysis of the arguments both in favor of and against cervical disc arthroplasty allows us to point out some evidence. First, the artificial cervical disc needs more homogeneity in biomedical data and in-vitro testing protocols. To be able to compare the different artificial devices and make a suitable choice for a patient, the neurosurgeon should be able to compare the biomedical characteristics of the different discs available on the market today. In their literature review of the biomechanical properties of artificial cervical disc prostheses, Bartels and colleagues[69] found several papers dedicated to the subject. They requested information from the manufacturers and tried to compare the biomechanical characteristics of the 11 artificial discs used in clinical practice. They discovered that the main clinical characteristics, such as range of motion, sheer resistance, compression fatigue, and wear, were not mentioned in the manufacturers' information for all these devices. But the outcome results are highly dependent on these biomechanical properties. In addition, the continuous evolution and adaptation of different prostheses makes the comparison difficult. For example, the Prestige disc on the market in 1998 was the Prestige I. The Prestige II appeared in 1999, the Prestige ST in 2002, the Prestige STLT in 2003, and finally the Prestige LP in 2004.[69] The same lack of homogeneity is found in the cadaveric studies testing the in-vitro motion of the prostheses. Some of these studies targeted the cervical spine from C2 to T1,[6,70] others from C3 to C1,[71,72] or from the occiput to T2.[73] The posterior longitudinal ligament was maintained intact in some tests, whereas in others it was removed through a conventional discectomy. The results of in-vivo tests of the immunologic response were available for only two disc prostheses.[73] With such a disparity of information about the biomechanical properties of the different devices and the results of their testing, whether in the laboratory or in vitro, choosing the appropriate artificial disc to implant can be difficult, and the neurosurgeon may have difficulty clearly advising the patient.

Second, the main reason favoring the use of artificial cervical discs is to maintain motion in the implanted segment and prevent the adjacent-level disease that may occur with ACDF.[40,43] This reason, however, is more theoretical, and the direct relationship between adjacent-level disease and the fusion is still a great subject of debate and has never been clinically documented. Furthermore, some studies of cervical arthroplasty show that a second surgery was also done for adjacent-level disease although the long-term follow-up in most of these series is limited to 24 months.[74] Proponents of artificial cervical disc implantation have not yet confirmed that long-term cervical mobility can be preserved or that adjacent-level disease can be definitely prevented.[48]

Third, the clinical measurements and tests that show the superiority of cervical arthroplasty compared with ACDF are subject to criticism. In many randomized clinical trials, the clinical results of disc prosthesis compared with ACDF were based on the fact that, in follow-up, patients with arthroplasty have less arm and neck pain and return to work earlier than those treated with ACDF. The difference was even statistically significant after a 6-month follow-up, but at 24 months none of these outcome measures favored arthroplasty for arm pain or neck pain. A potential explanation of this difference in arm pain in short-term follow-up is that patients undergoing arthroplasty may be pleased with their immediate positive results. Theoretically, the decompression of the nerve root is the same in either procedure. Therefore, the results of arm pain should be the same in both postoperative groups, and the differ-

ence cannot be explained theoretically by the use of the disc prosthesis. The neck pain in patients undergoing ACDF can be explained by the need for an adjustment period after surgery, during which other segments (discs, facets, joints, muscles) accommodate extra motion to compensate for the motion lost at the fused segment, and this can result in some pain. This does not happen in arthroplasty, but at 24 months the adaptation is already done and the neck pain disappears. Regarding an earlier return to work, it should be pointed out that most patients with ACDF are advised to wear a cervical collar, which may be a reason to delay the return to work. So although many cervical artificial discs are implanted worldwide, the clinical evidence of the superiority of cervical arthroplasty compared with ACDF has never yet been documented.

Fourth, there is no doubt today that the implantation of artificial cervical discs is being promoted very aggressively. Neurosurgeons should not forget that the manufacturers of the implants and instruments used are in business, and they want to make money by bringing new products on the market. They encourage and support randomized trials to take advantage of evidence-based medicine as a powerful marketing tool. Of course, the influence of financial interests is not always easy for some investigators to resist. Therefore, the price of the artificial disc is a big issue mainly in developing countries; in Rabat, Morocco, the current price is 3,000 Euros.

Conclusion

The many papers, articles, reports, and studies on cervical disc replacement should be interpreted with great care. It is important not only to report on the significant statistical differences, but also to insist on a discussion of the implication these differences have in clinical relevance. Reviewers of such articles should have nothing to disclose and be able either to judge the methodology or clarify the clinical relevance.

To continue the long-term evaluation of cervical arthroplasty, the following optimal indications may be acceptable: young patients who would benefit from preserved motion for a long period, and patients with proven symptomatic adjacent-level degeneration. All these patients should be randomized for long-term follow-up to clarify the real advantages of cervical arthroplasty.

References

1. Hilibrand AS, Carlson GD, Palumbo MA, Jones PK, Bohlman HH. Radiculopathy and myelopathy at segments adjacent to the site of a previous anterior cervical arthrodesis. J Bone Joint Surg Am 1999;81:519–528
2. Goffin J, Geusens E, Vantomme N, et al. Long-term follow-up after interbody fusion of the cervical spine. J Spinal Disord Tech 2004;17:79–85
3. Bartolomei JC, Theodore N, Sonntag VK. Adjacent level degeneration after anterior cervical fusion: a clinical review. Neurosurg Clin N Am 2005;16:575–587, v
4. Eck JC, Humphreys SC, Lim TH, et al. Biomechanical study on the effect of cervical spine fusion on adjacent-level intradiscal pressure and segmental motion. Spine 2002;27:2431–2434

5. Fuller DA, Kirkpatrick JS, Emery SE, Wilber RG, Davy DT. A kinematic study of the cervical spine before and after segmental arthrodesis. Spine 1998;23:1649–1656

6. DiAngelo DJ, Foley KT, Morrow BR, et al. In vitro biomechanics of cervical disc arthroplasty with the ProDisc-C total disc implant. Neurosurg Focus 2004;17:E7

7. Phillips FM, Garfin SR. Cervical disc replacement. Spine 2005;30:27–33

8. Bertagnoli R, Duggal N, Pickett GE, et al. Cervical total disc replacement, part two: clinical results. Orthop Clin North Am 2005;36:355–362

9. Yoon DH, Yi S, Shin HC, Kim KN, Kim SH. Clinical and radiological results following cervical arthroplasty. Acta Neurochir (Wien) 2006;148:943–950

10. Yang S, Wu X, Hu Y, et al. Early and intermediate follow-up results after treatment of degenerative disc disease with the Bryan cervical disc prosthesis: single- and multiple-level. Spine 2008;33:E371–E377

11. Porchet F, Metcalf NH. Clinical outcomes with the Prestige II cervical disc: preliminary results from a prospective randomized clinical trial. Neurosurg Focus 2004;17:E6

12. Sasso RC, Smucker JD, Hacker RJ, Heller JG. Artificial disc versus fusion: a prospective, randomized study with 2-year follow-up on 99 patients. Spine 2007;32:2933–2940, discussion 2941–2942

13. Heller JG, Sasso RC, Papadopoulos SM, et al. Comparison of BRYAN cervical disc arthroplasty with anterior cervical decompression and fusion: clinical and radiographic results of a randomized, controlled, clinical trial. Spine 2009;34:101–107

14. Sasso RC, Best NM. Cervical kinematics after fusion and Bryan disc arthroplasty. J Spinal Disord Tech 2008;21:19–22

15. McAfee PC, Cunningham BW, Devine J, Williams E, Yu-Yahiro J. Classification of heterotopic ossification (HO) in artificial disk replacement. J Spinal Disord Tech 2003;16:384–389

16. Mehren C, Suchomel P, Grochulla F, et al. Heterotopic ossification in total cervical artificial disc replacement. Spine 2006;31:2802–2806

17. Goffin J, Van Calenbergh F, van Loon J, et al. Intermediate follow-up after treatment of degenerative disc disease with the Bryan cervical disc prosthesis: single-level and bi-level. Spine 2003;28:2673–2678

18. Sola S, Hebecker R, Knoop M, Mann S. Bryan cervical disc prosthesis—three years' follow-up. Eur Spine J 2005;14 (Suppl 1):38

19. Pickett GE, Mitsis DK, Sekhon LH, Sears WR, Duggal N. Effects of a cervical disc prosthesis on segmental and cervical spine alignment. Neurosurg Focus 2004;17:E5

20. Johnson JP, Lauryssen C, Cambron HO, et al. Sagittal alignment and the Bryan cervical artificial disc. Neurosurg Focus 2004;7:E14

21. Fong SY, DuPlessis SJ, Casha S, Hurlbert RJ. Design limitations of Bryan disc arthroplasty. Spine J 2006;6:233–241

22. Sears WR, Sekhon LH, Duggal N, Williamson OD. Segmental malalignment with the Bryan cervical disc prosthesis—does it occur? J Spinal Disord Tech 2007;20:1–6

23. Pickett GE, Sekhon LH, Sears WR, Duggal N. Complications with cervical arthroplasty. J Neurosurg Spine 2006;4:98–105

24. Kawakami M, Tamaki T, Yoshida M, Hayashi N, Ando M, Yamada H. Axial symptoms and cervical alignments after cervical anterior spinal fusion for patients with cervical myelopathy. J Spinal Disord 1999;12:50–56

25. Katsuura A, Hukuda S, Saruhashi Y, Mori K. Kyphotic malalignment after anterior cervical fusion is one of the factors promoting the degenerative process in adjacent intervertebral levels. Eur Spine J 2001;10:320–324

26. van Ooij A, Oner FC, Verbout AJ. Complications of artificial disc replacement: a report of 27 patients with the SB Charité disc. J Spinal Disord Tech 2003;16:369–383

27. Sekhon LH, Duggal N, Lynch JJ, et al. Magnetic resonance imaging clarity of the Bryan, Prodisc-C, Prestige LP, and PCM cervical arthroplasty devices. Spine 2007;32:673–680

28. Putzier M, Funk JF, Schneider SV, et al. Charité total disc replacement—clinical and radiographical results after an average follow-up of 17 years. Eur Spine J 2006;15:183–195

29. Bertagnoli R, Schönmayr R. Surgical and clinical results with the PDN prosthetic disc-nucleus device. Eur Spine J 2002;11(Suppl 2):S143–S148

30. Huang RC, Girardi FP, Cammisa FP Jr, Lim MR, Tropiano P, Marnay T. Correlation between range of motion and outcome after lumbar total disc replacement: 8.6-year follow-up. Spine 2005;30:1407–1411

31. Scoville WB, Dohrmann GJ, Corkill G. Late results of cervical disc surgery. J Neurosurg 1976;45:203–210

32. Murphey F, Simmons JC, Brunson B. Surgical treatment of laterally ruptured cervical disc. Review of 648 cases, 1939 to 1972. J Neurosurg 1973;38:679–683

33. Henderson CM, Hennessy RG, Shuey HM Jr, Shackelford EG. Posterior-lateral foraminotomy as an exclusive operative technique for cervical radiculopathy: a review of 846 consecutively operated cases. Neurosurgery 1983;13:504–512

34. Kumar GR, Maurice-Williams RS, Bradford R. Cervical foraminotomy: an effective treatment for cervical spondylotic radiculopathy. Br J Neurosurg 1998;12:563–568

35. Clarke MJ, Ecker RD, Krauss WE, McClelland RL, Dekutoski MB. Same-segment and adjacent-segment disease following posterior cervical foraminotomy. J Neurosurg Spine 2007;6:5–9

36. Mummaneni PV, Burkus JK, Haid RW, Traynelis VC, Zdeblick TA. Clinical and radiographic analysis of cervical disc arthroplasty compared with allograft fusion: a randomized controlled clinical trial. J Neurosurg Spine 2007;6:198–209

37. Murrey D, Janssen M, Delamarter R, et al. Results of the prospective, randomized, controlled multicenter Food and Drug Administration investigational device exemption study of the ProDisc-C total disc replacement versus anterior discectomy and fusion for the treatment of 1-level symptomatic cervical disc disease. Spine J 2009;9:275–286

38. Bhadra AK, Raman AS, Casey AT, Crawford RJ. Single-level cervical radiculopathy: clinical outcome and cost-effectiveness of four techniques of anterior cervical discectomy and fusion and disc arthroplasty. Eur Spine J 2009;18:232–237

39. Menzin J, Zhang B, Neumann PJ, et al. A health-economic assessment of cervical disc arthroplasty compared with allograft fusion. Tech Orthop 2010;25:133–137

40. Baba H, Furusawa N, Imura S, Kawahara N, Tomita K. Laminoplasty following anterior cervical fusion for spondylotic myeloradiculopathy. Int Orthop 1994;18:1–5

41. Gore DR, Sepic SB. Anterior discectomy and fusion for painful cervical disc disease. A report of 50 patients with an average follow-up of 21 years. Spine 1998;23:2047–2051

42. Ishihara H, Kanamori M, Kawaguchi Y, Nakamura H, Kimura T. Adjacent segment disease after anterior cervical interbody fusion. Spine J 2004;4:624–628

43. Robertson JT, Papadopoulos SM, Traynelis VC. Assessment of adjacent-segment disease in patients treated with cervical fusion or arthroplasty: a prospective 2-year study. J Neurosurg Spine 2005;3:417–423

44. Winder MJ, Thomas KC. Minimally invasive versus open approach for cervical laminoforaminotomy. Can J Neurol Sci 2011;38:262–267

45. Figueiredo EG, Castillo De la Cruz M, Theodore N, Deshmukh P, Preul MC. Modified cervical laminoforaminotomy based on anatomic landmarks reduces need for bony removal. Minim Invasive Neurosurg 2006;49:37–42

46. Zeidman SM, Ducker TB. Posterior cervical laminoforaminotomy for radiculopathy: review of 172 cases. Neurosurgery 1993;33:356–362

47. Ducker TB, Zeidman SM. The posterior operative approach for cervical radiculopathy. Neurosurg Clin N Am 1993;4: 61–74

48. Matz PG, Ryken TC, Groff MW, et al; Joint Section on Disorders of the Spine and Peripheral Nerves of the American Association of Neurological Surgeons and Congress of Neurological Surgeons. Techniques for anterior cervical decompression for radiculopathy. J Neurosurg Spine 2009;11: 183–197

49. Korinth MC, Krüger A, Oertel MF, Gilsbach JM. Posterior foraminotomy or anterior discectomy with polymethyl methacrylate interbody stabilization for cervical soft disc disease: results in 292 patients with monoradiculopathy. Spine 2006;31:1207–1214, discussion 1215–1216

50. Davis RAA. A long-term outcome study of 170 surgically treated patients with compressive cervical radiculopathy. Surg Neurol 1996;46:523–530, discussion 530–533

51. Tomaras CR, Blacklock JB, Parker WD, Harper RL. Outpatient surgical treatment of cervical radiculopathy. J Neurosurg 1997;87:41–43

52. Rodrigues MA, Hanel RA, Prevedello DM, Antoniuk A, Araújo JC. Posterior approach for soft cervical disc herniation: a neglected technique? Surg Neurol 2001;55:17–22, discussion 22

53. Grieve JP, Kitchen ND, Moore AJ, Marsh HT. Results of posterior cervical foraminotomy for treatment of cervical spondylitic radiculopathy. Br J Neurosurg 2000;14:40–43

54. Adamson TE. Microendoscopic posterior cervical laminoforaminotomy for unilateral radiculopathy: results of a new technique in 100 cases. J Neurosurg 2001;95(1, Suppl): 51–57

55. Fessler RG, Khoo LT. Minimally invasive cervical microendoscopic foraminotomy: an initial clinical experience. Neurosurgery 2002;51(5, Suppl):S37–S45

56. Ruetten S, Komp M, Merk H, Godolias G. Full-endoscopic cervical posterior foraminotomy for the operation of lateral disc herniations using 5.9-mm endoscopes: a prospective, randomized, controlled study. Spine 2008;33:940–948

57. O'Toole JE, Sheikh H, Eichholz KM, Fessler RG, Perez-Cruet MJ. Endoscopic posterior cervical foraminotomy and discectomy. Neurosurg Clin N Am 2006;17:411–422

58. Heary RF, Ryken TC, Matz PG, et al; Joint Section on Disorders of the Spine and Peripheral Nerves of the American Association of Neurological Surgeons and Congress of Neurological Surgeons. Cervical laminoforaminotomy for the treatment of cervical degenerative radiculopathy. J Neurosurg Spine 2009;11:198–202

59. Fager CA. Posterolateral approach to ruptured median and paramedian cervical disk. Surg Neurol 1983;20:443–452

60. Southwick WO, Robinson RA. Surgical approaches to the vertebral bodies in the cervical and lumbar regions. J Bone Joint Surg Am 1957;39-A:631–644

61. Bohlman HH, Emery SE, Goodfellow DB, Jones PK. Robinson anterior cervical discectomy and arthrodesis for cervical radiculopathy. Long-term follow-up of one hundred and twenty-two patients. J Bone Joint Surg Am 1993;75:1298–1307

62. Gore DR, Sepic SB. Anterior cervical fusion for degenerated or protruded discs. A review of one hundred forty-six patients. Spine 1984;9:667–671

63. Robinson RA, Walker AE, Ferlic DC, Wiecking DK. The results of anterior interbody fusion of the cervical spine. J Bone Joint Surg Am 1962;44:1569–1587

64. Brodke DS, Zdeblick TA. Modified Smith-Robinson procedure for anterior cervical discectomy and fusion. Spine 1992;17(10, Suppl):S427–S430

65. Emery SE, Bolesta MJ, Banks MA, Jones PK. Robinson anterior cervical fusion comparison of the standard and modified techniques. Spine 1994;19:660–663

66. Krag MH, Robertson PA, Johnson CC, Stein AC. Anterior cervical fusion using a modified tricortical bone graft: a radiographic analysis of outcome. J Spinal Disord 1997;10: 420–430

67. Yue WM, Brodner W, Highland TR. Long-term results after anterior cervical discectomy and fusion with allograft and plating: a 5- to 11-year radiologic and clinical follow-up study. Spine 2005;30:2138–2144

68. Reitz H, Joubert MJ. Intractable headache and cervico-brachialgia treated by complete replacement of cervical intervertebral disc with metal prosthesis. S Afr Med J 1964;7: 881–884

69. Bartels RH, Donk RD, Pavlov P, van Limbeek J. Comparison of biomechanical properties of cervical artificial disc prosthesis: a review. Clin Neurol Neurosurg 2008;110:963–967

70. DiAngelo DJ, Roberston JT, Metcalf NH, McVay BJ, Davis RC. Biomechanical testing of an artificial cervical joint and an anterior cervical plate. J Spinal Disord Tech 2003;16:314–323

71. Dmitriev AE, Cunningham BW, Hu N, Sell G, Vigna F, McAfee PC. Adjacent level intradiscal pressure and segmental kinematics following a cervical total disc arthroplasty: an in vitro human cadaveric model. Spine 2005;30:1165–1172

72. Duggal N, Rabin D, Chamberlain RH, Baek S, Crawford NR. Traumatic loading of the Bryan cervical disc prosthesis: an in vitro study. Neurosurgery 2007;60(4, Suppl 2):388–392, discussion 392–393

73. Kotani Y, Cunningham BW, Abumi K, et al. Multidirectional flexibility analysis of cervical artificial disc reconstruction: in vitro human cadaveric spine model. J Neurosurg Spine 2005;2:188–194

74. Anderson PA, Sasso RC, Rouleau JP, Carlson CS, Goffin J. The Bryan Cervical Disc: wear properties and early clinical results. Spine J 2004;4(6, Suppl):303S–309S

Chapter 23

Clinical Trials: Are They Authoritative or Flawed?

Participants

Clinical Trials are Authoritative: Shobhan Vachhrajani, Abhaya V. Kulkarni, and James T. Rutka

The Flaws of Randomized Clinical Trials: Benedicto Colli

Moderators: The Randomized Clinical Trial: A. John Popp, Urvashi Upadhyay, and Robert E. Harbaugh

Clinical Trials Are Authoritative

Shobhan Vachhrajani, Abhaya V. Kulkarni, and James T. Rutka

The past two decades have seen a paradigm shift in the practice of medicine away from anecdotal approaches toward evidence-based medicine (EBM). A landmark article by the EBM Working Group[1] published in 1992 laid the groundwork for dissemination of this concept. In the group's opinion, EBM "de-emphasizes intuition, unsystematic clinical experience, and pathophysiologic rationale as sufficient grounds for clinical decision making and stresses the examination of evidence from clinical research." The concept of EBM has since been refined, and its founders suggest that its scientific basis rests on three key principles. First, clinical decisions should be based on systematic summaries of the highest quality evidence available. Second, wise use of the literature must incorporate a hierarchy of evidence. Third, clinical decisions cannot be entirely based on evidence: they also require the trading of risks and benefits, inconvenience, and costs with consideration for patient values and preferences.[2] Critics of EBM argue that currently used evidence grading systems too often discount the value of studies that they deem inferior.[3] With a growing emphasis on the development of evidence-based clinical practice guidelines, which rely on systematic grading and interpretation of evidence, this debate only becomes more important.

Neurosurgery as a specialty has been slow to adopt the tenets of EBM.[4] In many cases, clinical decisions remain dogmatic, largely due to the emphasis placed on personal experience and a lack of education about EBM methodologies.[5] Nevertheless, many recent major advances in neurosurgery have resulted from randomized controlled trials (RCTs), which represent the ultimate expression of high-quality evidence. Further advancement of neurosurgical practice will require clinicians to embrace the scientific basis of EBM and to understand the relative hierarchy of medical evidence. This chapter discusses key methodological issues in the design of clinical trials, exposes some of their limitations, and describes the recent impact of RCTs on neurosurgical practice.

The Hierarchy of Medical Evidence

The hierarchy of medical evidence is based on the progressive minimization of bias. Bias is any process or factor that serves to systematically deviate study results away from the truth. Historically, grading of medical evidence has been based solely on study design. The Canadian Task Force on the Periodic Health Examination was the first such system, published in 1979, and the United States Preventive Services Task Force (USPSTF) followed suit thereafter.[6,7] Several refinements based on an improved understanding of study methodology and relative risks and benefits have occurred since then, and the Grade of Recommendations,

Assessment, Development and Evaluation (GRADE) scheme is now the most widely accepted hierarchical system. The GRADE scheme has defined quality of evidence as the confidence in the magnitude of effect for patient-important outcomes, with higher quality evidence conveying less uncertainty in the estimates of their results **(Tables 23.1, 23.2)**.[8,9] Well-designed and conducted RCTs represent the epitome of study design due to the minimal bias that results.[8] Other study methodologies, although able to convey acceptable results, generally do not carry the authority of RCTs.

Clinical Trials

Clinicians are accustomed to ascribing the RCT, in which interventions are compared between patient groups, as the most common and ideal form of trial methodology. Other types of trials, however, are often necessary before comparative studies of treatment can be conducted on human subjects. Phase 1 studies are safety studies in which toxicity profiles can be assessed, whereas phase 2 studies examine the efficacy of the treatment in question. Phase 3 studies are the typical clinical trial with which most clinicians are familiar, as they involve the study of an intervention compared with another treatment strategy or a placebo agent in two or more randomly allocated groups.[10]

Randomized controlled trials are considered to represent the highest level of evidence because they can minimize

Table 23.1 Criteria for Assigning Grade of Evidence

Type of evidence:
  Randomized trial = high
  Observational study = low
  Any other evidence = very low

Decrease grade if:
  Serious (– 1) or very serious (– 2) limitation to study quality
  Important inconsistency (– 1)
  Some (– 1) or major (– 2) uncertainty about directness
  Imprecise or sparse data (– 1)
  High probability of reporting bias (– 1)

Increase grade if:
  Strong evidence of association—significant relative risk of > 2 (< 0.5) based on consistent evidence from two or more observational studies, with no plausible confounders (+ 1)
  Very strong evidence of association—significant relative risk of > 5 (< 0.2) based on direct evidence with no major threats to validity (+ 2)
  Evidence of a dose–response gradient (+ 1)
  All plausible confounders would have reduced the effect (+ 1)

Source: Atkins D, Best D, Briss PA, et al; GRADE Working Group. Grading quality of evidence and strength of recommendations. BMJ 2004;328: 1490. Reprinted by permission.

Table 23.2 Definitions of Grades of Evidence

High	Further research is unlikely to change our confidence in the estimate of effect.
Moderate	Further research is likely to have an important impact on our confidence in the estimate of effect and may change the estimate.
Low	Further research is very likely to have an important impact on our confidence in the estimate of effect and is likely to change the estimate.
Very low	Any estimate of effect is very uncertain.

Source: Atkins D, Best D, Briss PA, et al; GRADE Working Group. Grading quality of evidence and strength of recommendations. BMJ 2004;328: 1490. Reprinted by permission.

bias more than any other study methodology; however, such a distinction is achieved only by meeting certain criteria. Arguably the most important of these is appropriate randomization, in which the allocation of study subjects to treatment arms occurs completely by chance. This aims to achieve a balance between the known and, more importantly, unknown confounders of outcome.[11] In theory, the only factor that consequently differs between study arms is the intervention under examination. No other type of study design achieves this objective. But for randomization to truly eliminate "treatment selection bias" (in which clinicians preferentially offer one treatment to certain types of patients), investigators and trial participants must not be able to predict what the results of randomization will be for the next patient. This is called concealment of allocation and it protects the integrity of the randomization process.[12,13] Similarly, blinding of study participants and physicians is also crucial to minimizing bias in the assessment of study outcomes. Historically, the study subject is unaware of allocation in a single-blinded study, whereas the subject and investigator are unaware of allocation in double-blinded studies. For studies in which a subjective assessment of outcome is required, triple blinding also masks the outcome assessor from treatment allocation. Authors of RCTs are now strongly encouraged to explicitly identify which groups were masked and how, because the terminology of single-, double-, and triple-blind is open to interpretation.[14] Finally, well-planned and appropriate statistical analyses, including the *a priori* determination of sample size, study power, and the use of an intention-to-treat analysis, are important in maintaining the internal validity of any RCT.[8,15,16] Other threats to the validity of an RCT include, for example, a large loss to follow-up, a large proportion of subject crossover between groups, or unplanned and inappropriate early stoppage of a trial. Proponents of the GRADE system argue that, because of these issues, RCTs may not always represent the highest level of evidence and that well-conducted, large observational studies may provide better evidentiary quality in some settings.[2]

The only way for a clinician to critically evaluate the integrity of an RCT is by evaluating the final published work. Therefore, it is crucial that published RCTs contain enough information so that they can be appropriately judged. The Consolidated Standards of Reporting Trials (CONSORT) statement is a widely endorsed protocol of all essential elements that must be reported in published RCTs. The most recent version of CONSORT lists 25 mandatory elements, with an accompanying flow diagram to show the passage of participants through a trial (**Table 23.3, Fig. 23.1**).[15,17,18] Many journals have officially adopted the CONSORT statement in their editorial assessment of trial reports, which has resulted in improvements in the quality of their trial reporting.[19,20] A more recent study found that, despite improved reporting of trial characteristics after the publication of the CONSORT statement, the attrition of study subjects continues to undermine the quality of RCTs.[21] It is clear that, although a well-designed and well-conducted RCT represents the most robust standard of medical evidence, each trial report must be subject to careful scrutiny.

Clinical Trials in Neurosurgery

The use of clinical trials for surgical research has lagged in comparison to medical research. Of the relatively few published RCTs in surgery, many suffer from methodological flaws that significantly compromise their validity.[5] For some surgeons, obstacles to participating in or conducting randomized trials include issues of personal prestige, commercial interest, or an inherent belief in the superiority of surgical therapy. Additionally, the surgical community often rapidly disseminates and then accepts a new procedure as a therapeutic standard, thus eliminating the community equipoise that is necessary for randomization. Even if randomization is considered, technical learning curves associated with new operations and problems with blinding represent unique scenarios not encountered in medical trials.[5] Also, patients are often reluctant to enter into surgical trials, particularly when the opposing arm is nonsurgical, due to the vast contrast between the treatment arms and the irreversibility of surgical treatment.[22] Further obstacles include lack of funding or infrastructure and a lack of epidemiological expertise.

Despite these concerns, however, the use of RCT methodology in neurosurgery has seen a surge in recent years. In a recent systematic review of 159 neurosurgical RCTs, more than two thirds had been published since 1995.[23] A 2004 systematic review of 108 neurosurgical RCTs, however, found that several design and reporting characteristics would benefit from improvement. These included the adequacy and reporting of sample size and power calculations, the appropriate concealment of allocation from involved investigators, and explicit reporting of randomization methods.[24] The authors of the study encouraged increased adherence to the CONSORT statement as a means of improving standardization in neurosurgical RCT reporting. As of this writing, however, the major neurosurgery journals

Table 23.3   CONSORT 2010 Checklist of Information to Include When Reporting a Randomized Trial[15]

Section/Topic	Item Number	Checklist Item	Reported on Page Number
Title and abstract	1a	Identification as a randomized trial in the title	
	1b	Structured summary of trial design, methods, results, and conclusions (for specific guidance, see CONSORT for abstracts)	
Introduction			
Background and objectives	2a	Scientific background and explanation of rationale	
	2b	Specific objectives or hypotheses	
Methods			
Trial design	3a	Description of trial design (such as parallel, factorial), including allocation ratio	
	3b	Important changes to methods after trial commencement (such as eligibility criteria), with reasons	
Participants	4a	Eligibility criteria for participants	
	4b	Settings and locations where the data were collected	
Interventions	5	The interventions for each group with sufficient details to allow replication, including how and when they were actually administered	
Outcomes	6a	Completely defined prespecified primary an secondary outcome measures, including how and when they were assessed	
	6b	Any changes to trial outcomes after the trial commenced, with reasons	
Sample size	7a	How sample size was determined	
	7b	When applicable, explanation of any interim analyses and stopping guidelines	
Randomization sequence generation	8a	Method used to generate the random allocation sequence	
	8b	Type of randomization; details of any restriction (such as blocking and block size)	
Allocation concealment mechanism	9	Mechanism used to implement the random allocation sequence (such as sequentially numbered containers), describing any steps taken to conceal the sequence until interventions were assigned	
Implementation	10	Who generated the random allocation sequence, who enrolled participants, and who assigned participants to interventions	
Blinding	11a	If done, who was blinded after assignment to interventions (for example, participants, care providers, those assessing outcomes), and how	
	11b	If relevant, description of the similarity of interventions	
Statistical methods	12a	Statistical methods used to compare groups for primary and secondary outcomes	
	12b	Methods for additional analyses, such as subgroup analyses and adjusted analyses	
Results			
Participant flow (a diagram is strongly recommended)	13a	For each group, the numbers of participants who were randomly assigned, received intended treatment, and were analyzed for the primary outcome	
	13b	For each group, losses and exclusions after randomization, together with reasons	
Recruitment	14a	Dates defining the periods of recruitment and follow-up	
	14b	Why the trial ended or was stopped	
Baseline data	15	A table showing baseline demographic and clinical characteristics for each	
Numbers analyzed	16	For each group, number of participants (denominator) included in each analysis and whether the analysis was by original assigned groups	

Table 23.3 (*Continued*)

Section/Topic	Item Number	Checklist Item	Reported on Page Number
Outcomes and estimation	17a	For each primary and secondary outcome, results for each group, and the estimated effect size and its precision (such as 95% confidence interval)	
	17b	For binary outcomes, presentation of both absolute and relative effect sizes is recommended	
Ancillary analyses	18	Results of any other analyses performed, including subgroup analyses and adjusted analyses, distinguishing prespecified from exploratory	
Harms	19	All important harms or unintended effects in each group (for specific guidance, see CONSORT for harms)	
Discussion			
Limitations	20	Trial limitations; addressing sources of potential bias; imprecision; and, if relevant, multiplicity of analyses	
Generalizability	21	Generalizability (external validity, applicability) of the trial findings	
Interpretation	22	Interpretation consistent with results, balancing benefits and harms, and considering other relevant evidence	
Other information			
Registration	23	Registration number and name of trial registry	
Protocol	24	Where the full trial protocol can be accessed, if available	
Funding	25	Sources of funding and other support (such as supply of drugs), role of funders	

Source: Schulz KF, Altman DG, Moher D; CONSORT Group. CONSORT 2010 statement: updated guidelines for reporting parallel group randomized trials. Ann Intern Med 2010;152:726–732. Also available at www.consort-statement.org. Reprinted by permission.

have not adopted CONSORT standards for reporting of RCTs. A systematic approach to trial design, such as one suggested by Kan and Kestle,[25] might also reduce the methodological problems often observed in neurosurgical trials.

Despite the limitations and obstacles, RCTs have had a significant impact on neurosurgical practice. Prominent examples of this include the International Subarachnoid Trial (ISAT), the North American Symptomatic Carotid Endarterectomy Trial (NASCET), the EC-IC Bypass Study, the National Acute Spinal Cord Injury Studies (NASCIS I–III), the Corticosteroid Randomisation After Significant Head Injury (CRASH) trial, and the Surgical Trial in Intracerebral Hemorrhage (STICH).[26–30] RCTs in allied fields, including the trial of temozolomide for patients with glioblastoma, have also contributed significantly to the treatment of neurosurgical patients.[31] Clearly, neurosurgeons must familiarize themselves with the nuances of trial design and reporting.

Conclusion

Minimizing bias in clinical studies forms the cornerstone of the EBM movement. Well-designed and well-conducted RCTs represent the pinnacle of minimized bias because they balance all possible confounding factors and ensure masked outcome assessment and treatment allocation. Clinicians evaluating RCTs for use in practice, or for the development of evidence-based clinical practice guidelines, must continue to scrutinize individual studies to ensure that trials meet the methodological rigor required to render the highest quality of medical evidence. As the specialty of neurosurgery continues to embrace EBM, the need for neurosurgeons to become intimately familiar with RCTs and their applications will only continue to grow.

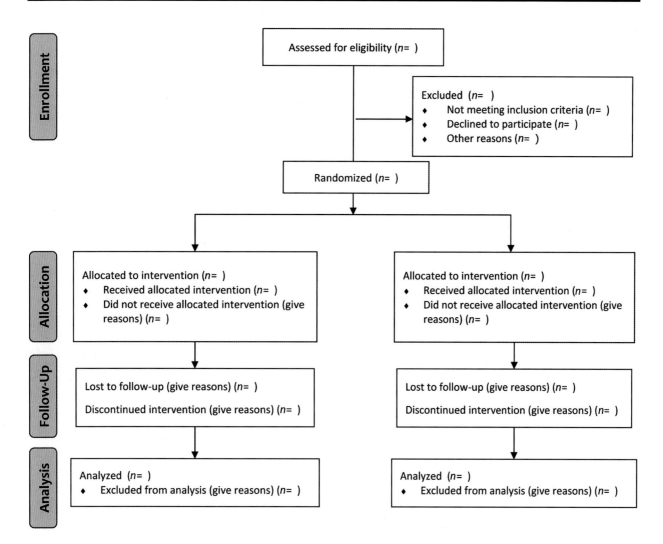

Fig. 23.1   CONSORT 2010 statement flow diagram. (From Schulz KF, Altman DG, Moher D; CONSORT Group. CONSORT 2010 statement: updated guidelines for reporting parallel group randomised trials. Ann Intern Med 2010;152:726–732. Also available at www .consort-statement.org. Reprinted by permission.)

The Flaws of Randomized Clinical Trials

Benedicto Colli

Because it provides the best evidence of the efficacy of health care interventions due to its great potential to show cause–effect relationships, a well-designed and properly executed RCT is the best type of scientific evidence and is considered the paradigm for clinical research for evidence-based medicine.[17,32,33]

Compared with other scientific research designs, RCTs have the advantage of experimental characteristics, in which a factor to be studied is deliberately introduced to the subject of the research as a preventive or therapeutic intervention. As an attribute of experimental research, the investigator has better control over the events of the research than have investigators in observational studies. In addition, the factor being studied is introduced at the beginning of the study, and the participants are followed as long as necessary to determine the outcome.[33]

Despite being the best scientific research design available, RCTs with inadequate methodological approaches are susceptible to flaws that generally are associated with exaggerated treatment effects.[32,34-36] Therefore, before accepting the results, readers should critically appraise the trial to exclude the most frequent causes of deviation from the truth. If the trial has eliminated flaws, there is a good chance that its results are reliable.[37]

Potential Flaws in Randomized Controlled Trials

A critical appraisal of RCTs should aim to find potential biases that can invalidate the reported results, but such an appraisal is possible only if the design, execution, and analysis of the trial is meticulously described in published articles.[34,38]

An important dimension of the quality of a clinical trial is the validity of the generated results,[35] and a useful distinction between internal and external validity was proposed in the middle of the last century.[39] *Internal validity* means that the differences observed between groups of patients allocated to different interventions may be attributed to the treatment under investigation instead of random error. *External validity* or *generalizability* is the extent to which the results of a clinical trial provide a correct basis for generalization to other circumstances. Therefore, internal validity is essential for external validity because there is no way to generalize invalid results.[35,39]

Internal validity can be affected by bias. Bias is the degree to which the result is skewed away from the truth, and it often reflects the human tendency to either consciously or subconsciously "help" things work out the way it seems they should go. For researchers, bias may happen to favor the results they want; for participants, a bias might be useful for their preconceptions of how the results will affect them, for example, getting better when they take the pill.[37] Biases are generally found at critical points when the trial is developed, and to determine whether biases have been reduced or eliminated, each stage of the study, especially the methodology, should be reviewed using simple questions.[33,37,38] In clinical trials, biases are classified into four categories: selection (occurring in the group allocation process), performance (observed when there is a difference in the provision of care apart from the treatment under evaluation), detection (also called observer, ascertainment, or assessment bias, which is verified in the assessment of outcomes), and attrition (due to handling of deviations from the protocol and loss of follow-up).[35]

Readers can do a critical assessment of the quality of an RCT by asking several fundamental questions regarding the methodology of the study[33]:

1. Were the characteristics of participants in both groups similar at the start of the study?
2. Was the allocation of participants randomized for both groups?
3. Were the participants concealed for the allocation of participants in both groups?
4. Were the researchers and participants blinded to treatment?
5. Were the results analyzed on an intent-to-treat basis?
6. Were participants lost to follow-up?

After the methodology has been analyzed and found adequate, the applicability of the results should be analyzed. With the intention of improving the quality of published clinical trials and facilitating critical appraisal and interpretation for readers, a group of scientists and editors of some leading medical journals developed the Consolidated Standards of Reporting Trials (CONSORT) statement,[17] which was later revised.[36,38,40]

The quality of RCTs can be practically assessed by using the Jada scale, which ranges from 0 to 5 points.[41] This tool aims to assess whether the study was described as randomized (including the use of words such as *randomly, random,* and *randomization*) and double-blind, and whether it includes a description of withdrawals or dropouts. A score of 1 point is given for each answer. An additional score of 1 point each is given if the method used to generate the sequence of randomization and the method of double-blinding were described and considered adequate. The method to generate randomization sequences was considered adequate if it allowed each study participant to have the same chance of receiving each intervention being assessed. Double-blinding was considered appropriate if it was stated or implied that neither the person doing the assessment nor the study participants could identify the intervention being assessed. The study is considered valid if it reaches a minimum final score of 3 points.

The main steps of RCTs that can be affected by biases are presented here with some classic examples.

Methods

Participants

Recruitment

How fairly were the participants recruited? Is the sample representative of the population?

Randomized controlled trials address an issue relevant to a particular population that has a characteristic condition of interest. A sample of participants is usually selected to restrict the source population by using eligibility criteria typically related to age, sex, clinical diagnosis, and comorbid conditions. The participants selected for study should appropriately represent the population of interest or source population. The ability to generalize the results of the RCT depends on its external validity, or how the population of the study represents the source population, the eligibility criteria, and the methods of recruitment. A trial that establishes many exclusion criteria selects a very specific population that compromises the application of its results to other contexts. To be representative, the study groups should have random recruitment and only relevant exclusion criteria.[33,37,38]

Potential participants sequentially or randomly recruited from the whole population of interest and the source of participants should be clearly described, for example, first presentation, emergency presentation due to subarachnoid hemorrhage, or participants with nonruptured aneurysms demonstrated on computed tomography or magnetic resonance imaging. The methods of recruitment, such as through referral or self-selection (for example, advertisements), are very important. Eligibility criteria do not affect the internal validity of the trial because they are applied before randomization. Nevertheless, they affect the external validity.[33,37,38] Obtaining a sequential or random sample of the population of interest for RCTs is difficult because of the need for consent. As these studies generally will not be representative of the whole population with a specific problem, a clear idea of who they do represent is necessary and should be described in the study as the severity, duration, and risk level of the participant to ensure that the target population was defined.[33]

The protocol should include only exclusion criteria relevant for the study methods, for example, the exclusion of small children or people with sensorial aphasia from a study requiring answering verbal questions. It should not include irrelevant criteria, such as weight or height, for the question to be answered.

The description of settings and locations of the trial should be precise because they can affect the external validity. Health care institutions vary greatly in their organization, experience, and resources. The baseline risk for the medical condition under investigation, as well as climate and other physical factors, economics, geography, and the social and cultural background, can all affect a study's external validity. If a trial aiming to assess the efficacy of treating cerebral aneurysms with clips or coils was done by experienced specialists in a referral neurovascular center, its results cannot be applied for participants treated by general neurosurgeons in a general hospital (performance bias). In a similar manner, when the study is a multicenter trial, the different centers should be well described because each one may have different levels of assistance or the assistant physicians may have different expertise, causing a performance bias. Several examples of possible performance biases appear in the ISAT, which compared the use of coils and clips for cerebral aneurysms.[26] Differences in the selected centers included the level of expertise in endovascular treatment, and the different contributions of each center, which suggest that an appreciation of the indications of clipping versus coiling differed from one center to another. These flaws were pointed out in many subsequent publications.[42–49] Therefore, a description of settings and locations should provide enough information to allow readers to judge whether the results of the trial are relevant to their own setting.[38]

Sample Size

The number of participants required for a significant study varies with the type of outcome studied, and for scientific and ethical reasons the sample size for a trial should be planned with a balance between clinical and statistical considerations.[37,38] The ideal number of samples should be large enough to have a high probability (power) of detect-

ing as statistically significant a clinically important difference of a given size if such a difference exists.[38] The size of effect considered important is inversely related to the size of the sample needed to detect it. Therefore, large samples are necessary to detect small differences. Elements to be included in sample size calculations are (1) the estimated outcome for each group (the clinically important target difference between groups); (2) the β-error level; (3) the statistical power of the β-type error level; and (4) for continuous outcomes, the standard deviation of the measurements.[37] How the sample size was determined should be clearly stated in the methods. If a formal method was used, the researchers should identify the primary outcome on which the calculation was based, all the quantities used in the calculation, and the resulting target sample size per comparison group.[37]

Frequently, studies with small samples arrive at the erroneous conclusion that the intervention groups are not different when too few participants were studied to make such a statement.[50,51] Reviews of published trials have consistently found that a high proportion of trials have very low statistical power to detect clinically significant treatment effects because they used small sample sizes, with some probability of missing an important therapeutic improvement.[52–54] When the study's conclusion is that "there is no evidence that *A* causes *B*," readers should first ask whether there is enough information to justify the absence of evidence or there is simply a lack of information.[50] An example is a trial that compared octreotide and sclerotherapy in participants with variceal bleeding, in which the authors reported calculations suggesting that 1,800 participants were needed, but they arbitrarily used a sample with only 100 participants, accepting the chance of a type II error.[54] If the stated clinically useful treatment difference truly existed, this trial had only a 5% chance of getting statistically significant results. As a consequence of this low power, the confidence interval for the treatment difference is too wide. Despite a 95% confidence interval including differences between the cure rates of the two treatments of up to 20 percentage points, the authors concluded that both treatments were equally effective.[50] Another example can be observed in an overview of RCTs evaluating fibrinolytic (mostly streptokinase) treatment to prevent the recurrence of myocardial infarction.[55] The overview showed a modest but clinically useful, highly significant, reduction in mortality of 22%, but only five of the 24 trials had shown a statistically significant effect with a *p* value of <0.05. Because of a lack of significance of many individual trials, the recognition of the true value of streptokinase was long delayed.[50]

Methods for calculating the sample size for different types of scientific research have been reviewed.[56] To quickly analyze the adequacy of the sample size of a specific trial, there are two rules of thumb to determine how many participants are needed.[57] For studies with a binary outcome, approximately 50 "events" are necessary in the control group to have an 80% power of detecting a 50% relative risk reduction. For example, if the expected event rate is 10%, 500 participants are necessary for each group. For studies with a continuous outcome (such as height, weight, or blood pressure measurements), in which each patient contributes information, 50 patients per group might be sufficient. For events such as a heart attack or episodes of ischemic stroke, the number of participants required depends on how common the event of interest is.[37]

Randomization

Did the allocation of participants allow similarity between the groups? Were the study groups comparable?

Besides the variables being measured, different basic characteristics among participants (confounding factors) can affect the outcome of the study. To reduce or eliminate these factors, the groups being studied should match as closely as possible in every way except for the intervention (or exposure or other indication) at the beginning of the study, and ideally participants should be assigned to each group on the basis of chance (a random process) characterized by unpredictability. If the groups are different from the beginning, any difference in outcomes can be due to nonmatched characteristics (or confounding factors) rather than the considered intervention (or exposure or other indicator).[12,33,37,38]

Simple randomization ensures that similar numbers are generated in both trial groups, and practically comparable groups are created for known and unknown prognostic variables. *Restricted randomization* uses procedures to control randomization to achieve a balance between groups. *Block randomization* aims to ensure similar numbers of patients in each group, and *stratified randomization* allows the groups to be balanced for some prognostic patient characteristics.[11,58,59]

Sequence Generation

Many methods of sequence generation are adequate, but it is not possible to judge the adequacy of generation from terms such as *random allocation, randomization,* or even *random.*[38] The methods used to generate the random allocation sequence, such as a random number or computerized random-number generation, should be explained so that the reader can better assess the possibility of bias in group allocation. Random allocation has a precise technical meaning, indicating that each participant of a clinical trial has a known probability of receiving each treatment before one is assigned, but the actual treatment is determined by a chance process and cannot be predicted.[11,38]

When nonrandom, "deterministic" allocation methods such as alternation, hospital number, or date of birth are used, the word *random* should not be used.[38,58] Empirical evidence indicates that these trials have a selection bias,[32,34,35] probably due to the inability to adequately conceal these allocation systems.[38] Examples of possible selection biases in the ISAT included the established opinions of investi-

gators as to which treatment would benefit patients with specific aneurysms; an endovascular approach was the favored treatment for basilar aneurysms because of the high surgical risks, whereas surgery was preferred for middle cerebral artery aneurysms. The same problem occurred with the size of aneurysms (92 to 93% were 10 mm or less in size and 50% were 5 mm or less), causing a bias that favored endovascular treatment.[45,47,49]

Allocation Concealment and Blinding

Were the participants, those administering the interventions, and those assessing the outcomes blinded to group allocation?

Methods to guarantee adequate comparison between groups vary according to the type of study. The experimental method (such as an RCT) is considered ideal because it allows the researcher to randomly allocate participants to groups, making these groups comparable.[33,58] Therefore, ideally, participants should be assigned to each group on the basis of chance (randomly), which is characterized by unpredictability, and this can be done using random allocation sequences. In some circumstances, however, randomization is not possible for ethical reasons or because few participants are willing to be randomized.[11,58] Unrandomized studies of concurrent groups treated differently on the basis of clinical judgment or patient preference, or both, will need careful analysis to take into account the differing characteristics of the participants and may still be of doubtful value. A failure to use randomization when it could be used may fatally compromise the credibility of the research.[11]

A generated allocation schedule must ideally guarantee allocation concealment to prevent investigators and participants from knowing the treatment before participants are assigned.[33,37,38,60,61] However, the randomization process should be carefully conducted to prevent a selection bias that renders the groups incomparable.[33,37]

In controlled trials, blinding keeps study participants, health care providers, and sometimes those collecting and analyzing clinical data uninformed of the assigned intervention, so that they will not be influenced by that knowledge.[38] Trials in which participants and assessors are blinded from groups the participants are allocated to are called *double-blind* studies, and trials in which either the participants or the outcome assessors are blinded to the group allocation are called *single-blind.*

Allocation concealment should not be confused with blinding. Allocation concealment aims to prevent a selection bias and protect the assignment sequence before and until allocation, and it can always be successfully applied. Blinding aims to prevent performance and ascertainment biases and protect the sequence after allocation, but it cannot always be implemented, for example, in a trial comparing the level of pain associated with sampling of blood from the ear versus the thumb.[12,34,38,60]

If the researchers or participants know which group subjects are allocated to before they consent, a selection allocation may occur and distort the groups.[34,58,61] Consent for participating should be obtained from the participants without knowledge of the next assignment, and this blinding of randomization could be as important as the blinding of therapy.[33,61] Inadequate allocation concealment, even random, unpredictable assignment sequences, can be undermined.[34,58,62] Decentralized or external assignment, such as the use of a pharmacy, a central telephone randomization system, or automated systems, is desirable for maintaining allocation concealment.[12,38,58,62] When this is not possible, the use of numbered containers is a good alternative. The assignments are enclosed in sequentially numbered, opaque, and sealed envelopes that are opened sequentially and only after the identification of the participant has been written on the appropriate envelope.[12,62] Nevertheless, neither external assignment nor sealed envelopes are completely undecipherable. Investigators must ensure the concealment of participants regarding the allocation sequence, and all pertinent details should be reported.[11,12,58-62]

Implementation

Who generated the allocation sequence, who enrolled participants, and who assigned participants to their groups?

Although the same persons may perform more than one process in a clinical trial, the generation of allocation sequences and implantation of allocation of participants to each group should not be done by the same person. Independent of the methodology used for randomization, a failure to separate generation of the allocation sequence from assignment to the group may introduce a selection bias. For example, the person who did the allocation sequence can keep a copy and consult it when participating in the allocation process, causing a selection bias regardless of the adequate generation of a random allocation sequence.[38]

If participants know they have been assigned to the group receiving a new treatment, their report of outcome can be influenced by favorable expectations or increased anxiety. On the other hand, patients who know they are receiving the standard treatment may feel discriminated against or reassured. Blinding of participants, health care providers, and other persons involved in the evaluation outcomes minimizes the risk of detection bias, also called observer, ascertainment or assessment bias.[38]

Evidence of bias has been detected in RCTs in which the allocated sequence was inadequate or not clearly concealed. These trials provided larger estimates of treatment effects (odds ratios were exaggerated, on average, by 30 to 40%) than did trials in which adequate allocation concealment was reported.[32,34,35,62]

Intervention

Intervention in a clinical trial is the treatment or other type of health course under investigation.[38] Interventions done in the experimental groups, and the experience of those who perform them, should be well described. For example,

with surgical interventions, in addition to the surgical procedure itself, it is important to know the training and experience of the surgeons who perform them, even including the number of similar interventions they do per year. When more than one person is involved in surgical interventions, as in a multicenter trial, these people should have equivalent training and experience. As an example, the inclusion of physicians from different centers and with different expertise to perform the interventions in the ISAT, which favored interventional radiologists, is the subject of many criticisms in many subsequent papers.[42,45-49]

Maintenance

Management

How fairly were the study groups maintained through equal management and follow-up of participants?

After comparable groups are established, it is important to keep this status during all follow-up and to provide the same management for both groups. The unique difference between the groups should be the factor being tested, for example, a drug's efficacy or exposure to a specific risk factor, such as obesity.[37,61] Unequal treatment invalidates the results (performance bias), as was observed in a trial in preterm infants in which vitamin E treatment was supposed to prevent retrolental dysplasia. Nevertheless, this effect was not due to the vitamin itself because participants of both groups were on 100% oxygen and the participants of the treatment group were frequently removed from the oxygen for doses of the vitamin whereas the participants in the control group were not.[37] Other examples of possible performance bias in the ISAT are the different treatments for patients with vasospasm when done by interventional radiologists in some centers or by neurosurgeons in others,[42] and the different approaches used for postinterventional angiography (done for all patients treated with coils and eventually for patients treated with clips).[42,46]

Intention-to-Treat

Was there migration between groups? Was there loss or dropout during the follow-up? Did the participants adhere to the intervention?

During any study, some participants quit or are lost to follow-up, which can render groups no longer comparable. Thus, it is important to assess whether the majority of participants who begin the study are present at the end, and whether participants are being analyzed in the same group they were allocated to at the beginning (intention-to-treat principle).[33,35,37,58,61] The main systematic deviations found in clinical trials are loss and abandonment of the trial by participants during the period of study. This is considered an attrition bias, and it alters the equilibrium in the distribution of participants in the experimental groups, breaks the similarity between the compared groups, and compromises the statistical power; despite using frustrating techniques for estimating values for the lost data, it cannot be controlled for in the analysis.[33,58] Attrition due to a loss of follow-up should be distinguished from investigator-determined exclusion for such reasons as ineligibility, withdrawal from treatment, and poor adherence to the trial protocol.[38] An example of a possible attrition bias was pointed out by many reviewers of the ISAT,[26] in which 9,559 patients with subarachnoid hemorrhage were assessed for eligibility and the trial aimed to recruit 2,500 participants. Nevertheless, only 2,143 patients (22.4%) were randomized, 9% refused, and 69% were excluded by the physicians, who explained neither why the set number was not obtained nor the causes of exclusion.[42,43,47–49]

Conventionally, the validity of a study's results is rejected when the loss of participants is equal to or greater than 20%.[33] Such an example is the loss of patients to follow-up observed in trials of traumatic brain injury, which reached 42% in the first year and 60% at the end of the second year. This dropout was more marked for participants who were socioeconomically disadvantaged, had a history of substance abuse, or had more severe injuries.[63] Because of this type of selection bias, studies involving participants with traumatic brain injury with prolonged follow-up are not likely to show valid results.[33] Another example is the long-term follow-up from the ISAT.[64] In this study, only 75% and 72% of the two groups in the original randomized cohort were eligible for follow-up, but the baseline characteristics were those reported for the original ISAT groups.[65] A related low rate of primary outcome and different baseline characteristics, including comorbidities, are potential sources of attrition biases.[65]

Providing the number of all participants randomized and allocated to their original groups (intention-to-treat analysis), as well as the number of participants who did not receive the intervention as allocated or who did not complete treatment, enables readers to evaluate how much the estimated efficacy of therapy might be underestimated in comparison to ideal circumstances.[38] The exclusion of participants from analysis can lead to erroneous conclusions, as is observed in a trial comparing medical and surgical treatment for carotid stenosis.[66] In this trial, the analysis restricted to participants available for follow-up showed a reduction of the risk of transient ischemic attack, stroke, and death by surgery. However, an intention-to-treat analysis based on all participants, as originally assigned, did not show the superiority of surgery.[38]

Outcomes

After readers assess the methods of a study using the previous questions, they can decide whether the study is suitable for further consideration. If the study is considered appropriate, the next step is to analyze whether the results could be obtained by chance and, if not, what these results mean. A presentation of the results should contain not only the analysis that was statistically significant but also all planned primary and secondary outcomes.[38]

Measurement

Were the outcome results measured with blinded participants and assessors, or objective measures, or both?

Results of a clinical trial can be presented as binary outcomes, that is, "yes or no" outcomes that happen or do not happen, such as cancer, heart attack, stroke, or death; or they can be presented as continuous outcomes when the measured data are continuous, such as height, weight, dosage of some substance in the blood, or intracranial pressure. Results should be reported as a summary of each outcome. For binary outcomes, the measure of effect could be the risk ratio (relative or absolute risk), risk difference, or odds ratio, which is a measure of probability instead of risk and is approximately equal to the relative risk. For continuous data, it is usually reported as the difference in means.[37,38] For binary and survival time data, the expression of results can be expressed as the number needed to treat to obtain the benefit or harm.[38]

Measurement biases (detection biases) are common problems found in clinical trials. Therefore, the measurement of outcomes warrants special attention and should be done by the same assessors, using the same methods and equipment for assessing participants of both groups. Variables assessed with some equipment, for example, blood pressure, should be measured by the same person every time and for all patients, using the same equipment, and the assessment is more reliable if more than one reading is obtained, using a random-zero instead of digital sphygmomanometer.[38]

Knowing which group they are in can affect participants' behavior in the trial and influence their report of symptoms. For clinicians who take measurements, this knowledge can influence the way they record the results. Blinding participants and assessors to which groups the participants are in (double-blinded studies) is the best way to overcome these biases. Double-blinded studies are less likely to be affected by bias than trials in which either the participants or the outcome assessors are blinded to the group allocation (single-blind studies). Trials that are not blinded either for participants or assessors are the least consistent because they have a high potential for bias. When it is impossible to blind the participants and treating doctors or researchers, at least the outcome assessors should be blinded to the groups' allocation.[37]

Using objective data (such as weight) instead of subjective information (such as feeling better) prevents a measurement bias. For recording objective measurements, the assessors may not need to be blinded, but for subjective measurements, blinding is critical.[37]

The placebo effect is the effect attributable to the expectation that a treatment will have an effect, and it is a common cause of measurement bias for experimental trials. The effects obtained in trials comparing treatment with no treatment may be due to the placebo effect instead of the treatment itself.[37] Therefore, a placebo treatment identical to the real treatment (placebo pill, sham intervention, etc.) should be administered to the control group in an RCT whenever possible.

Statistical Methods

Were the results obtained by chance? What do the results mean?

Once the results of the study show an effect, it is necessary to verify whether this effect is real or if it could have been obtained by chance. As it is impossible to determine the exact risk of a binary outcome in a population or the exact level of a continuous outcome, the best way is to estimate the true risk or level based on the sample of participants in a trial. This estimate can be done by using two statistical methods of assessing chance: *p* values (hypothesis testing) and confidence intervals (estimation).[37]

The *p* values measure the probability that a result occurred purely by chance. A small *p* value is desirable because it suggests a low probability that the difference between groups is due to chance. Scientific research tests a hypothesis that there will not be an effect ("null hypothesis"). If the results of the study indicate an effect, meaning the null hypothesis appears improbable, the *p* value shows the probability that this effect could be simply due to chance. A low *p* value (generally less than 0.05) indicates a low probability (less than 5%) that the result was caused by chance. If a bias was not detected before looking at the *p* value, the effect can be considered a real one. An effect with a low *p* value becomes a "statistically significant" result, which does not necessarily mean a clinically important result.[37,51]

The confidence interval is an estimate of the range of values that are supposed to contain the real value. Usually, this value is expressed as a 95% confidence interval, which means the range of values has a 95% chance of including the real value. If this interval is too small for a difference between the treatment and control groups and does not overlap the "no effect" point (0 for a difference or 1 for a ratio), this result can be considered real (that is, with a *p* value of less than 0.05).[37] Therefore, a confidence interval should be provided to indicate the precision (uncertainty) of the estimate.[38]

Narrower confidence intervals are more reliable in studies with large numbers of participants, and therefore larger studies give more consistent results than smaller studies. However, the size the study needs to be to obtain meaningful results depends on how rare is the event being measured.[37]

Clinical Importance

An intervention can only be considered useful if the 95% confidence interval includes clinically important treatment effects. Therefore, statistical significance does not mean clinical importance. Statistical significance is related to the size of the effect and the 95% confidence interval in relation to the null hypothesis; clinical importance is related to the size of the effect and the 95% confidence interval in relation

to a minimum effect that would be considered clinically important.[37] For example, a measurable and statistically significant reduction in a symptom (for example, back pain or hemiparesis) may not be considered clinically important if it is not enough to avoid the need for medication or to allow the patient to walk.

Generalizability (External Validity)

To whom can the results be applied?

External validity or generalizability is related to the extent to which the results of a study can be generalized to other populations, settings, treatments, variables, and measurement variables.[35] It is significant only under clearly specific conditions that were not directly examined in the trial. Generally, questions related to the external validity of results involve comparing the characteristics of specific participants or groups for whom the study results are intended with the characteristics of participants studied, or to identify similarities among drugs. As asked by the CONSORT group[38]:

> Can results be generalized to an individual patient or groups different from those enrolled in the trial with regard to age, sex, severity of disease, and comorbid conditions? Are the results applicable to other drugs within a class of similar drugs, to a different dosage, timing, and route of administration, and to different concomitant therapies? Can the same results be expected at the primary, secondary, and tertiary levels of care? What about the effect on related outcomes that were not assessed in the trial, and the importance of length of follow-up and duration of treatment?

An example of the difficulties in generalizability was pointed out in the long-term follow-up from the ISAT.[64] This study essentially reflects a population of the United Kingdom only, with 95.7%, 82.6%, and 89.3% of participants, respectively, in the endovascular group, the neurosurgical group, and the total population followed being from the United Kingdom.[65]

As some authors have noted, "External validity is a matter of judgment and depends on the characteristics of the participants included in the trial, the trial setting, the treatment regimens tested, and the outcomes assessed."[35] Therefore, for an adequate assessment of the applicability of trial results, researchers should provide adequate information about eligibility criteria, the setting and location, the interventions and how they were administered, the definition of outcomes, and the period of recruitment and follow-up.[35,38]

Conclusion

Well-designed and properly executed RCTs are the gold standard for producing evidence about the efficacy of health care interventions because of their great potential to establish cause-effect relationships. However, trials with inadequate methodological approaches are associated with exaggerated treatment effects, originating from ethical and methodological flaws. Since the development and implementation of the CONSORT statement, the quality of published RTCs has improved.[36] Therefore, before readers

accept the results of a trial as gospel, they should do a systematic critical appraisal of that trial. But critical appraisal is possible only if the design, conduct, and analysis of an RCT is meticulously and precisely described in published articles.

Moderators
The Randomized Clinical Trial
A. John Popp, Urvashi Upadhyay, and Robert E. Harbaugh

In this section, we analyze the debate generated by the authors of the two preceding sections. In the first section, Vachhrajani and colleagues discussed the methodology of RCT design that leads to the highest quality of evidence. The authors emphasize that EBM requires a minimization of bias and that the RCT is the best means to achieve this goal. In the next section, Colli highlighted the potential flaws in traditional RCT methodology and discussed how such trial design can be optimized.

Understanding what constitutes EBM and how the results of clinical trials are applied is paramount in any discussion of RCTs. EBM is an algorithm for clinical decision making that is largely constructed from evidence taken from peer-reviewed and published clinical research. EBM may be categorized and ordered based on the strength of evidence. The methodology of data collection defines this hierarchy, with RCTs as the accepted gold standard of clinical research. EBM thereby provides a framework for the treatment of a particular condition by generating a standard of care, guidelines, and options for the clinician. The rationale for embracing EBM is that it will improve patient care because medical decision making will be based on scientifically valid data rather than intuition. The logic extends to the concept that improving patient care should ultimately improve patient outcomes.

Evidence-based medicine is largely predicated on the notion that prospective RCTs are the gold standard of clinical research. They are accepted as the gold standard because they minimize errors from bias, confounding, and chance. The prospective nature of these trials is intended to decrease any recall bias from both subjects and investigators. The randomization process relies on the notion that an equal distribution of subjects should equally distribute any unidentified confounders and internal selection bias. Finally, these trials are subject to rigorous statistical review of the calculation of a trial's power and p-value analyses of the difference between various treatment groups. An ideal RCT allows for concurrent comparison of treatment groups, relies on objective outcome measures that eliminate ob-

server bias, and are of an adequate size to reduce the chance of sampling error.

Although the principal topic under discussion is the utility of the RCT, the practicality and cost of obtaining such information to address the demand for accurate information in our current health care environment is high, requiring that we explore other aspects of quality care delivery that may be equivalent to the RCT but more efficient and less costly to obtain. The importance of this discussion is heightened by the looming quest in the United States for cost-effective, value-based care that will diminish the three errors of health care delivery: overuse, underuse, and misuse. The RCT can produce evidence on which cohesive clinical practice standards can be developed, but the clinician must also recognize that results from large-scale RCTs should be adopted with care when applied to various clinical scenarios. It is the authors' stance that the value of information from the RCT can be enhanced if the clinician understands such issues as the challenges of the generalizability of the RCT, the influence of patient selection and comorbidities, the impact of differing processes of care, the importance of ongoing physician education, and the evolution of knowledge and therapeutics. Finally, and perhaps most importantly in an era of cost-consciousness in medicine, we describe a possible alternative to the RCT that will gather useful information but at a lower cost than the RCT.

Application of the Results of the Randomized Controlled Trial

Generalizability and Patient Selection

Using the results of an RCT in a clinical setting requires the physician to understand the concept of generalizability—the application of the results of the RCT to the general population. In an attempt to eliminate selection bias in the RCT, the trial is designed to enroll as uniform a patient population as possible—similar age groups, sexes, and, ideally, no confounding comorbid conditions. Although these aspects of the trial are important, the utility of the RCT results can change when applied in a setting where any of the trial parameters are not met. For example, a patient with a given neurosurgical condition previously studied in an RCT might not fit the RCT admission criteria, the intervention may be performed in an institution with less experience than a hospital enrolled in the RCT, or the intervention may be performed by a surgeon who might have less experience or use different techniques than those used by surgeons in the study.

In any of these scenarios, neither the clinician nor the patient should assume that the efficacious aspects of the RCT will apply. For example, in the case of carotid endarterectomy (CEA), the two large-scale RCTs, the North American Symptomatic Carotid Endarterectomy Trial (NASCET) and the European Carotid Surgery Trial (ECST), attempted to make the CEA intervention as uniform as possible by allowing only surgeons with less than 6% morbidity and mortality to participate in the trial.[67,68] Although the conclusions drawn by both trials have largely informed how patients presenting with symptomatic carotid stenosis will be treated, a central question posed by the issue of generalizability becomes apparent when comparing the results of CEA done by surgeons with less experience, in hospitals with lower volume, or both. A retrospective review of patients in New York State who underwent CEA between January 1990 and December 1995 found that patients who underwent CEA in low-volume centers (< 100) with procedures done by low-volume surgeons (< 5) were found to have higher inpatient mortality rates when compared with those treated in more experienced centers by more experienced surgeons.[69] Furthermore, experience has shown that outcomes may also be influenced because of differing techniques used for surgical interventions, although in some instances analysis of the influence of the process of care does not conclusively support this notion. A review of the Cochrane Library for techniques associated with CEA found results suggesting that variations in technique may have little effect on outcome; specifically, the use of local anesthesia compared with that of general anesthesia,[70] eversion CEA compared with conventional longitudinal arteriotomy,[71] and patch angioplasty compared with primary closure showed no significant differences.[72] Although conclusive data supporting one surgical technique over another may be difficult to obtain, what is missing from these analyses are such variables as the difference in experience, skill, and knowledge of the RCT surgeon who was selected to participate in the RCT and the surgeon who delivers care to patients when the results of the RCT are applied to the general population.

Patient sampling within an RCT is conducted on a selected subpopulation within the greater population so as to minimize the interference of nontreatment variables with the production of accurate, unbiased results, thereby predisposing to a lack of generalizability. This conflict between obtaining unbiased yet generalizable results is not an easy one to resolve for designers of an RCT and must be considered by the physician interested in applying the results to an untested population.

Ethics of Patient Selection

In addition to the challenge of identifying which patients to enroll in an RCT, some authors have raised ethical concerns about enrolling patients in an RCT at all and in the process of randomization in particular. Most clinical trials employ some form of randomization when determining a given patient's treatment assignment. However, although patients and physicians sign an informed consent contract in which patients acknowledge that they may or may not receive the experimental intervention, several studies have shown that patients have a poor understanding of the risks associated with no intervention in a RCT.[73] This situation increases the responsibility of the physician to ensure that the patient's best interest is being pursued, as the surgeon has an implicit contract with the patient to offer the best care available. This therapeutic imperative poses a challenge to the surgeon who may not believe that both treatment arms of the trial are equally efficacious. As a result, the process of randomization may not be free from bias; without clinical equipoise, the surgeon may offer surgery to patients thought to be more likely to benefit and randomize those who would be less likely to benefit.

Presumably, in any RCT, a new intervention is being compared with a prior standard of care or no treatment, and the starting assumption is that the two interventions are equivalent. Therefore, randomization, theoretically, should not put the patient at increased risk. Several authors argue the opposite; that is, all new treatments are inherently risky as their efficacy is unknown, but patients may prefer the "newer" intervention and investigators subjectively may often feel that one treatment is superior to others.[73,74] If one treatment is felt by the investigator or patient to be superior to another, it may be imprudent to subject any patient to an intervention thought to be less efficacious. Such ethical questions have been raised by multiple authors and have led some to consider alternative methods for choosing interventions worth subjecting to RCT. In 1980, Kadane and Sedransk[75] proposed a modification of the standard RCT in which the subjective Bayesian technique is employed to determine which interventions may be admissible in a trial. More specifically, using standard Bayesian probabilistic methods, multiple experts are polled to assess the treatment options and goals of treatment for a given condition; these treatment options then are reassessed in a conditional way, so that the expert's opinion (i.e., a probability distribution for the goal of treatment) can be determined as a function of predictor variables.[74] Only when a given treatment intervention withstands these tests is it included in a given RCT. Embracing this probabilistic methodology could mitigate the risk of including treatment interventions in which clinicians lack confidence. Ethical considerations in RCTs of surgical interventions may be even more challenging than those faced in medical RCTs. Often, a certain surgical intervention may be considered so intrinsically beneficial or necessary that some would argue that an RCT is unnecessary. This ethical challenge was articulated in 1987 by Freedman[76] as the principle of equipoise in RCTs.

Freedman describes two types of equipoise: theoretical and clinical. Theoretical equipoise exists when there is no evidence that one intervention is more or less beneficial than the other. Theoretical equipoise is tenuous, as any evidence that one intervention is superior will disrupt the equipoise. Clinical equipoise exists when well-informed clinicians have a difference of opinion about which intervention may be superior; in such cases, the need to resolve this conflict is what drives the RCT. These challenges were illustrated in the case of the Canadian Lung Volume Reduction Surgery Trial (CLVRT).[77] In a select group of patients with emphysema, lung volume reduction surgery appears to be highly beneficial, with an improvement in pulmonary function unmatched by the best medical interventions. In such a case, theoretical equipoise has been disturbed as many clinicians strongly believe in the pulmonary benefits of lung volume reduction surgery. However, the presence of clinical equipoise has prevented the universal adoption of lung volume reduction surgery because the procedure is associated with higher mortality rates and prolonged length-of-stay in intensive care units.[77] Given this dilemma, the study proceeded as a multicentered RCT. As illustrated by the CLVRT, designers of the surgical RCT must be conscious of the potential biases that exist toward surgical intervention and proceed only if clinical equipoise is present, necessitating an RCT to resolve the conflicting opinions.

Evolution of Knowledge and Therapeutics

Any discussion of providing quality care must take into account that medical knowledge is not static but constantly evolving, requiring the physician to be a lifelong learner. Although RCTs are designed and powered to be robust and without bias, subsequent research can often lead to knowledge that may require a change in the treatment paradigms established by the results of the RCT. Recent studies of CEA for both asymptomatic and symptomatic carotid stenosis have shown a higher operative mortality risk for women, thereby decreasing the overall improvement in outcome when NASCET criteria are applied to women, independent of age.[78,79] Furthermore, women with symptomatic carotid stenosis treated with CEA are at a higher risk of perioperative stroke, compared with symptomatic men, but are still within the normal and acceptable risks associated with the intervention.[79] This special case of women treated through CEA illustrates that what may appear to be the best treatment course defined by an RCT for a group of patients with a particular condition may ultimately change as new data emerge—a possibility that must be considered when inter-

preting any RCT results, especially those that are older than 5 years.

Although increasing knowledge may lead to modifications of the applicability of an RCT, an issue of greater concern is the likelihood of RCT conclusions to be known or accepted by practicing physicians. In a retrospective review of 2,124 patients who underwent CEA in six hospitals in 1997 and 1998, the authors found that a significant number of patients underwent non-indicated CEA when physicians used NASCET inclusion criteria for their patients.[80] The majority of these "inappropriate" cases were asymptomatic patients with 60 to 99% stenosis and high comorbidity. Perhaps more alarming is that nearly 9% of inappropriate cases were done on patients with less than 50% stenosis.[80] These findings highlight the limitation of any trial, not just RCTs—that the clinical application of trial results relies on the physician's awareness and understanding of the results of the RCT.

Economic Considerations

With rising costs in health care, attention must be paid to the cost of carrying out an RCT, especially when there may be evidence that will lead to the same results but at lower cost. Furthermore, it does not appear that common practices and philosophies underlying the planning of clinical trials will change; therefore, costs associated with any given clinical trial are unlikely to fall. Spending on clinical trials in the U.S. in 2005 was estimated at $24 billion and was projected to exceed $32 billion in 2011.[81] Given these staggering figures, the absolute necessity of conducting an RCT must be considered before embarking on a costly design and implementation process. For example, in certain clinical scenarios a particular surgical intervention is the only appropriate choice, such as shunting for acute communicating hydrocephalus. Placing these interventions under the burden of a large-scale clinical trial may place patients at undue risk as the alternative treatments (no treatment or a sham operation) would not only be fiscally irresponsible but also ethically ill-advised. Only in cases in which an intervention represents a potential improvement over existing interventions can the pursuit of a costly RCT be justified.

Given recent initiatives in health care reform calling for cost-effective approaches to delivering care, other forms of decision making, such as comparative effectiveness, are being promulgated as less expensive ways of gleaning meaningful information about the best practice for particular patient groups. In 2009, the American Recovery and Reinvestment Act committed over $1 billion to conducting new comparative effectiveness research (CER).[82–84] CER is predicated on the idea that assessing outcomes in a large, heterogeneous patient population will yield more generalizable results. At the heart of these initiatives is determining the value of a given surgical intervention. In the health care setting, value is defined as desired health outcomes achieved per dollar spent.[85] Determining the value of specific surgical interventions will require input from CER in which a population of patients with a given condition, undergoing a given surgical treatment, are compared with untreated patients. A comparative analysis of cost spent on each group, as well as analysis of their different outcomes, will help elucidate which treatment interventions provide the highest value.

Alternative Methods of Clinical Assessment

Alternatives to Randomized Controlled Trials

Although RCTs offer high-quality evidence of the benefits and risks of a particular intervention in a certain population of patients, they do not always address key questions that are important to clinicians and patients. For example, an RCT of a new medication may compare it to a placebo drug; however, physicians attempting to determine whether or not to switch from a current medication to the newly tested one may not find guidance from that specific trial data. As mentioned above, investigators conducting the RCT also tend to enroll a homogeneous group of patients, and therefore the trial does not reflect the diversity of the suitable clinical population. Given these limitations, researchers have placed new emphasis on designing "pragmatic" trials that attempt to answer more practical clinical dilemmas, such as the comparison of two interventions, and to employ broad eligibility for patient recruitment.[86–88] Such trials often compare a specific intervention to the current standard of care and do not employ blinding techniques.

Pragmatic trials do have limitations, particularly in adherence to the protocol, as most pragmatic trials allow patients to abort treatment as they might in normal clinical situations. This potential for poor adherence may minimize results of a pragmatic trial designed to assess the equivalence of two therapies.[86] Another challenge to pragmatic trials is that they require larger sample sizes than RCTs, often needing multiple care centers from which to enroll a suitable number of patients.[86,87] Finally, given that pragmatic trials tend to keep patients unblended, there is always a risk of bias introduced by both clinician and patient, especially when primary outcomes are subjective in nature.[89] A recent study of four treatments in patients with asthma found that albuterol, a sham inhaler, and sham acupuncture were equally efficacious in reducing patient-reported symptoms of asthma. However, lung function, as measured by forced expiratory volume in 1 second (FEV_1), was only improved by the albuterol.[89] When outcomes such as patient satisfaction or symptom improvement are sought, it becomes challenging to assess the quality and effectiveness of a particular intervention.[90] Thus, pragmatic trials, designed expressly to address some of the limitations of the RCT, may likewise be limited in their ability to guide clinical decision making.

Given these considerations, it is likely that the complete assessment of a new intervention may require both styles of clinical trials in a complementary way, in which the efficacy of an intervention is rigorously tested in an RCT and its generalizability is best assessed in a pragmatic trial. Reaching this totality of evidence is ideal; however, clinicians and health-policy makers often must make decisions in the face of less information.[82] It is therefore most important that clinicians understand the unique contributions from various types of trials to be able to interpret the trials and use the information gleaned most accurately and efficaciously.

Quality Measures

Assessing the quality of medical care delivered in various health care settings has proven difficult. In 1988, Donabedian highlighted[91] this dilemma when he suggested that quality of care depends on technical performance and an interpersonal factor, that is, the patient's expectation of a favorable outcome. He stated, "The goodness of technical care is proportional to its expected ability to achieve those improvements in health status that the current science and technology of health care have made possible." From this perspective, quality can then be seen as proportional to the effectiveness of a given intervention. Although Donabedian's model appears judicious, in fact evaluating effectiveness requires accounting for and assessing interpersonal aspects of health care, as he terms them. The challenge of evaluating quality in health care has spawned the field of CER, noted above, in which health care interventions are directly compared to determine which have the greatest benefits, harms, and costs. In the aforementioned asthma study, which found that albuterol treatment and sham treatments showed no difference in subjective outcomes, although objective lung function outcomes were different, it is difficult to assess which of these outcomes is more important.[89] A large factor in any subjective outcome measure is the patient's expectations, and so studies that rely exclusively on reports by patients may miss key aspects of surgical care. In such trials, it is even more challenging to define and quantify value.

Processes of care measures are one method by which the delivery of quality treatment by health care entities are assessed and compared. These measures often use chart review to quantify a given institution's ability to deliver care that follows national treatment guidelines and standards of care.[92] To promote transparent, high-quality patient care and accountability, the Centers for Medicare and Medicaid Services and Hospital Quality Alliance began publicly reporting outcome measures for several conditions, including 30-day mortality measures for acute myocardial infarction, heart failure, and pneumonia, as well as in-hospital adverse events and mortality.[92] One of the goals of publicly reporting such outcomes has been to assist medical centers in assessing the quality of the care they provide and to identify areas needing improvement. From this initiative, it has become clear that large-volume centers seem to have better outcomes than small-volume centers for the medical conditions mentioned here. This concept has been most clear in the case of trauma management; regionalization of care is based on the concept that high-volume centers are best equipped and experienced at dealing with acute trauma. In a large-scale prospective trial, one of the major factors associated with decreased mortality in trauma patients was transfer to a tertiary-care center.[93] Given the dependence of outcomes on the clinical care setting, applying the results of an RCT obtained in a large tertiary-care center becomes problematic if care predominately is delivered in a smaller clinical setting.

The use of prospective multispecialty registries has been proposed to generate an audited registry of patients with risk stratification, evaluation of processes of care, and attainment of meaningful clinical outcomes. An analysis of the pooled registry data would allow clinicians to determine best practices and refine surgical indications for the treatment of specific diagnoses. The analysis of these data would have to address the inherent lack of randomization of patients to different treatment arms. Propensity analysis, in which individuals with the same propensity score share the same multivariate distribution of covariates, is one strategy for controlling for *known* confounders. The key limitation is that this method does not control for unknown confounders.

Conclusion

Despite our specialty's recognition of the importance of research in delivering the best care for our patients, and other active initiatives such as designing evidence-based clinical

guidelines led by the American Association of Neurological Surgeons (AANS) and the Congress of Neurological Surgeons (CNS), compared with other specialties, neurosurgery historically has not had the benefit of as many large-scale RCTs. Therefore, efforts to generate clinical practice guidelines have been informed by a focus on effectiveness and a value assessment of particular surgical interventions.[83] In many cases, the neurosurgical treatment is determined on an institution-by-institution basis. Recent years have seen a change in this trend, with an increasing reliance on EBM in neurosurgery to establish appropriate treatment paradigms.

Although the move in all medical fields toward EBM represents a positive trend in patient care, the utility and cost-effectiveness of any given RCT must be examined critically. The neurosurgeon evaluating a patient and weighing treatment options must be aware of the fine points of the reported trial data. Knowledge of the patient demographics, conditions for surgeon inclusion, specific outcomes measured, and the extent of internal validity are all necessary to properly apply results from an RCT to a particular clinical setting. When the neurosurgeon approaches each patient as an individual and weighs the available data in the context of the unique situation of the patient, a truly informed decision can be made by both the physician and patient.[86] Most important, the best interests of the patient can be met when information and knowledge are thus united with clinical judgment. Although the use of the RCT appears to be at the pinnacle of EBM, modern value-based medical practice, of necessity, will require other forms of decision making that are less costly and more widely applicable.

References

1. Evidence-Based Medicine Working Group. Evidence-based medicine. A new approach to teaching the practice of medicine. JAMA 1992;268:2420–2425
2. Karanicolas PJ, Kunz R, Guyatt GH. Point: evidence-based medicine has a sound scientific base. Chest 2008;133:1067–1071
3. Tobin MJ. Counterpoint: evidence-based medicine lacks a sound scientific base. Chest 2008;133:1071–1074, discussion 1074–1077
4. Vachhrajani S, Kulkarni AV, Kestle JR. Clinical practice guidelines. J Neurosurg Pediatr 2009;3:249–256
5. McCulloch P, Taylor I, Sasako M, Lovett B, Griffin D. Randomised trials in surgery: problems and possible solutions. BMJ 2002; 324:1448–1451
6. Canadian Task Force on the Periodic Health Examination. The periodic health examination. Can Med Assoc J 1979;121:1193–1254
7. Harris RP, Helfand M, Woolf SH, et al; Methods Work Group, Third US Preventive Services Task Force. Current methods of the US Preventive Services Task Force: a review of the process. Am J Prev Med 2001;20(3, Suppl):21–35
8. Guyatt G, Gutterman D, Baumann MH, et al. Grading strength of recommendations and quality of evidence in clinical guidelines: report from an American College of Chest Physicians task force. Chest 2006;129:174–181

9. Atkins D, Best D, Briss PA, et al; GRADE Working Group. Grading quality of evidence and strength of recommendations. BMJ 2004;328:1490
10. Stanley K. Design of randomized controlled trials. Circulation 2007;115:1164–1169
11. Altman DG, Bland JM. Statistics notes. Treatment allocation in controlled trials: why randomise? BMJ 1999;318:1209
12. Altman DG, Schulz KF. Statistics notes: concealing treatment allocation in randomised trials. BMJ 2001;323:446–447
13. Schulz KF, Grimes DA. Allocation concealment in randomised trials: defending against deciphering. Lancet 2002;359:614–618
14. Devereaux PJ, Manns BJ, Ghali WA, et al. Physician interpretations and textbook definitions of blinding terminology in randomized controlled trials. JAMA 2001;285:2000–2003
15. Schulz KF, Altman DG, Moher D; CONSORT Group. CONSORT 2010 statement: updated guidelines for reporting parallel group randomized trials. Ann Intern Med 2010;152:726–732
16. Guyatt GH, Oxman AD, Kunz R, Vist GE, Falck-Ytter Y, Schünemann HJ; GRADE Working Group. What is "quality of evidence" and why is it important to clinicians? BMJ 2008;336:995–998
17. Begg C, Cho M, Eastwood S, et al. Improving the quality of reporting of randomized controlled trials. The CONSORT statement. JAMA 1996;276:637–639

18. Hopewell S, Clarke M, Moher D, et al; CONSORT Group. CONSORT for reporting randomized controlled trials in journal and conference abstracts: explanation and elaboration. PLoS Med 2008;5:e20

19. Moher D, Jones A, Lepage L; CONSORT Group (Consolitdated Standards for Reporting of Trials). Use of the CONSORT statement and quality of reports of randomized trials: a comparative before-and-after evaluation. JAMA 2001;285:1992–1995

20. Devereaux PJ, Manns BJ, Ghali WA, Quan H, Guyatt GH. The reporting of methodological factors in randomized controlled trials and the association with a journal policy to promote adherence to the Consolidated Standards of Reporting Trials (CONSORT) checklist. Control Clin Trials 2002;23:380–388

21. Kane RL, Wang J, Garrard J. Reporting in randomized clinical trials improved after adoption of the CONSORT statement. J Clin Epidemiol 2007;60:241–249

22. Fung EK, Loré JM Jr. Randomized controlled trials for evaluating surgical questions. Arch Otolaryngol Head Neck Surg 2002; 128:631–634

23. Schöller K, Licht S, Tonn JC, Uhl E. Randomized controlled trials in neurosurgery—how good are we? Acta Neurochir (Wien) 2009;151:519–527, discussion 527

24. Vranos G, Tatsioni A, Polyzoidis K, Ioannidis JP. Randomized trials of neurosurgical interventions: a systematic appraisal. Neurosurgery 2004;55:18–25, discussion 25–26

25. Kan P, Kestle JR. Designing randomized clinical trials in pediatric neurosurgery. Childs Nerv Syst 2007;23:385–390

26. Molyneux A, Kerr R, Stratton I, et al; International Subarachnoid Aneurysm Trial (ISAT) Collaborative Group. International Subarachnoid Aneurysm Trial (ISAT) of neurosurgical clipping versus endovascular coiling in 2143 patients with ruptured intracranial aneurysms: a randomised trial. Lancet 2002;360: 1267–1274

27. The EC/IC Bypass Study Group. Failure of extracranial-intracranial arterial bypass to reduce the risk of ischemic stroke. Results of an international randomized trial. N Engl J Med 1985; 313:1191–1200

28. Bracken MB, Shepard MJ, Holford TR, et al. Administration of methylprednisolone for 24 or 48 hours or tirilazad mesylate for 48 hours in the treatment of acute spinal cord injury. Results of the Third National Acute Spinal Cord Injury Randomized Controlled Trial. National Acute Spinal Cord Injury Study. JAMA 1997;277:1597–1604

29. Edwards P, Arango M, Balica L, et al; CRASH trial collaborators. Final results of MRC CRASH, a randomised placebo-controlled trial of intravenous corticosteroid in adults with head injury-outcomes at 6 months. Lancet 2005;365:1957–1959

30. Mendelow AD, Gregson BA, Fernandes HM, et al; STICH investigators. Early surgery versus initial conservative treatment in patients with spontaneous supratentorial intracerebral haematomas in the International Surgical Trial in Intracerebral Haemorrhage (STICH): a randomised trial. Lancet 2005;365: 387–397

31. Stupp R, Mason WP, van den Bent MJ, et al; European Organisation for Research and Treatment of Cancer Brain Tumor and Radiotherapy Groups; National Cancer Institute of Canada Clinical Trials Group. Radiotherapy plus concomitant and adjuvant temozolomide for glioblastoma. N Engl J Med 2005;352: 987–996

32. Moher D. CONSORT: an evolving tool to help improve the quality of reports of randomized controlled trials. Consolidated Standards of Reporting Trials. JAMA 1998;279:1489–1491

33. Nobre M, Bernardo W. Prática Clínica Baseada em Evidéncia, 2nd ed. Rio de Janeiro: Elsevier, 2006

34. Schulz KF, Chalmers I, Hayes RJ, Altman DG. Empirical evidence of bias. Dimensions of methodological quality associated with estimates of treatment effects in controlled trials. JAMA 1995; 273:408–412

35. Jüni P, Altman DG, Egger M. Systematic reviews in health care: assessing the quality of controlled clinical trials. BMJ 2001;323: 42–46

36. Moher D, Schulz KF, Altman D; CONSORT Group (Consolidated Standards of Reporting Trials). The CONSORT statement: revised recommendations for improving the quality of reports of parallel-group randomized trials. JAMA 2001;285:1987–1991

37. Glasziou P, Del Mar C, Salisbury J. Evidence-Based Practice Workbook (Evidence-Based Medicine), 2nd ed. Malden, MA: Blackwell, 2007

38. Altman DG, Schulz KF, Moher D, et al; CONSORT GROUP (Consolidated Standards of Reporting Trials). The revised CONSORT statement for reporting randomized trials: explanation and elaboration. Ann Intern Med 2001;134:663–694

39. Campbell DT. Factors relevant to the validity of experiments in social settings. Psychol Bull 1957;54:297–312

40. Egger M, Jüni P, Bartlett C; CONSORT Group (Consolidated Standards of Reporting of Trials). Value of flow diagrams in reports of randomized controlled trials. JAMA 2001;285:1996–1999

41. Jadad AR, Moore RA, Carroll D, et al. Assessing the quality of reports of randomized clinical trials: is blinding necessary? Control Clin Trials 1996;17:1–12

42. Ausman JI. ISAT study: is coiling better than clipping? [Commentary] Surg Neurol 2003;59:162–165, discussion 165–173, author reply 173–175

43. Kobayashi S. ISAT study: is coiling better than clipping? [Commentary] Surg Neurol 2003;59:168

44. Debrun G. ISAT study: is coiling better than clipping? [Commentary] Surg Neurol 2003;59:168

45. Batjer HH. ISAT study: is coiling better than clipping? [Commentary] Surg Neurol 2003;59:168–169

46. Salomon RA. ISAT study: is coiling better than clipping? [Commentary] Surg Neurol 2003;59:173

47. Britz GW, Newell DW, West GA, Lam A. The ISAT trial. Lancet 2003;361:431–432, author reply 432

48. Harbaugh RE, Heros RC, Hadley MN. More on ISAT. Lancet 2003;361:783–784, author reply 784

49. Sade B, Mohr G. Critical appraisal of the International Subarachnoid Aneurysm Trial (ISAT). Neurol India 2004;52:32–35

50. Altman DG, Bland JM. Absence of evidence is not evidence of absence. BMJ 1995;311:485

51. Goodman SN, Berlin JA. The use of predicted confidence intervals when planning experiments and the misuse of power when interpreting results. Ann Intern Med 1994;121:200–206

52. Freiman JA, Chalmers TC, Smith H Jr, Kuebler RR. The importance of beta, the type II error and sample size in the design and interpretation of the randomized control trial. Survey of 71 "negative" trials. N Engl J Med 1978;299:690–694

53. Moher D, Dulberg CS, Wells GA. Statistical power, sample size, and their reporting in randomized controlled trials. JAMA 1994;272:122–124

54. Sung JJ, Chung SC, Lai CW, et al. Octreotide infusion or emergency sclerotherapy for variceal haemorrhage. Lancet 1993; 342:637–641

55. Yusuf S, Collins R, Peto R, et al. Intravenous and intracoronary fibrinolytic therapy in acute myocardial infarction: overview of

results on mortality, reinfarction and side-effects from 33 randomized controlled trials. Eur Heart J 1985;6:556–585

56. Campbell MJ, Julious SA, Altman DG. Estimating sample sizes for binary, ordered categorical, and continuous outcomes in two group comparisons. BMJ 1995;311:1145–1148

57. Glasziou P, Doll H. Was the study big enough? Two café rules. Evid Based Med 2006;11:69–70

58. Altman DG. Randomisation. [Comment] BMJ 1991;302:1481–1482

59. Altman DG, Bland JM. How to randomise. BMJ 1999;319:703–704

60. Day SJ, Altman DG. Statistics notes: blinding in clinical trials and other studies. BMJ 2000;321:504

61. Chalmers TC, Levin H, Sacks HS, Reitman D, Berrier J, Nagalingam R. Meta-analysis of clinical trials as a scientific discipline. I: Control of bias and comparison with large co-operative trials. Stat Med 1987;6:315–328

62. Schulz KF. Subverting randomization in controlled trials. JAMA 1995;274:1456–1458

63. Corrigan JD, Harrison-Felix C, Bogner J, Dijkers M, Terrill MS, Whiteneck G. Systematic bias in traumatic brain injury outcome studies because of loss to follow-up. Arch Phys Med Rehabil 2003;84:153–160

64. Molyneux AJ, Kerr RS, Birks J, et al; ISAT Collaborators. Risk of recurrent subarachnoid haemorrhage, death, or dependence and standardised mortality ratios after clipping or coiling of an intracranial aneurysm in the International Subarachnoid Aneurysm Trial (ISAT): long-term follow-up. Lancet Neurol 2009;8:427–433

65. Raper DM, Allan R. International subarachnoid trial in the long run: critical evaluation of the long-term follow-up data from the ISAT trial of clipping vs coiling for ruptured intracranial aneurysms. Neurosurgery 2010;66:1166–1169, discussion 1169

66. Fields WS, Maslenikov V, Meyer JS, Hass WK, Remington RD, Macdonald M. Joint study of extracranial arterial occlusion. V. Progress report of prognosis following surgery or nonsurgical treatment for transient cerebral ischemic attacks and cervical carotid artery lesions. JAMA 1970;211:1993–2003

67. Beneficial effect of carotid endarterectomy in symptomatic patients with high-grade carotid stenosis. North American Symptomatic Carotid Endarterectomy Trial Collaborators. N Engl J Med 1991;325:445–453

68. European Carotid Surgery Trialists' Collaborative Group. Randomised trial of endarterectomy for recently symptomatic carotid stenosis: final results of the MRC European Carotid Surgery Trial (ECST). Lancet 1998;351:1379–1387

69. Hannan EL, Popp AJ, Tranmer B, Fuestel P, Waldman J, Shah D. Relationship between provider volume and mortality for carotid endarterectomies in New York state. Stroke 1998;29:2292–2297

70. Rerkasem K, Rothwell PM. Local versus general anaesthesia for carotid endarterectomy. Cochrane Database Syst Rev 2008;8:CD000126

71. Cao PG, de Rango P, Zannetti S, Giordano G, Ricci S, Celani MG. Eversion versus conventional carotid endarterectomy for preventing stroke. Cochrane Database Syst Rev 2001;1:CD001921

72. Rerkasem K, Rothwell PM. Patch angioplasty versus primary closure for carotid endarterectomy. Cochrane Database Syst Rev 2009;4:CD000160

73. Kadane JB. Introduction. In: Kadane JB, ed. Bayesian Methods and Ethics in a Clinical Trial Design. New York: Wiley-Interscience, 1996:3–18

74. Kairys D. The law of clinical testing with human subjects: legal implications of new and existing methodologies. In: Kadane JB, ed. Bayesian Methods and Ethics in a Clinical Trial Design. New York: Wiley-Interscience, 1996:223–249

75. Kadane J, Sedransk N. Toward a more ethical clinical trial. In: Bayesian Statistics. Valencia, Spain: University of Valencia, 1980:329–338

76. Freedman B. Equipoise and the ethics of clinical research. N Engl J Med 1987;317:141–145

77. Miller JD, Coughlin MD, Edey L, Miller P, Sivji Y. Equipoise and the ethics of the Canadian Lung Volume Reduction Surgery Trial study: should there be a randomized, controlled trial to evaluate lung volume reduction surgery? Can Respir J 2000;7:329–332

78. Bond R, Rerkasem K, Cuffe R, Rothwell PM. A systematic review of the associations between age and sex and the operative risks of carotid endarterectomy. Cerebrovasc Dis 2005;20:69–77

79. Rockman CB, Garg K, Jacobowitz GR, et al. Outcome of carotid artery interventions among female patients, 2004 to 2005. J Vasc Surg 2011;53:1457–1464

80. Halm EA, Chassin MR, Tuhrim S, et al. Revisiting the appropriateness of carotid endarterectomy. Stroke 2003;34:1464–1471

81. Fee R. The cost of clinical trials. Drug Discovery & Development Magazine. 2007;10:32

82. Hennekens CH, DeMets D. Statistical association and causation: contributions of different types of evidence. JAMA 2011;305:1134–1135

83. Ghogawala Z, Amin-Hanjani S. Comparative effectiveness research—what does it mean for you and your practice? Congress Q 2011;12:28; www.cns.org

84. American Recovery and Reinvestment Act of. 2009. http://www.gpo.gov/fdsys/pkg/BILLS-111hr1enr/pdf/BILLS-111hr1enr.pdf, pages 63–64

85. Porter ME. What is value in health care? N Engl J Med 2010;363:2477–2481

86. Ware JH, Hamel MB. Pragmatic trials—guides to better patient care? N Engl J Med 2011;364:1685–1687

87. Price D, Musgrave SD, Shepstone L, et al. Leukotriene antagonists as first-line or add-on asthma-controller therapy. N Engl J Med 2011;364:1695–1707

88. Dahlén SE, Dahlén B, Drazen JM. Asthma treatment guidelines meet the real world. N Engl J Med 2011;364:1769–1770

89. Moerman DE. Meaningful placebos—controlling the uncontrollable. N Engl J Med 2011;365:171–172

90. Donabedian A. Evaluating the quality of medical care. Milbank Mem Fund Q 1966;44(3, Suppl):166–206

91. Donabedian A. The quality of care. How can it be assessed? JAMA 1988;260:1743–1748

92. Hospital Quality Initiative Overview. Centers for Medicare & Medicaid Services. July 2008; https://www.cms.gov/Medicare/Quality-Initiatives-Patient-Assessment-Instruments/HospitalQualityInits/downloads/HospitalOverview.pdf

93. Sampalis JS, Denis R, Lavoie A, et al. Trauma care regionalization: a process-outcome evaluation. J Trauma 1999;46:565–579, discussion 579–581

Index